4. Osteomyelitis

5. Infectious Arthritis

6. Tuberculosis and Other Unusual Infections

7. General Principles of Tumors

坎贝尔骨科手术学
一般原则、感染与肿瘤

Campbell's Operative Orthopaedics

第 14 版
（影印版）

Frederick M. Azar, MD

James H. Beaty, MD

人民卫生出版社
·北 京·

图书在版编目（CIP）数据

坎贝尔骨科手术学 . 一般原则、感染与肿瘤：英文 /（美）弗雷德里克·M. 阿扎尔（Frederick M. Azar），（美）詹姆斯·H. 比蒂（James H. Beaty）主编 . —影印本 . —北京：人民卫生出版社，2021.12
ISBN 978-7-117-32522-6

Ⅰ. ①坎⋯ Ⅱ. ①弗⋯ ②詹⋯ Ⅲ. ①骨科学 – 外科手术 – 英文 Ⅳ. ①R68

中国版本图书馆 CIP 数据核字（2021）第 241256 号

人卫智网	www.ipmph.com	医学教育、学术、考试、健康，购书智慧智能综合服务平台
人卫官网	www.pmph.com	人卫官方资讯发布平台

图字：01–2021–6747 号

坎贝尔骨科手术学
一般原则、感染与肿瘤
Kanbeier Guke Shoushuxue
Yiban Yuanze、Ganran yu Zhongliu

主　　编：Frederick M. Azar　James H. Beaty
出版发行：人民卫生出版社（中继线 010-59780011）
地　　址：北京市朝阳区潘家园南里 19 号
邮　　编：100021
E - mail：pmph @ pmph.com
购书热线：010-59787592　010-59787584　010-65264830
印　　刷：三河市宏达印刷有限公司（胜利）
经　　销：新华书店
开　　本：889×1194　1/16　印张：30
字　　数：1428 千字
版　　次：2021 年 12 月第 1 版
印　　次：2022 年 1 月第 1 次印刷
标准书号：ISBN 978-7-117-32522-6
定　　价：399.00 元

坎贝尔骨科手术学
一般原则、感染与肿瘤

Campbell's Operative Orthopaedics

第 14 版
（影印版）

Frederick M. Azar, MD

Professor

Department of Orthopaedic Surgery and Biomedical Engineering University of Tennessee–Campbell Clinic

Chief of Staff, Campbell Clinic

Memphis, Tennessee

James H. Beaty, MD

Harold B. Boyd Professor and Chair

Department of Orthopaedic Surgery and Biomedical Engineering University of Tennessee–Campbell Clinic

Memphis, Tennessee

Editorial Assistance

Kay Daugherty *and* **Linda Jones**

人民卫生出版社

·北 京·

Elsevier (Singapore) Pte Ltd.
3 Killiney Road,
#08−01 Winsland House I,
Singapore 239519
Tel:（65）6349−0200; Fax:（65）6733−1817

This English Reprint of Parts Ⅰ, Ⅶ, and Ⅷ from Campbell's Operative Orthopaedics, 14E by Frederick M. Azar and James H. Beaty was undertaken by People's Medical Publishing House and is published by arrangement with Elsevier (Singapore) Pte Ltd.

Parts Ⅰ, Ⅶ, and Ⅷ from Campbell's Operative Orthopaedics, 14E by Frederick M. Azar and James H. Beaty由人民卫生出版社进行影印，并根据人民卫生出版社与爱思唯尔（新加坡）私人有限公司的协议约定出版。

Notice

Practitioners and researchers must always rely on their own experience and knowledge in evaluating and using any information, methods, compounds or experiments described herein. Because of rapid advances in the medical sciences, in particular, independent verification of diagnoses and drug dosages should be made. To the fullest extent of the law, no responsibility is assumed by Elsevier, authors, editors or contributors in relation to the adaptation or for any injury and/or damage to persons or property as a matter of products liability, negligence or otherwise, or from any use or operation of any methods, products, instructions, or ideas contained in the material herein.

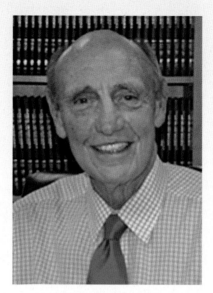

S. Terry Canale, MD

It is with humble appreciation and admiration that we dedicate this edition of *Campbell's Operative Orthopaedics* to Dr. S. Terry Canale, who served as editor or co-editor of five editions. He took great pride in this position and worked tirelessly to continue to improve "The Book." As noted by one of his co-editors, "Terry is probably the only person in the world who has read every word of multiple editions of *Campbell's Operative Orthopaedics.*" He considered *Campbell's Operative Orthopaedics* an opportunity for worldwide orthopaedic education and made it a priority to ensure that each edition provided valuable and up-to-date information. His commitment to and enthusiasm for this work will continue to influence and inspire every future edition.

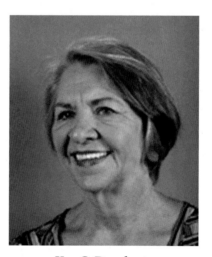

Kay C. Daugherty

It is with equal appreciation and regard that we dedicate this edition to Kay C. Daugherty, the managing editor of the last nine editions *Campbell's Operative Orthopaedics.* Over the last 40 years, she has faithfully and tirelessly edited, reshaped, and overseen all aspects of publication from manuscript preparation to proofing. She has a profound talent to put ideas and disjointed words into comprehensible text, ensuring that each revision maintains the gold standard in readability. Each edition is a testament to her dedication to excellence in writing and education. A favorite quote of Mrs. Daugherty to one of our late authors was, "I'll make a deal. I won't operate if you won't punctuate." We are grateful for her many years of continual service to the Campbell Foundation and for the publications yet to come.

FREDERICK M. AZAR, MD
Professor
Director, Sports Medicine Fellowship
University of Tennessee–Campbell Clinic
Department of Orthopaedic Surgery and
    Biomedical Engineering
Chief-of-Staff, Campbell Clinic
Memphis, Tennessee

JAMES H. BEATY, MD
Harold B. Boyd Professor and Chair
University of Tennessee–Campbell Clinic
Department of Orthopaedic Surgery and
    Biomedical Engineering
Memphis, Tennessee

MICHAEL J. BEEBE, MD
Instructor
University of Tennessee–Campbell Clinic
Department of Orthopaedic Surgery and
    Biomedical Engineering
Memphis, Tennessee

CLAYTON C. BETTIN, MD
Assistant Professor
Director, Foot and Ankle Fellowship
Associate Residency Program Director
University of Tennessee–Campbell Clinic
Department of Orthopaedic Surgery and
    Biomedical Engineering
Memphis, Tennessee

TYLER J. BROLIN, MD
Assistant Professor
University of Tennessee–Campbell Clinic
Department of Orthopaedic Surgery and
    Biomedical Engineering
Memphis, Tennessee

JAMES H. CALANDRUCCIO, MD
Associate Professor
Director, Hand Fellowship
University of Tennessee–Campbell Clinic
Department of Orthopaedic Surgery and
    Biomedical Engineering
Memphis, Tennessee

DAVID L. CANNON, MD
Associate Professor
University of Tennessee–Campbell Clinic
Department of Orthopaedic Surgery and
    Biomedical Engineering
Memphis, Tennessee

KEVIN B. CLEVELAND, MD
Instructor
University of Tennessee–Campbell Clinic
Department of Orthopaedic Surgery and
    Biomedical Engineering
Memphis, Tennessee

ANDREW H. CRENSHAW JR., MD
Professor Emeritus
University of Tennessee–Campbell Clinic
Department of Orthopaedic Surgery and
    Biomedical Engineering
Memphis, Tennessee

JOHN R. CROCKARELL, MD
Professor
University of Tennessee–Campbell Clinic
Department of Orthopaedic Surgery and
    Biomedical Engineering
Memphis, Tennessee

GREGORY D. DABOV, MD
Assistant Professor
University of Tennessee–Campbell Clinic
Department of Orthopaedic Surgery and
    Biomedical Engineering
Memphis, Tennessee

MARCUS C. FORD, MD
Instructor
University of Tennessee–Campbell Clinic
Department of Orthopaedic Surgery and
    Biomedical Engineering
Memphis, Tennessee

RAYMOND J. GARDOCKI, MD
Assistant Professor
University of Tennessee–Campbell Clinic
Department of Orthopaedic Surgery and
    Biomedical Engineering
Memphis, Tennessee

BENJAMIN J. GREAR, MD
Instructor
University of Tennessee–Campbell Clinic
Department of Orthopaedic Surgery and
    Biomedical Engineering
Memphis, Tennessee

JAMES L. GUYTON, MD
Associate Professor
University of Tennessee–Campbell Clinic
Department of Orthopaedic Surgery and
    Biomedical Engineering
Memphis, Tennessee

JAMES W. HARKESS, MD
Associate Professor
University of Tennessee–Campbell Clinic
Department of Orthopaedic Surgery and
    Biomedical Engineering
Memphis, Tennessee

ROBERT K. HECK JR., MD
Associate Professor
University of Tennessee–Campbell Clinic
Department of Orthopaedic Surgery and
    Biomedical Engineering
Memphis, Tennessee

MARK T. JOBE, MD
Associate Professor
University of Tennessee–Campbell Clinic
Department of Orthopaedic Surgery and
    Biomedical Engineering
Memphis, Tennessee

DEREK M. KELLY, MD
Professor
Director, Pediatric Orthopaedic Fellowship
Director, Resident Education
University of Tennessee–Campbell Clinic
Department of Orthopaedic Surgery and
    Biomedical Engineering
Memphis, Tennessee

SANTOS F. MARTINEZ, MD
Assistant Professor
University of Tennessee–Campbell Clinic
Department of Orthopaedic Surgery and
    Biomedical Engineering
Memphis, Tennessee

ANTHONY A. MASCIOLI, MD
Assistant Professor
University of Tennessee–Campbell Clinic
Department of Orthopaedic Surgery and
    Biomedical Engineering
Memphis, Tennessee

BENJAMIN M. MAUCK, MD
Assistant Professor
Director, Hand Fellowship
University of Tennessee–Campbell Clinic
Department of Orthopaedic Surgery and
    Biomedical Engineering
Memphis, Tennessee

MARC J. MIHALKO, MD
Assistant Professor
University of Tennessee–Campbell Clinic
Department of Orthopaedic Surgery and
    Biomedical Engineering
Memphis, Tennessee

WILLIAM M. MIHALKO, MD PhD
Professor, H.R. Hyde Chair of Excellence in
    Rehabilitation Engineering
Director, Biomedical Engineering
University of Tennessee–Campbell Clinic
Department of Orthopaedic Surgery and
    Biomedical Engineering
Memphis, Tennessee

ROBERT H. MILLER III, MD
Associate Professor
University of Tennessee–Campbell Clinic
Department of Orthopaedic Surgery and
    Biomedical Engineering
Memphis, Tennessee

G. ANDREW MURPHY, MD
Associate Professor
University of Tennessee–Campbell Clinic
Department of Orthopaedic Surgery and
    Biomedical Engineering
Memphis, Tennessee

ASHLEY L. PARK, MD
Clinical Assistant Professor
University of Tennessee–Campbell Clinic
Department of Orthopaedic Surgery and
    Biomedical Engineering
Memphis, Tennessee

EDWARD A. PEREZ, MD
Associate Professor
University of Tennessee–Campbell Clinic
Department of Orthopaedic Surgery and
    Biomedical Engineering
Memphis, Tennessee

BARRY B. PHILLIPS, MD
Professor
University of Tennessee–Campbell Clinic
Department of Orthopaedic Surgery and
    Biomedical Engineering
Memphis, Tennessee

DAVID R. RICHARDSON, MD
Associate Professor
University of Tennessee–Campbell Clinic
Department of Orthopaedic Surgery and
    Biomedical Engineering
Memphis, Tennessee

MATTHEW I. RUDLOFF, MD
Assistant Professor
Co-Director, Trauma Fellowship
University of Tennessee–Campbell Clinic
Department of Orthopaedic Surgery and
    Biomedical Engineering
Memphis, Tennessee

JEFFREY R. SAWYER, MD
Professor
Co-Director, Pediatric Orthopaedic
    Fellowship
University of Tennessee–Campbell Clinic
Department of Orthopaedic Surgery and
    Biomedical Engineering
Memphis, Tennessee

BENJAMIN W. SHEFFER, MD
Assistant Professor
University of Tennessee–Campbell Clinic
Department of Orthopaedic Surgery and
    Biomedical Engineering
Memphis, Tennessee

DAVID D. SPENCE, MD
Assistant Professor
University of Tennessee–Campbell Clinic
Department of Orthopaedic Surgery and
    Biomedical Engineering
Memphis, Tennessee

NORFLEET B. THOMPSON, MD
Instructor
University of Tennessee–Campbell Clinic
Department of Orthopaedic Surgery and
    Biomedical Engineering
Memphis, Tennessee

THOMAS W. THROCKMORTON, MD
Professor
Co-Director, Sports Medicine Fellowship
University of Tennessee–Campbell Clinic
Department of Orthopaedic Surgery and
    Biomedical Engineering
Memphis, Tennessee

PATRICK C. TOY, MD
Associate Professor
University of Tennessee–Campbell Clinic
Department of Orthopaedic Surgery and
    Biomedical Engineering
Memphis, Tennessee

WILLIAM C. WARNER JR., MD
Professor
University of Tennessee–Campbell Clinic
Department of Orthopaedic Surgery and
    Biomedical Engineering
Memphis, Tennessee

JOHN C. WEINLEIN, MD
Assistant Professor
Director, Trauma Fellowship
University of Tennessee–Campbell Clinic
Department of Orthopaedic Surgery and
    Biomedical Engineering
Memphis, Tennessee

WILLIAM J. WELLER, MD
Instructor
University of Tennessee–Campbell Clinic
Department of Orthopaedic Surgery and
    Biomedical Engineering
Memphis, Tennessee

A. PAIGE WHITTLE, MD
Associate Professor
University of Tennessee–Campbell Clinic
Department of Orthopaedic Surgery and
    Biomedical Engineering
Memphis, Tennessee

KEITH D. WILLIAMS, MD
Associate Professor
University of Tennessee–Campbell Clinic
Department of Orthopaedic Surgery and
    Biomedical Engineering
Memphis, Tennessee

DEXTER H. WITTE III, MD
Clinical Assistant Professor in
    Radiology
University of Tennessee–Campbell Clinic
Department of Orthopaedic Surgery and
    Biomedical Engineering
Memphis, Tennessee

When Dr. Willis Campbell published the first edition of *Campbell's Operative Orthopaedics* in 1939, he could not have envisioned that over 80 years later it would have evolved into a four-volume text and earned the accolade of the "bible of orthopaedics" as a mainstay in orthopaedic practices and educational institutions all over the world. This expansion from some 400 pages in the first edition to over 4,500 pages in this 14th edition has not changed Dr. Campbell's original intent: "to present to the student, the general practitioner, and the surgeon the subject of orthopaedic surgery in a simple and comprehensive manner." In each edition since the first, authors and editors have worked diligently to fulfill these objectives. This would have not been possible without the hard work of our contributors who always strive to present the most up-to-date information while retaining "tried and true" techniques and tips. The scope of this text continues to expand in the hope that the information will be relevant to physicians no matter their location or resources.

As always, this edition also is the result of the collaboration of a group of "behind the scenes" individuals who are involved in the actual production process. The Campbell Foundation staff—Kay Daugherty, Linda Jones, and Tonya Priggel—contributed their considerable talents to editing often confusing and complex author contributions, searching the literature for obscure references, and, in general, "herding the cats." Special thanks to Kay and Linda who have worked on multiple editions of *Campbell's Operative Orthopaedics* (nine editions for Kay and six for Linda). They probably know more about orthopaedics than most of us, and they certainly know how to make it more understandable. Thanks, too, to the Elsevier personnel who provided guidance and assistance throughout the publication process: John Casey, Senior Project Manager; Jennifer Ehlers, Senior Content Development Specialist; and Belinda Kuhn, Senior Content Strategist.

We are especially appreciative of our spouses, Julie Azar and Terry Beaty, and our families for their patience and support as we worked through this project.

The preparation and publication of this 14th edition was fraught with difficulties because of the worldwide pandemic and social unrest, but our contributors and other personnel worked tirelessly, often in creative and innovative ways, to bring it to fruition. It is our hope that these efforts have provided a text that is informative and valuable to all orthopaedists as they continue to refine and improve methods that will ensure the best outcomes for their patients.

Frederick M. Azar, MD
James H. Beaty, MD

CONTENTS

PART I

GENERAL PRINCIPLES

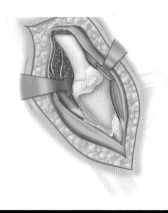

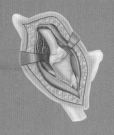

CHAPTER 1

SURGICAL TECHNIQUES
Andrew H. Crenshaw Jr.

SURGICAL TECHNIQUES

There are several surgical techniques especially important in orthopaedics: use of tourniquets, use of radiographs and image intensifiers in the operating room, positioning of the patient, local preparation of the patient, and draping of the appropriate part or parts. Operative techniques common to many procedures, fixation of tendons or fascia to bone, and bone grafting also are described.

TOURNIQUETS

Operations on the extremities are made easier using a tourniquet. The tourniquet is a potentially dangerous instrument that must be used with proper knowledge and care. In some procedures, a tourniquet is a luxury, whereas in others, such as delicate operations on the hand, it is a necessity. A pneumatic tourniquet is safer than an Esmarch tourniquet or a Martin sheet rubber bandage.

A pneumatic tourniquet with a hand pump and an accurate pressure gauge probably is the safest, but a constantly regulated pressure tourniquet is satisfactory if it is properly maintained and checked. A tourniquet should be applied by an individual experienced in its use.

Several sizes of pneumatic tourniquets are available for the upper and lower extremities. The upper arm or the thigh is wrapped with several thicknesses of smoothly applied cast padding. Rajpura et al. showed that application of more than two layers of padding resulted in a significant reduction in the actual transmitted pressure. When applying a tourniquet on an obese patient, an assistant manually grasps the flesh of the extremity just distal to the level of tourniquet application and firmly pulls this loose tissue distally before the cast padding is placed. Traction on the soft tissue is maintained while the padding and tourniquet are applied, and the latter is secured. The assistant's grasp is released, resulting in a greater proportion of the subcutaneous tissue remaining distal to the tourniquet. This bulky tissue tends to support the tourniquet and push it into an even more proximal position. All air is expressed from the sphygmomanometer or pneumatic tourniquet before application. When a sphygmomanometer cuff is used, it should be wrapped with a gauze bandage to prevent its slipping during inflation. The extremity is elevated for 2 minutes, or the blood is expressed by a sterile sheet rubber bandage or a cotton elastic bandage. Beginning at the fingertips or toes, the extremity is wrapped proximally to within 2.5 to 5 cm of the tourniquet. If a Martin sheet rubber bandage or an elastic bandage is applied up to the level of the tourniquet, the latter tends to slip distally at the time of inflation. The tourniquet should be inflated quickly to prevent filling of the superficial veins before the arterial blood flow has been occluded. Every effort is made to decrease tourniquet time; the extremity often is prepared and ready before the tourniquet is inflated. The conical, obese, or muscular lower extremity presents a special challenge. If a curved tourniquet is not available, a straight tourniquet may be used but is difficult to hold in place because it tends to slide distally during skin preparation. Application of adhesive drapes, extra cast padding, and pulling the fat tissue distally before applying the tourniquet generally works. A simple method has been described to keep a tourniquet in place on a large thigh. Surgical lubricating jelly is applied circumferentially to the thigh, and several layers of 6-inch cast padding are applied over the jelly. The tourniquet is then applied. The cast padding adheres to the lubricating jelly-covered skin and reduces the tendency of the tourniquet to slide.

If surgery is significantly delayed, both lower extremities should be studied with Doppler ultrasonography for the presence of deep venous thrombi. If present, the patient should receive full anticoagulation treatment and the procedure delayed. If the procedure is emergent, insertion of an inferior vena cava filter should be considered. There have been case reports describing fatal or near fatal pulmonary emboli after exsanguination of a leg.

The exact pressure to which the tourniquet should be inflated has not been determined (Table 1.1). The correct pressure depends on the age of the patient, the blood pressure, and the size of the extremity. Reid et al. used pneumatic tourniquet pressures determined by the pressure required to obliterate the peripheral pulse (limb occlusion pressure) using a Doppler stethoscope; they then added 50 to 75 mm Hg to allow for collateral circulation and blood pressure changes. Tourniquet pressures of 135 to 255 mm Hg for the upper extremity and 175 to 305 mm Hg for the lower extremity were satisfactory for maintaining hemostasis.

Wide tourniquet cuffs are more effective at lower inflation pressures than are narrow ones. Curved tourniquets on conical extremities require significantly lower arterial occlusion pressures than straight (rectangular) tourniquets (Fig. 1.1). The use of straight tourniquets on conical thighs should be avoided, especially in extremely muscular or obese individuals.

TABLE 1.1

Published Recommendations on Tourniquet Use

ORGANIZATION/STUDY	PRESSURE	DURATION (MIN)	REPERFUSION INTERVAL
Association of Surgical Technologists	Upper extremity, 50 mm Hg above SBP; lower extremity, 100 mm Hg above SBP	Upper extremity, 60; lower extremity, 90	15 min
Association of Perioperative Registered Nurses	40 mm Hg above LOP for LOP <130 mm Hg; 60 mm Hg above LOP for LOP <131-190 mm Hg; 80 mm Hg above LOP for LOP >190 mm Hg	Upper extremity, 60; lower extremity, 90	15 min deflation after every 1 h of tourniquet time
Wakai et al.	General recommendation, 50-75 mm Hg above LOP; upper extremity, 50-75 mm Hg above SBP; lower extremity, 90-150 mm Hg above SBP	120	30 min at 2-h point in surgery lasting >3 h
Kam et al.	50-150 mm Hg above SBP, using the lower end of the range for the upper extremity and the higher end for the lower extremity	120	10 min at the 2-h point for surgery lasting <2 h
Noordin et al.	Use LOP. No margin specified	120	NR

LOP, Limb occlusion pressure; *NR,* no recommendation; *SBP,* systolic blood pressure.
From Fitzgibbons PG, DiGiovanni C, Hares S, Akelman E: Safe tourniquet use: a review of the literature, *J Am Acad Orthop Surg* 20:310, 2012.

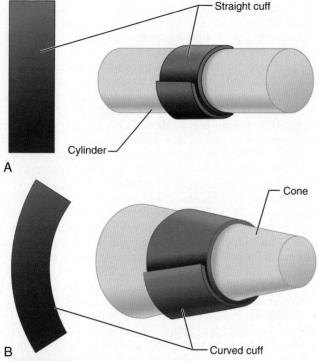

A

B

FIGURE 1.1 **A,** Straight (rectangular) tourniquets fit optimally on cylindrical limbs. **B,** Curved tourniquets best fit conical limbs. (From Pedowitz RA, Gershuni DH, Botte MJ, et al: The use of lower tourniquet inflation pressures in extremity surgery facilitated by curved and wide tourniquets and integrated cuff inflation system, *Clin Orthop Relat Res* 287:237, 1993.)

Any solution applied to skin must not be allowed to run beneath the tourniquet, or a chemical burn may result. A circumferential adhesive-backed plastic drape applied to the skin just distal to the tourniquet prevents solutions from running under the tourniquet. Sterile pneumatic tourniquets are available for operations around the elbow and knee. The limb may be prepared and draped before the tourniquet is applied. Rarely, a superficial slough of the skin may occur at the upper margin of the tourniquet in the region of the gluteal fold. This slough usually occurs in obese individuals and is probably related to the use of a straight, instead of a curved, tourniquet.

Pneumatic tourniquets should be kept in good repair, and all valves and gauges must be checked routinely. The inner tube should be completely enclosed in a casing to prevent the tube from ballooning through an opening, allowing the pressure to fall or causing a "blowout." The cuff also should be inspected carefully. Single-use sterile disposable tourniquets are preferable because reusable tourniquets must be thoroughly decontaminated after each use to prevent microbial colonization.

Any aneroid gauge must be calibrated frequently. Newer gauges carry instruction cards with them. They are sold with test gauges so that the gauges on the tourniquets can be tested for proper calibration. Many automatic tourniquet control units will self-test when turned on. If there is a discrepancy, the unit must be manually checked with a test gauge. If the discrepancy is more than 20 mm Hg, the unit should be repaired or replaced. One of the greatest dangers in the use of a tourniquet is an improperly registering gauge; gauges have

been found to be 300 mm off calibration. In many tourniquet injuries, the gauges were later checked and found to be grossly inaccurate, allowing excessive pressure.

Tourniquet paralysis can result from (1) excessive pressure; (2) insufficient pressure, resulting in passive congestion of the part, with hemorrhagic infiltration of the nerve; (3) keeping the tourniquet inflated too long; or (4) application without consideration of the local anatomy. There is no rule as to how long a tourniquet may be safely inflated. The time may vary with the age of the patient and the vascular supply of the extremity. In an average healthy adult younger than 50 years of age, we prefer to leave the tourniquet inflated for no more than 2 hours. If an operation on the lower extremity takes longer than 2 hours, it is better to finish it as rapidly as possible than to deflate the tourniquet for 10 minutes and then reinflate it. It has been found that 40 minutes is required for the tissues to return to normal after prolonged use of a tourniquet. Consequently, the previous practice of deflating the tourniquet for 10 minutes seems to be inadequate. Posttourniquet syndrome, as first recognized by Bunnell, is a common reaction to prolonged ischemia and is characterized by edema, pallor, joint stiffness, motor weakness, and subjective numbness. This complication is thought to be related to the duration of ischemia and not to the mechanical effect of the tourniquet. Posttourniquet syndrome interferes with early motion and results in increased requirement for narcotics. Spontaneous resolution usually occurs within 1 week.

Compartment syndrome, rhabdomyolysis, and pulmonary emboli are rare complications of tourniquet use. Rasmussen et al. found that muscle beneath the tourniquet had a greater ischemic response than muscle distal to the tourniquet. One study, using transesophageal echocardiography during arthroscopic knee surgery, showed that asymptomatic pulmonary embolism can occur within 1 minute after tourniquet release. The number of small emboli depended on the duration of tourniquet inflation. Vascular complications can occur in patients with severe arteriosclerosis or prosthetic grafts. A tourniquet should not be applied over a prosthetic vascular graft.

Pneumatic tourniquets usually are applied to the upper arm and thigh, and a well-padded proximal calf tourniquet is safe for foot and ankle surgery. General guidelines for the safe use of pneumatic tourniquets are outlined in Table 1.2.

The Esmarch tourniquet is still in use in some areas and is the safest and most practical of the elastic tourniquets. It is never used except in the middle and upper thirds of the thigh. This tourniquet has a definite, although limited, use in that it can be applied higher on the thigh than can the pneumatic tourniquet. The Esmarch tourniquet is applied in layers, one on top of the other; a wide band produces less tissue damage than does a narrow one.

A Martin rubber sheet bandage can be safely used as a tourniquet for short procedures on the foot. The leg is elevated and exsanguinated by wrapping the rubber bandage up over the malleoli of the ankle and securing it with a clamp. The distal portion of the bandage is released to expose the operative area.

Special attention should be given when using tourniquets on fingers and toes. A rubber ring tourniquet or a tourniquet made from a glove finger that is rolled onto the digit should not be used because it can be inadvertently left in place under a dressing, resulting in catastrophic loss of the digit. A glove finger or Penrose drain can be looped around the proximal

TABLE 1.2	
Braithwaite and Klenerman's Modification of Bruner's Ten Rules of Pneumatic Tourniquet Use	
APPLICATION	Apply only to a healthy limb or with caution to an unhealthy limb
SIZE OF TOURNIQUET	Arm, 10 cm; leg, 15 cm or wider in large legs
SITE OF APPLICATION	Upper arm; mid/upper thigh ideally
PADDING	At least two layers of orthopaedic felt
SKIN PREPARATION	Occlude to prevent soaking of wool. Use 50-100 mm Hg above systolic for the arm; double systolic for the thigh; or arm 200-250 mm Hg, leg 250-350 mm Hg (large cuffs are recommended for larger limbs instead of increasing pressure)
TIME	Absolute maximum 3 h (recovers in 5-7 days) generally not to exceed 2 h
TEMPERATURE	Avoid heating (e.g., hot lights), cool if feasible, and keep tissues moist
DOCUMENTATION	Duration and pressure at least weekly calibration and against mercury manometer or test maintenance gauge; maintenance every 3 months

Modified from Kutty S, McElwain JP: Padding under tourniquets in tourniquet controlled surgery: Bruner's ten rules revisited, *Injury* 33:75, 2002.

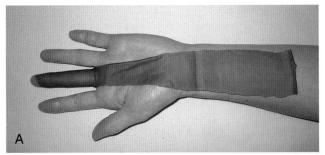
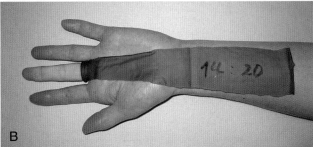

FIGURE 1.2 **A,** Cut 1 cm from the end of the corresponding glove finger, then cut through the palm half of the glove finger at the base and extend both ends of the cut longitudinally along the backside of the glove. Remove the remaining glove and finger and apply it to the palm side of the hand. **B,** Roll the glove finger back to serve as a tourniquet. Tourniquet start time can be written on the glove flap. (From Osanai T, Ogino T: Modified digital tourniquet designed to prevent the tourniquet from inadvertently being left in place after the end of the surgery, *J Orthop Trauma* 24:387, 2010.)

portion of the digit, stretched, and secured with a hemostat. It is difficult to include a hemostat inadvertently in a digital dressing. A modified glove finger with a volar flap will help prevent inadvertently leaving the tourniquet in place after surgery (Fig. 1.2).

The ForgetMeNot digital tourniquet (Arex, Palaiseau, France) is a reusable silicone tourniquet (Fig. 1.3) with long tails and a bright color (blue or yellow) that help prevent accidental incorporation of the tourniquet into a dressing. Sterile disposable rubber ring tourniquets are now available for use on the upper and lower extremities. These tourniquets are wrapped in stockinette and are applied by rolling the rubber ring and stockinette up the extremity, which exsanguinates the extremity. The stockinette is then cut away at the operative site. Rubber ring tourniquets are not indicated in the presence of malignancy, infections, significant skin lesions, unstable fractures or dislocations, poor peripheral blood flow, edema, or deep venous thrombosis. Sizing of these tourniquets is based on systolic blood pressure.

The use of preoperative prophylactic antibiotics in orthopaedic operations has been accepted practice for over 30 years and decreases the likelihood of postoperative infection. Most believe that these antibiotics should be given prior to inflation of the tourniquet to ensure that the antibiotic is present in the tissues before the incision is made. There has been no consensus as to the interval between antibiotic administration and tourniquet inflation, with variations in time from 5 to 20 minutes being reported. Our institution recommends administration of cefazolin within 1 hour of tourniquet inflation. Studies have shown that a 1-minute interval resulted in cefazolin concentration in soft tissue and bone at or greater than the minimum inhibitory concentrations for microorganisms encountered in orthopaedic surgery. A prospective randomized study found that the administration of antibiotics 1 minute after tourniquet inflation resulted in a significantly lower infection rate than the administration of antibiotics 5 minutes before tourniquet inflation, suggesting that administration before tourniquet inflation does not give better results.

RADIOGRAPHS IN THE OPERATING ROOM

Often it is necessary to obtain radiographs during an orthopaedic procedure. Radiography technicians who work in the operating room must wear the same clothing and masks as the circulating personnel. These technicians must have a clear understanding of aseptic surgical technique and draping to avoid contaminating the drapes in the operative field. Portable radiograph units used in the operating room should be cleaned regularly and ideally are not used in any other area of the hospital.

When an unsterile radiograph cassette is to be introduced into the sterile field, it should be placed inside a sterile double pillowcase or sterile plastic bag that is folded over so that the exterior remains sterile. The pillowcase or plastic bag is covered by a large sterile towel, ensuring at least two layers of sterile drapes on the cassette. The operative wound should be covered with a sterile towel when anteroposterior view

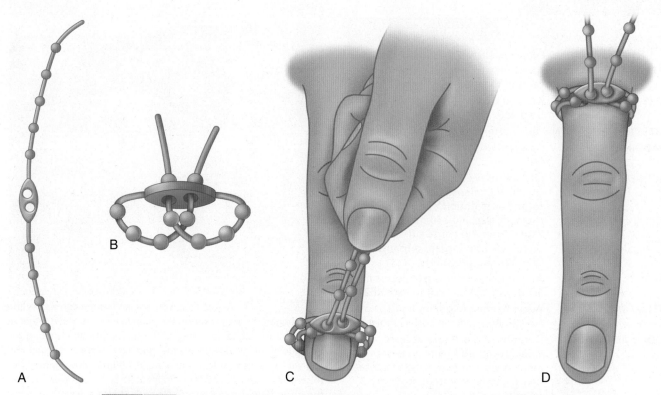

FIGURE 1.3 **A,** The ForgetMeNot tourniquet as supplied. **B,** Form two loops. **C,** Place the digit in the space between the two loops and pull proximally to exsanguinate the digit. **D,** Tourniquet in place. (Modified from Diaz HJJ, et al: The new digit tourniquet ForgetMeNot, *Orthop Traumatol Surg Res* 104:133, 2018.)

radiographs are made to avoid possible contamination from the machine as it is moved into position.

Portable C-arm image intensifier television fluoroscopy allows instantaneous evaluation of the position of fracture fragments and internal fixation devices. Many of these machines have the ability to make permanent radiographs. When used near the sterile field, the C-arm portion of the machine must be draped in a sterile fashion (Fig. 1.4A). Every time the C-arm is brought to the lateral position (Fig. 1.4B), a fresh or sterile, disposable drape should be applied over the end of the C-arm and dropped off the field when complete. This prevents the potentially contaminated lower half of the drape from getting near the patient and operating surgeon.

As with any electronic device, failure of an image intensifier can occur. In this event, backup plain radiographs are necessary. Two-plane radiographs can be made, even of the hip when necessary, using portable equipment (Fig. 1.4C, D). Closed intramedullary nailing or percutaneous fracture fixation techniques may need to be abandoned for an open technique if the image intensifier fails.

All operating room personnel should avoid exposure to radiation. Proper lead-lined aprons should be worn beneath sterile operating gowns. Thyroid shields, lead-impregnated eyeglasses, and rubber gloves are available to decrease exposure. C-arm imaging should be used as a 1- to 2-second pulse to produce a still image for viewing. Active fluoroscopy with the C-arm should be avoided to prevent excessive radiation exposure.

PREVENTING MISTAKES

Before entering the operating room, the surgeon and the awake, alert patient should agree on the planned procedure and the surgical site. The surgeon should mark this clearly with his or her initials to prevent a "wrong-site" error. Once the patient is under anesthesia, a designated member of the team should state the name of the patient, the procedure, and the correct site. All members of the team should be in agreement. This statement should be clear, concise, and not contain unnecessary information. A short statement is more likely to be closely heard. This statement should be preferably made after draping.

POSITIONING OF THE PATIENT

The position of a patient on the operating table should be adjusted to afford maximal safety to the patient and convenience for the surgeon. A free airway must be maintained at all times, and unnecessary pressure on the chest or abdomen should be avoided. This is of particular importance when the patient is prone; in this position, sandbags are placed beneath the shoulders, and a thin pillow is placed beneath the symphysis

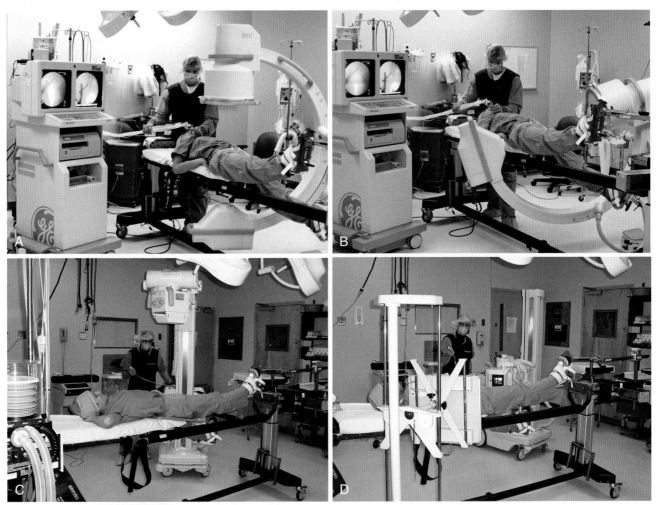

FIGURE 1.4   **A** and **B,** Portable C-arm image intensifier television fluoroscopy setup for fracture repair. C-arm rotates 90 degrees to obtain lateral view. **C** and **D,** Technique for two-plane radiographs during hip surgery with a portable machine for anteroposterior and lateral views. Film cassette for lateral view is positioned over superolateral aspect of hip.

pubis and hips to minimize pressure on the abdomen and chest. Large, moderately firm chest rolls extending from the iliac crests to the clavicular areas may serve the same purpose.

When the patient is supine, the sacrum must be well padded; and when the patient is lying on his or her side, the greater trochanter and the fibular neck should be similarly protected. When a muscle relaxant drug is used, the danger of stretching a nerve or a group of nerves is increased. Figure 1.5 shows traction on the brachial plexus from improper positioning of the arm. The brachial plexus can be stretched when the arm is on an arm board, particularly if it is hyperabducted to make room for the surgeon or an assistant or for administration of intravenous therapy. The arm should not be tied above the head in abduction and external rotation while a body cast is applied because this position may cause a brachial plexus paralysis. Rather, the arm should be suspended in flexion from an overhead frame, and the position should be changed frequently. Figure 1.6 shows the position of the arm on the operating table that may cause pressure on the ulnar nerve, particularly if someone on the operating team leans against the arm. The arm must never be allowed to hang over the edge of the table. Padding should be placed over the area

where a nerve may be pressed against the bone (i.e., the radial nerve in the arm, the ulnar nerve at the elbow, and the peroneal nerve at the neck of the fibula).

LOCAL PREPARATION OF THE PATIENT

Superficial oil and skin debris are removed with a thorough 10-minute soap-and-water scrub. We prefer a skin cleanser containing 7.5% povidone-iodine solution that is diluted approximately 50% with sterile saline solution or Hexachlorophene-containing skin cleanser when allergy to shellfish or iodine is present or suspected. After scrubbing, the skin is blotted dry with sterile towels.

After a tourniquet has been fitted, if one is required, the sterile sheets applied during the earlier preparation should be removed. Care should be taken that the operative field does not become contaminated because the effectiveness of the preparation would be partially lost. With the patient in the proper position, the solutions are applied, each with a separate sterile sponge stick, beginning in the central area of the

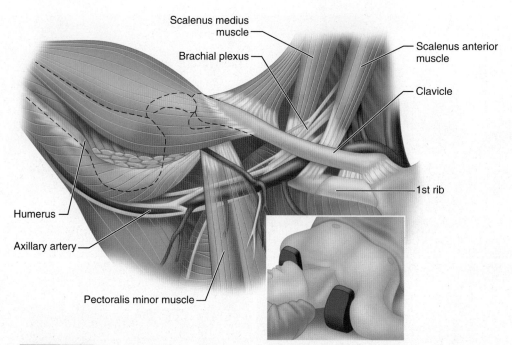

Scalenus medius muscle

Brachial plexus

Scalenus anterior muscle

Clavicle

1st rib

Humerus

Axillary artery

Pectoralis minor muscle

FIGURE 1.5 Anatomic relationships of brachial plexus when limb is hyperabducted. *Inset,* With patient in Trendelenburg position, brace at shoulder is in poor position because limb has been abducted and placed on arm board.

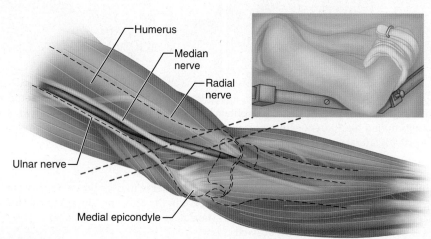

Humerus

Median nerve

Radial nerve

Ulnar nerve

Medial epicondyle

FIGURE 1.6 Points at which nerves of arm may be damaged by pressure *(dashed lines). Inset,* Pressure is applied to medial side of arm because patient is poorly positioned on operating table.

site of the incision and proceeding peripherally. Once painted on, it is allowed to dry and then is taken off with plain alcohol. Some surgeons routinely use povidone-iodine solution, especially when the risk of a chemical burn from tincture of iodine is significant. The immediate operative field is prepared first; the area is enlarged to include ample surrounding skin. The sponges used to prepare the lumbar spine are carried toward the gluteal cleft and anus rather than in the opposite direction. Sponges should not be saturated because the solution would extend beyond the operative field and must be removed. If the linen on the table or the sterile drape becomes saturated with strong antiseptic solutions, they should be replaced by fresh linen or drapes. Solutions should not be allowed to flow

underneath a tourniquet. Pooled alcohol-based solutions should be removed from the field because they can be ignited by a spark from a cautery unit.

When traumatic wounds are present, tincture of iodine and other alcohol-containing solutions should not be used for antiseptic wound preparation. Povidone-iodine or hexachlorophene solutions without alcohol should be used instead to avoid tissue death.

In operations around the upper third of the thigh, the pelvis, or the lower lumbar spine in male patients, the genitalia should be displaced and held away from the operative field with adhesive tape. A long, wide strip of tape similarly helps cover the gluteal cleft, from which there is the potential of infection.

In female patients, the genital area and gluteal cleft also are covered longitudinally by strips of adhesive tape. Adherent, sterile, plastic drapes can be used for these purposes.

Before the operative field in the region of the lower lumbar spine, sacroiliac joints, or buttocks is prepared, the gluteal cleft is sponged with alcohol and sterile dry gauze is inserted around the anus so that iodine or other solutions are prevented from running down to this region, causing dermatitis.

Brown et al. and others recommended that before total joint arthroplasty, the extremity should be held by a scrubbed and gowned assistant because this reduces bacterial air counts by almost half. They also recommended that instrument packs not be opened until skin preparation and draping are completed.

When these preparations are done in haste, the gown or gloves of the sterile assistant preparing the area may become contaminated without the assistant's knowledge. To prevent this, a nurse or anesthetist should be appointed to watch this stage of preparation.

WOUND IRRIGATING SOLUTIONS

At our institution, we routinely irrigate clean surgical wounds to keep them moist with sterile isotonic saline or lactated Ringer solution. Occasionally, if the risk of wound contamination is high, antimicrobial irrigating solutions are used. A triple antibiotic solution of bacitracin, neomycin, and polymyxin is recommended because it provides the most complete coverage in clean and contaminated wounds. Antibiotic solutions should remain in the wound for at least 1 minute. Pulsatile lavage systems and basting-type syringes blow debris into the soft tissues and are being replaced with cystoscopy tubing for irrigation and debridement, especially in treatment of open fractures and infections.

DRAPING

Draping is an important step in any surgical procedure and should not be assigned to an inexperienced assistant. Haphazard draping that results in exposure of unprepared areas of skin in the middle of an operation can be catastrophic. Considerable experience is required in placing the drapes, not only to prevent them from becoming disarranged during the operation but also to avoid contamination of the surgeon and the drapes. If there is the least doubt as to the sterility of the drapes or the surgeon when draping is complete, the entire process should be repeated. Unless assistants are well trained, the surgeon should drape the patient.

In the foundation layer of drapes, towel clips or skin staples are placed not only through the drapes but also through the skin to prevent slipping of the drapes and exposure of the contaminated skin. In every case, the foundation drapes should be placed to overlap the prepared area of skin at least 3 inches (7.5 cm). During draping, the gloved hands should not come in contact with the prepared skin.

Cloth drapes are being replaced with disposable paper and plastic drape packages specifically designed for the area to be draped (Figs. 1.7 and 1.8). A disposable drape package should have at least one layer made of waterproof plastic to prevent fluids from soaking through to unprepared areas of the body. Drape packages for bilateral knee and foot surgery also are available. Paper drapes shed lint that collects on exposed horizontal surfaces in the operating room if those surfaces are not cleaned daily.

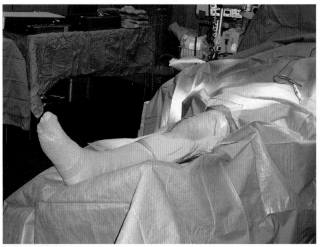

FIGURE 1.7   Disposable drape package for knee surgery.

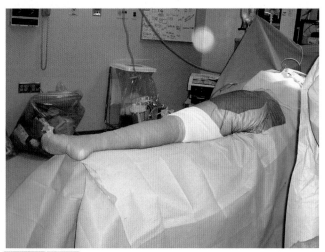

FIGURE 1.8   Disposable drape package for hip surgery.

DRAPING THE EDGES OF THE INCISION

The gloved hand should not come in contact with the skin before the incision is made. For the extremities, a section of sterile stockinette is drawn proximally over the operative field. The stockinette is grasped proximally and distally and cut with scissors to uncover the area of the proposed incision. Its cut edges are pulled apart, and the area is covered by a transparent adhesive-coated material (Fig. 1.9). A large transparent plastic adhesive drape may be wrapped entirely around the extremity or over the entire operative field so that the stockinette is not needed. The incision is made through the material and the skin at the same time. The edges of the incision are neatly draped, and the operative field is virtually waterproof; this prevents the drapes in some areas from becoming soaked with blood, which can be a source of contamination. The plastic adhesive drape minimizes the need for towel clips or staples around the wound edge and allows the entire undraped field to be seen easily. Visibility is especially important when there are scars from previous injuries or surgery that must be accommodated by a new incision. Old incisions should be traced with a sterile marking pen before application of plastic adhesive drape material.

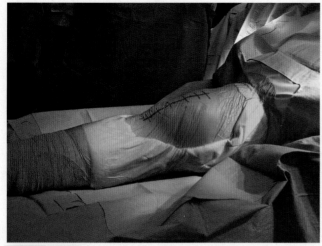

FIGURE 1.9   Iodoform-impregnated plastic adhesive drape.

PREVENTION OF HUMAN IMMUNODEFICIENCY VIRUS AND HEPATITIS VIRUS TRANSMISSION

At our institution, we follow the American Academy of Orthopaedic Surgeons (AAOS) Task Force recommendations on acquired immunodeficiency syndrome (HIV), hepatitis B virus (HBV), and hepatitis C virus (HCV), which go beyond those recommended for health care personnel by the Centers for Disease Control and Prevention (CDC) and the American Hospital Association. Every effort should be made to prevent further transmission of these diseases in all areas of medical care. For specific recommendations, the reader is referred to the AAOS Task Force guidelines. We strongly agree with the following AAOS recommendations regarding HIV, HBV, and HCV precautions in the operating room:

1. Do not hurry an operation. Excess speed results in injury. The most experienced surgeon should be responsible for the surgical procedure if the risk of injury to operating room personnel is high.
2. Wear surgical garb that offers protection against contact with blood. Knee-high, waterproof, surgical shoe covers, water-impervious gowns or undergarments, and full head covers should be worn.
3. Double gloves should be worn at all times.
4. Surgical masks should be changed if they become moist or splattered.
5. Protective eyewear (goggles or full face shields) that covers exposed skin and mucous membranes should be used.
6. To avoid inadvertent injury to surgical personnel, the surgeon should:
   - Use instrument ties and other "no-touch" suturing and sharp instrument techniques when possible.
   - Avoid tying with a suture needle in hand.
   - Avoid passing sharp instruments and needles from hand to hand; instead, they should be placed on an intermediate tray.
   - Announce when sharp instruments are about to be passed.
   - Avoid having two surgeons suture the same wound.
   - Take extra care when performing digital examinations of fracture fragments or wounds containing wires or sharp instrumentation.
   - Avoid contact with osteotomes, drill bits, and saws.
   - Use of full protective gowns, hoods, and surgical facemasks with eyeshields when splatter is inevitable, such as when irrigating large wounds or using power equipment.
   - Routinely check gowns, masks, and shoe covers of operating room personnel for contamination during the surgical procedure and change as necessary.
7. Incidents of exposure of health care personnel to potentially infected fluids should be reported to a person designated by the health care facility to be responsible for managing occupational exposures. Relevant histories and incident information should be documented, and the source patient and exposed health care worker appropriately tested within applicable laws as recommended by the CDC. Follow-up testing of exposed personnel should be performed as recommended by the CDC. Patients exposed to a potentially infected health care provider should be immediately informed of the incident and the above recommendations for exposed health care providers must be followed.
8. Postexposure prophylaxis for HBV and HIV should be provided as recommended by the U.S. Public Health Service. There is no postexposure prophylaxis for HCV.

Protective gowns and full hoods with surgical facemask should be routinely used for total joint arthroplasty and for large trauma and elective cases. Blood spatter should be avoided and at a minimum protective eyewear and gloves should be worn by all members of the team including observers. Kevlar impregnated gloves worn under rubber gloves will not prevent puncture wounds but will prevent scalpel lacerations and should be worn when operating on patients with HIV, HBV, or HBC.

REVERSING PROPHYLACTIC ANTICOAGULATION PRIOR TO SURGERY

Patients on anticoagulants will usually need reversal prior to major surgery. Anticoagulation in electively scheduled patients can easily be reversed with medical management prior to surgery. Tables 1.3 and 1.4 outline procedures for urgent reversal of anticoagulants and give the half-lives of the various anticoagulants in use if reversal is not as urgent.

BLOOD LOSS CONTROL DURING SURGERY

When a tourniquet cannot be used because of the location of the surgical site or when blood loss is expected to be high after tourniquet release, routine blood loss control measures should be readily available. These include electrocautery, gel foam, thrombin, and epinephrine. Preoperative planning for larger procedures should include expected blood loss, and preparation should be made to have donor or autologous blood, or both, available and a blood recycling system (cell-saver) present if needed.

The use of the fibrinolytic, tranexamic acid (TXA) has become popular in large joint arthroplasty surgery for reducing blood loss. Luo et al. performed a prospective, randomized, double-blind, controlled study that showed equal efficacy in reducing blood loss in primary total hip surgery when TXA was used orally, topically, or by intravenous infusion. TXA was administered 2 g orally 2 hours before surgery, 2 g into the wound, or 20 mg/kg intravenously.

VENOUS THROMBOEMBOLISM PROPHYLAXIS

Patients with acute lower extremity injuries or other injuries requiring bed rest should have prophylactic anticoagulation with a readily reversible anticoagulant (heparin or a low-molecular weight heparin) before surgery. Anticoagulation should be continued after surgery until the patient is mobile. Subcutaneous low-molecular-weight heparin for 10 to 14 days after discharge followed by 4 to 6 weeks of aspirin works well. Patients having elective lower extremity surgery may receive prophylactic anticoagulation immediately after surgery, and this should be continued for 6 to 8 weeks after discharge as outlined above. Patients with bilateral lower extremity injuries that prevent ambulation for a longer period of time require bridging from low-molecular-weight heparin to warfarin, and this is continued with prothrombin time monitoring until the patient is mobile. All patients requiring surgery should have lower extremity segmental compression devices applied to unoperated lower extremities during surgery and while in bed before and after surgery.

POSTOPERATIVE PAIN CONTROL

The use of local anesthetic infiltration of surgical wounds and regional anesthetic blocks has increased with the popularity of outpatient total joint surgery. Specific modalities for these procedures can be found in the arthroplasty sections of this edition. Local infiltration in layers with bupivacaine or bupivacaine liposome suspension (Pacira, Parsippany, NJ) helps decrease use of opioids in the immediate postoperative period. The suspension is expensive but can last up to 72 hours. The maximal dose is 266 mg and should be infiltrated in divided doses in a layered approach from deep musculature and fascia up into subcutaneous tissue.

Regional blocks can be administered before or after the procedure. A team approach between the orthopaedic surgeon and the anesthesiologist regarding the use of regional blocks and postanesthesia intravenous nonnarcotic pain medications also helps to decrease the need for opioid pain medication. Patients should be advised on how much reliance on narcotic pain medication is expected after surgery. Other nonnarcotic medications are just as effective and not addictive. If patients know the surgeon's narcotic prescribing boundaries on the front end, the postoperative period will be less stressful for all. Drug testing should be performed if warranted, and the anesthesiologist notified of the results.

Careful attention must be paid to patients treated by pain management specialists. Their postoperative care should be

TABLE 1.3
Anticoagulant Reversal

ANTITHROMBOTIC	REVERSAL AGENT(S)	COMMENTS
DIRECT THROMBIN INHIBITORS (DTIs) *PO:* ■ Dabigatran (Pradaxa) Half-life 12-17 hr in normal renal function	**Idarucizumab (Praxbind)**—*only used for reversal of dabigatran (Pradaxa)* *Restrictions:* patients confirmed to have recent dabigatran use who: ■ Require anticoagulant reversal for life-threatening hemorrhage, *OR* ■ Require urgent/emergent invasive procedure within the next 8 hours *Dose:* 5 g *Administration:* Infuse *two* 2.5 g/50 mL vials undiluted over 5-10 min each, consecutively ■ Line should be flushed with NS prior to infusion ■ Second vial should be infused within 15 min of first vial *Onset:* Immediate **Kcentra—4 Factor PCC** **(May be considered for dabigatran reversal if idarucizumab not available)** *Dose*:* 1500 units × 1 (optional rescue dose of 1500 units available if hemostasis not achieved) *Administration:* Send Kcentra Kit for bedside reconstitution and administer via IV push over 5 min ■ Use within 4 hr of reconstitution *Onset:* <30 min *Caution:* thrombotic risk *Kcentra contains trace amounts of heparin (to mitigate thrombotic potential) and should not be used in bleeding patients with active or recent (last 100 days) heparin-induced thrombocytopenia (HIT). In this instance, please contact pharmacy to discuss possible use of the alternative procoagulant FEIBA for reversal.*	*Use of PCC Idarucizumab:* ■ **REQUIRES ATTENDING APPROVAL** ■ Document attending name in the order comments *Additional options:* ■ If dabigatran ingested within 1 hour, consider activated charcoal. ■ Mechanical methods, such as dialysis, may be considered as a last resort *Laboratory measurement:* ■ A normal thrombin time (TT) rules out clinically relevant dabigatran effect ■ Do not use INR

Continued

TABLE 1.3		
Anticoagulant Reversal—cont'd		
ANTITHROMBOTIC	**REVERSAL AGENT(S)**	**COMMENTS**
IV: - Argatroban - Bivalirudin (Angiomax) Half-life 10-90 min	**IV DTIs:** - Short half-life and discontinuation of IV DTIs are primary means of attenuating bleed. - Support with crystalloid and blood products to facilitate rapid renal clearance of drug. - IV DTIs should be discontinued immediately upon bleeding discovery and rarely require other means of reversal.	

FACTOR XA INHIBITORS
- Fondaparinux (Arixtra)
Half-life 17-21 hr in normal renal function
- Rivaroxaban (Xarelto)
Half-life 5-9 hr
- Apixaban (Eliquis)
Half-life 8-15 hr
- Edoxaban (Savaysa)
Half-life 10-14 hr
	Kcentra - 4 Factor PCC
	Dose*: 1500 units × 1 (optional rescue dose of 1500 units available if hemostasis not achieved)
	Administration: Send Kcentra Kit for bedside reconstitution and administer via IV push over 5 min
	  - Use within 4 hr of reconstitution
	Onset: <30 min
	Caution: thrombotic risk
	Kcentra contains trace amounts of heparin (to mitigate thrombotic potential) and should not be used in bleeding patients with active or recent (last 100 days) heparin-induced thrombocytopenia (HIT). In this instance, please contact pharmacy to discuss possible use of the alternative procoagulant FEIBA for reversal.
	rFVIIa (if refractory to Kcentra)
	Dose*: 100 mcg/kg (dose cap at 100 kg to mitigate thrombotic risk)
	  - May repeat in 2 hr if continued bleeding
	Administration: IV bolus over 3-5 min
	  - Use within 3 hr of reconstitution
	Onset: <30 min
	Caution: thrombotic risk
		Use of PCC/rFVIIa:
		- **REQUIRES ATTENDING APPROVAL**
		- Document attending name in the order comments
		Additional options:
		- If rivaroxaban, apixaban, or edoxaban ingested within 1 hr, consider activated charcoal.
		- NOT DIALYZABLE
		Laboratory measurement:
		- A normal anti-Factor Xa level rules out clinically relevant drug effect
		- Do not use INR

HEPARIN Half-life:1-2 hr	**Protamine** *Dose:* 1 mg reverses 100 units of IV-administered UFH | TIME SINCE UFH	DOSE PER 100 UNITS UFH OVER LAST 3 HR | |---|---| | <30 min | 1.0 mg | | 30-120 min | 0.5 mg | | >120 min | 0.25 mg | - Do not exceed 50 mg in a single dose: high doses can have an undesirable ANTIcoagulant effect - **In clinical practice, give 50 mg IV x 1 over 10 min. May redose if bleeding continues.** *Administration:* Slow IV push not to exceed 5 mg/min *Onset:* 5-15 min *Caution:* Rapid administration can cause severe hypotension and anaphylaxis	- Prophylactic SQ doses of UFH do not lead to increased risk of hemorrhage. - Look for other causes of hemorrhage

LMWHs (enoxaparin)
Half-life 2-8 hr
	Protamine (Does not reverse LMWH as effectively as it does UFH)
	Dose: **1 mg for each 1 mg** of enoxaparin in last 8 hr
	  - If > 12 hr have elapsed since LMWH administration, protamine may not be needed
	  - Do not exceed 50 mg in a single dose; high doses can have an undesirable ANTIcoagulant effect
	  - In clinical practice, give 50 mg IV × 1 over 10 min. May redose if bleeding continues
	Administration: Slow IV push not to exceed 5 mg/min
	Onset: 5-15 min
	Caution: Rapid administration can cause severe hypotension and anaphylaxis
		- If aPTT remains prolonged, may give second dose of 0.5 mg protamine per 1 mg LMWH
		- Consider FFP and other blood product support

TABLE 1.3

Anticoagulant Reversal—cont'd

ANTITHROMBOTIC	REVERSAL AGENT(S)		COMMENTS

WARFARIN
Half-life 36 hr (5 days for INR normalization)
	SUPRATHERAPEUTIC INR
	■ INR 5-9: Omit 1-2 warfarin doses ±1-2.5 mg PO Vit K
	■ INR >9 (NO BLEED): omit 1-2 warfarin doses ± 2.5-5 mg PO Vit K
	ACTIVE BLEEDING AT ANY INR:
	■ Hold warfarin and give Vit K 5-10 mg IV (may repeat q 12 h based on repeat INR)
	MAJOR OR LIFE-THREATENING BLEED:
	■ Hold warfarin and give Vit K 10 mg IV (may repeat q 12 h based on repeat INR)
	   PLUS either Kcentra (preferred) or FFP
	■ Kcentra 1500 units × 1 **OR**
	■ FFP 10-30 mL/kg
	SURGERY REVERSAL
	■ INR >1.5-2.5
	   Surgery <24 hr:
	    ■ 0.5-1 mg IV Vit K × 1; ±5-8 mL/kg FFP
	   Surgery 24-96 hr:
	    ■ 0.5-1 mg PO Vit K ×1; monitor INR q12-24hr
	■ INR >2.5-5
	   Surgery <24 hr:
	    ■ 1-2.5 mg IV Vit K × 1; ±5-8 mL/kg FFP
	   Surgery 24-96 hr:
	    ■ 1-2.5 mg PO Vit K × 1; monitor INR q12-24hr
		Phytonadione (Vitamin K)
		Dose: See box on left
		Administration: IV-dilute in 50 mL NS and give over 30 min
		Onset: PO=24 hr; IV=12 hr
		Caution: IV—may be associated with very small risk of anaphylaxis
		FFP
		Dose: See box on left
		Administration: At least 10 mL/min
		Onset: 2-6 hr
		Caution: Carries risk of infection, must be thawed and a large volume is required (often >1 L)
		Kcentra
		Dose: 1500 units × 1 (optional rescue dose of 1500 units available if hemostasis or desired target INR not achieved)
		Administration: Send Kcentra Kit for bedside reconstitution and administer via IV push over 5 min
		■ Use within 4 hr of reconstitution
		Onset: <30 min
		Caution: thrombotic risk
		Kcentra contains trace amounts of heparin (to mitigate thrombotic potential) and should not be used in bleeding patients with active or recent (last 100 days) heparin-induced thrombocytopenia (HIT). In this instance, please contact pharmacy to discuss possible use of the alternative procoagulant FEIBA for reversal.
				Use of Kcentra:
				■ **REQUIRES ATTENDING APPROVAL**
				■ Document attending name in the order comments
				■ **REPEAT INR 30 MIN AFTER END OF Kcentra/FFP INFUSION**

*Doses are NOT based on high-quality evidence and are intended as suggestions only.
DDAVP, Desmopressin; *FFP*, fresh frozen plasma; *INR*, International Normalized Ratio; *IV*, intravenous; *LMWH*, low-molecular-weight heparin; *PCC*, prothrombin complex concentrates (Kcentra); *rVIIa*, recombinant active factor VIIa (NovoSeven); *SIVP*, slow intravenous push; *UFH*, unfractionated heparin.

Consider the following agents if patient refractory to standard therapies:

DDAVP:
  Mechanism: increases release of vWF and enhances platelet adhesion and aggregation
  Dose: 0.3 mcg/kg in 50 mL NS IV over 15 min
  Caution: Serial doses associated with tachyphylaxis, hyponatremia, and seizures

Aminocaproic acid:
  Mechanism: antifibrinolytic
  Dose: 4-5 g loading dose in 250 mL NS over 15 min followed by infusion of 1 g/hr infusion until bleeding subsides (max 30 g/day)
  Caution: May require renal adjustment.

Tranexamic acid:
  Mechanism: antifibrinolytic
  Dose: 1 g loading dose in 50 mL NS IV over 10 min followed by 1 g in 250 mL NS infused over the next 8 hr
  Caution: May require renal adjustment

From Dilworth T, Burnett A, Tawil I, Garcia D, Fletcher: Guideline for antithrombotic reversal. UNM Health System. Anticoagulation Subcommittee, UNMH P&T Committee. Updated October 2016. PDF downloads from here: https://hospitals.health.unm.edu/intranet7/apps/doc_management/index.cfm?document_id=198547.

TABLE 1.4			
Antiplatelet Reversal			
	HALF-LIFE	**REVERSAL AGENT**	**COMMENTS**
ASPIRIN	15-30 min 5-10 days for platelet recovery	**DDVAP** *Dose:* 0.3 mcg/kg IV × 1 *Administration:* over 15 min *Onset:* Immediate *Caution:* Serial doses associated with tachyphylaxis, hyponatremia, and seizures	▪ Short half-life and discontinuation of GP IIb-IIIa are primary means of attenuating bleed ▪ May consider transfusion of functioning platelets to attenuate bleeding ▪ Mechanical methods, such as dialysis, may be considered as a last resort
CLOPIDOGREL (Plavix)	8 hr ~5 days for platelet recovery		
PRASUGREL (Effient)	7 hr ≤7 days for platelet recovery		
TICAGRELOR (Brilinta)	~9 hr 3 days for platelet recovery		
GP IIb-IIIa Eptifibatide (Integrilin) Abciximab (ReoPro) Tirofiban (Aggrastat)	30-120 min		

*Doses are NOT based on high-quality evidence.
DDAVP, Desmopressin; *FFP*, fresh frozen plasma; *LMWH*, low-molecular-weight heparin; *PCC*, prothrombin complex concentrates (Bebulin); *rVIIa*, recombinant active factor VIIa (NovoSeven); *SIVP*, slow intravenous push; *UFH*, unfractionated heparin.
From Dilworth T, Burnett A, Tawil I, Garcia D, Fletcher: Guideline for antithrombotic reversal. UNM Health System. Anticoagulation Subcommittee, UNMH P&T Committee. Updated October 2016. https://hospitals.health.unm.edu/intranet7/apps/doc_management/index.cfm?document_id=198547

coordinated with their specialist in regard to who is responsible for postoperative pain management and for how long. Patients under pain management contracts should be handled carefully because most pain management specialists will stop caring for patients who violate their contract.

SPECIAL OPERATIVE TECHNIQUES

Special operative techniques are used in a variety of procedures and are described here so that repetition in other chapters will be unnecessary. The methods of tendon or fascia fixation and bone grafting are discussed here. The methods of tendon suture are discussed in other chapter.

METHODS OF TENDON-TO-BONE FIXATION

The principles of tendon suture are described in other chapter for the hand; in other chapter, in which disorders of muscles and tendons are discussed; and under the discussion of tendon transfers in other chapter. The following discussion deals only with the methods of attaching a tendon to bone.

Attaching tendon to bone can be a fairly easy task. Healing of tendon to bone with something close to biologically normal tissue is the challenge. Multiple modalities such as osteoinductive growth factors, periosteal grafts, osteoconductive factors, platelet-rich plasma, biodegradable scaffolds, ultrasound, and extracorporeal shockwave therapy are being studied.

FIXATION OF TENDON TO BONE

TECHNIQUE 1.1

▪ Scarify the apposing surfaces of bone and tendon to hasten attachment by incising the periosteum and elevating it enough to expose the bony surface. After completion of the tendon fixation, an attempt should be made to close the periosteum over the tendon, although this usually is impossible. Instead, the periosteum may be sutured to the edges of the tendon.
▪ Place a suture in the end of the tendon by one of the techniques described in other chapter. With this suture, pull the tendon distally, removing all slack, and determine the point of attachment.
▪ Drill a hole transversely into the bone just distal to this point.
▪ Pass the sutures on each side of the tendon through this hole in opposite directions and tie them tightly over the shaft of the bone (Fig. 1.10A).
▪ If the tendon is long enough, pass the end through the hole in the bone and suture the tendon to itself (Fig. 1.10B). If passing the tendon or piece of fascia through the hole drilled in bone is difficult, construct a homemade Chinese finger trap from two pieces of suture woven around the tendon (Fig. 1.11).
▪ If a distally based strip of iliotibial band is to be inserted into bone, roll the part of the band that is to be inserted into a cylindrical shape and wrap a suitable length

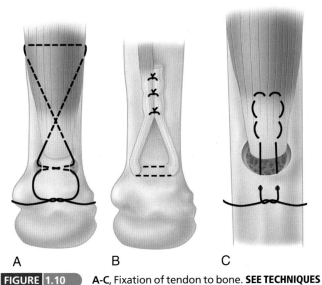

A   B   C

FIGURE 1.10   A-C, Fixation of tendon to bone. **SEE TECHNIQUES 1.1 AND 1.5.**

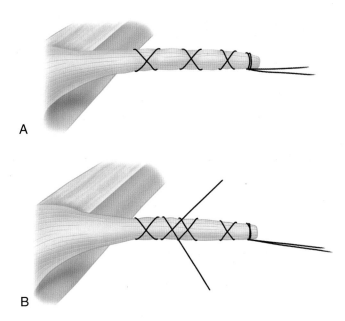

A

B

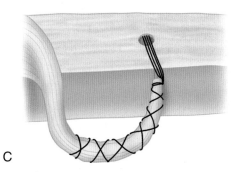

C

of strong, nonabsorbable suture around the fascia in a crisscross fashion, beginning about 4 cm proximal to the end of the strip. At the end of the strip, tie the suture into a knot, leaving the ends long (Fig. 1.11A).

- Wrap a second piece of suture around the fascia in the same way but out of phase with the first piece of suture (Fig. 1.11B) and tie it at the end.
- Pass the ends of the suture through the hole in the bone (Fig. 1.11C), followed by the rolled up fascial strip.
- Finally, cut the sutures just proximal to the knots at the apex of the finger trap and remove them one at a time.

For larger muscles, a broad, firm, bony attachment must be ensured (Fig. 1.10C). The advantage of this method is that drilling a transverse hole through the shaft of the bone is unnecessary; such a procedure is sometimes difficult in deep wounds, and exposure requires considerable stripping of soft tissues from the bone.

FIGURE 1.11   Krackow and Cohn technique for passing tendon or fascia through hole in bone. **A,** Suture is wrapped in crisscross fashion around the distal end of the tendon or fascia and is tied in a knot, leaving the ends of the suture long. **B,** A second suture is wrapped in similar fashion but out of phase with the first suture. **C,** A Chinese finger-trap suture fits tightly around the tendon or fascia and allows it to enter the hole without difficulty. (Redrawn from Krackow KA, Cohn BT: A new technique for passing tendon through bone: brief note, *J Bone Joint Surg* 69A:922, 1987.) **SEE TECHNIQUE 1.1.**

TENDON FIXATION INTO THE INTRAMEDULLARY CANAL

TECHNIQUE 1.2

- After placing the suture in the end of the tendon and leaving two long, free strands, create a trapdoor in the bone, exposing the medullary canal at the predetermined point of attachment.
- Just distal to the trapdoor, drill two holes through the cortex into the medullary canal.
- Pass the free ends of the suture through the trapdoor and out through the two holes.
- Pull the sutures taut and draw the end of the tendon through the trapdoor into the medullary canal.
- Partially replace the trapdoor or break into small fragments and pack it into the defect as grafts.

TENDON TO BONE FIXATION USING LOCKING LOOP SUTURE

Krackow et al. have devised a locking loop suture that is relatively simple to use and is especially suited to attaching flat structures, such as the tibial collateral ligament, joint capsule, or patellar tendon, to bone. It allows the application of tension to the structure, resists pulling out, and does not cause major purse-stringing or bunching. A doubled suture of strong suture material is nearly twice as strong as staple fixation to bone. When the suture is used in combination with a staple, fixation is significantly improved.

TECHNIQUE 1.3   *Figure 1.12*

(KRACKOW, THOMAS, JONES)
- Approach the tendon or ligament from the raw end, and place three or more locking loops along each side of the structure.
- Apply tension during the procedure to remove excess suture material within the locking loops. This suture may be reinforced proximal to the first suture.
- Attach the tendon or ligament and the suture to bone through holes drilled in the bone, or tie the suture over a screw or staple fixed in the bone.

TENDON TO BONE FIXATION USING WIRE SUTURE

Because of the scarcity of surrounding soft tissue and the nature of the bone, Cole's method is especially applicable to the fixation of tendons to the dorsum of the tarsus, to the calcaneus, or to the phalanges of the fingers.

TECHNIQUE 1.4   *Figure 1.13*

(COLE)
- Prepare the tendon and place a pull-out suture in the end of the tendon, as described for end-to-end sutures (Chapter 66).

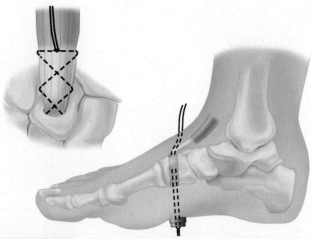

FIGURE 1.13   The Cole method of anchoring tendons to bone. Ends of wire suture are passed on a straight skin needle through a hole drilled in bone. The needle is drawn through the skin on the opposite side. Wire sutures are anchored over a rubber tube or button. To prevent necrosis of the skin when the suture is under considerable tension, ends of wire may be passed through the bottom of the cast. Subsequently, wire is anchored over the button on the outside of the cast. **SEE TECHNIQUE 1.4.**

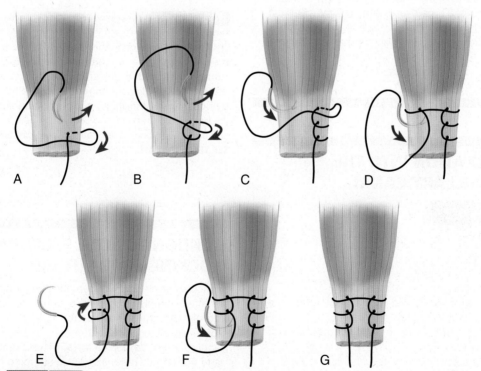

FIGURE 1.12   Krackow, Thomas, and Jones technique for ligament or tendon fixation to bone. **A-G,** Detail of placement of suture in wide tendon. (Redrawn from Krackow KA, Thomas SC, Jones LC: Ligament-tendon fixation: analysis of a new stitch and comparison with standard techniques, *Orthopedics* 11:909, 1988.) **SEE TECHNIQUE 1.3.**

- Reflect a small flap of bone with a chisel, and at the apex of the flap drill a tunnel through the bone.
- Place both ends of the wire suture on a long, straight skin needle.
- Pass the needle through the hole in the bone and out through the skin on the opposite side, drawing the end of the tendon into the tunnel.
- Anchor the wire snugly over a loop of gauze or a padded button. If considerable tension is necessary, as in Achilles tendon, the skin should be padded with heavy felt.
- Apply a cast with the wires protruding through the bottom of the cast. After the plaster sets, anchor the wire over a button on the outside of the cast.

SUTURE ANCHORS

Suture-anchoring devices also are useful in securing tendon, ligament, or capsule to bone (Fig. 1.14). The pull-out strength of these devices is at least equal to that of a suture passed through drill holes in bone, and these devices are especially useful in deep wounds with limited room, such as in the shoulder. Tingart et al. found that metal suture anchors withstand a significantly higher load to failure than biodegradable anchors. Bottoni et al. found that the suture used usually failed before the suture anchor in an animal model. Suture anchors made from methyl methacrylate cement are useful in osteopenic bone (Fig. 1.15). Giori et al. found that augmenting suture anchors with methyl methacrylate greatly improved pull-out strength in osteopenic cadaver bone.

A tendon or ligament also can be secured to bone through a drill hole using a screw for an interference fit as in anterior cruciate ligament reconstruction procedures. Allograft cortical bone is now being commercially machined into screws for such a purpose.

FIXATION OF OSSEOUS ATTACHMENT OF TENDON TO BONE

When larger muscles are transferred, such as the quadriceps or the abductor muscles of the hip, better fixation is secured if the tendon is removed with a portion of its bony attachment.

TECHNIQUE 1.5

- Remove sufficient bone to ensure a cancellous surface.
- Draw the bony segment distally and determine the location of its reattachment.
- Elevate the periosteum, scarify the surface of the shaft, and fix the attachment of the tendon to the raw area by two threaded pins inserted obliquely or by a screw (Fig. 1.16A). Staples also are useful for anchoring a ligament or a tendon to bone (Figs. 1.17 and 1.18), and wire loops passed through holes drilled into the bone (Fig. 1.16B,C) are efficient. Heavy sutures may be used instead of metal for fixation of tendons in the less powerful muscles.
- If desired, create a trapdoor in the shaft of the bone, and countersink the osseous attachment of the tendon into the defect and hold with a suture, as illustrated in Figure 1.10.

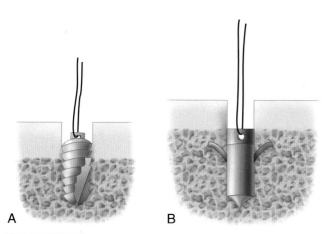

FIGURE 1.14 Suture-anchoring implants. **A,** Statak (Zimmer) suture-anchoring device is drilled into bone. **B,** QuickAnchor (Mitek) suture anchor consists of a hook device with suture that is anchored into drill hole in the bone.

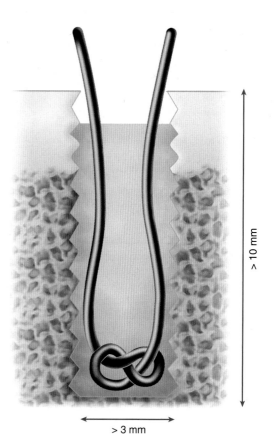

FIGURE 1.15 Methyl methacrylate suture anchor. Figure-of-eight knot increases load to failure.

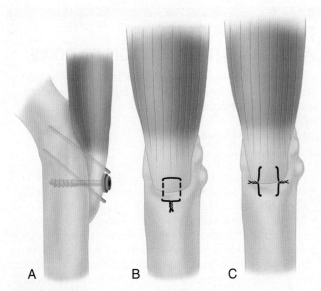

FIGURE 1.16 Fixation of osseous attachment of tendon to bone. **A,** Fixation by screw or threaded pins. **B,** Fixation by mattress suture of wire through holes drilled in bone. **C,** Fixation by wire loops. **SEE TECHNIQUE 1.5.**

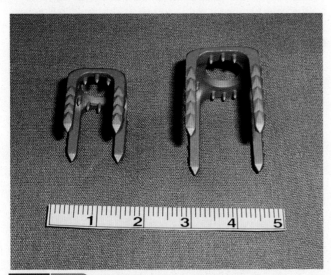

FIGURE 1.17 Stone table staple, used most frequently for anchoring tendinous tissue to bone. **SEE TECHNIQUE 1.5.**

SUTURE BUTTONS

Suture-button devices are now available for minimally invasive tendon-to-bone, ligament-to-bone, and fracture fixation. The Endobutton (Smith and Nephew, York, UK) and the TightRope Fixation System (Arthrex, Naples, Florida) can be inserted through a single incision and drill hole. These devices have been successfully used in acromioclavicular joint dislocations, Neer II distal clavicular fractures, ankle syndesmosis disruptions, and high-energy os calcis fractures with compromised skin (Fig. 1.19).

BONE GRAFTING

The indications for bone grafting are to:
- Fill cavities or defects resulting from cysts, tumors, or other causes

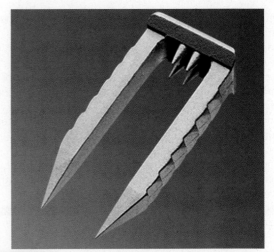

FIGURE 1.18 Arthrex low-profile bridge staple. (Courtesy Arthrex, Naples, FL.) **SEE TECHNIQUE 1.5.**

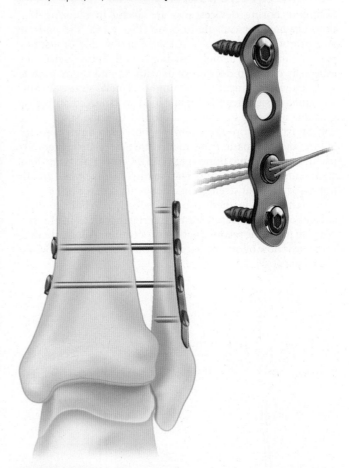

FIGURE 1.19 TightRope Syndesmosis Buttress Plate Kit (Arthrex, Naples, FL). One suture strand is used to "flip" the medial button so a second incision is unnecessary.

- Bridge joints to perform arthrodesis
- Bridge major defects or re-establish the continuity of a long bone
- Provide bone blocks to limit joint motion (arthroereisis)
- Establish union of a pseudarthrosis
- Promote union or fill defects in delayed union, malunion, fresh fractures, or osteotomies

STRUCTURE OF BONE GRAFTS

Cortical bone grafts are used primarily for structural support, and cancellous bone grafts are used for osteogenesis. Structural support and osteogenesis may be combined; this is one of the prime advantages of using bone graft. These two factors vary, however, with the structure of the bone. Probably all or most of the cellular elements in grafts (particularly cortical grafts) die and are slowly replaced by creeping substitution, the graft merely acting as a scaffold for the formation of new bone. In hard cortical bone, this process of replacement is considerably slower than in cancellous bone. Although cancellous bone is more osteogenic, it is not strong enough to provide efficient structural support. When selecting the graft or combination of grafts, the surgeon must be aware of these two fundamental differences in bone structure. When a graft has united with the host and is strong enough to permit unprotected use of the part, remodeling of the bone structure takes place commensurate with functional demands.

SOURCES OF BONE GRAFTS
■ AUTOGENOUS GRAFTS

When the bone grafts come from the patient, the grafts usually are removed from the tibia, fibula, or ilium. These three bones provide cortical grafts, whole-bone transplants, and cancellous bone.

When internal or external fixation appliances are not used, which is currently rare, strength is necessary in a graft used for bridging a defect in a long bone or even for the treatment of pseudarthrosis. The subcutaneous anteromedial aspect of the tibia is an excellent source for structural autografts. In adults, after removal of a cortical graft, the plateau of the tibia supplies cancellous bone. Apparently, leaving the periosteum attached to the graft has no advantage; however, suturing to the periosteum over the defect has definite advantages. The periosteum seems to serve as a limiting membrane to prevent irregular callus when the defect in the tibia fills in with new bone. The few bone cells that are stripped off with the periosteum can help in the formation of bone needed to fill the defect.

Disadvantages to the use of the tibia as a donor area include (1) a normal limb is jeopardized; (2) the duration and magnitude of the procedure are increased; (3) ambulation must be delayed until the defect in the tibia has partially healed; and (4) the tibia must be protected for 6 to 12 months to prevent fractures. For these reasons, structural autografts from the tibia are now rarely used.

A good source for bulk cancellous autogenous graft is material from a reamer-irrigator-aspirator (RIA) used in the canal of the femoral and tibial shafts. A complication rate of less than 2% has been reported in approximately 200 patients with a mean volume harvested of 47 ± 22 mL. Debris harvested during RIA and bone graft harvested from iliac crest have similar RNA transcriptional profiles for genes that act in bone repair and formation, suggesting that material harvested by RIA is a viable alternative to iliac crest autogenous cancellous graft.

Marchand et al. compared 61 patients who had a graft harvested by RIA with 47 patients who had a graft harvested from the iliac crest and found that 44% of the patients undergoing RIA bone graft harvest required transfusion. Only 21% of the group with graft harvested from the iliac crest required transfusion.

The entire proximal two thirds of the fibula can be removed without disabling the leg. Most patients have complaints and mild muscular weakness after removal of a portion of the fibula. The configuration of the proximal end of the fibula is an advantage. The proximal end has a rounded prominence that is partially covered by hyaline cartilage and forms a satisfactory transplant to replace the distal third of the radius or the distal third of the fibula. After transplantation, the hyaline cartilage probably degenerates rapidly into a fibrocartilaginous surface; even so, this surface is preferable to raw bone.

The middle one third of the fibula also can be used as a vascularized free autograft based on the peroneal artery and vein pedicle using microvascular technique. Portions of the iliac crest also can be used as free vascularized autograft. The use of free vascularized autografts has limited indications, requires expert microvascular technique, and is not without donor site morbidity particularly at the ankle.

The management of segmental bone loss can be difficult. Taylor et al. described a two-stage induced membrane technique using a methyl methacrylate spacer. The spacer is placed into the defect to induce the formation of a bioactive membrane. Four to 8 weeks later the spacer is removed and cancellous autograft is placed in the now membrane surrounded defect. The membrane helps prevent graft resorption, promote revascularization, and consolidation of new bone. We have had good results with this technique.

■ ALLOGENIC GRAFTS

An allogenic graft, or allograft, is one that is obtained from an individual other than the patient. In small children, the usual donor sites do not provide cortical grafts large enough to bridge defects or the available cancellous bone may not be enough to fill a large cavity or cyst; the possibility of injuring a physis also must be considered. Allograft is preferred in this situation. Allografts are also indicated in the elderly, patients who are poor operative risks, and patients from whom not enough acceptable autogenous bone can be harvested. Larger structural allografts have been used successfully for many years in revision total joint surgery, periprosthetic long bone fractures, and reconstruction after tumor excision. Osteochondral allografts are now being used with some success in a few centers to treat distal femoral osteonecrosis. Large osteochondral allografts, such as the distal femur, are used in limb salvage procedures after tumor resection. Autogenous cancellous bone can be mixed in small amounts with allograft bone as "seed" to provide osteogenic potential. Mixed bone grafts of this type incorporate more rapidly than allograft bone alone. Increased allograft union rates and less resorption have been noted in large acetabular defects when allografts were loaded with bone marrow derived mesenchymal stem cells. The various properties of autogenous and allogenic bone grafts are summarized in Table 1.5.

■ BONE BANK

To provide safe and useful allograft material efficiently, a bone banking system is required that uses thorough donor screening, rapid procurement, and safe, sterile processing. Standards outlined by the U.S. Food and Drug Administration (FDA) and American Association of Tissue Banks must be followed. Donors must be screened for bacterial, viral (including HIV and hepatitis), and fungal infections. Malignancy (except basal cell carcinoma of the skin), collagen vascular

TABLE 1.5
Bone Graft Activity by Type

GRAFT	OSTEOGENESIS	OSTEOCONDUCTION	OSTEOINDUCTION	MECHANICAL PROPERTIES	VASCULARITY
AUTOGRAFT					
Bone marrow	++	±	+	−	−
Cancellous	++	++	+	+	−
Cortical	+	+	±	++	−
Vascularized	++	++	+	++	++
ALLOGRAFT					
Cancellous	−	++	+	+	−
Cortical	−	±	±	++	−
Demineralized	−	++	+++	−	−

From Kahn SN, et al: The biology of bone grafting, *J Am Acad Orthop Surg* 13:80, 2005.

disease, metabolic bone disease, and the presence of toxins are all contraindications to donation. No system is perfect, and the transmission of disease by allograft material has been reported from single donors to multiple recipients.

Bone and ligament and bone and tendon are now banked for use as allografts. The use of allograft ligaments and tendons in knee surgery is discussed in other chapter. Bone can be stored and sterilized in several forms. It can be harvested in a clean, nonsterile environment; sterilized by irradiation, strong acid, or ethylene oxide; and freeze-dried for storage. Bone under sterile conditions can be deep frozen (−70°C to −80°C) for storage. Fresh frozen bone is stronger than freeze-dried bone and better as structural allograft material. Articular cartilage and menisci also can be cryopreserved in this manner. Cancellous allografts incorporate to host bone, as do autogenous cancellous grafts. These allografts are mineralized and are not osteoinductive, although they are osteoconductive. Cancellous allografts can be obtained in a demineralized form that increases osteogenic potential but greatly decreases resistance to compressive forces.

Cortical allografts are invaded by host blood vessels and substituted slowly with new host bone to a limited degree, especially in massive allografts. This probably accounts for the high incidence of fracture in these grafts because dead bone cannot remodel in response to cyclic loading and then fails.

CANCELLOUS BONE GRAFT SUBSTITUTES

Interest in bone graft substitutes has mushroomed in recent years. Dozens of products are in general use or in clinical trials. To understand better the properties of these products, the following bone synthesis processes need to be understood (see Table 1.5). *Graft osteogenesis* is the ability of cellular elements within a graft that survive transplantation to synthesize new bone. *Graft osteoinduction* is the ability of a graft to recruit host mesenchymal stem cells into the graft that differentiate into osteoblasts. Bone morphogenetic proteins and other growth factors in the graft facilitate this process. *Graft osteoconduction* is the ability of a graft to facilitate blood vessel ingrowth and bone formation into a scaffold structure.

Bone graft substitutes can replace autologous or allogenic grafts or expand an existing amount of available graft material. Autologous cancellous and cortical grafts are still the "gold standards" against which all other graft forms are judged. Bone

TABLE 1.6
Classification of Bone Graft Substitutes

PROPERTY	DESCRIPTION	CLASSES
Osteoconduction	Provides a passive porous scaffold to support or direct bone formation	Calcium sulfate, ceramics, calcium phosphate cements, collagen, bioactive glass, synthetic polymers
Osteoinduction	Induces differentiation of stem cells into osteogenic cells	Demineralized bone matrix, bone morphogenic proteins, growth factors, gene therapy
Osteogenesis	Provides stem cells with osteogenic potential, which directly lays down new bone	Bone marrow aspirate
Combined	Provides more than one of the above mentioned properties	Composites

From Parikh SN: Bone graft substitutes in modern orthopedics, *Orthopedics* 25:1301, 2002.

graft substitutes are classified based on properties outlined in Table 1.6. FDA-approved applications for these products are variable and ever changing. Table 1.7 lists bone graft substitutes that are FDA approved with published, peer-reviewed, level I or II human studies as burden of proof. Surgeons must carefully review the manufacturers' stated indications and directions for use. For more in-depth discussions of the biologic events in bone graft incorporation, see the reviews by Khan et al. and Gardiner and Weitzel. The Orthopaedic Trauma Association Orthobiologics Committee (DeLong et al.) reported a review of the literature on bone grafts and bone graft substitutes and provided recommendations to the orthopaedic community based on levels of evidence. Kurien et al. reviewed 59 bone

TABLE 1.7

Commercially Available FDA-Approved Bone Graft Substitutes With Peer-Reviewed Published Level I-II Human Studies as Burden of Proof (2010)

PRODUCT	COMPOSITION AND MECHANISM OF ACTION	FDA STATUS
HEALOS DePuy Spine	Mineralized collagen matrix in strips of varying sizes Mechanisms of action: osteoinduction/conduction, creeping substitution, osteogenesis when mixed with autogenous bone graft	Cleared as bone filler but must be used with autogenous bone marrow
Vitoss Orthovita	100% beta TCP; 80% beta TCP/20% collagen; 70% beta TCP/20% collagen/10% bioactive glass as putty, strip, flow, morsels, or shapes Mechanism of action: osteoconduction/bioresorbable, bioactive, osteostimulation, osteogenesis, and osteoinduction when mixed with bone marrow aspirate	Cleared as bone void filler
NovaBone NovaBone/MTF	Bioactive silicate in particulate or putty or morsel form Mechanism of action: osteoconduction, bioresorbable, osteostimulation	Cleared as a bone void filler
GRAFTON A-FLEX, Flex, Matrix Scoliosis Strips, Putty Osteotech	DBM fiber technology in flexible sheets of varying shapes and sizes or moldable or packable graft Mechanism of action: osteoinduction/conduction, incorporation, osteogenesis when mixed with autogenous bone graft or bone marrow aspirate	Cleared as bone graft substitute, bone graft extender, and bone void filler
GRAFTON Crunch Orthoblend Large Defect Orthoblend Small Defect Osteotech	DBM fibers with demineralized cortical cubes or crushed cancellous chips as packable or moldable graft Mechanism of action: osteoinduction/conduction, incorporation, osteogenesis when mixed with autogenous bone graft or bone marrow aspirate	Cleared as bone graft substitute, bone graft extender, and bone void filler
GRAFTON Gel Osteotech	DBM in a syringe for MIS and percutaneous injectable graft Mechanism of action: osteoinduction/conduction, incorporation, osteogenesis when mixed with autogenous bone graft or bone marrow aspirate	Cleared as bone graft substitute, bone graft extender, and bone void filler
GRAFTON Plus Paste Osteotech	DBM in a syringe for MIS injectable graft that resists irrigation Mechanism of action: osteoinduction/conduction, incorporation, osteogenesis when mixed with autogenous bone graft or bone marrow aspirate	Cleared as bone graft substitute, bone graft extender, and bone void filler

DBM, Demineralized bone matrix; *MIS*, minimally invasive surgery; *TCP*, tricalcium phosphate.

graft substitutes available for use in the United Kingdom, only 22 of which had peer-reviewed published clinical literature. They questioned the need for so many products and called for more prospective randomized trials. They also provided a good review of uses of various bone graft substitutes.

Bone graft substitutes are not without complications, however. Recombinant human bone morphogenic protein-2 (rh BMP-2) has been associated with an increased cancer risk. Data from a randomized trial involving over 500 patients who had spine fusion with single-level lumbar fusion using rh BMP-2 in a compression-resistant material showed a significant increase of cancer events in the rh BMP-2 group. A 16% complication rate involving soft-tissue inflammation also was noted in another study of 31 patients after the use of tricalcium phosphate and calcium sulfate. An increased risk for retrograde ejaculation also has been reported after anterior lumbar interbody fusion using rh BMP-2.

The use of bone graft substitutes containing recombinant proteins or synthetic peptides in younger patients with developing skeletons has not been approved by the U.S. FDA. The extra stimulation for bone growth can lead to injury. The

agency has received reports of fluid accumulation, excessive bone growth, delayed bone healing, and swelling from the off-label use of these products in juveniles.

The use of stem cells in bone graft substitutes is considered investigational. The FDA has recently stated: "A major challenge posed by SC [stem cell] therapy is the need to ensure their efficacy and safety. Cells manufactured in large quantities outside their natural environment in the human body can become ineffective or dangerous and produce significant adverse effects, such as tumors, severe immune reactions, or growth of unwanted tissue."

Demineralized bone matrix (DBM) is considered minimally processed allograft tissue and, therefore, does not require approval from the FDA for use. The use of mesenchymal stem-cell (autograft or allograft) therapy alone or in combination with bone graft substitutes is considered investigational. There is controversy as to whether or not the combination of DBM plus stem cells constitutes a minimally processed tissue. Some believe that since these products require the metabolic activity of living cells, they should be considered biologic products and, therefore, be required to demonstrate safety and efficacy and be considered investigational drugs that require a biologic application license.

INDICATIONS FOR VARIOUS BONE GRAFT TECHNIQUES
■ ONLAY CORTICAL GRAFTS

Until relatively inert metals became available, the onlay bone graft was the simplest and most effective treatment for most ununited diaphyseal fractures. Usually the cortical graft was supplemented by cancellous bone for osteogenesis. The onlay graft is applicable to a limited group of fresh, malunited, and ununited fractures and after osteotomies.

Cortical grafts also are used when bridging joints to produce arthrodesis, not only for osteogenesis but also for fixation. Fixation as a rule is best furnished by internal or external metallic devices. Only in an extremely unusual situation would a cortical onlay graft be indicated for fixation, and then only in small bones and when little stress is expected. For osteogenesis, the thick cortical graft has largely been replaced by thin cortical and cancellous bone from the ilium. Dual onlay bone grafts are useful when treating difficult and unusual nonunions or for bridging massive defects. The treatment of a nonunion near a joint is difficult because the fragment nearest the joint is usually small, osteoporotic, and largely cancellous, having only a thin cortex. It often is so small and soft that fixation with a single graft is impossible because screws tend to pull out of it and wire sutures cut through it. Dual grafts provide stability because they grip the small fragment-like forceps.

The advantages of dual grafts for bridging defects are as follows: (1) mechanical fixation is better than fixation by a single onlay bone graft; (2) the two grafts add strength and stability; (3) the grafts form a trough into which cancellous bone may be packed; and (4) during healing, the dual grafts, in contrast to a single graft, prevent contracting fibrous tissue from compromising transplanted cancellous bone. A whole fibular graft usually is better than dual grafts for bridging defects in the upper extremity except when the bone is osteoporotic or when the nonunion is near a joint.

The disadvantages of dual grafts are the same as those of single cortical grafts: (1) they are not as strong as metallic fixation devices; (2) an extremity usually must serve as a donor site if autogenous grafts are used; and (3) they are not as osteogenic as autogenous iliac grafts, and the surgery necessary to obtain them has more risk.

■ INLAY GRAFTS

By the inlay technique, a slot or rectangular defect is created in the cortex of the host bone, usually with a power saw. A graft the same size or slightly smaller is fitted into the defect. In the treatment of diaphyseal nonunions, the onlay technique is simpler and more efficient and has almost replaced the inlay graft. The latter still is occasionally used in arthrodesis, particularly at the ankle.

■ MULTIPLE CANCELLOUS CHIP GRAFTS

Multiple chips of cancellous bone are widely used for grafting. Segments of cancellous bone are the best osteogenic material available. They are particularly useful for filling cavities or defects resulting from cysts, tumors, or other causes; for establishing bone blocks; and for wedging in osteotomies. Being soft and friable, this bone can be packed into any nook or crevice. The ilium is a good source of cancellous bone; and if some rigidity and strength are desired, the cortical elements may be retained. In most bone grafting procedures that use cortical bone or metallic devices for fixation, supplementary cancellous bone chips or strips are used to hasten healing. Cancellous grafts are particularly applicable to arthrodesis of the spine because osteogenesis is the prime concern.

Iliac crest cancellous grafts can be easily harvested from the anterior crest, using an acetabular reamer as described by Dick with excellent results and no graft-related complications as reported by Brawley and Simpson.

Large-volume cancellous bone grafts can be harvested from the femoral canal using a RIA as described by Newman et al.

■ HEMICYLINDRICAL GRAFTS

Hemicylindrical grafts are suitable for obliterating large defects of the tibia and femur. A massive hemicylindrical cortical graft from the affected bone is placed across the defect and is supplemented by cancellous iliac bone. A procedure of this magnitude has only limited use, but it is applicable for resection of bone tumors when amputation is to be avoided.

■ WHOLE-BONE TRANSPLANT

The fibula provides the most practical graft for bridging long defects in the diaphyseal portion of bones of the upper extremity, unless the nonunion is near a joint. A fibular graft is stronger than a full-thickness tibial graft. When soft tissue is scant, a wound that cannot be closed over dual grafts can be closed over a fibular graft. Disability after removing a fibular graft is less than after removing a larger tibial graft. In children, the fibula can be used to span a long gap in the tibia, usually by a two-stage procedure. The shape of the proximal end of the fibula makes it a satisfactory substitute for the distal end of the fibula or distal end of the radius.

A free vascularized fibular autograft has greater osteogenic potential for incorporation but is technically much more demanding to use. Bone transplants consisting of whole segments of the tibia or femur, usually freeze dried or fresh frozen, are available. Their greatest use is in the treatment of defects of the long bones produced by massive resections for bone tumors or complex total joint revisions.

CONDITIONS FAVORABLE FOR BONE GRAFTING

For a bone grafting procedure to be successful, patient factors, such as patient overall condition and recipient site preparation, must be optimal, as outlined in Table 1.8.

PREPARATION OF BONE GRAFTS

REMOVAL OF A TIBIAL GRAFT

TECHNIQUE 1.6

- To avoid excessive loss of blood, use a tourniquet (preferably pneumatic) when the tibial graft is removed. After removal of the graft, the tourniquet may be released without disturbing the sterile drapes.

TABLE 1.8

Local and Systemic Factors Influencing Graft Incorporation

POSITIVE FACTORS	NEGATIVE FACTORS
LOCAL	**LOCAL**
Electrical stimulation	Denervation
Good vascular supply at the graft site	Infection
	Local bone disease
Growth factors	Radiation
Large surface area	Tumor mechanical instability
Mechanical loading	
Mechanical stability	
SYSTEMIC	**SYSTEMIC**
Growth hormone	Chemotherapy
Insulin	Corticosteroids
Parathyroid hormone	Diabetes
Somatomedins	Malnutrition
Thyroid hormone	Metabolic bone disease
Vitamins A and D	Nonsteroidal antiinflammatory drugs
	Sepsis
	Smoking

- Make a slightly curved longitudinal incision over the anteromedial surface of the tibia, placing it to prevent a painful scar over the crest.
- Without reflecting the skin, incise the periosteum to the bone.
- With a periosteal elevator, reflect the periosteum, medially and laterally, exposing the entire surface of the tibia between the crest and the medial border. For better exposure at each end of the longitudinal incision, incise the periosteum transversely; the incision through the periosteum is I shaped.
- Because of the shape of the tibia, the graft usually is wider at the proximal end than at the distal end. This equalizes the strength of the graft because the cortex is thinner proximally than distally (Fig. 1.20). Before cutting the graft, drill a hole at each corner of the anticipated area.
- With a single-blade saw, remove the graft by cutting through the cortex at an oblique angle, preserving the anterior and medial borders of the tibia. Do not cut beyond the holes, especially when cutting across at the ends; overcutting here weakens the donor bone and may serve as the starting point of a future fracture. This is particularly true at the distal end of the graft.
- As the graft is pried from its bed, have an assistant grasp it firmly to prevent it from dropping to the floor.
- Before closing the wound, remove additional cancellous bone from the proximal end of the tibia with a curet. Take care to avoid the articular surface of the tibia or, in a child, the physis.
- The periosteum over the tibia is relatively thick in children and usually can be sutured as a separate layer. In adults, it is often thin, and closure may be unsatisfactory; suturing the periosteum and the deep portion of the subcutaneous tissues as a single layer usually is wise.

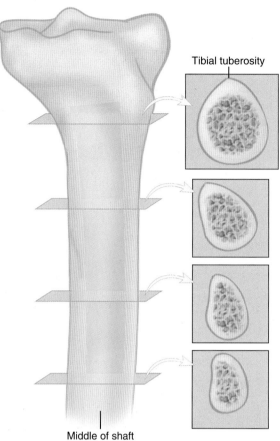

Tibial tuberosity

Middle of shaft

FIGURE **1.20**   Method of removing tibial graft. Graft is wider proximally than distally. A hole is drilled at each corner before cutting to decrease stress riser effect of sharp corner after removal of graft. Cortex is cut through at an oblique angle. **SEE TECHNIQUE 1.6.**

- If the graft has been properly cut, little shaping is necessary. Our practice is to remove the endosteal side of the graft because (1) the thin endosteal portion provides a graft to be placed across from the cortical graft; and (2) the endosteal surface, being rough and irregular, should be removed to ensure good contact of the graft with the host bone.

REMOVAL OF FIBULAR GRAFTS

Three points should be considered in the removal of a fibular graft: (1) the peroneal nerve must not be damaged; (2) the distal fourth of the bone must be left to maintain a stable ankle; and (3) the peroneal muscles should not be cut.

TECHNIQUE 1.7   *FIGURES 1.21 and 1.22*

- For most grafting procedures, resect the middle third or middle half of the fibula through a Henry approach.
- Dissect along the anterior surface of the septum between the peroneus longus and soleus muscles.

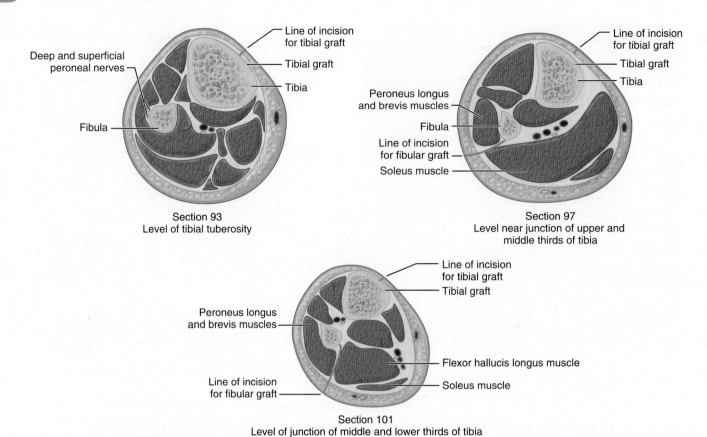

Section 93
Level of tibial tuberosity

Section 97
Level near junction of upper and
middle thirds of tibia

Section 101
Level of junction of middle and lower thirds of tibia

FIGURE 1.21 Cross-sections of leg showing line of approach for removal of whole fibular transplants or tibial grafts. *Colored* segment shows portion of tibia to be removed. Thick, strong angles of tibia are not violated. **SEE TECHNIQUE 1.7.**

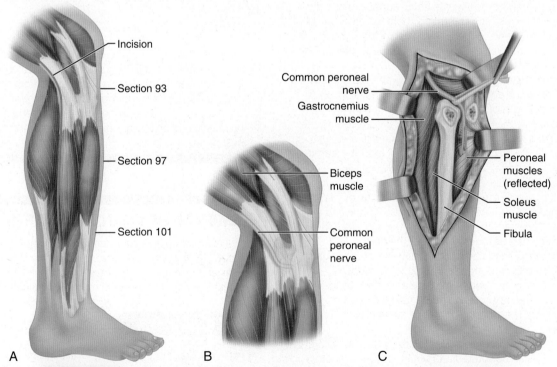

FIGURE 1.22 Resection of fibula for transplant. **A,** Line of skin incision; levels of cross-sections shown in Figure 1.21 are indicated. **B,** Relation of common peroneal nerve to fibular head and neck. **C,** Henry method of displacing peroneal nerve to expose fibular head and neck. **SEE TECHNIQUE 1.7.**

- Reflect the peroneal muscles anteriorly after subperiosteal dissection.
- Begin the stripping distally and progress proximally so that the oblique origin of the muscle fibers from the bone tends to press the periosteal elevator toward the fibula.
- Drill small holes through the fibula at the proximal and distal ends of the graft.
- Connect the holes by multiple small bites with the bone-biting forceps to osteotomize the bone; otherwise, the bone may be crushed. A Gigli saw, an oscillating power saw, or a thin, air-powered cutting drill can be used. An osteotome may split or fracture the graft. *The nutrient artery enters the bone near the middle of the posterior surface and occasionally may require ligation.*
- If the transplant is to substitute for the distal end of the radius or for the distal end of the fibula, resect the proximal third of the fibula through the proximal end of the Henry approach and take care to avoid damaging the peroneal nerve.
- Expose the nerve first at the posteromedial aspect of the distal end of the biceps femoris tendon and trace it distally to where it winds around the neck of the fibula. In this location, the nerve is covered by the origin of the peroneus longus muscle. With the back of the knife blade toward the nerve, divide the thin slip of peroneus longus muscle bridging it. Displace the nerve from its normal bed into an anterior position.
- As the dissection continues, protect the anterior tibial vessels that pass between the neck of the fibula and the tibia by subperiosteal dissection.
- After the resection is complete, suture the biceps tendon and the fibular collateral ligament to the adjacent soft tissues.

CANCELLOUS ILIAC CREST BONE GRAFTS

Unless considerable strength is required, the cancellous graft fulfills almost any requirement. Regardless of whether the cells in the graft remain viable, clinical results indicate that cancellous grafts incorporate with the host bone more rapidly than do cortical grafts.

Large cancellous and corticocancellous grafts may be obtained from the anterior superior iliac crest and the posterior iliac crest. Small cancellous grafts may be obtained from the greater trochanter of the femur, femoral condyle, proximal tibial metaphysis, medial malleolus of the tibia, olecranon, and distal radius. At least 2 cm of subchondral bone must remain to avoid collapse of the articular surface.

If form and rigidity are unnecessary, multiple sliver or chip grafts may be removed. When preservation of the iliac crest is desirable, the outer cortex of the ilium may be removed along with considerable cancellous bone. If a more rigid piece of bone is desirable, the posterior or anterior one third of the crest of the ilium is a satisfactory donor site. For wedge grafts, the cuts are made at a right angle to the crest. Jones et al. found that full-thickness iliac grafts harvested with a power saw are stronger than grafts harvested with an osteotome, presumably because of less microfracturing of bone with the saw.

If the patient is prone, the posterior third of the ilium is used; if the patient is supine, the anterior third is available (Fig. 1.23). In children, the physis of the iliac crest is ordinarily

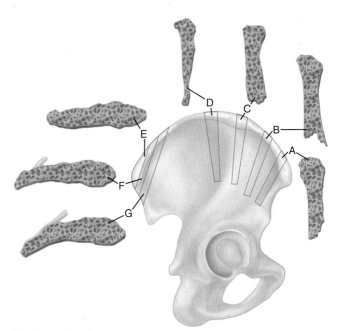

FIGURE 1.23 Coronal sections *(A-D)* from anterior portion of ilium. Accompanying cross-sections show width of bone and its cancellous structure. Iliac grafts for fusion of spine are ordinarily removed from posterior third of crest *(E-G)*.

preserved together with the attached muscles. To accomplish this, a cut is made parallel to and below the apophysis, and this segment is fractured in greenstick fashion at the posterior end. Ordinarily, only one cortex and the cancellous bone are removed for grafts, and the fractured crest, along with the apophysis, is replaced in contact with the remnant of the ilium and is held in place with heavy nonabsorbable sutures. When full-thickness grafts are removed from the ilium in adults, a similar procedure may be used, preserving the crest of the ilium and its external contour. The patient cannot readily detect the absence of the bone, and the cosmetic result is superior. This method also is less likely to result in a "landslide" hernia. Wolfe and Kawamoto reported a method of taking full-thickness bone from the anterior ilium; the iliac crest is split off obliquely medially and laterally so that the edges of the crest may be reapproximated after the bone has been excised (Fig. 1.24). They also used this method in older children without any evidence of growth disturbance of the iliac crestal physis.

REMOVAL OF AN ILIAC BONE GRAFT

Harvesting autograft bone from the ilium is not without complications. Hernias have been reported to develop in patients from whom massive full-thickness iliac grafts were taken. Muscle-pedicle grafts for arthrodesis of the hip (see other chapter for hip arthrodesis techniques) also have resulted in a hernia when both cortices were removed. With this graft, the abductor muscles and the layer of periosteum laterally are removed with the graft. Careful repair of the supporting structures remaining after removal of an iliac graft is important and probably the best method of preventing these hernias. Full-thickness windows made below the iliac crest are less likely to lead to hernia formation. In addition

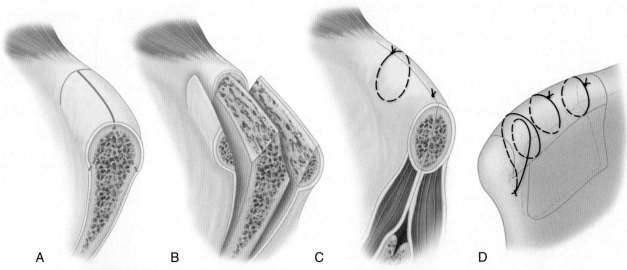

A   B   C   D

FIGURE 1.24 Wolfe-Kawamoto technique of taking iliac bone graft. **A** and **B,** Outer ridges of iliac crest are split off obliquely with retention of muscular and periosteal attachments. **C** and **D,** Closure of donor site. Note offset anteriorly for reattachment of crest to anterior superior iliac spine **(D)**. (Redrawn from Wolfe SA, Kawamoto HK: Taking the iliac-bone graft: a new technique, *J Bone Joint Surg* 60A:411, 1978.)

to hernia formation, nerve injury, arterial injury, or cosmetic deformity can be a problem after harvesting of iliac bone. The lateral femoral cutaneous and ilioinguinal nerves are at risk during harvest of bone from the anterior ilium. The superior cluneal nerves are at risk if dissection is carried farther than 8 cm lateral to the posterior superior iliac spine (Fig. 1.25). The superior gluteal vessels can be damaged by retraction against the roof of the sciatic notch. Removal of large full-thickness grafts from the anterior ilium can alter the contour of the anterior crest, producing significant cosmetic deformity. Arteriovenous fistula, pseudoaneurysm, ureteral injury, anterior superior iliac spine avulsion, and pelvic instability have been reported as major complications of iliac crest graft procurement.

TECHNIQUE 1.8

- Make an incision along the subcutaneous border of the iliac crest at the point of contact of the periosteum with the origins of the gluteal and trunk muscles; carry the incision down to the bone.
- When the crest of the ilium is not required as part of the graft, split off the lateral side or both sides of the crest in continuity with the periosteum and the attached muscles. To avoid hemorrhage, dissect subperiosteally.
- If a cancellous graft with one cortex is desired, elevate only the muscles from either the inner or the outer table of the ilium. The inner cortical table with underlying cancellous bone may be preferable, owing to body habitus.
- For full-thickness grafts, also strip the iliacus muscle from the inner table of the ilium (Fig. 1.26).
- When chip or sliver grafts are required, remove them with an osteotome or gouge from the outer surface of the wing of the ilium, taking only one cortex.
- After removal of the crest, considerable cancellous bone may be obtained by inserting a curet into the cancellous space between the two intact cortices.

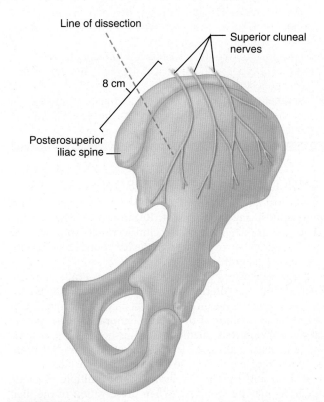

Line of dissection

Superior cluneal nerves

8 cm

Posterosuperior iliac spine

FIGURE 1.25 Posteroanterior view of pelvis showing superior cluneal nerves crossing over posterior iliac crest beginning 8 cm lateral to posterior superior iliac spine. **SEE TECHNIQUE 1.8.**

- When removing a cortical graft from the outer table, first outline the area with an osteotome or power saw. Then peel the graft up with slight prying motions with a broad osteotome. Wedge grafts or full-thickness grafts may be removed more easily with a power saw; this technique

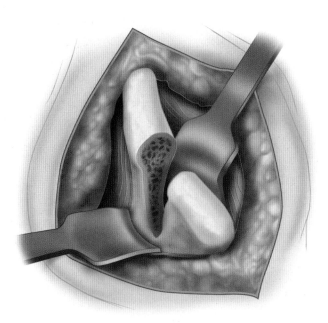

FIGURE 1.26 Method of removing full-thickness coronal segment of ilium. **SEE TECHNIQUE 1.8.**

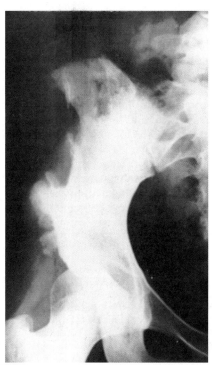

FIGURE 1.27 Defect in ilium after large graft was removed. Anterior border of ilium that included the anterior superior iliac spine was preserved, but because the defect was so large, deformity was visible even under clothing. Unsightly contour was improved by removing more bone from the crest posteriorly. **SEE TECHNIQUE 1.8.**

also is less traumatic than when an osteotome and mallet are used. For this purpose, an oscillating saw or an air-powered cutting drill is satisfactory. Avoid excessive heat by irrigating with saline at room temperature. Avoid removing too much of the crest anteriorly and leaving an unsightly deformity posteriorly (Fig. 1.27).

- After removal of the grafts, accurately appose and suture the periosteum and muscular origins with strong interrupted sutures.
- Bleeding from the ilium is sometimes profuse; avoid using Gelfoam and bone wax and depend on wound packing and local pressure. Gelfoam and bone wax are foreign materials. Bone wax is said to impair bone healing, and Gelfoam in large amounts has been associated with sterile serous drainage from wounds. Microcrystalline collagen has been reported to be more efficient in reducing blood loss from cancellous bone than either thrombin powder or thrombin-soaked gelatin foam. Gentle wound suction for 24 to 48 hours combined with meticulous obliteration of dead space is satisfactory for the management of these wounds.
- When harvesting bone from the posterior ilium, Colterjohn and Bednar recommended making the incision parallel to the superior cluneal nerves and perpendicular to the posterior iliac crest (see Fig. 1.25).

SURGICAL APPROACHES

A surgical approach should provide easy access to all structures sought. The incision should be long enough not to hinder any part of the operation. When practical, it should parallel or at least consider the natural creases of the skin to avoid undesirable scars. A longitudinal incision on the flexor or extensor surface of a joint may cause a large, unsightly scar or even a keloid that may permanently restrict motion. A longitudinal midlateral incision, especially on a finger or thumb or on the ulnar border of the hand, produces little scarring because it is located where movements of the skin are relatively slight. The approach also should do as little damage as possible to the deeper structures. It should follow lines of cleavage and planes of fascia and when possible should pass between muscles rather than through them. Important nerves and vessels must be spared by locating and protecting them or by avoiding them completely; when an important structure is in immediate danger, it should be exposed. In addition to learning approaches described by others, the surgeon should know the anatomy so well that an approach can be modified when necessary.

Not all approaches are described in this chapter, but rather only those found suitable for most of the orthopaedic operations now in use. Additional approaches are described in other sections of this book. There has been recent interest in less invasive total joint arthroplasties. These approaches are outlined in other chapters.

Making a long incision parallel to the scar of a previous long incision is unjustified. An incision through an old scar heals as well as a new incision; and even though the scar may not be ideally located, the deeper structures may be reached by retracting the skin and subcutaneous tissues. A second incision made parallel to and near an old scar may impair the circulation in the strip of skin between the two, leading to skin slough.

The position of the patient for surgery also is important. It should be properly established before the operation is begun, and provisions should be made to prevent undesirable changes in position during the operation. The surgeon should be able to reach all parts of the surgical field easily. If there is a chance that intraoperative fluoroscopy will be needed, a radiolucent table should be used.

A tourniquet, unless specifically contraindicated, should always be used in surgery on the extremities; the dry field it provides makes the dissection easier, the surgical technique less traumatic, and the time required for the operation shorter. Also, in a dry field, the cutaneous nerves are identified and protected more easily, and they often may be used as guides to deeper structures. The identification, dissection, and ligation of vessels are also made easier. Although the extremity is temporarily ischemic, an electrocautery unit should be used to cauterize small vessels that cross the incision. An electrocautery unit is even more useful in surgical sites where a tourniquet cannot be employed, such as the shoulder, hip, spine, or pelvis.

TOES

APPROACH TO THE INTERPHALANGEAL JOINTS

TECHNIQUE 1.9

- For procedures on the interphalangeal joint of the great toe, make an incision 2.5 cm long on the medial aspect of the toe.
- For the interphalangeal joints of the fifth toe, make a lateral incision.
- Approach the interphalangeal joints of the second, third, and fourth toes through an incision just lateral to the corresponding extensor tendon.
- Carry the dissection through the subcutaneous tissue and fascia to the capsule of the joint.
- Reflect the edges of the incision with care to avoid damaging the dorsal or plantar digital vessels and nerves; retract the dorsal nerves and vessels dorsally and the plantar nerves and vessels plantarward.
- To expose the articular surfaces, open the capsule transversely or longitudinally.

APPROACHES TO THE METATARSOPHALANGEAL JOINT OF THE GREAT TOE

The metatarsophalangeal joint of the great toe may be exposed in one of several ways. Two ways are described.

MEDIAL APPROACH TO THE GREAT TOE METATARSOPHALANGEAL JOINT

TECHNIQUE 1.10

- Make a curved incision 5 cm long on the medial aspect of the joint (Fig. 1.28A). Begin it just proximal to the interphalangeal joint, curve it over the dorsum of the metatarsophalangeal joint medial to the extensor hallucis longus

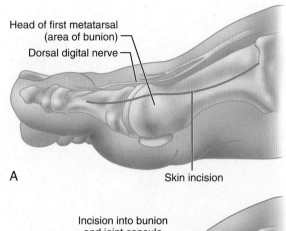

A

Head of first metatarsal (area of bunion)

Dorsal digital nerve

Skin incision

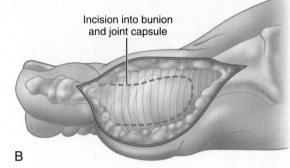

B

Incision into bunion and joint capsule

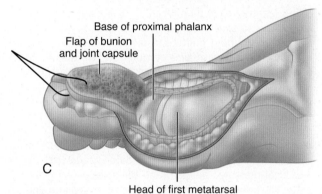

C

Base of proximal phalanx

Flap of bunion and joint capsule

Head of first metatarsal

FIGURE 1.28　**A-C,** Medial approach to metatarsophalangeal joint of great toe (see text). (Modified from Hoppenfeld S, deBoer P: *Surgical exposures in orthopaedics: the anatomic approach*, Philadelphia, 2003, Lippincott Williams & Wilkins.) **SEE TECHNIQUE 1.10.**

tendon, and end it on the medial aspect of the first metatarsal 2.5 cm proximal to the joint.
- As the deep fascia is incised, laterally retract the medial branch of the first dorsal metatarsal artery and the medial branch of the dorsomedial nerve (a branch of the superficial peroneal nerve), which supplies the medial side of the great toe.
- Dissect the fascia from the dorsum down to the bursa over the medial aspect of the metatarsal head.
- Make a curved incision through the bursa and capsule of the joint (Fig. 1.28B); begin the incision over the dorsomedial aspect of the joint, continue it proximally dorsal to the metatarsal head and plantarward and distally around the joint, and end it distally on the medioplantar aspect of the metatarsophalangeal joint. This incision forms an elliptical, racquet-shaped flap attached at the base of the

proximal phalanx (Fig. 1.28C). Although distal reflection of this flap amply exposes the first metatarsophalangeal joint, the use of a dorsomedial approach is preferable because healing of the skin flap may be delayed.

DORSOMEDIAL APPROACH TO GREAT TOE METATARSOPHALANGEAL JOINT

TECHNIQUE 1.11

- Begin the incision just proximal to the interphalangeal joint and continue it proximally for 5 cm parallel with and medial to the extensor hallucis longus tendon.
- To expose the capsule, divide the fascia and retract the tendon.
- The capsule can be incised by forming a flap with its attachment at the base of the first phalanx, as in the preceding approach, or by continuing the dissection in the plane of the skin incision.

APPROACH TO THE LESSER TOE METATARSOPHALANGEAL JOINTS

TECHNIQUE 1.12

- The second, third, and fourth metatarsophalangeal joints are reached by a dorsolateral incision parallel to the corresponding extensor tendon (Fig. 1.29).
- The fifth metatarsophalangeal joint is best exposed by a straight or curved dorsal or dorsolateral incision.
- The joint capsules may be opened transversely or longitudinally, as necessary.

CALCANEUS

Approaches to the calcaneus are carried out most easily with the patient prone. The medial approach, however, can be made with the patient supine, the knee flexed, and the foot crossed over the opposite leg. The lateral approach also can be made with the patient supine by placing a sandbag under the ipsilateral buttock, internally rotating the hip, and everting the foot.

MEDIAL APPROACH TO THE CALCANEUS

TECHNIQUE 1.13   *Figure 1.30*

- Begin the incision 2.5 cm anterior to and 4 cm inferior to the medial malleolus, carrying it posteriorly along the medial surface of the foot to the Achilles tendon.

- Divide the fat and fascia and define the inferior margin of the abductor hallucis.
- Mobilize the muscle belly and retract it dorsally to expose the medial and inferomedial aspects of the body of the calcaneus.
- Continue the dissection distally by dividing the plantar aponeurosis and the muscles attaching to the calcaneus or by stripping these from the bone with an osteotome. Carefully avoid the medial calcaneal nerve and the nerve to the abductor digiti minimi.
  The inferior surface of the body of the calcaneus can be exposed subperiosteally.

LATERAL APPROACH TO THE CALCANEUS

TECHNIQUE 1.14

- Begin the incision on the lateral margin of the Achilles tendon near its insertion and pass it distally to a point 4 cm inferior to and 2.5 cm anterior to the lateral malleolus (Fig. 1.31).
- Divide the superficial and deep fasciae, isolate the peroneal tendons and incise and elevate the periosteum below the tendons to expose the bone.
- If necessary, and if no infection is present, divide the tendons by Z-plasty and repair them later.

EXTENDED LATERAL APPROACH TO THE CALCANEUS

The extended lateral approach was developed for open fixation of calcaneal fractures. The condition of the skin is most important. Swelling and bruised skin are factors leading to superficial and deep infections. The initial trauma impairs the microvasculature of the skin and subcutaneous tissues. A single-layer interrupted absorbable subcuticular suture is recommended for closure. This is less traumatic to the skin and subcutaneous tissues than a two-layer closure. An inverse relationship between surgeon experience and wound complications has been demonstrated, and patient age and use of nicotine in any form are also important factors.

TECHNIQUE 1.15

- Beginning several centimeters proximal to the posterior tuberosity and the lateral edge of the Achilles tendon, begin the incision and carry it to the smooth skin just above the heel pad. Curve the incision anteriorly following the contour of the heel and carry it to below the tip of the fifth metatarsal base (Fig. 1.31A).
- Develop a full-thickness flap containing the peroneal tendons and sural nerve.

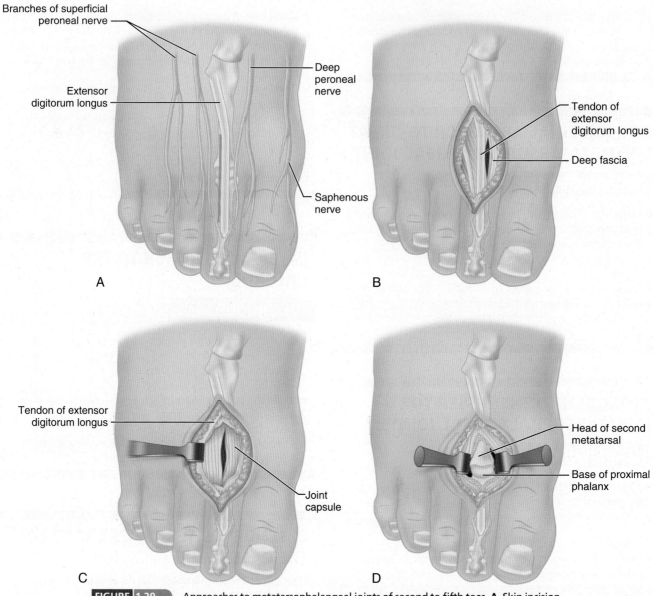

Branches of superficial peroneal nerve

Extensor digitorum longus

Deep peroneal nerve

Saphenous nerve

A

Tendon of extensor digitorum longus

Deep fascia

B

Tendon of extensor digitorum longus

Joint capsule

C

Head of second metatarsal

Base of proximal phalanx

D

FIGURE 1.29 Approaches to metatarsophalangeal joints of second to fifth toes. **A,** Skin incision. **B,** Incision through deep fascia medial to tendons. **C,** Longitudinal incision in joint capsule. **D,** Joint is exposed. (Modified from Hoppenfeld S, deBoer P: *Surgical exposures in orthopaedics: the anatomic approach,* Philadelphia, 2003, Lippincott Williams & Wilkins.) **SEE TECHNIQUE 1.12.**

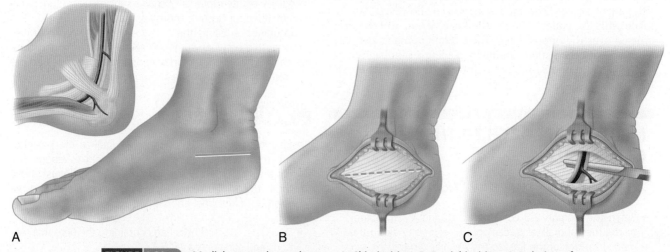

A

B

C

FIGURE 1.30 Medial approach to calcaneus. **A,** Skin incision. **B,** Fascial incision. **C,** Isolation of neurovascular bundle. (Modified from Burdeaux BD: Reduction of calcaneal fractures by the McReynolds medial approach technique and its experimental basis, *Clin Orthop Relat Res* 177:93, 1983.) **SEE TECHNIQUE 1.13.**

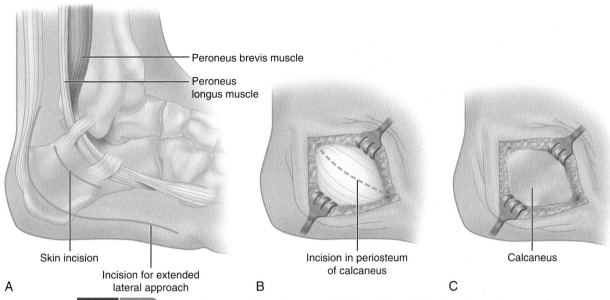

Peroneus brevis muscle
Peroneus longus muscle

Skin incision
Incision for extended lateral approach

Incision in periosteum of calcaneus

Calcaneus

A   B   C

FIGURE 1.31 Lateral approach to calcaneus. **A,** Skin incision. **B,** Incision in periosteum of calcaneus. **C,** Calcaneus is exposed. **SEE TECHNIQUES 1.14 AND 1.15.**

- Reflect it anteriorly and hold it in place with one or two Kirschner wires drilled into the lateral talus.
- At closure, use a single layer of interrupted 2-0 absorbable sutures.
- Use a single tube vacuum drain and apply a sterile Jones-type compression dressing.

SINUS TARSI APPROACH

The extended lateral approach is usually considered the approach of choice for intra-articular os calcis fractures. Soft-tissue problems are the major concern because the lateral calcaneal flap is thin. A limited lateral approach such as the sinus tarsi approach is a good alternative to reduce soft-tissue complications and is preferred at this time.

TECHNIQUE 1.16

(PARK AND CHO)
- Place the patient in the lateral decubitus position on a radiolucent table.
- Make an oblique incision just beneath the tip of the lateral malleolus and carry it toward the fourth metatarsal base (Fig. 1.32).
- Deepen the dissection while preserving the sural nerve.
- Reflect the peroneal tendons inferiorly and open the subtalar joint.
- Incise the calcaneofibular ligament if needed for exposure.

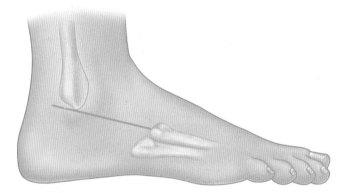

FIGURE 1.32 Sinus tarsi approach. Oblique skin incision under tip of lateral malleolus directed toward the fourth metatarsal base. **SEE TECHNIQUE 1.16.**

U-SHAPED APPROACH TO THE CALCANEUS

TECHNIQUE 1.17

- With the patient prone, support the leg on a large sandbag.
- For access to the entire plantar surface of the calcaneus, make a large U-shaped incision around the posterior four fifths of the bone (Fig. 1.33).
- After the dissections described, retract a flap consisting of skin, the fatty heel pad, and the plantar fascia.

32

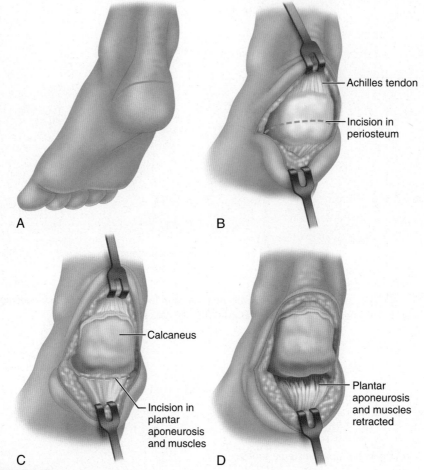

B — Achilles tendon / Incision in periosteum

C — Calcaneus / Incision in plantar aponeurosis and muscles

D — Plantar aponeurosis and muscles retracted

FIGURE 1.33 U-shaped approach to calcaneus. **A,** Skin incision. **B,** Periosteal incision. **C,** Incision in plantar aponeurosis and muscles. **D,** Plantar aponeurosis and muscles are retracted. **SEE TECHNIQUE 1.17.**

KOCHER APPROACH (CURVED L) TO THE CALCANEUS

TECHNIQUE 1.18

- The Kocher approach is suitable for complete excision of the calcaneus in cases of tumor or infection (see Fig. 1.36B).
- Incise the skin over the medial border of the Achilles tendon from 7.5 cm proximal to the tuberosity of the calcaneus to the inferoposterior aspect of the tuberosity, continuing it transversely around the posterior aspect of the calcaneus and distally along the lateral surface of the foot to the tuberosity of the fifth metatarsal.
- Divide the Achilles tendon at its insertion and carry the dissection down to the bone.
- To reach the superior surface, free all tissues beneath the severed Achilles tendon.
- The calcaneus may be enucleated with or without its periosteal attachments.
- The central third of the incision is ideal for fixation of posterior tuberosity avulsion fractures.

TARSUS AND ANKLE
ANTERIOR APPROACHES

ANTEROLATERAL APPROACH TO CHOPART JOINT

The anterolateral approach gives excellent access to the ankle joint, the talus, and most other tarsal bones and the anterior tuberosity of the calcaneal joints, and it avoids all important vessels and nerves. Because so many reconstructive operations and other procedures involve the structures exposed, it may well be called the "universal incision" for the foot and ankle. It permits excision of the entire talus, and the only tarsal joints that it cannot reach are those between the navicular and the second and first cuneiforms. This approach is good for a single-incision "triple" arthrodesis and a pantalar arthrodesis, as the tibiotalar, talonavicular, subtalar, and calcaneocuboid joints are exposed.

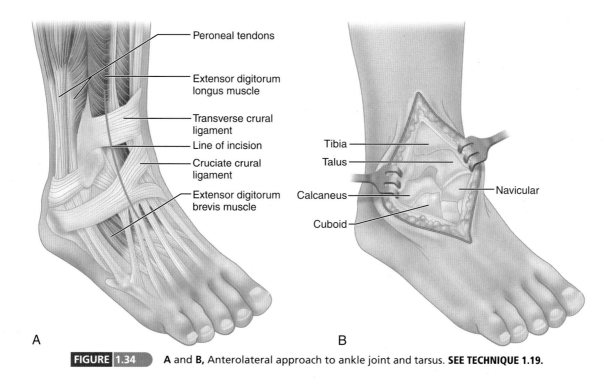

A and B, Anterolateral approach to ankle joint and tarsus. **SEE TECHNIQUE 1.19.**

TECHNIQUE 1.19

- Begin the incision over the anterolateral aspect of the leg medial to the fibula and 5 cm proximal to the ankle joint, carrying it distally over the joint, the anterolateral aspect of the body of the talus, and the calcaneocuboid joint, and end it at the base of the fourth metatarsal (Fig. 1.34A). The incision may begin more proximally or end more distally, or any part may be used, as needed.
- Incise the fascia and the superior and inferior extensor retinacula down to the periosteum of the tibia and the capsule of the ankle joint. This dissection usually divides the anterolateral malleolar and lateral tarsal arteries.
- While retracting the edges of the wound, identify and protect the intermediate dorsal cutaneous branches of the superficial peroneal nerve.
- Divide the extensor digitorum brevis muscle in the direction of its fibers or detach it from its origin and reflect it distally.
- Retract the extensor tendons, the dorsalis pedis artery, and the deep peroneal nerve medially and incise the capsule.
- Expose the talonavicular joint by dissecting deep to the tendons and incise its capsule transversely.
- Continue the dissection laterally through the capsule of the calcaneocuboid joint, which lies on the same plane as the talonavicular joint.
- Incise the mass of fat lateral to and inferior to the neck of the talus to bring the subtalar joint into view.
- Extend the dissection distally to provide access to the articulation between the cuboid and the fourth and fifth metatarsals and between the navicular and the third cuneiform (Fig. 1.34B).

ANTERIOR APPROACH TO EXPOSE THE ANKLE JOINT AND BOTH MALLEOLI

Gaining access to the part of the ankle joint between the medial malleolus and the medial articular facet of the body of the talus often is difficult when fusing the ankle through the anterolateral approach. Through the anterior approach, however, both malleoli may be exposed easily. Usually the approach is developed between the extensor hallucis longus and extensor digitorum longus tendons (Fig. 1.35), but it also can be developed between the anterior tibial and extensor hallucis longus tendons. In this case, the neurovascular bundle is retracted laterally with the long extensor tendons of the toes, and the anterior tibial tendon is retracted medially.

TECHNIQUE 1.20

- Begin the incision on the anterior aspect of the leg 7.5 to 10 cm proximal to the ankle and extend it distally to about 5 cm distal to the joint. Its length varies with the surgical indication (Fig. 1.36A).
- Divide the deep fascia in line with the skin incision.
- Isolate, ligate, and divide the anterolateral malleolar and lateral tarsal arteries, and carefully expose the neurovascular bundle and retract it medially.
- Incise the periosteum, capsule, and synovium in line with the skin incision, and expose the full width of the ankle joint anteriorly by subcapsular and subperiosteal dissection.

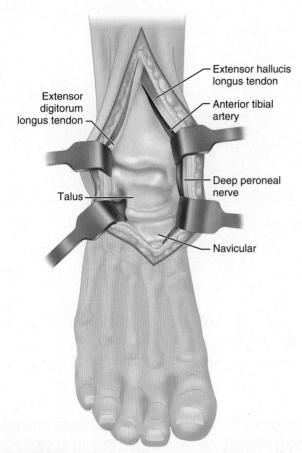

Extensor hallucis longus tendon
Anterior tibial artery
Extensor digitorum longus tendon
Deep peroneal nerve
Talus
Navicular

FIGURE 1.35 Anterior approach to ankle joint. Extensor hallucis longus and anterior tibial tendons, along with neurovascular bundle, are retracted medially. Tendons of extensor digitorum longus muscle are retracted laterally. **SEE TECHNIQUE 1.20.**

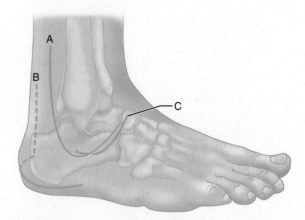

FIGURE 1.36 **A,** Kocher approach to ankle. **B,** Kocher approach to calcaneus. **C,** Ollier approach to midtarsal and subtalar joints. **SEE TECHNIQUES 1.18, 1.20, 1.21, AND 1.22.**

- Incise the fascia down to the peroneal tendons and retract them posteriorly, protecting the lesser saphenous vein and sural nerve lying immediately posterior to the incision.
- If a larger operative field is necessary, divide the tendons by Z-plasty and retract them.
- Deepen the dissection distally, divide the calcaneofibular ligament, and expose the subtalar joint. The calcaneocuboid and talonavicular joints may be reached through the distal part of this incision.
- After dividing the talofibular ligaments, dislocate the ankle by medial traction if access to its entire articular surface is desired.

LATERAL APPROACHES TO THE TARSUS AND ANKLE

KOCHER LATERAL APPROACH TO THE TARSUS AND ANKLE

The Kocher approach gives excellent exposure of the midtarsal, subtalar, and ankle joints (Fig. 1.36A). The disadvantage of this procedure is that the skin may slough around the margins of the incision, especially if dislocation of the ankle has been necessary, as in a talectomy. The peroneal tendons usually must be divided. In most instances, the anterolateral incision is more satisfactory.

TECHNIQUE 1.21

- From a point just lateral and distal to the head of the talus, curve the incision 2.5 cm inferior to the tip of the lateral malleolus, then posteriorly and proximally, and end it 2.5 cm posterior to the fibula and 5 cm proximal to the tip of the lateral malleolus or, if desired, 5 or 7 cm further proximally, parallel with and posterior to the fibula (Fig. 1.36A).

OLLIER APPROACH TO THE TARSUS

The Ollier approach is excellent for a triple arthrodesis: the three joints are exposed through a small opening without much retraction, and the wound usually heals well because the proximal flap is dissected full thickness and the skin edges are protected during retraction.

TECHNIQUE 1.22

- Begin the skin incision over the dorsolateral aspect of the talonavicular joint, extend it obliquely inferoposteriorly, and end it about 2.5 cm inferior to the lateral malleolus (Fig. 1.36C).
- Divide the inferior extensor retinaculum in the line of the skin incision.
- In the superior part of the incision, expose the long extensor tendons to the toes and retract them medially, preferably without opening their sheaths.
- In the inferior part of the incision, expose the peroneal tendons and retract them inferiorly.
- Divide the origin of the extensor digitorum brevis muscle, retract the muscle distally, and bring into view the sinus tarsi.
- Extend the dissection to expose the subtalar, calcaneocuboid, and talonavicular joints.

SINGLE-INCISION POSTEROLATERAL APPROACH TO THE LATERAL AND POSTERIOR MALLEOLI

Choi et al. described a single-incision oblique posterolateral approach for posterior malleolar fracture with an associated lateral malleolar fracture.

TECHNIQUE 1.23

(CHOI ET AL.)
- Place the patient in the prone or lateral position.
- Make a 10-cm incision following the posterior edge of the lateral malleolus and curve it posteriorly at the level of the syndesmosis to end at the Achilles tendon insertion on the os calcis. Carefully dissect out the sural nerve (Fig. 1.37). The incision can be extended proximally if necessary.
- Take down the peroneal tendons from the posterior aspect of the lateral malleolus, and expose the lateral malleolar fracture.
- Develop the interval between the peroneal tendons and the flexor hallucis longus.
- Retract both the flexor hallucis longus and the Achilles tendon medially, exposing the posterior malleolus.

POSTEROLATERAL APPROACH TO THE ANKLE

The Gatellier and Chastang posterolateral approach permits open reduction and internal fixation of fractures of the ankle in which the fragment of the posterior tibial lip (posterior malleolus) is large and laterally situated. It makes use of the fact that the fibula usually is fractured in such injuries; should it be intact, it is osteotomized about 10 cm proximal to the tip of the lateral malleolus. The approach also is used for osteochondritis dissecans involving the lateral part of the dome of the talus and for osteochondromatosis of the ankle.

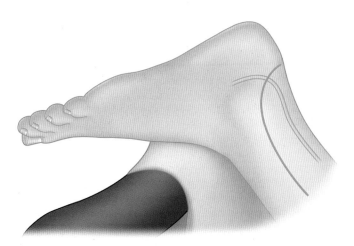

FIGURE 1.37 Yellow line shows the course of the sural nerve. Green line shows the incision. **SEE TECHNIQUE 1.23.**

TECHNIQUE 1.24

(GATELLIER AND CHASTANG)
- Begin the incision about 12 cm proximal to the tip of the lateral malleolus and extend it distally along the posterior margin of the fibula to the tip of the malleolus. Curve the incision anteriorly for 2.5 to 4 cm in the line of the peroneal tendons (Fig. 1.38).
- Expose the fibula, including the lateral malleolus subperiosteally, and incise the sheaths of the peroneal retinacula and tendons, permitting the tendons to be displaced anteriorly.
- If the fibula is not fractured, divide it 10 cm proximal to the tip of the lateral malleolus and free the distal fragment by dividing the interosseous membrane and the anterior and posterior tibiofibular ligaments.
- Carefully preserve the calcaneofibular and talofibular ligaments to serve as a hinge and to maintain the integrity of the ankle after operation. Turn the fibula laterally on this hinge and expose the lateral and posterior aspects of the distal tibia and the lateral aspect of the ankle joint. Great care should be used in children to avoid creating a fracture through the distal fibular physis when reflecting the fibula.
- When closing the incision, replace the fibula and secure it with a screw extending transversely from the proximal part of the lateral malleolus through the tibiofibular syndesmosis into the tibia just proximal and parallel to the ankle joint.
- Overdrill the hole made in the fibula to allow for compression across the syndesmosis. Dorsiflex the ankle joint as the screw is tightened because the talar dome is wider at its anterior half than its posterior half. Failure to overdrill the fibula can result in widening of the syndesmosis and ankle mortise, with resulting arthritic degeneration of the tibiotalar joint. Add additional fixation with a small plate and screws if desired.
- Replace the tendons, repair the tendon sheaths and retinacula, and close the incision.
- After the osteotomy or fracture has healed, remove the screw to prevent its becoming loose or breaking.

ANTEROLATERAL APPROACH TO THE LATERAL DOME OF THE TALUS

As an alternative to lateral malleolar osteotomy, Tochigi et al. described an anterolateral approach to the lateral dome of the talus for extensive lateral osteochondral lesions. All but the posterior one fourth of the lateral talus can be exposed. An osteotomy of the anterolateral tibia is required.

TECHNIQUE 1.25

(TOCHIGI, AMENDOLA, MUIR, AND SALTZMAN)
- Make a vertical 10-cm incision along the anterolateral corner of the ankle, avoiding the lateral branch of the superficial peroneal nerve.

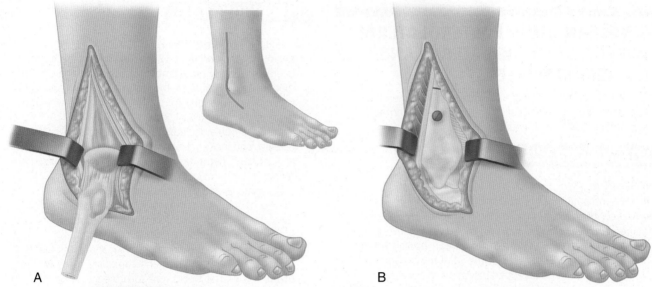

FIGURE 1.38   Posterolateral approach of Gatellier and Chastang. **A,** Peroneal tendons have been displaced anteriorly, and fibula has been divided; distal fragment has been turned laterally after interosseous membrane and anterior and posterior tibiofibular ligaments have been divided. **B,** Distal fibula has been replaced and fixed to tibia with syndesmosis screw. **SEE TECHNIQUE 1.24.**

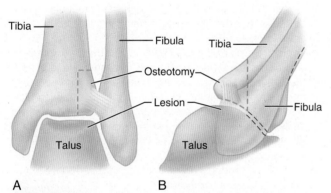

FIGURE 1.39   Tochigi, Amendola, Muir, and Saltzman antero- lateral approach to talus. **A,** Anterior view of osteotomy. **B,** Lateral view of osteotomy. (From Tochigi Y, Amendola A, Muir D, et al: Surgical approach for centrolateral talar osteochondral lesions with an anterolateral osteotomy, *Foot Ankle Int* 23:1038, 2002.) **SEE TECHNIQUE 1.25.**

- Outline the osteotomy of the anterolateral tibia to include the anterior tibiofibular ligament. The cortical surface of the fragment should be at least 1 cm² (Fig. 1.39). Predrill the fragment to accept a 4-mm cancellous screw.
- Use a micro-oscillating saw to begin the osteotomy in two planes. Complete the osteotomy with a small, narrow os- teotome by gently levering it in an externally rotated di- rection. The cartilaginous surface of the tibia is "cracked" as the fragment is rotated.
- At wound closure, rotate the fragment back into position and secure it with a 4-mm cancellous screw and washer.

POSTERIOR APPROACH TO THE ANKLE

If only the anterolateral distal tibia needs to be exposed, the anterolateral tibial osteotomy is omitted and the super- ficial peroneal nerve is protected until its position becomes more posterior entering deep fascia.

TECHNIQUE 1.26

- With the patient prone, make a 12-cm incision along the posterolateral border of the Achilles tendon down to the insertion of the tendon on the calcaneus (Fig. 1.40A).
- Divide the superficial and deep fasciae, divide the Achil- les tendon by Z-plasty or retract it, and incise the fat and areolar tissue to the posterior surface of the tibia in the space between the flexor hallucis longus and the peroneal tendons (Fig. 1.40B).
- Retract the flexor hallucis longus tendon medially to ex- pose 2.5 cm of the distal end of the tibia, the posterior aspect of the ankle joint, the posterior end of the talus, the subtalar joint, and the posterior part of the superior surface of the calcaneus (Fig. 1.40C).
- If the dissection is kept lateral to the flexor hallucis longus tendon, the posterior tibial vessels and the tibial nerve will not be at risk because this tendon protects them.
- Alternatively, the Achilles tendon can be split from just above the ankle joint distally to its insertion on the os calcis. Hammit et al. found a lower wound complication rate with- out sacrificing exposure using this technique rather than standard posteromedial and posterolateral approaches.

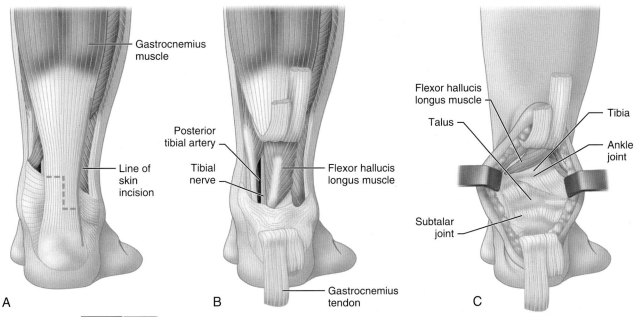

FIGURE 1.40 Posterior approach to ankle. **A,** Skin incision. **B,** Z-plasty division and reflection of Achilles tendon. **C,** Exposure of ankle and subtalar joints after retraction of flexor hallucis longus tendon and posterior capsulotomy. **SEE TECHNIQUE 1.26.**

MEDIAL APPROACHES

MEDIAL APPROACH TO THE TARSUS

Knupp et al. described a medial approach to the subtalar joint that is useful for hindfoot arthrodesis in posterior tibial tendon dysfunction.

TECHNIQUE 1.27

(KNUPP ET AL.)
- Place the patient supine with the involved foot externally rotated.
- Make a 4-cm long incision from the center of the medial malleolus toward the navicular 5 mm above and parallel to the posterior tibial tendon (Fig. 1.41). Extend the incision as necessary to reach as far as the cuneiform.
- Open the subtalar joint capsule being careful not to damage the anterior fibers of the deltoid ligament.

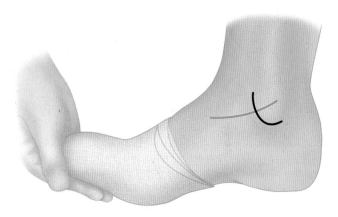

FIGURE 1.41 Medial approach to the subtalar joint. **SEE TECHNIQUE 1.27.**

TECHNIQUE 1.28

(KOENIG AND SCHAEFER)
- Curve the incision just proximal to the medial malleolus (Fig. 1.42A) and divide the malleolus with an osteotome or small power saw; preserve the attachment of the deltoid ligament.
- Subluxate the talus and malleolus laterally to reach the joint surfaces.
- Later replace the malleolus and fix it with one or two cancellous screws. To make replacement easier, drill the holes for the screws before the osteotomy, insert the screw, and then remove it. At the end of the operation, reinsert the screws and close the wound.

MEDIAL APPROACH TO THE ANKLE

Koenig and Schaefer approached the ankle from the medial side by a method similar in principle to the Gatellier and Chastang exposure of the posterolateral side. It is not a popular method because, despite utmost care, it is possible to injure the tibial vessels and nerve. Nevertheless, it may be useful for fracture-dislocations of the talus, other traumatic lesions of the ankle joint, and osteochondritis dissecans of the talus.

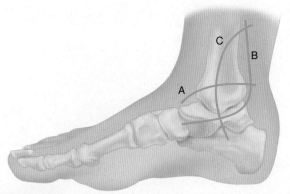

FIGURE 1.42 Incisions for medial approaches to ankle joint: Koenig and Schaefer *(A)*, Broomhead *(B)*, and Colonna and Ralston *(C)*. **SEE TECHNIQUES 1.28 AND 1.29.**

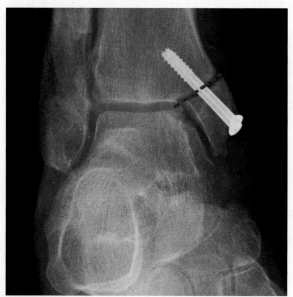

FIGURE 1.43 Osteotomy of medial malleolus for access to medial dome of talus. Note line of osteotomy. **SEE TECHNIQUE 1.28.**

- The surfaces of the osteotomized bone are smooth, and the malleolus can rotate on a single screw. Two screws are used to prevent rotation of the osteotomized medial malleolus (Fig. 1.43). Interfragmentary technique should be used for screw fixation of the medial malleolus to provide compression across the osteotomy site.

MEDIAL APPROACH TO THE POSTERIOR LIP OF THE TIBIA

Broomhead advised a curved medial incision for fractures of the medial part of the posterior lip of the tibia that require open reduction. The line of approach lies midway between the posterior border of the tibia and the medial border of the Achilles tendon, curves inferior to the medial malleolus to the medial border of the foot, and permits exposure

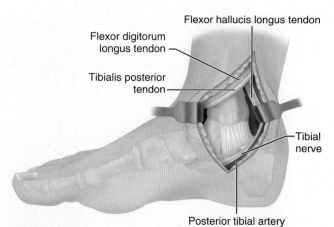

FIGURE 1.44 Colonna and Ralston posteromedial approach to distal tibia. Posterior tibial and flexor digitorum longus tendons have been retracted anteriorly, and flexor hallucis longus tendon, posterior tibial vessels, and tibial nerve have been retracted posteriorly and laterally. **SEE TECHNIQUE 1.29.**

of medial and posterior malleoli (Fig. 1.42*B*). The latter is exposed by reflecting the capsule and periosteum and retracting the tendons of the posterior tibial, flexor digitorum longus, and flexor hallucis longus muscles together with the neurovascular bundle posteriorly and medially.

Colonna and Ralston described the following modification of Broomhead's approach.

TECHNIQUE 1.29

(COLONNA AND RALSTON)

- Begin the incision at a point about 10 cm proximal and 2.5 cm posterior to the medial malleolus and curve it anteriorly and inferiorly across the center of the medial malleolus and inferiorly and posteriorly 4 cm toward the heel (Fig. 1.42*C*).
- Expose the medial malleolus by reflecting the periosteum, but preserve the deltoid ligament.
- Divide the flexor retinaculum and retract the flexor hallucis longus tendon and the neurovascular bundle posteriorly and laterally.
- Retract the tibial posterior and flexor digitorum longus tendons medially and anteriorly to expose the posterior tibial fracture (Fig. 1.44).

In addition to the approaches described, short medial, lateral, and dorsal approaches may be used to expose small areas of the tarsal and metatarsal joints. In all, the vessels, nerves, and tendons must be protected.

TIBIA

The tibia is a superficial bone that can be easily exposed anteriorly without damaging any important structure except the tendons of the anterior tibial and extensor hallucis longus muscles, which cross the tibia anteriorly in its lower fourth.

ANTEROLATERAL APPROACH TO THE TIBIA

TECHNIQUE 1.30

- Make a longitudinal incision 1 to 2 cm lateral to the anterior border of the bone. This will provide an adequate skin bridge.
- Sharply incise the fascia the entire length of the wound. Incise and elevate the periosteum over the desired area. Strip the periosteum as little as possible because its circulation is a source of nutrition for the bone.

MEDIAL APPROACH TO THE TIBIA

In some delayed unions and nonunions, Phemister inserted a bone graft in a bed prepared on the posterior surface of the tibia.

TECHNIQUE 1.31

(PHEMISTER)
- Make a longitudinal incision along the posteromedial border of the tibia.
- Incise the subcutaneous tissues and deep fascia and reflect the periosteum from the posterior surface for the required distance.

POSTEROLATERAL APPROACH TO THE TIBIAL SHAFT

The posterolateral approach is valuable in the middle two thirds of the tibia when the anterior and anteromedial aspects of the leg are badly scarred. It also is satisfactory for removing a portion of the fibula for transfer.

TECHNIQUE 1.32

(HARMON, MODIFIED)
- Position the patient prone or on the side, with the affected extremity uppermost.
- Make the skin incision the desired length along the lateral border of the gastrocnemius muscle on the posterolateral aspect of the leg (Fig. 1.45A).
- Develop the plane between the gastrocnemius, the soleus, and the flexor hallucis longus muscles posteriorly and the peroneal muscles anteriorly (Fig. 1.45B).
- Find the lateral border of the soleus muscle and retract it and the gastrocnemius muscle medially and posteriorly; arising from the posterior surface of the fibula is the flexor hallucis longus (Fig. 1.45C).
- Detach the distal part of the origin of the soleus muscle from the fibula and retract it posteriorly and medially (Fig. 1.45D).

- Continue the dissection medially across the interosseous membrane, detaching those fibers of the posterior tibial muscle arising from it (Fig. 1.45E). The posterior tibial artery and the tibial nerve are posterior and separated from the dissection by the posterior tibial and flexor hallucis longus muscles (Fig. 1.45F).
- Follow the interosseous membrane to the lateral border of the tibia and detach subperiosteally the muscles that arise from the posterior surface of the tibia (Fig. 1.45G, and H).
- The posterior half of the fibula lies in the lateral part of the wound; its entire shaft can be explored. The flat posterior surface of the tibial shaft can be completely exposed except for its proximal fourth, which lies in close relation to the popliteus muscle and to the proximal parts of the posterior tibial vessels and the tibial nerve.
- When the operation is completed, release the tourniquet, secure hemostasis, and let the posterior muscle mass fall back into place.
- Loosely close the deep fascia on the lateral side of the leg with a few interrupted sutures.

TIBIAL PLATEAU APPROACHES

It is recommended that all these approaches be made on a radiolucent operating table.

ANTEROLATERAL APPROACH TO THE LATERAL TIBIAL PLATEAU

The anterolateral approach is commonly used because most tibial plateau fractures involve the lateral tibial plateau.

TECHNIQUE 1.33

(KANDEMIR AND MACLEAN)
- Place the patient supine on a radiolucent table.
- Begin the incision 2 to 3 cm proximal to the joint line and extend it 3 cm below the inferior margin of the tibial tubercle crossing Gerdy's tubercle at the midpoint of the incision (Fig. 1.46).
- Detach the iliotibial band and develop the interval between it and the joint capsule.
- Reflect the origin of the tibialis anterior muscle from the anterolateral tibia and reflect it posteriorly exposing the anterolateral surface of the tibial plateau.
- If direct exposure of the articular surface is necessary, perform a submeniscal arthrotomy incising the meniscotibial ligaments. Leave the anterior horn of the meniscus intact.
- Place three or four sutures in the periphery of the meniscus to serve as retractors and for later repair. If a repairable vertical meniscal tear is present, pass the necessary number of sutures in a vertical fashion through the inner part of the meniscus for later attachment to the capsule.
- If a submeniscal arthrotomy is not planned, a hockey-stick skin incision can be used for minimally invasive procedures. Make the proximal limb of the incision parallel to the lateral joint line and cross Gerdy's tubercle.

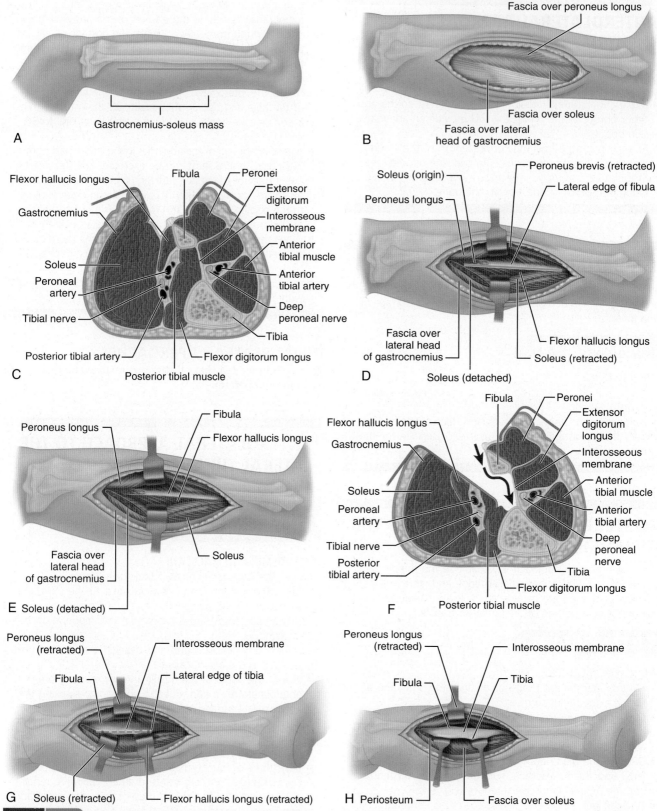

A, Gastrocnemius-soleus mass

B, Fascia over peroneus longus · Fascia over soleus · Fascia over lateral head of gastrocnemius

C, Flexor hallucis longus · Fibula · Peronei · Gastrocnemius · Extensor digitorum · Interosseous membrane · Soleus · Anterior tibial muscle · Peroneal artery · Anterior tibial artery · Tibial nerve · Deep peroneal nerve · Posterior tibial artery · Tibia · Flexor digitorum longus · Posterior tibial muscle

D, Soleus (origin) · Peroneus brevis (retracted) · Peroneus longus · Lateral edge of fibula · Fascia over lateral head of gastrocnemius · Flexor hallucis longus · Soleus (retracted) · Soleus (detached)

E, Peroneus longus · Fibula · Flexor hallucis longus · Soleus · Fascia over lateral head of gastrocnemius · Soleus (detached)

F, Fibula · Peronei · Flexor hallucis longus · Extensor digitorum longus · Gastrocnemius · Interosseous membrane · Soleus · Anterior tibial muscle · Peroneal artery · Anterior tibial artery · Tibial nerve · Deep peroneal nerve · Posterior tibial artery · Tibia · Flexor digitorum longus · Posterior tibial muscle

G, Peroneus longus (retracted) · Interosseous membrane · Fibula · Lateral edge of tibia · Soleus (retracted) · Flexor hallucis longus (retracted)

H, Peroneus longus (retracted) · Interosseous membrane · Fibula · Tibia · Periosteum · Fascia over soleus

FIGURE 1.45 Posterolateral approach to tibia. **A,** Skin incision. **B,** Plane between gastrocnemius, soleus, and flexor hallucis longus posteriorly and peroneal muscles anteriorly is developed. **C,** Flexor hallucis longus arising from posterior surface of fibula. **D,** Distal part of origin of soleus is detached from fibula and retracted posteriorly and medially. **E,** Dissection medially across interosseous membrane, detaching fibers of posterior tibial muscle. **F,** Posterior tibial artery and tibial nerve are protected by posterior tibial and flexor hallucis longus muscles. **G** and **H,** Muscles are detached subperiosteally from posterior surface of tibia. (Modified from Hoppenfeld S, deBoer P: *Surgical exposures in orthopaedics: the anatomic approach*, Philadelphia, 2003, Lippincott Williams & Wilkins.) **SEE TECHNIQUE 1.32.**

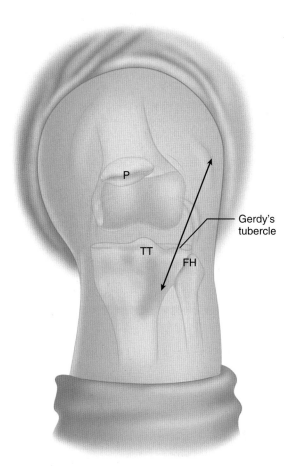

FIGURE 1.46 Anterolateral approach to the tibial plateau. Begin the incision 2 to 3 cm proximal to the joint line and carry it obliquely across Gerdy's tubercle aiming for a point 1 cm off the lateral aspect of the tibial tubercle. Extend it as far distally as needed. *FH,* Fibular head; *P,* patella; *TT,* tibial tubercle. **SEE TECHNIQUE 1.33.**

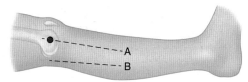

FIGURE 1.47 Medial and posteromedial approaches to the tibial plateau. *A,* Begin the skin incision for the medial approach 2 to 3 cm above the joint line at the medial epicondyle and extend it distally, bisecting the posteromedial border of the tibia and tibial crest. *B,* Begin the skin incision for the posteromedial approach 2 to 3 cm above the joint line and follow the posteromedial border of the tibia. **SEE TECHNIQUES 1.34 AND 1.35.**

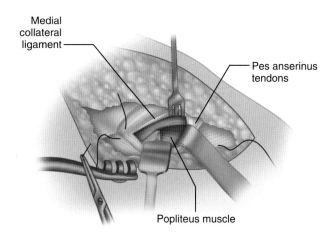

FIGURE 1.48 Posteromedial approach (supine). Retract the tendons of the pes anserinus distal and posterior. Incise the posterior edge of the medial collateral ligament and reflect the popliteus muscle insertion from the posterior border of the tibia. **SEE TECHNIQUE 1.35.**

MEDIAL APPROACH TO THE MEDIAL TIBIAL PLATEAU

This approach is useful for isolated medial plateau fractures and for medial half of bicondylar plateau fractures.

TECHNIQUE 1.34

- With the patient supine, make an incision 1 to 2 cm proximal to the joint line in line with the medial femoral epicondyle and extend it over the pes anserinus insertion (Fig. 1.47). Avoid the saphenous vein and nerve that usually are posterior.
- Take the pes anserinus tendons down sharply from the tibia, exposing the superficial and deep medial collateral ligaments.
- Indirectly reduce the fracture and apply a plate over the medial collateral ligaments.

POSTEROMEDIAL APPROACH TO THE MEDIAL TIBIAL PLATEAU

This approach is useful for shear fractures of the medial plateau. It can be performed with the patient supine or prone.

TECHNIQUE 1.35

(SUPINE)
- Externally rotate and slightly flex the knee.
- Make a longitudinal incision along the posteromedial aspect of the tibia, beginning 3 cm above the joint line and extend it as far distally as needed (Fig. 1.47*B*). Avoid the great saphenous vein and saphenous nerve anterior to the incision.
- Mobilize and retract the pes anserinus tendons proximally and anteriorly or distally and posteriorly.
- Retract the medial gastrocnemius and soleus muscles posteriorly, exposing the junction of popliteal fascia, the semimembranosus insertion, and the medial collateral ligaments.
- Incise the periosteum longitudinally and subperiosteally elevate the popliteus muscle insertion off the posterior tibia (Fig. 1.48).

POSTEROMEDIAL APPROACH (PRONE) TO THE SUPEROMEDIAL TIBIA

The posterior approach to the superomedial region of the tibia is useful for fixation of posteromedial split fractures of the tibial plateau. This is also known as the "reversed L" posteromedial approach.

TECHNIQUE 1.36

(BANKS AND LAUFMAN)

- With the patient positioned prone, begin the transverse segment of a hockey-stick incision (Fig. 1.49A) at the lateral end of the flexion crease of the knee, and extend it across the popliteal space. Turn the incision distally along the medial side of the calf for 7 to 10 cm.
- Develop the angular flap of skin and subcutaneous tissue and incise the deep fascia in line with the skin incision (Fig. 1.49B). Identify and protect the cutaneous nerves and superficial vessels.
- Define the interval between the tendon of the semitendinosus muscle and the medial head of the gastrocnemius muscle.
- Retract the semitendinosus proximally and medially and the gastrocsoleus component distally and laterally; the popliteus and flexor digitorum longus muscles lie in the floor of the interval (Fig. 1.49C).
- Elevate subperiosteally the flexor digitorum longus muscle distally and laterally and the popliteus muscle proximally and medially, and expose the posterior surface of the proximal fourth of the tibia (Fig. 1.49D). Further elevation of the popliteus will expose the posterior cruciate ligament fossa.
- If necessary, extend the incision distally along the medial side of the calf by continuing the dissection in the same intermuscular plane. The tibial nerve and posterior tibial artery lie beneath the soleus muscle.

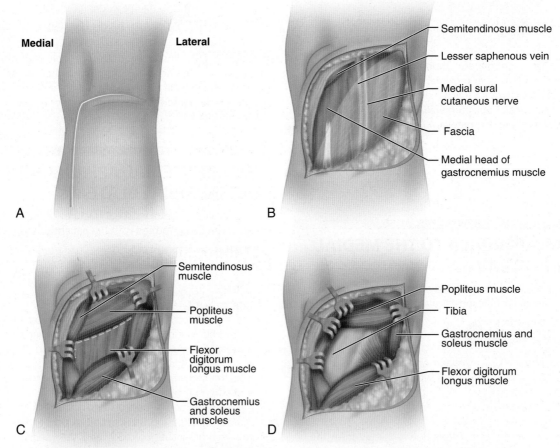

FIGURE 1.49   Banks and Laufman posterior approach to superomedial region of tibia. **A,** Incision extends transversely across popliteal fossa and then turns distally on medial side of calf. **B,** Skin and deep fascia have been incised and reflected. **C,** *Broken line* indicates incision to be made between popliteus and flexor digitorum longus. **D,** Popliteus and flexor digitorum longus have been elevated subperiosteally to expose tibia. **SEE TECHNIQUE 1.36.**

POSTEROLATERAL APPROACH TO THE TIBIAL PLATEAU

This approach is useful for lateral and posterolateral plateau fractures. This approach with a fibular osteotomy is useful for fractures of the posterolateral plateau.

TECHNIQUE 1.37

(SOLOMON ET AL.)

- Position the patient supine with the knee extended. Make a 6-cm longitudinal incision anterior to the biceps femoris tendon contour on the fibular head. The incision can be extended distally as needed.
- Flex the knee to 60 degrees.
- Incise the subcutaneous fat in line with the skin incision, exposing the deep fascia.
- Incise the fascia lata over the biceps tendon and the common peroneal nerve. Identify the common peroneal nerve in the adipose tissue of the popliteal fossa (Fig. 1.50A).
- Knee flexion relaxes the common peroneal nerve. Expose the nerve down to the fibular head. Protect the sural nerve branch from the common peroneal nerve in the popliteal fossa.

- Transect the branch of the common peroneal nerve to the proximal tibiofibular joint.
- Release the common peroneal nerve from the posterior intermuscular septum posterior to the peroneus longus muscle as it enters the lateral compartment.
- Expose the deep peroneal nerve by detaching the peroneus longus and tibialis anterior muscles from the posterior and anterior aspects of the anterior intermuscular septum, respectively.
- Release the deep peroneal nerve as it enters the anterior compartment and goes through the anterior septum.
- Pre-drill the fibular head and neck just lateral to the biceps femoris insertion.
- Osteotomize the fibular neck with an osteotome just above the peroneal nerve (Fig. 1.50B).
- Release the joint capsule from the proximal tibiofibular joint and reflect the fibular head proximally with attached biceps femoris tendon and lateral collateral ligament complex, exposing the postural corner of the knee joint.
- Mobilize the lateral meniscus by detaching the coronary ligament from the posterior cruciate ligament medially to the iliotibial band laterally, and elevate it to expose the tibial articular surfaces.

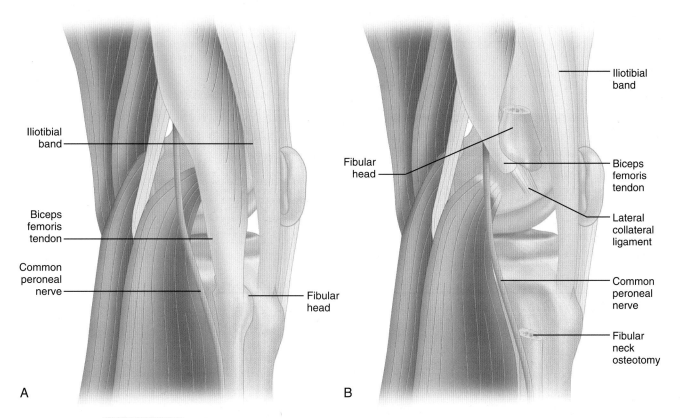

FIGURE 1.50 Posterolateral approach with osteotomy of the fibular neck. **A,** Superficial dissection of posterolateral corner. **B,** Osteotomy and reflection of fibular head proximally with attached biceps femoris tendon and lateral collateral ligament. Flex the knee to relax the common peroneal nerve, lateral head of gastrocnemius muscle, and popliteus muscle. Visualize the joint between to posterior cruciate ligament and posterior border of the iliotibial band. (Redrawn from Solomon LB, Stevenson AW, Baird RPV, Pohl AP. Posterolateral transfibular approach to tibial plateau fracture: technique, results, and rationale, *J Orthop Trauma* 24:505, 2010.) **SEE TECHNIQUE 1.37.**

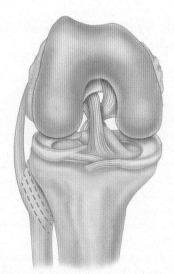

FIGURE `1.51` Posterolateral approach with osteotomy of fibular head. Make the plane of the osteotomy parallel to fibular articular surface. Remove the entire fibular head if needed but leave the attachments of the fibular collateral ligament and biceps femoris intact. (Redrawn from Yu B, Han K, Zhan C, et al: Fibular head osteotomy: a new approach for the treatment of lateral or posterolateral tibial plateau fractures, *The Knee* 17:313, 2010.) **SEE TECHNIQUE 1.37.**

- At closure, repair the osteotomy with a longitudinal screw.
- Alternatively, the fibular head can be osteotomized in a longitudinal direction as described by Yu et al. One third of the fibular head or the entire fibular head can be removed, depending on the exposure required (Fig. 1.51). The biceps femoris and lateral collateral ligament insertions are left intact.

POSTEROLATERAL APPROACH TO THE TIBIAL PLATEAU WITHOUT FIBULAR OSTEOTOMY

TECHNIQUE 1.38

(FROSCH ET AL.)
- Place the patient in the lateral decubitus position with the operative side up.
- Support the knee with a thick, rolled pillow.
- Make a 15-cm posterolateral incision starting 3 cm above the joint line then following the fibula distally.
- Incise the posterior portion of the iliotibial band from Gerdy's tubercle and perform a lateral arthrotomy.
- Bluntly dissect into the popliteal fossa between the lateral origin of the gastrocnemius muscle and soleus muscle, exposing the popliteus muscle.
- Ligate the inferior geniculate vessels if necessary.
- Develop the interval between the biceps femoris muscle and the popliteus muscle (Fig. 1.52).
- Detach the soleus muscle from the posterior aspect of the fibula exposing the posterolateral plateau.

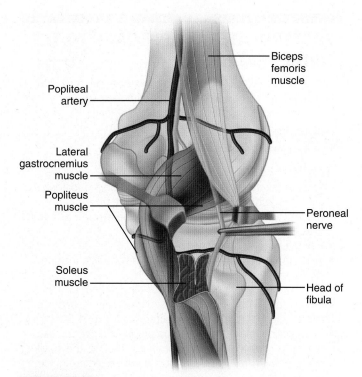

FIGURE `1.52` Posterolateral corner of tibia. Develop the interval between the popliteus muscle and the biceps femoris muscle. Reflect the soleus muscle origin from the proximal tibia. (Redrawn from Frosch KH, Balcarek P, Walde T, Stürmer KM: A new posterolateral approach without fibular osteotomy for the treatment of tibial plateau fractures, *J Orthop Trauma* 24:515, 2010.) **SEE TECHNIQUE 1.38.**

TSCHERNE-JOHNSON EXTENSILE APPROACH TO THE LATERAL TIBIAL PLATEAU

This approach is useful for depressed lateral plateau fractures.

TECHNIQUE 1.39

(JOHNSON ET AL.)
- Position the patient supine with a bump under the ipsilateral hip.
- Flex the knee over a large bump so that the leg will rest just off the edge of the table.
- Perform a lateral parapatellar incision from the supracondylar area of the distal femur to below and lateral to the tibial tubercle.
- Develop a lateral soft-tissue flap from the wound edge to the posterolateral corner of the tibial plateau.
- Identify Gerdy's tubercle and the anterior and posterior edges of the iliotibial band.
- Flex the knee to 40 degrees and incise the central portion of the iliotibial band distally from a point 4 cm above the joint line to the joint line and continue it anteriorly, dividing the anterior half of the band (Fig. 1.53A). Carry the incision anteriorly to the patellar tendon.
- Retract the anterior half of the iliotibial band exposing the lateral joint line.

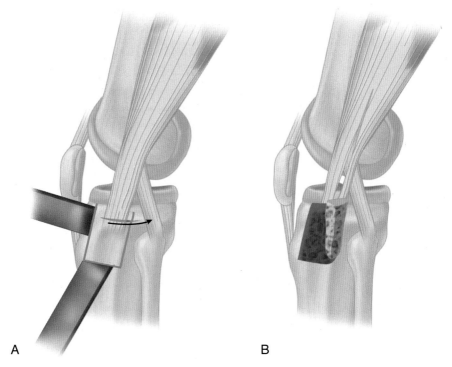

A   B

FIGURE 1.53   Tscherne-Johnson extensile approach to the lateral tibial plateau. **A,** Elevate Gerdy's tubercle with two osteotomies with bone cuts 90 degrees to each other. Base it on a posterior hinge behind Gerdy's tubercle. **B,** Externally rotate the fragment leaving the posterior insertion of the iliotibial band attached. (Redrawn from Johnson EE, Timon S: Tscherne-Johnson extensile approach for tibial plateau fractures, *Clin Orthop Relat Res* 471:2760, 2013.) **SEE TECHNIQUE 1.39.**

- Incise the meniscal coronary ligament from posterior to anterior ending at the level of the patellar tendon.
- Place three 2-0 absorbable sutures in the meniscal edge and elevate it. The sutures will be used to later repair the meniscus to the lateral plateau rim.
- Incise the origin of the tibialis anterior muscle along the lateral tibial metaphyseal flair and elevate it distally.
- Perform two osteotomies anterior and distal to Gerdy's tubercle with a narrow osteotome (Fig. 1.53A).
- Rotate Gerdy's tubercle fragment posteriorly on its posterior soft-tissue hinge to expose the undersurface of the lateral plateau (Fig. 1.53B).
- At closure, repair the osteotomy with an overlying plate and screws with one of the screws directly repairing the osteotomy.

TECHNIQUE 1.40

(SUN ET AL.)
- Place the patient in the lateral decubitus position.
- Make a 15-cm longitudinal incision 1.5-cm lateral to the tibial crest, and extend it between Gerdy's tubercle and the fibular head.
- Raise a full-thickness myocutaneous flap, and reflect the iliotibial tract from Gerdy's tubercle.
- Perform an osteotomy of the lateral tibial plateau, beginning at the anterolateral quadrant and moving posteriorly medial to the proximal tibiofibular joint (Fig. 1.54).
- The depressed posterolateral corner can now be exposed.
- Repair the osteotomy after elevation and grafting of the depressed segment.

ANTEROLATERAL APPROACH FOR ACCESS TO POSTEROLATERAL CORNER

Sun et al. described an anterolateral approach to gain access to the posterolateral corner when a depressed fracture involves this area.

Yoon et al. described an approach to the posterolateral corner by taking down the lateral collateral ligament with a piece of the lateral femoral epicondyle. The osteotomized piece should be large enough to allow repair with a large screw and washer.

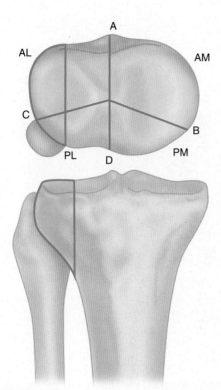

FIGURE 1.54 Osteotomy of the lateral tibial plateau. *A*, Knee center. *B*, Posteromedial ridge. *C*, Anterior edge of fibula. *D*, Posterior sulcus. *PL*, Posterolateral corner. *AL*, anterolateral; *AM*, anteromedial; *PM*, posteromedial. **SEE TECHNIQUE 1.40.**

FIBULA

POSTEROLATERAL APPROACH TO THE FIBULA

TECHNIQUE 1.41

(HENRY)

- Beginning 13 cm proximal to the lateral malleolus, incise the skin proximally along the posterior margin of the fibula to the posterior margin of the head of the bone and continue farther proximally for 10 cm along the posterior aspect of the biceps tendon.
- Divide the superficial and deep fasciae. Isolate the common peroneal nerve along the posteromedial aspect of the biceps tendon in the proximal part of the wound, and free it distally to its entrance into the peroneus longus muscle (Fig. 1.55).
- Pointing the knife blade proximally and anteriorly, detach the part of the peroneus longus muscle that arises from the lateral surface of the head of the fibula proximal to the common peroneal nerve. Retract the nerve over the head of the fibula.
- Locate the fascial plane between the soleus muscle posteriorly and the peroneal muscles anteriorly and deepen the dissection along the plane to the fibula.
- Expose the bone by retracting the peroneal muscles anteriorly and incising the periosteum. When retracting these muscles, avoid injuring the branches of the deep peroneal nerve that lie on their deep surfaces and are in close contact with the neck of the fibula and proximal 5 cm of the shaft.
- The distal fourth of the fibula is subcutaneous on its lateral aspect and may be exposed by a longitudinal incision through the skin, fascia, and periosteum.

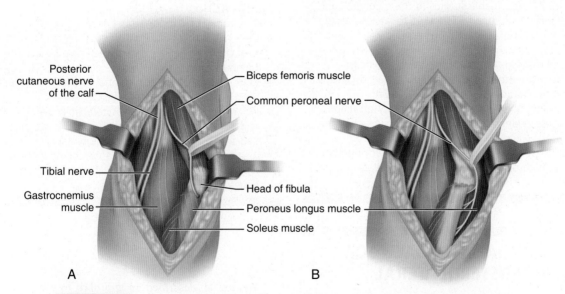

FIGURE 1.55 Method of mobilizing and retracting common peroneal nerve when approaching proximal fibula posterolaterally. **A,** Anatomic relationships. **B,** Part of peroneus longus that arises from lateral surface of fibular head proximal to common peroneal nerve has been detached, allowing nerve to be retracted over fibular head. **SEE TECHNIQUE 1.41.**

KNEE

ANTEROMEDIAL AND ANTEROLATERAL APPROACHES

ANTEROMEDIAL PARAPATELLAR APPROACH

When any anteromedial approach is made, including one for meniscectomy, the infrapatellar branch of the saphenous nerve should be protected (Fig. 1.56). The saphenous nerve courses posterior to the sartorius muscle and then pierces the fascia lata between the tendons of the sartorius and gracilis muscles and becomes subcutaneous on the medial aspect of the leg; on the medial aspect of the knee it gives off a large infrapatellar branch to supply the skin over the anteromedial aspect of the knee. Several variations exist in the location and distribution of this infrapatellar branch. Consequently, no single incision on the anteromedial aspect of the knee can avoid it for certain. The nerve should be located and protected if possible.

TECHNIQUE 1.42   *Figure 1.57*

(VON LANGENBECK)

- Begin the incision at the medial border of the quadriceps tendon 7 to 10 cm proximal to the patella, curve it around the medial border of the patella and back toward the midline, and end it at or distal to the tibial tuberosity. As a more cosmetically pleasing alternative, a longitudinal incision centered over the patella can be made, reflecting the subcutaneous tissue and superficial fascia over the patella medially by blunt dissection to the medial border of the patella.
- Divide and retract the fascia.
- Deepen the dissection between the vastus medialis muscle and the medial border of the quadriceps tendon and incise the capsule and synovium along this medial border and along the medial border of the patella and patellar tendon.

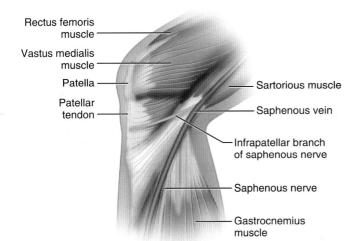

Rectus femoris muscle
Vastus medialis muscle
Patella
Patellar tendon
Sartorious muscle
Saphenous vein
Infrapatellar branch of saphenous nerve
Saphenous nerve
Gastrocnemius muscle

FIGURE 1.56   Anatomic relationships of superficial structures on medial aspect of knee. **SEE TECHNIQUE 1.42.**

- Retract the patella laterally and flex the knee to gain a good view of the anterior compartment of the joint and the suprapatellar bursa. Divide the ligamentum mucosa if necessary.
- Attain wider access to the joint in the following ways: (1) extending the incision proximally, (2) extending the proximal part of the incision obliquely medially and separating the fibers of the vastus medialis, (3) dividing the medial alar fold and adjacent fat pad longitudinally, and (4) mobilizing the medial part of the insertion of the patellar tendon subperiosteally.

If contracture of the quadriceps prevents sufficient exposure, detach the tibial tuberosity and reattach later with a screw. Fernandez described an extensive osteotomy of the tibial tuberosity and reattachment of the tuberosity with three lag screws engaging the posterior tibial cortex. This technique achieves rigid fixation and allows early postoperative rehabilitation. Keshmiri et al. recommended repair of the medial patellofemoral ligament at closure of a medial parapatellar approach during total knee arthroplasty (nonresurfaced patella). This is to prevent significant medial capsular dehiscence and resultant loading of the lateral patellar facet and increased anterior knee pain.

SUBVASTUS (SOUTHERN) ANTEROMEDIAL APPROACH TO THE KNEE

Problems with patellar dislocation, subluxation, and osteonecrosis after total knee arthroplasty performed through an anteromedial parapatellar approach led to the rediscovery of the subvastus, or Southern, anteromedial approach first described by Erkes in 1929. According to Hofmann et al., this approach preserves the vascularity of the patella by sparing the intramuscular articular branch of the descending genicular artery and preserves the quadriceps tendon, providing more stability to the patellofemoral joint in total knee arthroplasty. This approach also is useful for lesser anteromedial and medial knee procedures. The relative contraindications to this approach are previous major knee arthroplasty and weight greater than 200 lb, which makes eversion of the patella difficult. In a retrospective study of 143 knees in 96 patients, In et al. found that in patients with a thigh girth of larger than 55 cm the patella could not be everted when using a subvastus approach for total knee arthroplasty.

TECHNIQUE 1.43

(ERKES, AS DESCRIBED BY HOFMANN, PLASTER, AND MURDOCK)

- Exsanguinate the limb and inflate the tourniquet with the knee flexed to at least 90 degrees to prevent tenodesis of the extensor mechanism.
- Make a straight anterior skin incision, beginning 8 cm above the patella, carrying it distally just medial and 2 cm distal to the tibial tubercle.

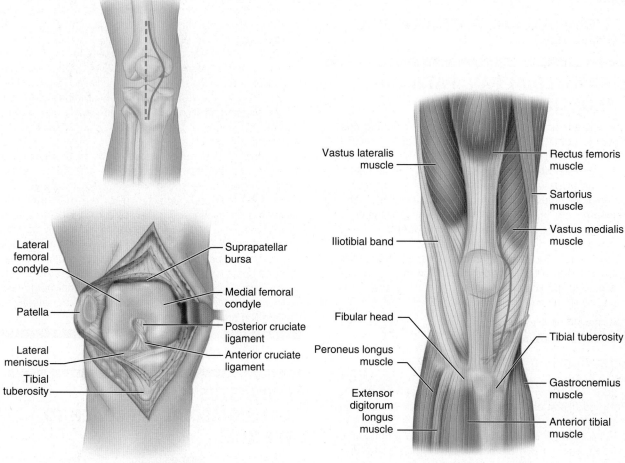

Lateral femoral condyle

Patella

Lateral meniscus

Tibial tuberosity

Suprapatellar bursa

Medial femoral condyle

Posterior cruciate ligament

Anterior cruciate ligament

Vastus lateralis muscle

Iliotibial band

Fibular head

Peroneus longus muscle

Extensor digitorum longus muscle

Rectus femoris muscle

Sartorius muscle

Vastus medialis muscle

Tibial tuberosity

Gastrocnemius muscle

Anterior tibial muscle

FIGURE 1.57 Anteromedial approach to knee joint. **SEE TECHNIQUE 1.42.**

- Incise the superficial fascia slightly medial to the patella (Fig. 1.58A) and bluntly dissect it off the vastus medialis muscle fascia down to the muscle insertion (Fig. 1.58B).
- Identify the inferior edge of the vastus medialis and bluntly dissect it off the periosteum and intermuscular septum for a distance of 10 cm proximal to the adductor tubercle.
- Identify the tendinous insertion of the muscle on the medial patellar retinaculum (Fig. 1.58C) and lift the vastus medialis muscle anteriorly and perform an L-shaped arthrotomy beginning medially through the vastus insertion on the medial patellar retinaculum and carrying it along the medial edge of the patella.
- Partially release the medial edge of the patellar tendon and evert the patella laterally with the knee extended (Fig. 1.58D).

ANTEROLATERAL APPROACH TO THE KNEE

Usually the anterolateral approach is not as satisfactory as the anteromedial one, primarily because it is more difficult to displace the patella medially than laterally. It also requires a longer incision, and often the patellar tendon must be

partially freed subperiosteally or subcortically. The iliotibial band can be released or lengthened, and the tight posterolateral corner can be released easily. The fibular head can be resected through the same incision to decompress the peroneal nerve if necessary.

TECHNIQUE 1.44   *Figure 1.59*

(KOCHER)

- Begin the incision 7.5 cm proximal to the patella at the insertion of the vastus lateralis muscle into the quadriceps tendon; continue it distally along the lateral border of this tendon, the patella, and the patellar tendon; and end it 2.5 cm distal to the tibial tuberosity.
- Deepen the dissection through the joint capsule.
- Retract the patella medially, with the tendons attached to it, and expose the articular surface of the joint.

Satish et al. found the modified Keblish approach useful in total knee arthroplasty in patients with fixed valgus knees. The approach relies on a quadriceps snip and coronal Z-plasty of lateral retinacular capsule complex. The lateral retinacular complex is separated into two layers, deep (capsule and synovium) and superficial. The lateral parapatellar arthrotomy is performed 3 to 7 cm lateral to the patella, and the

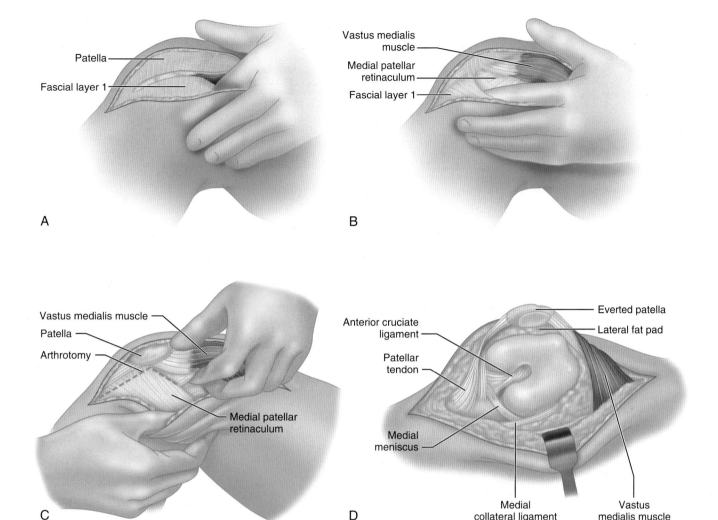

FIGURE 1.58   Subvastus anteromedial approach. **A,** Superficial fascia is incised medial to patella. **B,** Superficial fascia is bluntly elevated from perimuscular fascia of vastus medialis down to its insertion on medial patellar retinaculum. **C,** Tendinous insertion elevated by blunt dissection. *Dashed line* indicates arthrotomy. **D,** Patella is everted, and knee is flexed. **SEE TECHNIQUE 1.43.**

deep and superficial layers are separated with dissection carried medially toward the patella. The superficial layer is kept attached to the patella, and the deep layer remains attached to the iliotibial band. At closure, the layers are approximated in an expanded fashion (Fig. 1.60).

POSTEROLATERAL AND POSTEROMEDIAL APPROACHES TO THE KNEE

In some patients, a median septum separates the posterior aspect of the knee into two compartments. The posterior cruciate ligament is extrasynovial and projects anteriorly in the septum; it contributes to the partition between the two posterior compartments. The middle genicular artery courses anteriorly in the septum to nourish the tissues of the intercondylar notch of the femur (Fig. 1.61). The presence of this septum may assume great importance when exploring the posterior aspect of the knee for a loose body or when draining the joint in the rare instances in which pyogenic arthritis of the knee requires posterior drainage. In the latter, both posterior compartments must be opened for drainage, not one alone.

POSTEROLATERAL APPROACH TO THE KNEE

TECHNIQUE 1.45   *Figure 1.62*

(HENDERSON)
- With the knee flexed between 60 and 90 degrees, make a curved incision on the lateral side of the knee, just anterior to the biceps femoris tendon and the head of the fibula, and avoid the common peroneal nerve, which passes over the lateral aspect of the neck of the fibula.
- In the proximal part of the incision, trace the anterior surface of the lateral intermuscular septum to the linea aspera 5 cm proximal to the lateral femoral condyle.
- Expose the lateral femoral condyle and the origin of the fibular collateral ligament.
- The tendon of the popliteus muscle lies between the biceps tendon and the fibular collateral ligament; mobilize

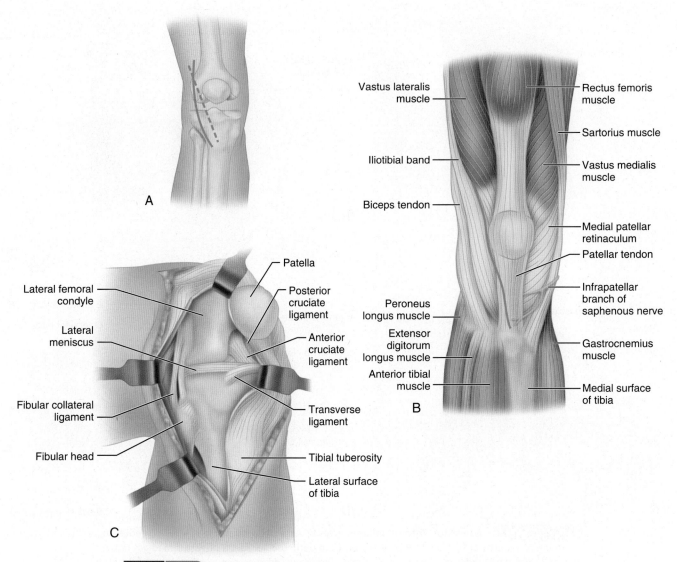

Lateral femoral condyle

Patella

Posterior cruciate ligament

Lateral meniscus

Anterior cruciate ligament

Fibular collateral ligament

Transverse ligament

Fibular head

Tibial tuberosity

Lateral surface of tibia

A

Vastus lateralis muscle

Rectus femoris muscle

Iliotibial band

Sartorius muscle

Biceps tendon

Vastus medialis muscle

Medial patellar retinaculum

Patellar tendon

Peroneus longus muscle

Infrapatellar branch of saphenous nerve

Extensor digitorum longus muscle

Gastrocnemius muscle

Anterior tibial muscle

Medial surface of tibia

B

C

FIGURE 1.59 **A-C,** Kocher anterolateral approach to knee joint. **SEE TECHNIQUE 1.44.**

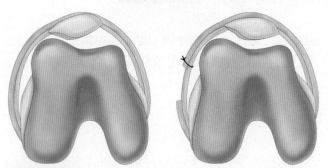

FIGURE 1.60 Coronal Z-plasty of lateral retinaculum capsule complex. (Redrawn from Satish BRJ, Ganesan JC, Chandran P, et al: Efficacy and mid-term results of lateral parapatellar approach without tibial tubercle osteotomy for primary total knee arthroplasty in fixed valgus knees, *J Arthroplasty* 28:1751, 2013.)

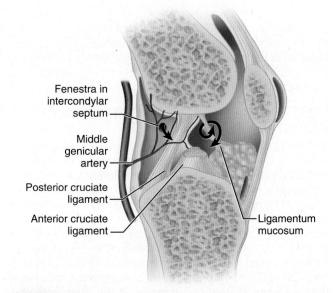

Fenestra in intercondylar septum

Middle genicular artery

Posterior cruciate ligament

Anterior cruciate ligament

Ligamentum mucosum

FIGURE 1.61 Median septum separating two posterior compartments of knee. Note fenestra at proximal pole. Synovial septum invests cruciate ligaments and contains branch of middle genicular artery.

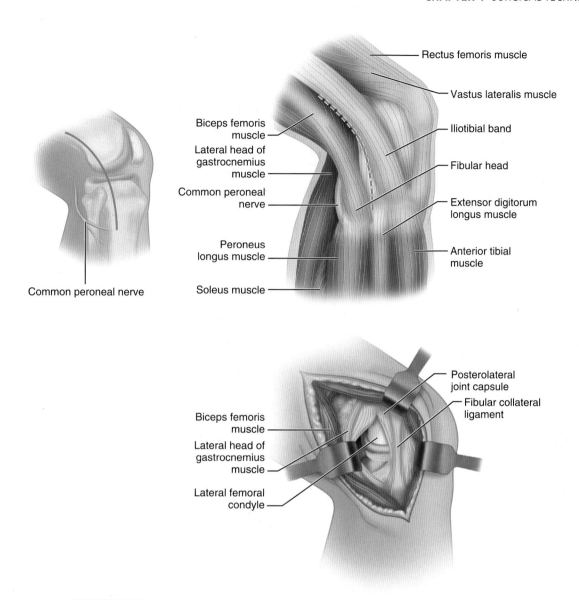

Rectus femoris muscle

Vastus lateralis muscle

Iliotibial band

Fibular head

Extensor digitorum longus muscle

Anterior tibial muscle

Biceps femoris muscle

Lateral head of gastrocnemius muscle

Common peroneal nerve

Peroneus longus muscle

Soleus muscle

Common peroneal nerve

Posterolateral joint capsule

Fibular collateral ligament

Biceps femoris muscle

Lateral head of gastrocnemius muscle

Lateral femoral condyle

FIGURE 1.62   Henderson posterolateral approach to knee joint. **SEE TECHNIQUE 1.45.**

and retract it posteriorly, and expose the posterolateral aspect of the joint capsule.

- Make a longitudinal incision through the capsule and synovium of the posterior compartment. To see the insertion of the muscle fibers of the short head of the biceps muscle onto the long head of the biceps, develop the interval between the lateral head of the quadriceps muscle and the long head of the biceps tendon. To isolate the common peroneal nerve, dissect directly posterior to the long head of the biceps. These intervals are useful in repair of the posterolateral corner of the knee.

Bowers and Huffman found the Hughston and Jacobson technique for exposure of the posterolateral corner by wafer osteotomy of the lateral collateral ligament insertion on the lateral femoral epicondyle with reflection of the ligament distally useful. Alternatively, if a fracture of the lateral femoral

condyle needs to be treated, an osteotomy of Gerdy's tubercle can be performed with reflection of the iliotibial band proximally as described by Liebergall et al.

POSTEROMEDIAL APPROACH TO THE KNEE

TECHNIQUE 1.46   *Figure 1.63*

(HENDERSON)

- With the knee flexed 90 degrees, make a curved incision, slightly convex anteriorly and approximately 7.5 cm long, distally from the adductor tubercle and along the course of the tibial collateral ligament, anterior to the relaxed tendons of the semimembranosus, semitendinosus, sartorius, and gracilis muscles.

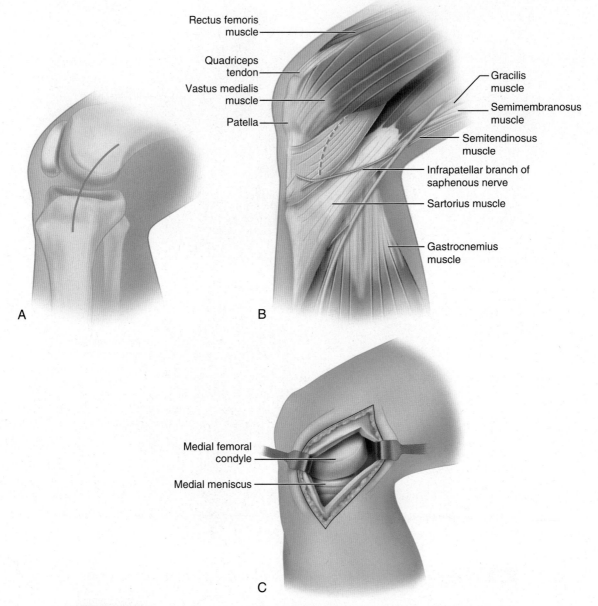

Rectus femoris muscle

Quadriceps tendon

Vastus medialis muscle

Patella

Gracilis muscle

Semimembranosus muscle

Semitendinosus muscle

Infrapatellar branch of saphenous nerve

Sartorius muscle

Gastrocnemius muscle

A

B

Medial femoral condyle

Medial meniscus

C

FIGURE **1.63**   A-C, Henderson posteromedial approach to knee joint. **SEE TECHNIQUE 1.46.**

- Expose and incise the oblique part of the tibial collateral ligament and incise the capsule longitudinally and enter the posteromedial compartment of the knee posterior to the tibial collateral ligament, retracting the hamstring tendons posteriorly.

MEDIAL APPROACHES TO THE KNEE AND SUPPORTING STRUCTURES

Usually the entire medial meniscus can be excised through a medial parapatellar incision about 5 cm long. If the posterior horn of the meniscus cannot be excised through this incision, a separate posteromedial Henderson approach can be made (Fig. 1.63). The anterior and posterior compartments may be entered, however, through an approach in which only one incision is made through the skin but two incisions are used

through the deeper structures; this type of approach is rarely indicated.

MEDIAL APPROACH TO THE KNEE

The Cave approach is a curved incision that allows exposure of the anterior and posterior compartments.

TECHNIQUE 1.47

(CAVE)
- With the knee flexed at a right angle, identify the medial femoral epicondyle and begin the incision 1 cm posterior to and on a level with it approximately 1 cm proximal to the joint line. Carry the incision distally and anteriorly to

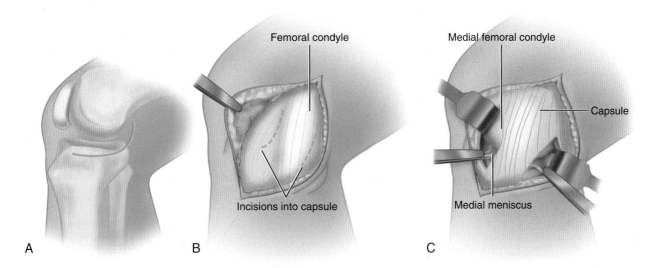

FIGURE 1.64 Exposure of anterior and posterior compartments of knee joint through one skin incision, according to Cave. **A,** Single skin incision. **B,** Two incisions through deep structures. **C,** Removal of meniscus. **SEE TECHNIQUE 1.47.**

a point 0.5 cm distal to the joint line and anterior to the border of the patellar tendon.

- After reflecting the subcutaneous tissues, expose the anterior compartment through an incision that begins anterior to the tibial collateral ligament, continues distally and anteriorly in a curve similar to that of the skin incision, and ends just distal to the joint line (Fig. 1.64).
- To expose the posterior compartment, make a second deep incision posterior to the tibial collateral ligament, from the level of the femoral epicondyle straight distally across the joint line.

MEDIAL APPROACH TO THE KNEE

TECHNIQUE 1.48

(HOPPENFELD AND DEBOER)
- With the patient supine and the affected knee flexed about 60 degrees, place the foot on the opposite shin and abduct and externally rotate the hip.
- Begin the incision 2 cm proximal to the adductor tubercle of the femur, curve it anteroinferiorly about 3 cm medial to the medial border of the patella, and end it 6 cm distal to the joint line on the anteromedial aspect of the tibia (Fig. 1.65A).
- Retract the skin flaps to expose the fascia of the knee and extend the exposure from the midline anteriorly to the posteromedial corner of the knee (Fig. 1.65B).
- Cut the infrapatellar branch of the saphenous nerve and bury its end in fat; preserve the saphenous nerve itself and the long saphenous vein.
- Longitudinally incise the fascia along the anterior border of the sartorius, starting at the tibial attachment of the

muscle and extending it to 5 cm proximal to the joint line.

- Flex the knee further and allow the sartorius to retract posteriorly, exposing the semitendinosus and gracilis muscles (Fig. 1.65C).
- Retract all three components of the pes anserinus posteriorly and expose the tibial attachment of the tibial collateral ligament, which inserts 6 to 7 cm distal to the joint line (Fig. 1.65D).
- To open the joint anteriorly, make a longitudinal medial parapatellar incision through the retinaculum and synovium (Fig. 1.65E).
- To expose the posterior third of the medial meniscus and the posteromedial corner of the knee, retract the three components of the pes anserinus posteriorly (Fig. 1.65F) and separate the medial head of the gastrocnemius muscle from the posterior capsule of the knee almost to the midline by blunt dissection (Fig. 1.65G).
- To open the joint posteriorly, make an incision through the capsule posterior to the tibial collateral ligament.

TRANSVERSE APPROACH TO THE MENISCUS

Using a transverse approach to the medial meniscus has the advantage that the scar has no contact with the femoral articular surface.

TECHNIQUE 1.49

- Make a transverse incision 5 cm long at the level of the articular surface of the tibia, extending laterally from the medial border of the patellar tendon to the anterior border of the tibial collateral ligament (Fig. 1.66).

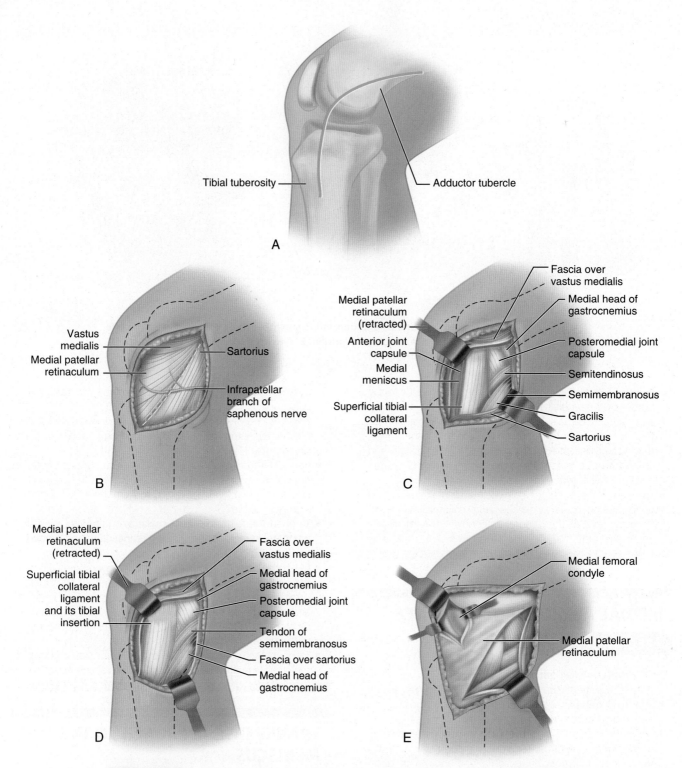

FIGURE 1.65 Medial approach to knee and supporting structures. **A,** Skin incision. **B,** Skin flaps have been retracted. **C,** Sartorius has been retracted posteriorly, exposing semitendinosus and gracilis. **D,** All three components of pes anserinus have been retracted posteriorly to expose tibial attachment of tibial collateral ligament. **E,** Medial parapatellar incision has been made through retinaculum and synovium.

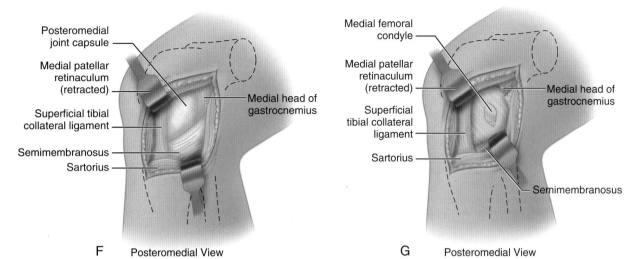

F Posteromedial View   G Posteromedial View

FIGURE 1.65, Cont'd **F,** Three components of pes anserinus have been retracted posteriorly to expose posteromedial corner. **G,** Medial head of gastrocnemius has been separated from posterior capsule of knee and has been retracted. Capsulotomy is made posterior to tibial collateral ligament. (Modified from Hoppenfeld S, deBoer P: *Surgical exposures in orthopaedics: the anatomic approach*, Philadelphia, 2003, Lippincott Williams & Wilkins.) **SEE TECHNIQUE 1.48.**

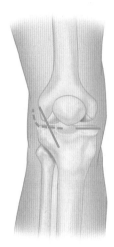

FIGURE 1.66 Transverse approaches to menisci. Medial meniscus is approached through transverse incisions in skin and capsule; lateral meniscus is approached through oblique incision in skin and hockey-stick incision in capsule. **SEE TECHNIQUE 1.49.**

- Incise the capsule along the same line and dissect the proximal edge of the divided capsule from the underlying synovium and retract it proximally.
- Open the synovium along the proximal border of the medial meniscus. Charnley advised making a preliminary 1.5-cm opening into the small synovial sac beneath the meniscus, introducing a blunt hook into it, and turning the hook so that its end rests on the proximal surface of the meniscus. By cutting down on the point of the hook, one can make the synovial incision at the most distal level.
- Divide the anterior attachment of the meniscus, retract the tibial collateral ligament, and complete the excision of the meniscus in the usual way.

- When closing the incision, place the first suture in the synovium at the medial side near the collateral ligament while the knee is still flexed; if the joint is extended before the first suture is inserted, the posterior part of the synovial incision retracts under the tibial collateral ligament. To complete the suture line, extend the joint.
- The transverse incision is not satisfactory for removing the lateral meniscus because it would require partial division of the iliotibial band. To avoid this, make an oblique incision 7.5 cm long centered over the joint line (Fig. 1.67).
- In the capsule, make a hockey-stick incision that runs transversely along the joint line and curves obliquely proximally along the anterior border of the iliotibial band for a short distance.
- Undermine and retract the capsule and incise the synovial membrane transversely as previously described.

LATERAL APPROACHES TO THE KNEE AND SUPPORTING STRUCTURES

Lateral approaches permit good exposure for complete excision of the lateral meniscus. They do not require division or release of the fibular collateral ligament.

LATERAL APPROACH TO THE KNEE

TECHNIQUE 1.50

(BRUSER)
- Place the patient supine and drape the limb to permit full flexion of the knee. Flex the knee fully so that the foot rests flat on the operating table.

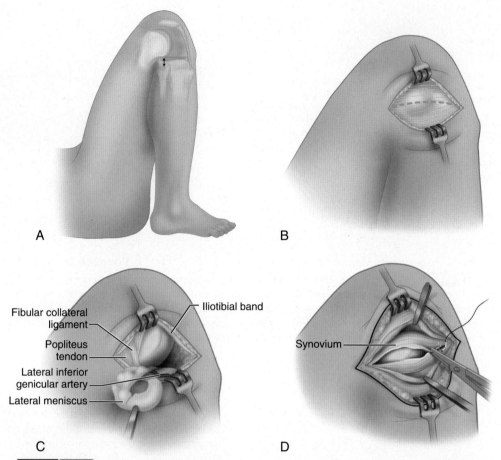

FIGURE 1.67 Bruser lateral approach to knee. **A,** Skin incision (see text). **B,** *Broken line* indicates proposed incision in iliotibial band, whose fibers, when knee is fully flexed, are parallel with skin incision. **C,** Knee has been extended slightly, and lateral meniscus is being excised. **D,** Lateral meniscus has been excised, and synovium is being closed. (Modified from Bruser DM: A direct lateral approach to the lateral compartment of the knee joint, *J Bone Joint Surg* 42B:348, 1960.) **SEE TECHNIQUES 1.49 AND 1.50.**

- Begin the incision anteriorly where the patellar tendon crosses the lateral joint line, continue it posteriorly along the joint line, and end it at an imaginary line extending from the proximal end of the fibula to the lateral femoral condyle (Fig. 1.67A).
- Incise the subcutaneous tissue and expose the iliotibial band, whose fibers are parallel with the skin incision when the knee is fully flexed (Fig. 1.67B). Split the band in line with its fibers. Posteriorly, take care to avoid injuring the relaxed fibular collateral ligament; it is protected by areolar tissue, which separates it from the iliotibial band.
- Retract the margins of the iliotibial band; this is possible to achieve without much force because the band is relaxed when the knee and hip are flexed.
- Locate the lateral inferior genicular artery, which lies outside the synovium between the collateral ligament and the posterolateral aspect of the meniscus.
- Incise the synovium. The lateral meniscus lies in the depth of the incision and can be excised completely (Fig. 1.67C).
- With the knee flexed 90 degrees, close the synovium (Fig. 1.67D); and with the knee extended, close the deep fascia.

LATERAL APPROACH TO THE KNEE

Brown et al. have developed an approach for lateral meniscectomy in which the knee is flexed to allow important structures to fall posteriorly as in the Bruser approach. In addition, a varus strain is created to open the lateral joint space.

TECHNIQUE 1.51

(BROWN ET AL.)

- Place the patient supine with the extremity straight and with a small sandbag under the ipsilateral hip.
- Make a vertical, oblique, or transverse skin incision on the anterolateral aspect of the knee.
- Identify the anterior border of the iliotibial band and make an incision in the fascia 0.5 to 1 cm anterior to the band in line with its fibers.
- Incise the synovium in line with this incision and inspect the joint.
- By sharp dissection, free the anterior horn of the meniscus.
- Flex the knee, cross the foot over the opposite knee, and push firmly toward the opposite hip, applying a varus

force to the knee. Ensure the thigh on the involved side is in line with the sagittal plane of the trunk; the hip is flexed about 45 degrees and externally rotated about 40 degrees. Push, as described, until the joint space opens up 3 to 5 mm. If necessary, internally rotate the tibia to bring the lateral tibial plateau into better view; however, this tends to close the joint space.

■ With proper retractors, expose the entire meniscus, which can be excised completely by sharp dissection.

LATERAL APPROACH TO THE KNEE

TECHNIQUE 1.52

(HOPPENFELD AND DEBOER)

■ Place the patient supine with a sandbag beneath the ipsilateral buttock and flex the knee 90 degrees.
■ Begin the incision 3 cm lateral to the middle of the patella, extend it distally over Gerdy's tubercle on the tibia, and

end it 4 to 5 cm distal to the joint line. Complete the incision proximally by curving it along the line of the femur (Fig. 1.68A).
■ Widely mobilize the skin flaps anteriorly and posteriorly.
■ Incise the fascia between the iliotibial band and biceps femoris, carefully avoiding the common peroneal nerve on the posterior aspect of the biceps tendon (Fig. 1.68B).
■ Retract the iliotibial band anteriorly and the biceps femoris and common peroneal nerve posteriorly to expose the fibular collateral ligament and the posterolateral corner of the knee capsule (Fig. 1.68C).
■ To expose the lateral meniscus, make a separate lateral parapatellar incision through the fascia and joint capsule (Fig. 1.68B).
■ To avoid cutting the meniscus, begin the arthrotomy 2 cm proximal to the joint line.
■ To expose the posterior horn of the lateral meniscus, locate the origin of the lateral head of the gastrocnemius muscle on the posterior surface of the lateral femoral condyle.
■ Dissect between it and the posterolateral corner of the joint capsule; ligate or cauterize the lateral superior genicular arterial branches located in this area.

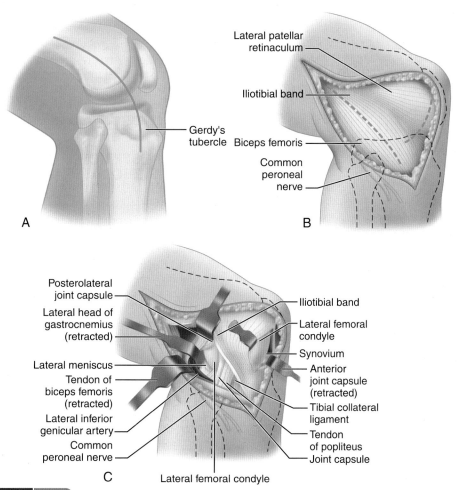

FIGURE 1.68 Lateral approach to knee and supporting structures. **A,** Skin incision. **B,** Incision between biceps femoris and iliotibial band. **C,** Deep dissection (see text). (Modified from Hoppenfeld S, deBoer P: *Surgical exposures in orthopaedics: the anatomic approach*, Philadelphia, Lippincott Williams & Wilkins, 2003.) **SEE TECHNIQUE 1.52.**

- Make a longitudinal incision in the capsule, beginning well proximal to the joint line to avoid damaging the meniscus or the popliteus tendon. Inspect the posterior half of the lateral compartment posterior to the fibular collateral ligament (Fig. 1.68C).

EXTENSILE APPROACH TO THE KNEE

Fernandez described an extensile anterior approach to the knee based on an anterolateral approach that allows easy access to the medial and lateral compartments in the following ways: (1) by an extensive osteotomy of the tibial tuberosity that allows proximal reflection of the patella, patellar tendon, and retropatellar fat pad and (2) by transecting the anterior horn and anterior portion of the coronary ligament of the medial meniscus or the lateral meniscus or both as necessary to achieve adequate exposure. This approach may be used for tumor resection, ligament reconstruction, fracture reduction and fixation, and adult reconstructive procedures. Part or all of this approach may be used as necessary to achieve the required exposure. Rigid screw fixation of the tibial tuberosity engaging the posterior cortex of the tibia allows early postoperative knee motion.

Perry et al. first reported transection of the anterior horn of the lateral meniscus to aid exposure of lateral tibial plateau fractures. Alternatively, the articular surface of either tibial plateau can be approached with a submeniscal exposure by releasing the peripheral attachment of the meniscus at the coronary ligament and by elevating the meniscus, as described by Gossling and Peterson.

TECHNIQUE 1.53

(FERNANDEZ)
- Place the patient supine and drape the limb to allow at least 60 degrees of knee flexion.
- Begin a lateral parapatellar incision 10 cm proximal to the lateral joint line; continue it distally along the lateral border of the patella, patellar tendon, and tibial tuberosity; and end it 15 cm distal to the lateral joint line (Fig. 1.69A).
- Develop skin flaps deep in the subcutaneous tissue, extending medially to the anterior edge of the tibial collateral ligament and laterally, exposing the iliotibial band and the proximal origins of the anterior tibial and peroneal muscles (Fig. 1.69B).
- To expose the lateral tibial metaphysis, detach the anterior tibial muscle and retract it distally, and elevate the iliotibial band by dividing it transversely at the joint line or by performing a flat osteotomy of Gerdy's tubercle (Fig. 1.69C). If exposure of the posteromedial portion of the tibial metaphysis is necessary, divide the tibial insertion of the pes anserinus or elevate it as an osteoperiosteal flap.
- Fernandez advocates an extended osteotomy into the tibial crest in the presence of a bicondylar tibial plateau fracture to ensure that the osteotomy fragment is securely fixed into the tibial diaphysis below the level of the fracture. A less extensive osteotomy may be used as appropriate.

- Perform an extended trapezoidal osteotomy of the tibial tuberosity as follows:
  1. Mark with an osteotome a site 5 cm in length, 2 cm in width proximally, and 1.5 cm in width distally.
  2. Drill three holes for later reattachment of the tibial tuberosity.
  3. Complete the osteotomy with a flat osteotome.
- Elevate the tibial tuberosity and patellar tendon and incise the joint capsule transversely, medially, and laterally at the joint line.
- Carry each limb of the capsular incision proximally to the level of the anterior border of the vastus medialis and vastus lateralis (Fig. 1.69C,D).
- If further exposure of the articular surface of the tibial plateaus is needed, detach one or both menisci by transection of the anterior horn, cutting the transverse ligament and dividing the anterior portion of the coronary ligament. The meniscus may be elevated and held with a stay suture (Fig. 1.69E).
- At wound closure, repair the anterior meniscus, coronary ligament, and transverse ligament with 2-0 nonabsorbable sutures. Use square stitches to repair the meniscus and two or three U-shaped stitches to stabilize the periphery of the meniscus.
- Tie the stitches over the joint capsule after closure of the medial and lateral arthrotomies (Fig. 1.69F).
- Reattach the anterior tibial muscle and pes anserinus to bone with interrupted sutures.
- Reattach Gerdy's tubercle with a lag screw.
- Rigidly fix the tibial tuberosity osteotomy with lag screws obtaining good purchase in the posterior cortex of the tibia.
- Close the arthrotomy with interrupted sutures (Fig. 1.69G).

DIRECT POSTERIOR, POSTEROMEDIAL, AND POSTEROLATERAL APPROACHES TO THE KNEE

The posterior midline approach involves structures that, if damaged, can produce a permanent, serious disability. Thorough knowledge of the anatomy of the popliteal space is essential. Figure 1.70 shows the relationship of the flexion crease to the joint line, and Figure 1.71 shows the collateral circulation around the knee posteriorly. The approach provides access to the posterior capsule of the knee joint, the posterior part of the menisci, the posterior compartments of the knee, the posterior aspect of the femoral and tibial condyles, and the origin of the posterior cruciate ligament. All posterior approaches are done with the patient supine.

DIRECT POSTERIOR APPROACH TO THE KNEE

TECHNIQUE 1.54

(BRACKETT AND OSGOOD; PUTTI; ABBOTT AND CARPENTER)
- Make a curvilinear incision 10 to 15 cm long over the popliteal space (Fig. 1.72A), with the proximal limb following

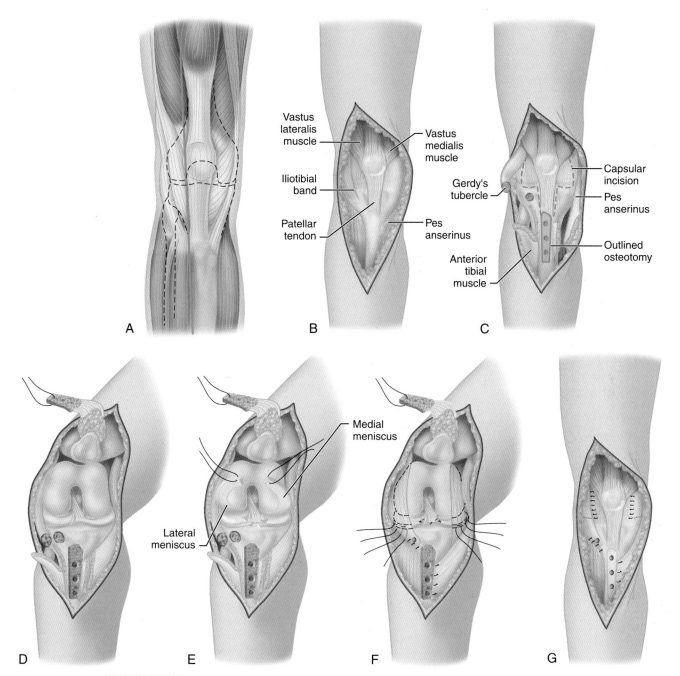

FIGURE 1.69 Fernandez extensile anterior approach. **A,** Anterolateral incision. **B,** Extensor mechanism exposed. **C,** Iliotibial band is reflected with Gerdy's tubercle. Anterior compartment and pes anserinus are detached and elevated as necessary. Osteotomy of tibial tuberosity is outlined, and screw holes are predrilled (see text). **D,** Patella, patellar tendon, and tibial tuberosity are elevated. **E,** Medial and lateral menisci are detached anteriorly and peripherally and are elevated. **F,** Meniscal repair is performed with 2-0 nonabsorbable sutures (see text). Gerdy's tubercle is reattached with lag screw. Anterior tibial and pes anserinus are reattached. **G,** Tibial tuberosity is secured with lag screws engaging posterior cortex of tibia. Capsule is closed with interrupted sutures. Sutures in periphery of menisci are now tied (see text). (Modified from Fernandez DL: Anterior approach to the knee with osteotomy of the tibial tubercle for bicondylar tibial fractures, *J Bone Joint Surg* 70A:208, 1988.) **SEE TECHNIQUE 1.53.**

the tendon of the semitendinosus muscle distally to the level of the joint. Curve it laterally across the posterior aspect of the joint for about 5 cm and distally over the lateral head of the gastrocnemius muscle.

■ Reflect the skin and subcutaneous tissues to expose the popliteal fascia.

■ Identify the posterior cutaneous nerve of the calf (the medial sural cutaneous nerve) lying beneath the fascia and between the two heads of the gastrocnemius muscle because it is the clue to the dissection. Lateral to it, the short saphenous vein perforates the popliteal fascia to join the popliteal vein at the middle of the fossa. Trace the posterior cutaneous nerve of the calf (the medial sural cutaneous nerve) proximally to its origin from the tibial

nerve because the contents of the fossa can be dissected accurately and safely once this nerve is located. Trace the tibial nerve distally and expose its branches to the heads of the gastrocnemius, the plantaris, and the soleus muscles; these branches are accompanied by arteries and veins. Follow the tibial nerve proximally to the apex of the fossa where it joins the common peroneal nerve (Fig. 1.72B). Dissect the common peroneal nerve distally along the medial border of the biceps muscle and tendon, and protect the lateral cutaneous nerve of the calf and the anastomotic peroneal nerve.

■ Expose the popliteal artery and vein, which lie directly anterior and medial to the tibial nerve. Gently retract the artery and vein and locate and trace the superolateral and superomedial genicular vessels passing beneath the hamstring muscles on either side just proximal to the heads of origin of the gastrocnemius (Fig. 1.71).

■ Open the posterior compartments of the joint with the knee extended and explore them with the knee slightly flexed. The medial head of the gastrocnemius arises at a more proximal level from the femoral condyle than does the lateral head, and the groove it forms with the semimembranosus forms a safe and comparatively avascular approach to the medial compartment (Fig. 1.72C). Turn the tendinous origin of the medial head of the gastrocnemius laterally to serve as a retractor for the popliteal vessels and nerves (Fig. 1.72D).

■ Greater access can be achieved by ligating one or more genicular vessels. If the posterolateral aspect of the joint is to be exposed, elevate the lateral head of the gastrocnemius muscle from the femur and approach the lateral compartment between the tendon of the biceps femoris and the lateral head of the gastrocnemius muscle.

■ When closing the wound, place interrupted sutures in the capsule, the deep fascia, and the skin. The popliteal fascia is best closed by placing all sutures before drawing them tight. Tie the sutures one by one.

Nicandri et al. reported that the medial head of the gastrocnemius can be left intact by identifying and ligating the anterior branches of the middle geniculate artery and

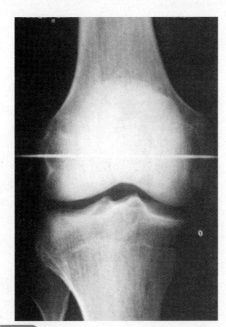

FIGURE 1.70 Knee with Kirschner wire taped along flexion crease. Note relation of wire to joint line. Flexion crease sags distally in elderly or obese individuals.

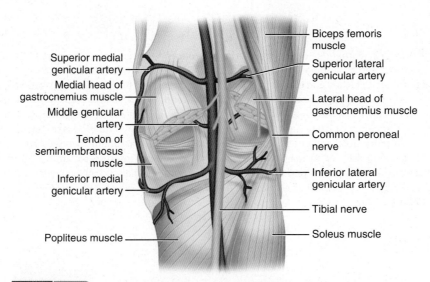

Biceps femoris muscle

Superior medial genicular artery

Medial head of gastrocnemius muscle

Middle genicular artery

Tendon of semimembranosus muscle

Inferior medial genicular artery

Popliteus muscle

Superior lateral genicular artery

Lateral head of gastrocnemius muscle

Common peroneal nerve

Inferior lateral genicular artery

Tibial nerve

Soleus muscle

FIGURE 1.71 Collateral circulation around knee posteriorly. **SEE TECHNIQUE 1.54.**

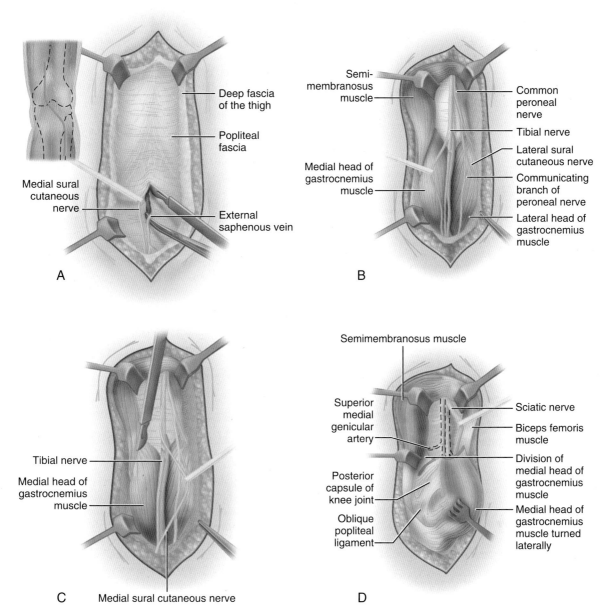

FIGURE 1.72 Posterior approach to knee joint. **A,** Posterior curvilinear incision. Posterior cutaneous nerve of calf exposed and retracted. **B,** Sciatic nerve and its division defined. **C,** Medial head of gastrocnemius muscle exposed. **D,** Tendon of origin of medial head of gastrocnemius muscle divided, exposing capsule of knee joint. If further exposure is necessary, lateral head of gastrocnemius is defined, incised, and retracted in similar fashion. **SEE TECHNIQUE 1.54.**

dissecting free the tibial motor branches to the medial head of the gastrocnemius. This allows enough mobilization of the medial head of the gastrocnemius to expose the posterior cruciate ligament insertion on the posterior tibia.

DIRECT POSTEROMEDIAL APPROACH TO THE KNEE FOR TIBIAL PLATEAU FRACTURE

Galla and Lobenhoffer described a direct posteromedial approach for managing medial tibial plateau fractures.

This approach does not involve dissection of the popliteal neurovascular structures and uses the interval between the semimembranosus complex and the medial head of the gastrocnemius muscle.

TECHNIQUE 1.55

(GALLA AND LOBENHOFFER AS DESCRIBED BY FAKLER ET AL.)
- Make a straight 6- to 8-cm-long longitudinal skin incision along the medial border of the medial head of the gastrocnemius muscle, beginning at the level of the joint line.
- Incise the subcutaneous tissue and popliteal fascia sharply.

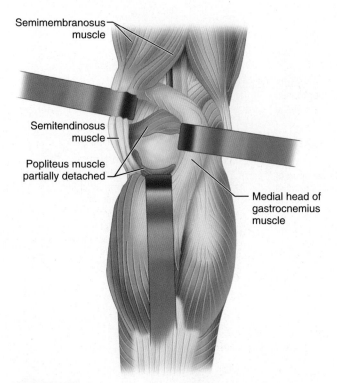

Semimembranosus muscle

Semitendinosus muscle

Popliteus muscle partially detached

Medial head of gastrocnemius muscle

FIGURE 1.73 Galla and Lobenhoffer posteromedial approach. (Modified from Fakler JKM, Ryzewicz M, Hartshorn C, et al: Optimizing the management of Moore type I posteromedial split fracture-dislocations of the tibial head: description of the Lobenhoffer approach, *J Orthop Trauma* 21:330, 2007.) **SEE TECHNIQUE 1.55.**

- Free up the medial head of the gastrocnemius muscle without detaching it and retract it laterally.
- Bluntly dissect the semimembranosus complex and retract it medially (Fig. 1.73).
- Identify the upper edge of the popliteus muscle and detach it subperiosteally, exposing the posteromedial tibial plateau.
- If more exposure is needed, incise the tibial insertion of the semimembranosus muscle in a subperiosteal fashion.

DIRECT POSTEROLATERAL APPROACH TO THE KNEE

Minkoff et al. described a limited posterolateral approach to the proximal lateral tibia and knee. It uses the interval between the popliteus and soleus muscles and exposes the uppermost lateral portion of the posterior tibial metaphysis and the proximal tibiofibular joint. Although this approach was developed to excise an osteoid osteoma from the lateral tibial plateau, it can be used for other conditions affecting the posterior aspect of the knee.

TECHNIQUE 1.56

(MINKOFF, JAFFE, AND MENENDEZ)
- Begin the skin incision 1 to 2 cm below the popliteal crease slightly medial to the midline of the knee, carrying

it transversely and curving it distally just medial and parallel to the head of the fibula, ending 5 to 6 cm distal to it.
- Reflect the skin and subcutaneous flap inferomedially.
- Isolate the lateral cutaneous nerve of the calf, retract it laterally, and preserve it.
- Identify the short saphenous vein superficial to the fascia and divide and ligate it.
- Open the fascia carefully in line with the incision. The sural nerve lies deep to the fascia just superficial to the heads of the gastrocnemius muscle and must be protected (Fig. 1.74A).
- Identify the common peroneal nerve and retract it laterally.
- Develop the interval between the lateral head of the gastrocnemius and the soleus muscles and retract the lateral head of the gastrocnemius medially.
- Retract the popliteal artery and vein and the tibial nerve along with the lateral head of the gastrocnemius (Fig. 1.74B). Dissect free the fibular origin of the soleus muscle and retract it distally.
- Retract the underlying popliteus muscle medially to expose the posterior aspect of the lateral tibial plateau and proximal tibiofibular joint (Fig. 1.74C).

FEMUR

ANTEROLATERAL APPROACH TO THE FEMUR

The anterolateral approach exposes the middle third of the femur, but postoperative adhesions between the individual muscles of the quadriceps group and between the vastus intermedius and the femur may limit knee flexion. The quadriceps mechanism must be handled gently. Infections of the middle third of the shaft are best approached posterolaterally. When the shaft must be approached from the medial side, this anterolateral approach, rather than an anteromedial one, is indicated.

TECHNIQUE 1.57

(THOMPSON)
- Incise the skin over the middle third of the femur in a line between the anterior superior iliac spine and the lateral margin of the patella (Fig. 1.75A).
- Incise the superficial and deep fasciae and separate the rectus femoris and vastus lateralis muscles along their intermuscular septum. The vastus intermedius muscle is brought into view.
- Divide the vastus intermedius muscle in the line of its fibers down to the femur.
- Expose the femur by subperiosteal reflection of the incised vastus intermedius muscle (Fig. 1.75B).
  Henry exposed the entire femoral shaft by extending this incision proximally and distally. The approach is not recommended for operations on the proximal third of the femur because exposing the bone here is difficult without injuring the lateral femoral circumflex artery and the nerve to the vastus lateralis muscle. Distally, the incision may be

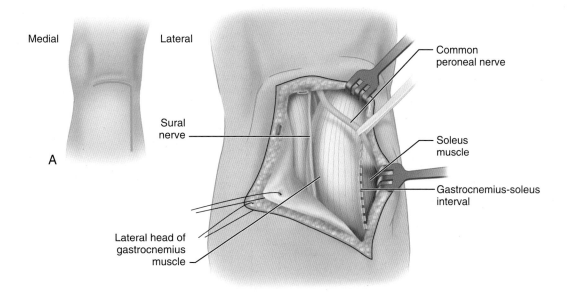

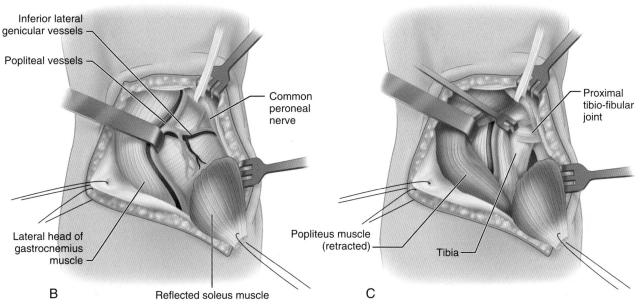

FIGURE 1.74 Minkoff, Jaffe, and Menendez posterolateral approach. **A,** Superficial dissection. **B,** Gastrocnemius and popliteal vessels are retracted medially, and fibular origin of soleus is reflected distally. **C,** Popliteus is retracted medially, exposing the posterior aspect of tibial plateau and proximal tibiofibular joint. (Modified from Minkoff J, Jaffe L, Menendez L: Limited posterolateral surgical approach to the knee for excision of osteoid osteoma, *Clin Orthop Relat Res* 223:237, 1987.) **SEE TECHNIQUE 1.56.**

extended to within 12 to 15 cm of the knee joint; at this point, however, the insertion of the vastus lateralis muscle into the quadriceps tendon is encountered, as is the more distal suprapatellar bursa.

LATERAL APPROACH TO THE FEMORAL SHAFT

Anatomically, the entire femoral shaft may be exposed by the lateral approach, but only its less extensive forms are

recommended. The posterolateral approach is preferred whenever possible to avoid splitting the vastus lateralis.

TECHNIQUE 1.58

- Make an incision of the desired length over the lateral aspect of the thigh along a line from the greater trochanter to the lateral femoral condyle (Fig. 1.76A).
- Incise the superficial and deep fasciae.
- Divide the vastus lateralis and vastus intermedius muscles in the direction of their fibers and open and reflect the periosteum for the proper distance.

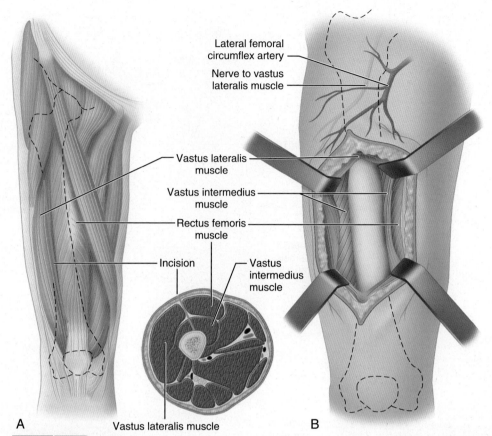

Lateral femoral
circumflex artery

Nerve to vastus
lateralis muscle

Vastus lateralis
muscle

Vastus intermedius
muscle

Rectus femoris
muscle

Incision

Vastus
intermedius
muscle

A

B

Vastus lateralis muscle

FIGURE 1.75 Anterolateral approach to femur. **A,** Skin incision. **B,** Femur exposed by separation of rectus femoris and vastus lateralis muscles and division of vastus intermedius muscle. **SEE TECHNIQUE 1.57.**

- A branch of the lateral femoral circumflex artery is encountered when exposing the proximal fourth of the femur and the lateral superior genicular artery in the distal fourth; these may be clamped, divided, and ligated without harm.

POSTEROLATERAL APPROACH TO THE FEMORAL SHAFT

TECHNIQUE 1.59

- Turn the patient slightly to elevate the affected side.
- Make the incision from the base of the greater trochanter distally to the lateral condyle (Fig. 1.76B).
- Incise the superficial fascia and fascia lata along the anterior border of the iliotibial band.
- Expose the posterior part of the vastus lateralis muscle and retract it anteriorly (in muscular individuals this retraction may be difficult); continue the dissection down to bone along the anterior surface of the lateral intermuscular septum, which is attached to the linea aspera.
- Retract the deep structures and split the periosteum in the line of the incision.
- With a periosteal elevator, free the attachment of the vastus intermedius muscle as far as necessary.

- In the middle third of the thigh, the second perforating branch of the profunda femoris artery and vein run transversely from the biceps femoris to the vastus lateralis. Ligate and divide these vessels.
- To avoid damaging the sciatic nerve and the profunda femoris artery and vein, do not separate the long and short heads of the biceps femoris muscle.

POSTERIOR APPROACH TO THE FEMUR

TECHNIQUE 1.60

(BOSWORTH)
- With the patient prone, incise the skin and deep fascia longitudinally in the middle of the posterior aspect of the thigh, from just distal to the gluteal fold to the proximal margin of the popliteal space.
- Use the long head of the biceps as a guide. By blunt dissection with the index finger, palpate the posterior surface of the femur at the middle of the thigh. To expose the middle three fifths of the linea aspera, use the fingers to retract the attachment of the vastus medialis and lateralis muscles.

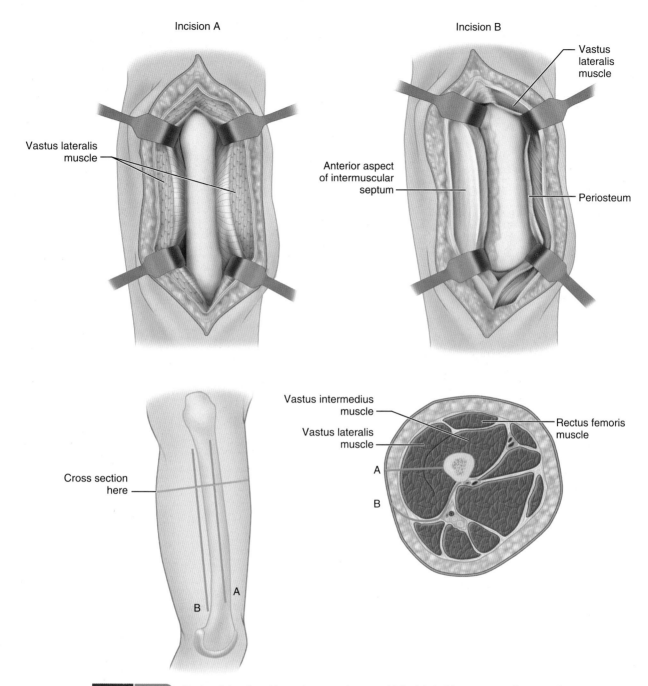

Incision A

Incision B

Vastus lateralis
muscle

Vastus lateralis
muscle

Anterior aspect
of intermuscular
septum

Periosteum

Vastus intermedius
muscle

Vastus lateralis
muscle

Rectus femoris
muscle

A

B

Cross section
here

A

B

FIGURE 1.76   Posterolateral and lateral approaches to middle third of femur. Lateral approach
(A). Vastus lateralis and vastus intermedius have been incised in line with their fibers. Cross-section
shows these approaches. Posterolateral approach *(B)* along lateral intermuscular septum. **SEE
TECHNIQUES 1.58 AND 1.59.**

- To expose the proximal part of the middle three fifths of
  the femur, continue the blunt dissection along the lateral
  border of the long head of the biceps, developing the
  fascial plane between the long head of the biceps and the
  vastus lateralis muscle, and reflect the long head of the
  biceps *medially* (Fig. 1.77A).
- To expose the distal part of the middle three fifths of
  the femur, carry the dissection along the medial surface
  of the long head of the biceps, developing the fascial
  plane between the long head of the biceps and the

semitendinosus, and retract the long head of the biceps
and the sciatic nerve *laterally* (Fig. 1.77B).
- To expose the entire middle three fifths of the femur,
  carry the blunt dissection to the linea aspera lateral to
  the long head of the biceps, divide the latter muscle in
  the distal part of the wound, and displace it *medially,*
  together with the sciatic nerve (Fig. 1.77C).
- Part of the nerve supply to the short head of the biceps
  crosses the exposure near its center; this branch of the
  sciatic nerve may be saved or divided, depending on the

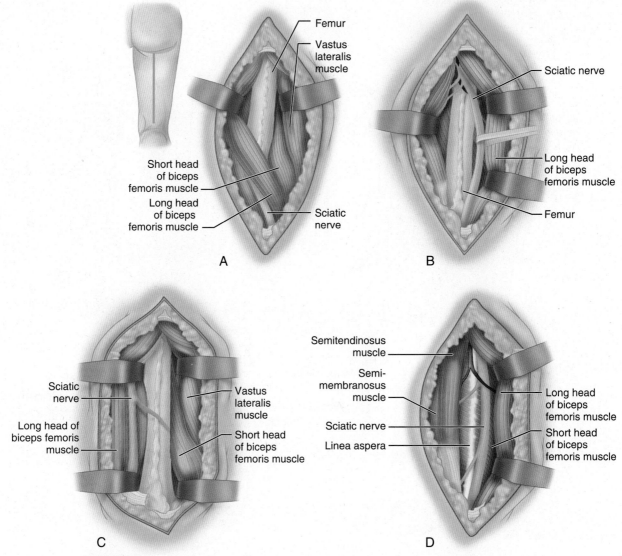

FIGURE 1.77 Bosworth posterior approach to femur. **A,** To expose proximal part of middle three fifths of femur, long head of biceps femoris has been retracted medially. *Inset,* Skin incision. **B,** To expose distal part of middle three fifths of femur, long head of biceps femoris and sciatic nerve have been retracted laterally. **C,** To expose entire middle three fifths of femur, long head of biceps femoris has been divided in distal part of wound, and this muscle and sciatic nerve have been retracted medially. **D,** Sciatic nerve would be subject to injury if entire middle three fifths of femur were exposed by retracting biceps femoris laterally. **SEE TECHNIQUE 1.60.**

requirements of the incision because it does not make up the entire nerve supply of this part of the biceps.

■ After exposing the linea aspera, free the muscle attachments by sharp dissection and expose the femur by subperiosteal dissection.

■ Bosworth points out that the entire middle three fifths of the femur should *never* be exposed by retracting the long head of the biceps and sciatic nerve *laterally* because this unnecessarily endangers the sciatic nerve (Fig. 1.77D).

■ When the distal end of the long head of the biceps is to be divided, place sutures in the distal segment of the muscle before the division is carried out; this makes suturing the muscle easier when the wound is being closed.

■ After suturing the biceps, close the wound by suturing only the skin and subcutaneous tissue because the other structures fall into position.

■ When developing this approach, the surgeon must keep in mind the possibility of damaging the sciatic nerve. Rough handling and prolonged or strenuous retraction of the nerve may cause distressing symptoms after surgery or possibly a permanent disability in the leg.

MEDIAL APPROACH TO THE POSTERIOR SURFACE OF THE FEMUR IN THE POPLITEAL SPACE

When possible, the medial approach to the posterior surface of the femur in the popliteal space should be used in preference to an anteromedial approach because in the latter the vastus medialis must be separated from the rectus femoris and the vastus intermedius must be split.

TECHNIQUE 1.61

(HENRY)
- With the knee slightly flexed, begin the incision 15 cm proximal to the adductor tubercle and continue it distally along the adductor tendon, following the angle of the knee to 5 cm distal to the tubercle (Fig. 1.78A).
- In the distal part of the incision, carry the dissection posteriorly to the anterior edge of the sartorius muscle just proximal to the level of the adductor tubercle.
- Free the deep fascia proximally over this muscle, taking care to avoid puncturing the synovial membrane, which is beneath the muscle when the joint is flexed. After this procedure, the sartorius falls posteriorly, exposing the tendon of the adductor magnus muscle. Protect the

saphenous nerve, which follows the sartorius on its deep surface; the great saphenous vein is superficial and is not in danger if the incision is made properly.
- Divide the thin fascia posterior to the adductor tendon by blunt dissection to the posterior surface of the femur at the popliteal space.
- Retract the large vessels and nerves posteriorly; branches from the muscles to the bone may be isolated, clamped, and divided.
- Retract the adductor magnus tendon and a part of the vastus medialis muscle anteriorly and expose the bone. The tibial and common peroneal nerves are not encountered because they lie lateral and posterior to the line of incision.

LATERAL APPROACH TO THE POSTERIOR SURFACE OF THE FEMUR IN THE POPLITEAL SPACE

TECHNIQUE 1.62

(HENRY)
- With the knee slightly flexed, incise the skin and superficial fascia for 15 cm along the posterior edge of the ilio-

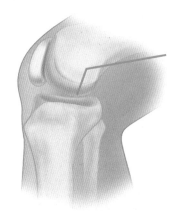

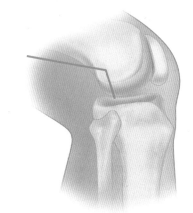

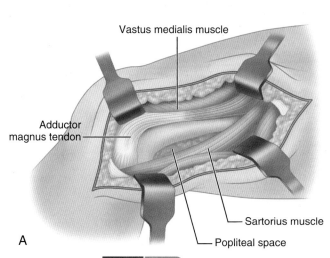

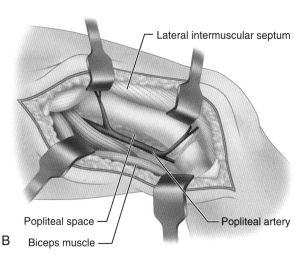

A

Vastus medialis muscle

Adductor magnus tendon

Sartorius muscle

Popliteal space

B

Lateral intermuscular septum

Popliteal space

Biceps muscle

Popliteal artery

FIGURE 1.78 Henry medial and lateral approaches to posterior surface of femur in popliteal space. **A,** Medial approach. **B,** Lateral approach. **SEE TECHNIQUES 1.61 AND 1.62.**

tibial band and follow the angle of the knee to the head of the fibula (Fig. 1.78B).

- Divide the deep fascia immediately posterior to the iliotibial band.
- Just proximal to the condyle, separate the attachment of the short head of the biceps from the posterior surface of the lateral intermuscular septum; reach the popliteal space by blunt dissection between these structures.
- Ligate and divide the branches of the perforating vessels and retract the popliteal vessels posteriorly in the posterior wall of the wound. The tibial nerve lies posterior to the popliteal vessels, and the common peroneal nerve follows the medial edge of the biceps.
- Expose the surface of the femur by incising and elevating the periosteum.

LATERAL APPROACH TO THE PROXIMAL SHAFT AND THE TROCHANTERIC REGION

The lateral approach is excellent for reduction and internal fixation of trochanteric fractures or for subtrochanteric osteotomies under direct vision.

TECHNIQUE 1.63

- Begin the incision about 5 cm proximal and anterior to the greater trochanter, curving it distally and posteriorly over the posterolateral aspect of the trochanter and distally along the lateral surface of the thigh, parallel with the femur, for 10 cm or more, depending on the desired exposure (Fig. 1.79A).

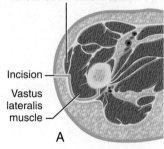

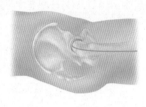

Tensor fascia latae muscle

Incision

Vastus lateralis muscle

A

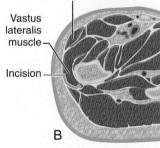

Tensor fascia latae muscle

Vastus lateralis muscle

Incision

B

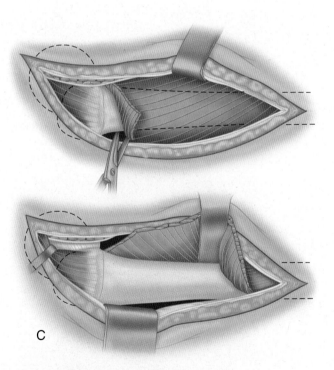

C

FIGURE 1.79 Lateral approach to proximal shaft and trochanteric region of femur. **A,** Cross-section shows level of approach at lesser trochanter. Fascia lata has been incised in line with skin incision. Vastus lateralis has been incised transversely just distal to greater trochanter and is being incised longitudinally 0.5 cm from linea aspera. *Inset,* Skin incision. **B,** Cross-section shows approach at level of distal end of skin incision. **C,** Approach has been completed by dissecting vastus lateralis subperiosteally from femur. Hip joint may be exposed by continuing approach proximally as in Watson-Jones approach. **SEE TECHNIQUE 1.63.**

- Deepen the dissection in the line of the incision down to the fascia lata.
- In the distal part of the wound, incise the fascia lata with a scalpel and split it proximally with scissors. In the proximal part of the wound, divide the fascia just posterior to the tensor fasciae latae muscle to avoid splitting this muscle.
- By retraction, bring into view the vastus lateralis muscle and its origin from the inferior border of the greater trochanter. Divide the origin of the muscle transversely along this border down to the posterolateral surface of the femur.
- Divide the vastus lateralis and its fascia longitudinally with scissors, beginning on its posterolateral surface, 0.5 cm from its attachment to the linea aspera.
- Alternatively, first split the muscle fascia alone laterally instead of posterolaterally, dissect the muscle from its deep surface posteriorly, and divide the muscle near the linea aspera (closing the fascia lata then is easier). The muscle is divided where it is thin rather than thick, as is necessary in a direct lateral muscle-splitting approach (Fig. 1.79A,B). Section no more than 0.5 cm of the muscle at one time. Keep the body of the vastus retracted anteriorly; by this means, if one of the perforating arteries is divided, it may be clamped and tied before it retracts beyond the linea aspera.
- After dividing the muscle along the femur for the required distance, elevate it with a periosteal elevator and expose the lateral and anterolateral surfaces of the femoral shaft (Fig. 1.79C).
- By further subperiosteal elevation of the proximal part of the vastus lateralis and intermedius muscles, expose the intertrochanteric line and the anterior surface of the femur just below this line.
- The base of the femoral neck may be exposed by dividing the capsule of the joint at its attachment to the intertrochanteric line.
- If a wider exposure is desired, elevate the distal part of the gluteus minimus from its insertion on the trochanter.
- In closure, the vastus lateralis muscle falls over the lateral surface of the femur. Suture the fascia lata and close the remainder of the wound routinely.

HIP

Numerous new approaches to the hip have been described since the 1990s; most are based on older approaches and are modified for a specific surgical procedure. In this section, the general approaches we have found most useful are described. The specific approaches used in revision total hip arthroplasty are described in other chapter. Approaches used for minimally invasive hip arthroplasty procedures are described in other chapter.

The approach selected should be based on access needed, the potential for complications, the procedure to be performed, and the experience of the surgeon. The need for maintaining the primary blood supply to the femoral head (medial femoral circumflex artery and its ascending branches) must be considered before the procedure (Fig. 1.80). In total hip arthroplasty, disruption of the ascending branches of the medial circumflex femoral artery is of

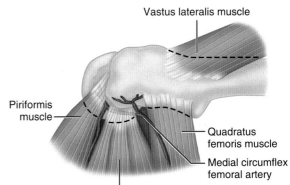

Vastus lateralis muscle

Piriformis muscle

Quadratus femoris muscle

Medial circumflex femoral artery

Obturator internus and gemelli muscles

FIGURE 1.80 The relevant deep anatomic structures of posterior aspect of the hip shows the course of medial circumflex femoral artery to the femoral head. (From Nork SE, Schär M, Pfander G, et al: Anatomic considerations for the choice of surgical approach for hip resurfacing arthroplasty, *Orthop Clin North Am* 36:163, 2005.)

no consequence. If hip resurfacing, femoral neck fracture repair, or osteotomy is to be performed, lateral anterolateral, anterior, or medial approaches are more desirous to prevent osteonecrosis of the femoral head. Lateral approaches requiring osteotomy of the greater trochanter have a significant nonunion rate of that osteotomy, which should also be considered.

Mednick et al. demonstrated consistent occlusion of the femoral vein when using a Hohmann-like retractor over the anterior wall of the acetabulum during an anterior approach. Anterior approaches risk injury to the lateral femoral cutaneous nerve, which can lead to significant patient dissatisfaction (Fig. 1.81). The superior gluteal nerve can be injured in the process of ligating or cauterizing the ascending branch of the lateral femoral circumflex artery where it enters the tensor fascia latae muscle. Ohmori et al. used computed tomography on normal volunteers to determine the distance to the center of the femoral head and found that it is shortest in an anterior approach regardless of body mass index or gender and is longest in a posterior approach.

ANTERIOR APPROACHES TO THE HIP

ANTERIOR ILIOFEMORAL APPROACH TO THE HIP

Nearly all surgery of the hip joint may be carried out through this approach, or separate parts can be used for different purposes. The entire ilium and hip joint can be reached through the iliac part of the incision; all structures attached to the iliac crest from the posterior superior iliac spine to the anterior superior iliac spine are freed and are reflected from the lateral surface of the ilium; dissection is carried distally to the anterior inferior iliac spine. Smith-Petersen also modified and improved this approach for extensive surgery of the hip by reflecting the iliacus muscle from the medial surface of the anterior part of the ilium and by detaching the rectus femoris muscle from its origin. All or part of this approach can be used depending on how much of the ilium or acetabulum needs to be exposed.

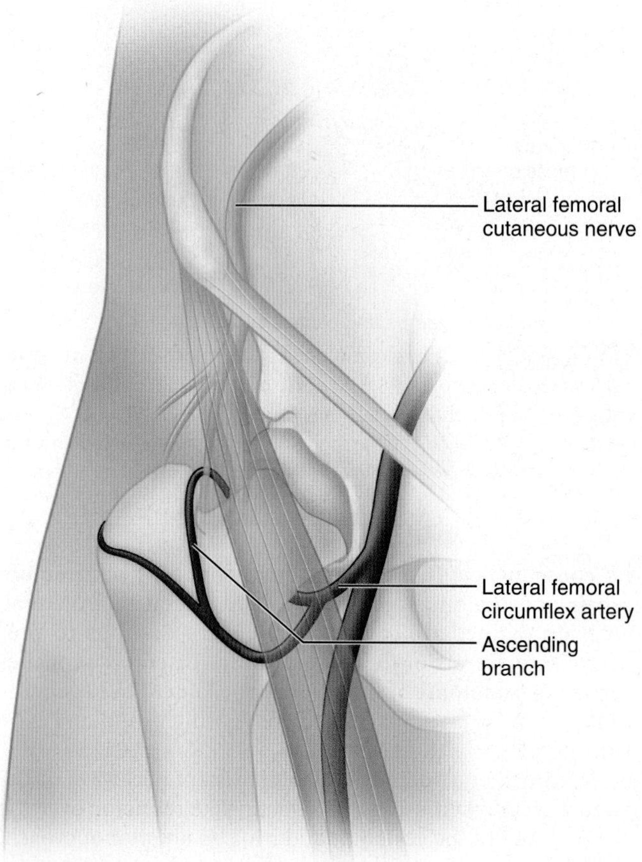

Lateral femoral
cutaneous nerve

Lateral femoral
circumflex artery

Ascending
branch

FIGURE 1.81 Relationship between the lateral femoral cutaneous nerve and ascending branch of the lateral femoral circumflex artery. (Modified from York PJ, Smack CT, Judet T, Mauffrey C: Total hip arthroplasty via anterior approach: tips and tricks for primary and revision surgery, *Int Orthop* 40:2041, 2016.)

TECHNIQUE 1.64   *Figure 1.82*

(SMITH-PETERSEN)

- Begin the incision at the middle of the iliac crest or, for a larger exposure, as far posteriorly on the crest as desired. Carry it anteriorly to the anterior superior iliac spine and distally and slightly laterally 10 to 12 cm.
- Divide the superficial and deep fasciae and free the attachments of the gluteus medius and the tensor fasciae latae muscles from the iliac crest.
- With a periosteal elevator, strip the periosteum with the attachments of the gluteus medius and minimus muscles from the lateral surface of the ilium. Control bleeding from the nutrient vessels by packing the interval between the ilium and the reflected muscles.
- Carry the dissection through the deep fascia of the thigh and between the tensor fasciae latae laterally and the sartorius and rectus femoris medially.
- Clamp and ligate the ascending branch of the lateral femoral circumflex artery, which lies 5 cm distal to the hip joint.
- The lateral femoral cutaneous nerve passes over the sartorius 2.5 cm distal to the anterior superior spine; retract it to the medial side.
- If the structures at the anterior superior spine are contracted, free the spine with an osteotome and allow it to retract with its attached muscles to a more distal level.
- Expose and incise the capsule transversely and reveal the femoral head and the proximal margin of the acetabulum. The capsule also may be sectioned along its attachment to the acetabular labrum (cotyloid ligament) to give the required exposure.
- If necessary, the ligamentum teres may be divided with a curved knife or with scissors and the femoral head dislocated, giving access to all parts of the joint.

Schaubel modified the Smith-Petersen anterior approach after finding reattachment of the fascia lata to the fascia on

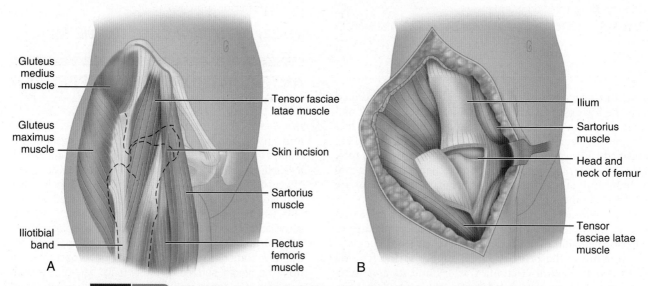

Gluteus
medius
muscle

Gluteus
maximus
muscle

Iliotibial
band

Tensor fasciae
latae muscle

Skin incision

Sartorius
muscle

Rectus
femoris
muscle

Ilium

Sartorius
muscle

Head and
neck of femur

Tensor
fasciae latae
muscle

A   **B**

FIGURE 1.82 Smith-Petersen anterior iliofemoral approach to hip. **A,** Line of skin incision. **B,** Exposure of joint after reflection of tensor fasciae latae and gluteal muscles from lateral surface of ilium and division of capsule. **SEE TECHNIQUE 1.64.**

the iliac crest difficult. Instead of dividing the fascia lata at the iliac crest, an osteotomy of the overhang of the iliac crest is performed between the attachments of the external oblique muscle medially and the fascia lata. The osteotomy may be carried posteriorly as far as the origin of the gluteus maximus. The tensor fasciae latae, gluteus medius, and gluteus minimus muscle attachments are subperiosteally dissected distally to expose the hip joint capsule. The abductors and short external rotators may be dissected from the greater trochanter as necessary for total hip arthroplasty, prosthetic replacement of the femoral head, or arthrodesis of the hip. At closure, the iliac osteotomy fragment is reattached with 1-0 nonabsorbable sutures passed through holes drilled in the fragment and the ilium. Zahradnicek extended the skin incision along the anterolateral aspect of the thigh and developed an interval between the tensor fascia lata (superior gluteal nerve) laterally and the sartorius and rectus femoris (femoral nerve) medially. This is useful when both acetabulum and proximal femoral shaft exposure are necessary.

ANTERIOR APPROACH TO THE HIP USING A TRANSVERSE INCISION

Somerville described an anterior approach using a transverse "bikini" incision for irreducible congenital dislocation of the hip in a young child. This approach allows sufficient exposure of the ilium, and access to the acetabulum is satisfactory even when it is in an abnormal location. For reduction of a congenitally dislocated hip, the following sequential steps must be performed: psoas tenotomy, complete medial capsulotomy including the transverse acetabular ligament, excision of hypertrophied ligamentum teres, and reduction of the femoral head into the true acetabulum. Specific indications and postoperative care for congenital dislocation of the hip are discussed in other chapter.

TECHNIQUE 1.65

(SOMERVILLE)
- Place a small bump beneath the affected hip.
- Make a straight skin incision, beginning anteriorly inferior and medial to the anterior superior spine and coursing obliquely superiorly and posteriorly to the middle of the iliac crest (Fig. 1.83A). Deepen the incision to expose the crest.
- Reflect the abductor muscles subperiosteally from the iliac wing distally to the capsule of the joint. Increase exposure of the capsule by separating the tensor fasciae latae from the sartorius for about 2.5 cm inferior to the anterior superior spine.
- Expose the reflected head of the rectus femoris and separate it from the acetabulum and capsule, leaving the straight head attached to the anterior inferior spine (Fig. 1.83B). The straight head may be detached to increase exposure.
- Near the acetabular rim, make a small incision in the capsule and extend it anteriorly to a point deep to the rectus

and posteriorly to the posterosuperior margin of the joint (Fig. 1.83C).
- Exert enough traction on the limb to distract the cartilage of the femoral head from that of the acetabulum about 0.7 cm.
- Examine the inside of the acetabulum visually (Fig. 1.83D). If no inverted labrum is seen, insert a blunt hook and palpate the joint for the free edge of an inverted labrum. If one is found, place the tip of the hook deep to the labrum and force it through its base; separate from its periphery that part of the labrum lying anterior to the hook until the hook comes out.
- With Kocher forceps, grasp the labrum by the end thus freed and excise it with strong curved scissors or make radial T-shaped incisions to evert the limbs and allow reduction of the femoral head (Fig. 1.83E).
- Reduce the head into the acetabulum by abducting the thigh 30 degrees and internally rotating it. Hold the joint in this position and close the capsule (Fig. 1.83F).
- Reattach the muscles to the iliac crest, close the skin, and apply a spica cast.

MODIFIED ANTEROLATERAL ILIOFEMORAL APPROACH TO THE HIP

Smith-Petersen described a modification of the anterior iliofemoral approach that he used for open reduction and internal fixation of fractures of the femoral neck. This approach retains the advantages of the anterior iliofemoral approach but exposes the trochanteric region laterally; this makes aligning a fracture or osteotomy of the femoral neck and inserting pins, screws, or nails under direct vision easier. This approach also is useful in reconstructive procedures such as osteotomy for slipping of the proximal femoral epiphysis and procedures for nonunions of the femoral neck. It gives a continuous exposure of the anterior aspect of the hip from the acetabular labrum to the base of the trochanter.

TECHNIQUE 1.66

(SMITH-PETERSEN)
- Make the skin incision along the anterior third of the iliac crest and along the anterior border of the tensor fasciae latae muscle; curve it posteriorly across the insertion of this muscle into the iliotibial band in the subtrochanteric region (usually at a point 8 to 10 cm below the base of the greater trochanter) and end it there.
- Incise the fascia along the anterior border of the tensor fasciae latae muscle. Identify and protect the lateral femoral cutaneous nerve, which usually is medial to the medial border of the tensor fasciae latae and close to the lateral border of the sartorius.
- Cleanly incise the muscle attachments to the lateral aspect of the ilium along the iliac crest to make reflection of the periosteum easier. Reflect it as a continuous structure, without fraying, distally to the superior margin of the acetabulum.

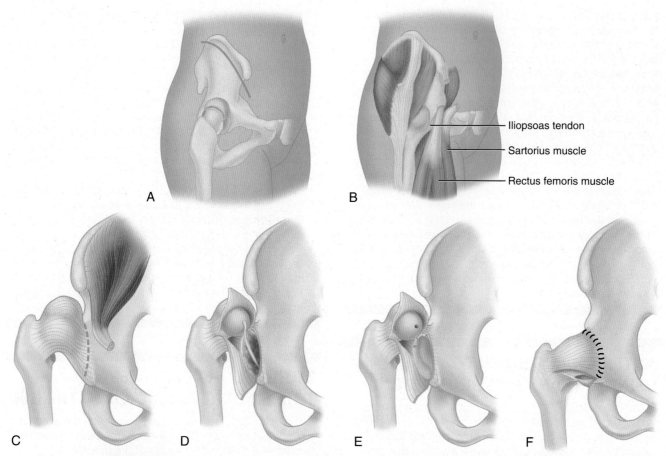

Iliopsoas tendon

Sartorius muscle

Rectus femoris muscle

A

B

C

D

E

F

FIGURE 1.83 Somerville technique of open reduction. **A,** Bikini incision. **B,** Division of sartorius and rectus femoris tendons and iliac epiphysis. **C,** Incision of capsule. **D,** Capsulotomy of hip and use of ligamentum teres to find true acetabulum. **E,** Radial incisions in acetabular labrum and removal of all tissue from depth of true acetabulum. **F,** Capsulorrhaphy after excision of redundant capsule. **SEE TECHNIQUE 1.65.**

■ Divide the muscle attachments between the anterior superior iliac spine and the acetabular labrum. The posterior flap thus reflected consists of the tensor fasciae latae, the gluteus minimus, and the anterior part of the gluteus medius (Fig. 1.84).

■ Inferiorly carry the fascial incision across the insertion of the tensor fasciae latae into the iliotibial band and expose the lateral part of the rectus femoris and the anterior part of the vastus lateralis muscles.

■ Begin the capsular incision on the inferior aspect of the capsule just lateral to the acetabular labrum; from this point, extend it proximally, parallel with the acetabular labrum, to the superior aspect of the capsule, and curve it laterally, continuing on beyond the capsule to the base of the greater trochanter. This incision divides that part of the reflected head of the rectus femoris that blends into the capsule inferior to its insertion into the superior margin of the acetabulum. By reflecting it with the capsule, the capsular flap is reinforced, and repair is made easier.

Ishimatsu et al. reported significant reversible femoral nerve amplitude reduction when a retractor is placed between the anterior wall of the acetabulum and the iliopsoas

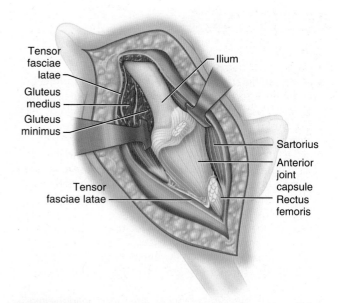

Tensor fasciae latae

Gluteus medius

Gluteus minimus

Tensor fasciae latae

Ilium

Sartorius

Anterior joint capsule

Rectus femoris

FIGURE 1.84 Modified Smith-Petersen anterolateral iliofemoral approach. **SEE TECHNIQUE 1.66.**

and sartorius muscles. This was observed in 77% of 22 patients undergoing total hip arthroplasty even with careful placement of the retractor. As mentioned earlier the femoral vein can be easily occluded with this maneuver.

LATERAL APPROACHES TO THE HIP

LATERAL APPROACH TO THE HIP

TECHNIQUE 1.67

(WATSON-JONES)
- Begin an incision 2.5 cm distal and lateral to the anterior superior iliac spine and curve it distally and posteriorly over the lateral aspect of the greater trochanter and lateral surface of the femoral shaft to 5 cm distal to the base of the trochanter (Fig. 1.85A).
- Locate the interval between the gluteus medius and tensor fasciae latae. The delineation of this interval often is difficult. Brackett pointed out that it can be done more easily by beginning the separation midway between the anterior superior spine and the greater trochanter, before the tensor fasciae latae blends with its fascial insertion. The coarse grain and the direction of the fibers of the gluteus medius help to distinguish them from the finer structure of the tensor fasciae latae muscle (Fig. 1.85B).
- Carry the dissection proximally to expose the inferior branch of the superior gluteal nerve, which innervates the tensor fasciae latae muscle.
- Incise the capsule of the joint longitudinally along the anterosuperior surface of the femoral neck. In the distal part of the incision, the origin of the vastus lateralis may be reflected distally or split longitudinally to expose the

base of the trochanter and proximal part of the femoral shaft.
- If a wider field is desired, detach the anterior fibers of the gluteus medius tendon from the trochanter or reflect the anterosuperior part of the greater trochanter proximally with an osteotome, together with the insertion of the gluteus medius muscle. This preserves the insertion of the gluteus medius in such a way that it can be easily reattached later.

LATERAL APPROACH FOR EXTENSIVE EXPOSURE OF THE HIP

Harris recommends the following lateral approach for extensive exposure of the hip. It permits dislocation of the femoral head anteriorly and posteriorly. This approach requires an osteotomy of the greater trochanter, however, with the resulting risk of nonunion or trochanteric bursitis. Also, as reported by Testa and Mazur, the incidence of significant or disabling heterotopic ossification is increased after total hip arthroplasty using a transtrochanteric lateral approach compared with a direct lateral approach.

TECHNIQUE 1.68

(HARRIS)
- Place the patient on the unaffected hip and elevate the affected one 60 degrees; maintain this position by using sandbags or a long, thick blanket roll extending from beneath the scapula to the sacrum.
- Make a U-shaped skin incision, with its base at the posterior border of the greater trochanter as follows (Fig. 1.86A, inset). Begin the incision about 5 cm posterior and slightly proximal to the anterior superior iliac spine, curve it distally and posteriorly to the posterosuperior corner of the greater trochanter, extend it longitudinally for about 8 cm, and finally curve it gradually anteriorly and distally, making the two limbs of the U symmetrical.
- Beginning distally, divide the iliotibial band in line with the skin incision; at the greater trochanter, place a finger deep to the band, feel the femoral insertion of the gluteus maximus on the gluteal tuberosity, and guide the incision in the fascia lata posteriorly, but stay one fingerbreadth anterior to this insertion.
- Continue the incision in the fascia lata proximally in line with the skin incision, releasing the fascia overlying the gluteus medius.
- Exposure of the posterior aspect of the greater trochanter, the insertion of the short external rotators, and the posterior part of the joint capsule is limited by the posterior part of the fascia lata and the gluteus maximus fibers that insert into it. To obtain wide exposure posteriorly and to provide a space into which the femoral head can be dislocated, make a short oblique incision in the deep surface of the posteriorly reflected fascia lata, extending into the substance of the gluteus maximus (Fig. 1.86A). Begin this incision at the level of the middle of the greater

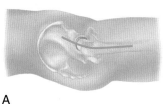

A

Tensor fasciae
latae muscle

B   Gluteus medius muscle   Vastus lateralis muscle

FIGURE 1.85 Watson-Jones lateral approach to hip joint. **A,** Skin incision. **B,** Approach has been completed except for incision of joint capsule. **SEE TECHNIQUE 1.67.**

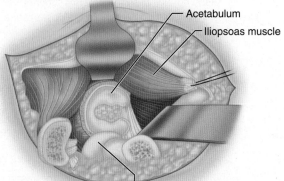

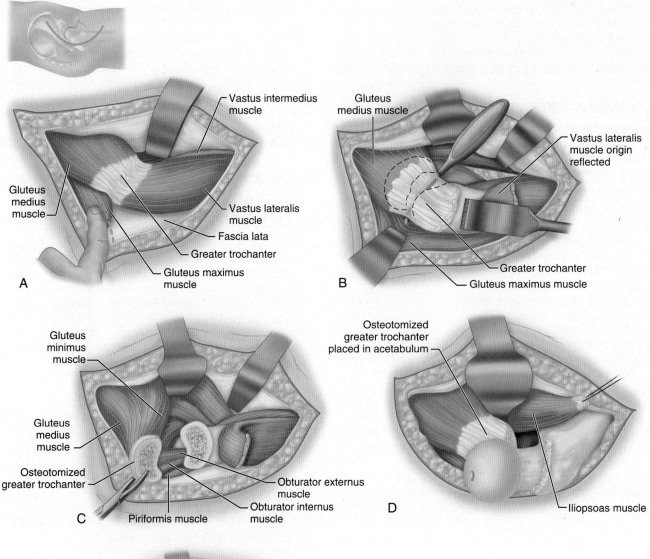

A, Vastus intermedius muscle

Gluteus medius muscle

Vastus lateralis muscle

Fascia lata

Greater trochanter

Gluteus maximus muscle

B, Gluteus medius muscle

Vastus lateralis muscle origin reflected

Greater trochanter

Gluteus maximus muscle

C, Gluteus minimus muscle

Gluteus medius muscle

Osteotomized greater trochanter

Piriformis muscle

Obturator externus muscle

Obturator internus muscle

D, Osteotomized greater trochanter placed in acetabulum

Iliopsoas muscle

E, Acetabulum

Iliopsoas muscle

Femoral head dislocated posterior to acetabulum

FIGURE 1.86 Harris lateral approach to hip. **A,** Iliotibial band has been divided proximal to greater trochanter. A finger has been placed on insertion of gluteus maximus deep to band, and fascia lata is to be incised 1 fingerbreadth anterior to insertion *(broken line)* without cutting into insertion of gluteus maximus. **B,** To obtain wide exposure posteriorly and to provide space into which femoral head can be dislocated, a short oblique incision has been made in posteriorly reflected fascia lata, extending into gluteus maximus (see text). Greater trochanter is to be osteotomized (see text). **C,** Greater trochanter has been osteotomized and retracted superiorly; superior part of joint capsule has been freed; and insertions of piriformis, obturator externus, and obturator internus are to be divided. **D,** Full circumference of femoral head has been exposed by placing greater trochanter and its muscle pedicle into acetabulum and externally rotating femur. **E,** Entire acetabulum has been exposed by retracting the greater trochanter superiorly and dislocating the femoral head posteriorly. **SEE TECHNIQUE 1.68.**

trochanter and extend it medially and proximally into the gluteus maximus parallel to its fibers for 4 cm.

- Reflect anteriorly the anterior part of the iliotibial band and the tensor fasciae latae, which form the anterior flap, passing a periosteal elevator along the anterior capsule to the acetabulum.
- Free the abductor muscles by osteotomizing the greater trochanter as follows (Fig. 1.86B): reflect distally the origin of the vastus lateralis; place an instrument between the abductor muscles and the superior surface of the joint capsule, and direct the osteotomy superiorly and medially from a point 1.5 cm distal to the tubercle of the vastus lateralis to the superior surface of the femoral neck.
- Free the superior part of the joint capsule from the greater trochanter. During these maneuvers, protect the sciatic nerve by using a smooth retractor.
  1. Divide the piriformis, obturator externus, and obturator internus at their femoral insertions (Fig. 1.86C).
  2. Excise the anterior and posterior parts of the capsule under direct vision as far proximally as the acetabulum.
- Proceed with the operation anteriorly. Deep to the rectus femoris insert a small, blunt-pointed Bennett retractor so that its hook is placed over the anterior inferior iliac spine.
- Reflect superiorly the greater trochanter and its attached abductor muscles to expose the superior and anterior parts of the capsule.
- Place a thin retractor between the capsule and the iliopsoas to expose the anterior and inferior parts of the capsule. Working from the anterior and posterior aspects of the joint, excise as much of the capsule as desired; if the iliopsoas muscle is to be transplanted, leave the stump of the anterior part of the capsule intact.
- Dislocate the femoral head anteriorly by extending, adducting, and externally rotating the femur. Before or after the hip has been dislocated, bring the lesser trochanter into view by flexing and externally rotating the femur and, if desired, divide the iliopsoas under direct vision.
- Expose the full circumference of the femoral head by placing the greater trochanter and its muscle pedicle into the acetabulum and externally rotating the femur (Fig. 1.86D).
- To expose the entire acetabulum, retract the greater trochanter superiorly and dislocate the femoral head posteriorly (Fig. 1.86E) by flexing the knee and adducting, flexing, and internally rotating the hip. Flexing the knee reduces tension on the sciatic nerve while the head is dislocated posteriorly.
- When closing the wound, position the limb in almost full abduction and in about 10 degrees of external rotation. Transplant the greater trochanter distally, and fix it directly to the lateral side of the femoral shaft with two wire loops, screws, or a cable grip. For a more detailed description of fixation of the greater trochanter, see other chapter.

LATERAL APPROACH TO THE HIP PRESERVING THE GLUTEUS MEDIUS

McFarland and Osborne described a lateral approach to the hip that preserves the integrity of the gluteus medius muscle. They noted that the gluteus medius and vastus lateralis muscles can be regarded as being in direct functional continuity through the thick periosteum covering the greater trochanter.

TECHNIQUE 1.69

(MCFARLAND AND OSBORNE)
- Make a midlateral skin incision (Fig. 1.87A) centered over the greater trochanter; its length depends on the amount of subcutaneous fat. Expose the gluteal fascia and the iliotibial band, and divide them in a straight midlateral line along the entire length of the skin incision (Fig. 1.87B).
- Retract the gluteus maximus posteriorly and the tensor fasciae latae anteriorly.
- Expose the gluteus medius and separate it from the piriformis and gluteus minimus by blunt dissection.
- Identify the prominent posterior border of the gluteus medius where it joins the posterior edge of the greater trochanter. From this point, make an incision down to the bone through the periosteum and fascia obliquely and distally across the greater trochanter to the middle of the lateral aspect of the femur; continue it further distally in the vastus lateralis to the distal end of the skin incision (Fig. 1.87C).
- With a knife or a sharp chisel, peel from the bone, in one piece, the attachment of the gluteus medius, the periosteum, the tendinous junction of the gluteus medius and vastus lateralis, and the origin of the vastus lateralis. The portion of the vastus lateralis peeled off includes that attached to the proximal part of the linea aspera, the distal border of the greater trochanter, and part of the shaft of the femur.
- Anteriorly retract the whole combined muscle mass, consisting of the gluteus medius and vastus lateralis with their tendinous junction (Fig. 1.87D). Split, divide, and proximally retract the tendon of the gluteus minimus to expose the capsule of the hip joint (Fig. 1.87E). Incise the capsule as desired (Fig. 1.87F).
- During closure, suture the capsule and gluteus minimus as one structure. Abduct the hip, return the gluteus medius and vastus lateralis to their original position, and suture them to the undisturbed part of the vastus lateralis, to the deep insertion of the gluteus maximus, and to the proximal part of the quadratus femoris.

LATERAL TRANSGLUTEAL APPROACH TO THE HIP

Hardinge described a useful transgluteal modification of the McFarland and Osborne direct lateral approach based on the observation that the gluteus medius inserts on the greater trochanter by a strong, mobile tendon that curves around the apex of the trochanter. This approach can be easily made with the patient supine. Osteotomy of the greater trochanter is avoided.

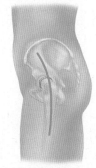

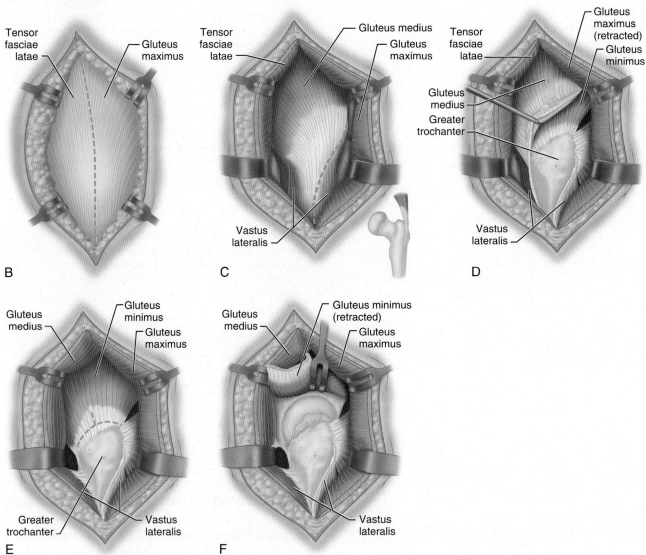

FIGURE 1.87 McFarland and Osborne lateral or posterolateral approach to hip. **A,** Skin incision. **B,** Gluteal fascia and iliotibial band are divided in midlateral line. **C,** Incision is made to bone obliquely across trochanter and distally in vastus lateralis. **D,** Combined muscle mass consisting of gluteus medius and vastus lateralis with their tendinous junction is elevated and retracted anteriorly. **E,** Tendon of gluteus minimus is split and divided before retraction proximally. **F,** Capsule has been opened to expose joint. (From McFarland B, Osborne G: Approach to the hip: a suggested improvement on Kocher's method, *J Bone Joint Surg* 36B:364, 1954.) **SEE TECHNIQUE 1.69.**

TECHNIQUE 1.70

(HARDINGE)

- Place the patient supine with the greater trochanter at the edge of the table and the muscles of the buttocks freed from the edge.
- Make a posteriorly directed lazy-J incision centered over the greater trochanter (Fig. 1.88A).
- Divide the fascia lata in line with the skin incision and centered over the greater trochanter.
- Retract the tensor fasciae latae anteriorly and the gluteus maximus posteriorly, exposing the origin of the vastus lateralis and the insertion of the gluteus medius (Fig. 1.88B).
- Incise the tendon of the gluteus medius obliquely across the greater trochanter, leaving the posterior half still attached to the trochanter. Carry the incision proximally in line with the fibers of the gluteus medius at the junction of the middle and posterior thirds of the muscle. This gluteus medius split should be no farther than 4 to 5 cm from the tip of the greater trochanter to avoid damage to the superior gluteal nerve and artery. Distally, carry the incision anteriorly in line with the fibers of the vastus lateralis down to bone along the anterolateral surface of the femur (Fig. 1.88B).
- Elevate the tendinous insertions of the anterior portions of the gluteus minimus and vastus lateralis muscles. Abduction of the thigh exposes the anterior capsule of the hip joint (Fig. 1.88C).
- Incise the capsule as desired.

- During closure, repair the tendon of the gluteus medius with nonabsorbable braided sutures.

Frndak et al. modified the Hardinge direct lateral transgluteal approach by placing the abductor "split" more anterior, directly over the femoral head and neck (Fig. 1.89). The "split" must not extend more than 2 cm above the lateral lip of the acetabulum to avoid damage to the gluteal neurovascular bundle. Because the abductor "split" is more anterior, exposure of the femoral head and neck requires less retraction.

LATERAL TRANSGLUTEAL APPROACH TO THE HIP

McLauchlan described a direct lateral transgluteal approach to the hip through the gluteus medius used for many years by Hay at the Stracathro Hospital. It also is based on the anatomic observation made by McFarland and Osborne mentioned earlier that the gluteus medius and vastus lateralis are in functional continuity through the thick periosteum covering the greater trochanter.

TECHNIQUE 1.71

(HAY AS DESCRIBED BY MCLAUCHLAN)

- Place the patient in the Sims position with the affected hip uppermost.

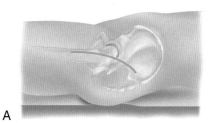

A

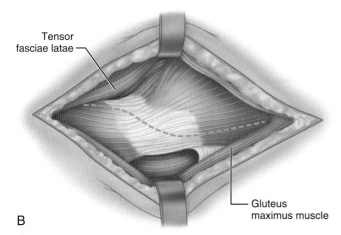

Tensor fasciae latae

Gluteus maximus muscle

B

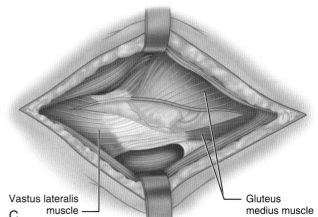

Vastus lateralis muscle

Gluteus medius muscle

C

FIGURE 1.88 Hardinge direct lateral transgluteal approach. **A,** Lazy-J lateral skin incision. **B,** Tensor fasciae latae retracted anteriorly, and gluteus maximus is retracted posteriorly. Incision through gluteus medius tendon is outlined. Posterior half is left attached to greater trochanter. **C,** Anterior joint capsule is exposed. (Modified from Hardinge K: The direct lateral approach to the hip, *J Bone Joint Surg* 64B:17, 1982.) **SEE TECHNIQUE 1.70.**

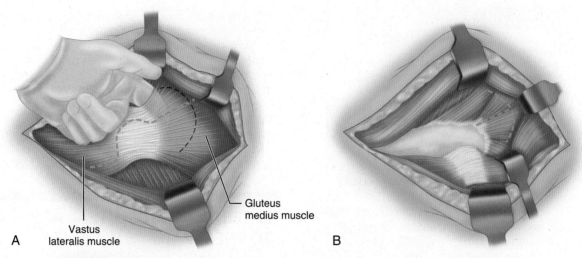

A
Vastus
lateralis muscle

Gluteus
medius muscle

B

FIGURE 1.89 Modified direct lateral transgluteal approach. **A,** Abductor "split" is determined by location of the femoral neck. **B,** Capsular incision parallels superior border. **SEE TECHNIQUE 1.70.**

- Make a lateral longitudinal skin incision (Fig. 1.90A) centered midway between the anterior and posterior borders of the greater trochanter and extending an equal distance proximal and distal to the tip of the trochanter. In lateral rotational deformities of the hip, place the incision more posteriorly.
- Incise the deep fascia and the tensor fasciae latae in line with the skin incision.
- Retract these structures anteriorly and posteriorly to expose the greater trochanter with the gluteus medius attached to it proximally and the vastus lateralis attached distally (Fig. 1.90B).
- Split the gluteus medius in the line of its fibers for a distance of no more than 4 to 5 cm to avoid damage to the superior gluteal neurovascular bundle. Elevate two rectangular slices of greater trochanter, one anteriorly and one posteriorly with an osteotome. These slices of trochanter have gluteus medius attached to them proximally and vastus lateralis attached distally (Fig. 1.90C).
- Retract anteriorly and posteriorly to reveal the gluteus minimus.
- Rotate the hip externally and split the gluteus minimus in the line of its fibers or detach it from the greater trochanter.
- Incise the capsule of the hip joint, insert spike retractors anteriorly and posteriorly over the edges of the acetabulum, and dislocate the hip anteriorly by flexion and external rotation (Fig. 1.90D). The femoral neck and acetabulum are well exposed for routine total hip arthroplasty or for difficult revisions.
- When closing, suture the capsule if enough of it is left.
- Internally rotate the hip and suture the trochanteric slices to the periosteum and the other soft tissue covering the trochanter. The trochanteric slices unite without any problem, and abductor function returns rapidly.
- Carefully close the deep fascia with interrupted sutures.

POSTEROLATERAL APPROACH

Alexander Gibson is responsible for the rediscovery in North America of the posterolateral approach to the hip

first described and recommended by Kocher and Langenbeck. Because detaching the gluteal muscles from the ilium and interfering with the function of the iliotibial band are unnecessary, rehabilitation after surgery is rapid.

TECHNIQUE 1.72

(GIBSON)
- Place the patient in a lateral position.
- Begin the proximal limb of the incision at a point 6 to 8 cm anterior to the posterior superior iliac spine and just distal to the iliac crest, overlying the anterior border of the gluteus maximus muscle. Extend it distally to the anterior edge of the greater trochanter and farther distally along the line of the femur for 15 to 18 cm (Fig. 1.91A).
- By blunt dissection, reflect the flaps of skin and subcutaneous fat from the underlying deep fascia a short distance anteriorly and posteriorly.
- Incise the iliotibial band in line with its fibers, beginning at the distal end of the wound and extending proximally to the greater trochanter.
- Abduct the thigh, insert the gloved finger through the proximal end of the incision in the band, locate by palpation the sulcus at the anterior border of the gluteus maximus muscle, and extend the incision proximally along this sulcus. Adduct the thigh, reflect the anterior and posterior masses, and expose the greater trochanter and the muscles that insert into it (Fig. 1.91B).
- Separate the posterior border of the gluteus medius muscle from the adjacent piriformis tendon by blunt dissection.
- Divide the gluteus medius and minimus muscles at their insertions, but leave enough of their tendons attached to the greater trochanter to permit easy closure of the wound. Reflect these muscles (innervated by the superior gluteal nerve) anteriorly (Fig. 1.91C). The anterior and superior parts of the joint capsule now can be seen.
- Incise the capsule superiorly in the axis of the femoral neck from the acetabulum to the intertrochanteric line; incise as much of the capsule as desired along the joint line anteriorly and along the anterior intertrochanteric line laterally. The hip now can be dislocated by flexing the hip

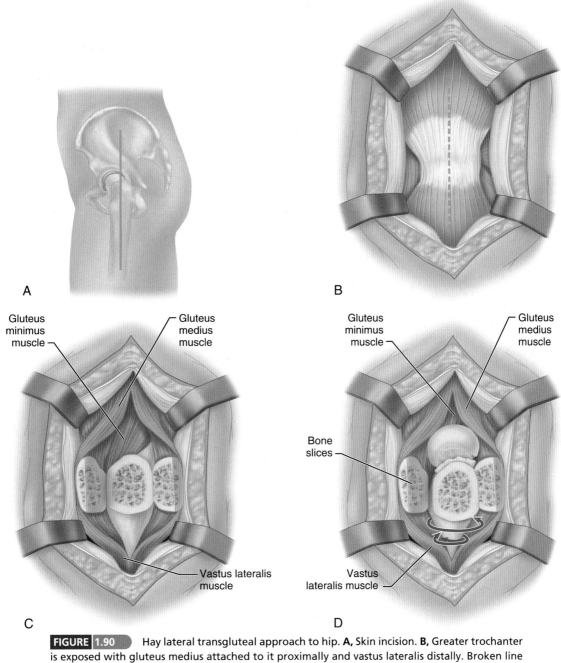

Gluteus minimus muscle — Gluteus medius muscle

Gluteus minimus muscle — Gluteus medius muscle

Bone slices —

Vastus lateralis muscle

Vastus lateralis muscle —

A

B

C

D

FIGURE 1.90 Hay lateral transgluteal approach to hip. **A,** Skin incision. **B,** Greater trochanter is exposed with gluteus medius attached to it proximally and vastus lateralis distally. Broken line indicates incision to be made in soft tissues. **C,** Rectangular slices of greater trochanter have been elevated anteriorly and posteriorly. **D,** Hip joint has been opened and can be dislocated as described. (Modified from McLauchlan J: The Stracathro approach to the hip, *J Bone Joint Surg* 66B:30, 1984.) **SEE TECHNIQUE 1.71.**

and knee and abducting and externally rotating the thigh (Fig. 1.91D).
- Sufficient exposure of the hip often can be obtained with less extensive division of the muscles inserting on the trochanter; the extent of division depends on the type of operation proposed, the amount of exposure required, the tightness of the soft tissues, and the presence or absence of contractures around the joint. Conversely, when wide exposure of the joint, especially of the acetabulum,

is needed, more extensive division of the muscles may be necessary. Gibson thought that reattaching the muscles to the greater trochanter by interrupted sutures is adequate.
- To preserve the insertion of the abductor muscles, osteotomize the trochanter and later reattach it with two wire loops, 6.5-mm lag screws, or cable grip. Wire loops are passed through the insertion of the muscles proximal to

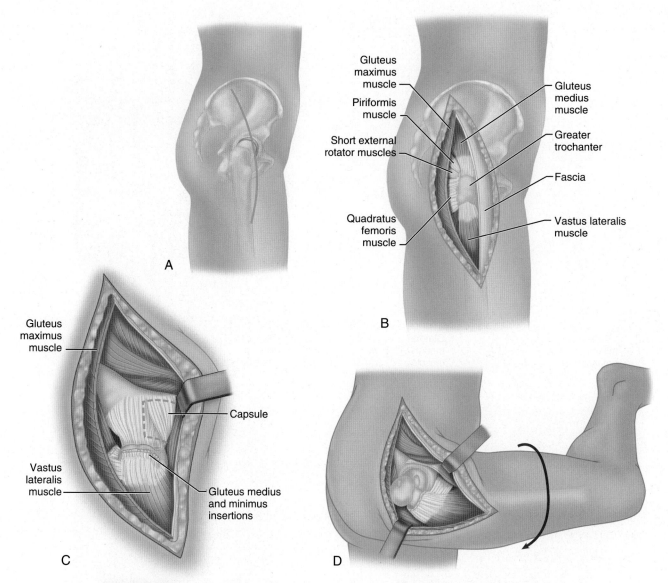

FIGURE 1.91 Gibson posterolateral approach to hip joint. **A,** Skin incision. **B,** Anterior and posterior muscle masses have been retracted to expose greater trochanter and muscles that insert into it. **C,** Gluteus medius and minimus have been divided near their insertions into greater trochanter and retracted. Incision in capsule is shown. **D,** Hip joint has been dislocated by flexing, abducting, and externally rotating thigh. **SEE TECHNIQUE 1.72.**

the trochanter and through a hole drilled in the femoral shaft 4 cm distal to the osteotomy.

Figure 1.92 shows a modification of the Gibson approach by Marcy and Fletcher for insertion of a prosthesis in which the hip is dislocated by internal rotation and the anterior part of the joint capsule is preserved to keep the hip from dislocating anteriorly after surgery.

The piriformis, obturator internus, and gemelli muscles must be separated well away from the posterior aspect of the greater trochanter (Fig. 1.93) and the attachments of the obturator externus and quadriceps femoris muscles must be preserved. Other, more anterior approaches often are better suited for these procedures.

POSTERIOR APPROACHES TO THE HIP

Posterior approaches are ideally suited for procedures in which femoral head viability is unnecessary, such as resection arthroplasty and insertion of a proximal femoral prosthesis. If femoral head viability is necessary, such as in hip resurfacing arthroplasty or fracture repair, the medial femoral circumflex artery and its ascending branches must be protected (Fig. 1.80).

POSTERIOR APPROACH TO THE HIP

TECHNIQUE 1.73

(OSBORNE)

■ Begin the incision 4.5 cm distal and lateral to the posterior superior iliac spine and continue it laterally and distally,

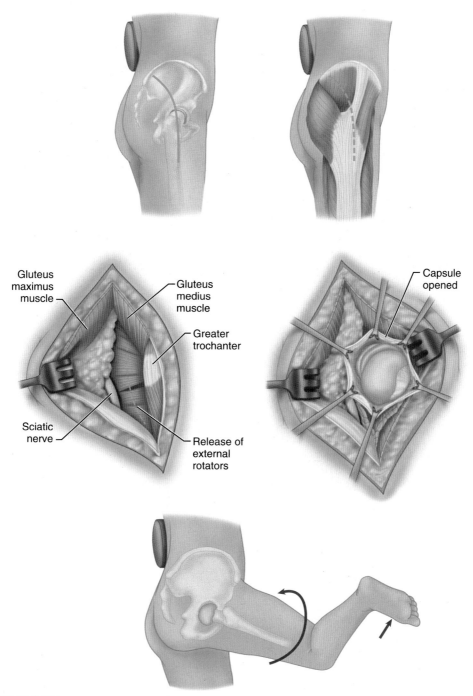

FIGURE 1.92 Modification of Gibson posterolateral approach to hip. Anterior part of joint capsule is preserved to keep hip from dislocating after surgery. Acetabulum is not well exposed, but approach is sufficient for removing femoral head and inserting prosthesis. **SEE TECHNIQUE 1.72.**

remaining parallel with the fibers of the gluteus maximus muscle, to the posterosuperior angle of the greater trochanter, and distally along the posterior border of the trochanter for 5 cm (Fig. 1.93A).

■ Separate the fibers of the gluteus maximus parallel with the line of incision, no more than 7 cm to protect the branches of the inferior gluteal artery and nerve (Fig. 1.93B).

■ Divide the insertion of the gluteus maximus into the fascia lata for 5 cm, corresponding to the longitudinal limb of the incision.

■ Rotate the thigh internally, detach the tendons of the piriformis and gemellus muscles near their insertions into the trochanter, and retract the muscles medially. The gemelli protect the sciatic nerve (Fig. 1.93C).

■ The capsule of the joint is now in view and may be incised longitudinally to expose the posterior surface of the femoral neck and posterior border of the acetabulum. Further exposure may be obtained by retracting the gluteus medius muscle proximally and the quadratus femoris muscle distally.

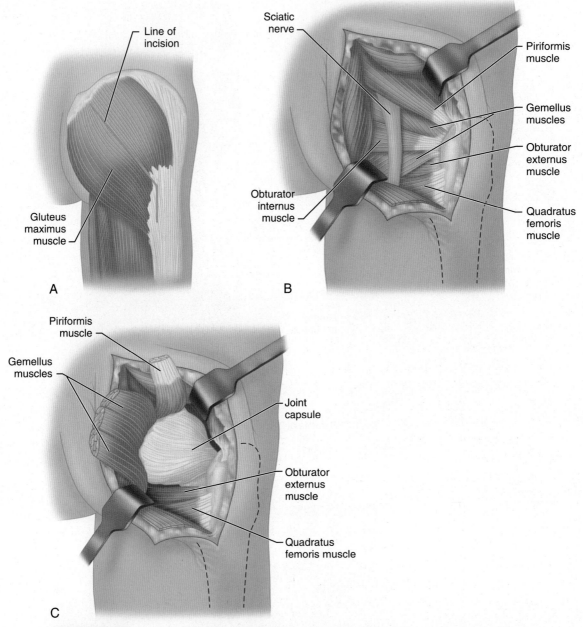

FIGURE 1.93 Osborne posterior approach to hip joint. **A,** Skin incision. **B,** Gluteus maximus has been opened in line with its fibers and retracted. **C,** Piriformis, gemellus, and obturator internus muscles have been divided at their insertions and reflected medially to expose posterior aspect of joint capsule. **SEE TECHNIQUE 1.73.**

POSTERIOR APPROACH TO THE HIP

TECHNIQUE 1.74

(MOORE)
- Moore's approach has been facetiously labeled "the southern exposure." Place the patient on the unaffected side.
- Start the incision approximately 10 cm distal to the posterior superior iliac spine and extend it distally and laterally parallel with the fibers of the gluteus maximus to the posterior

margin of the greater trochanter. Direct the incision distally 10 to 13 cm parallel with the femoral shaft (Fig. 1.94A).
- Expose and divide the deep fascia in line with the skin incision.
- By blunt dissection, separate the fibers of the gluteus maximus no more than 7 cm from the tip of the trochanter to avoid injury to the branches of the inferior gluteal artery and nerve (Fig. 1.94B).
- Retract the proximal fibers of the gluteus maximus proximally and expose the greater trochanter. Retract the distal fibers distally, and partially divide their insertion into the linea aspera in line with the distal part of the incision.

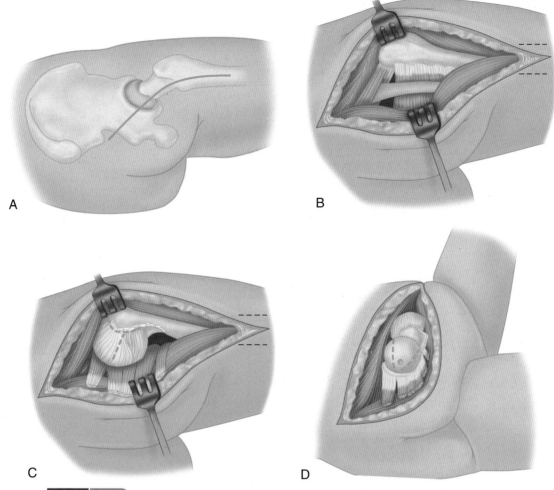

FIGURE 1.94 Moore posterior approach to hip joint. **A,** Skin incision. **B,** Gluteus maximus has been split in line with its fibers and retracted to expose sciatic nerve, greater trochanter, and short external rotator muscles. **C,** Short external rotator muscles have been freed from femur and retracted medially to expose joint capsule. **D,** Joint capsule has been opened, and hip joint has been dislocated by flexing, adducting, and internally rotating thigh. **SEE TECHNIQUE 1.74.**

- Expose the sciatic nerve and retract it carefully. After the surgeon becomes familiar with this approach, the sciatic nerve rarely needs to be exposed. Divide a small branch of the sacral plexus to the quadratus femoris and inferior gemellus, which contains sensory fibers to the joint capsule.
- Expose and divide the gemelli and obturator internus and, if desired, the tendon of the piriformis at their insertion on the femur, and retract the muscles medially. Tag these for later reattachment to the trochanter if desired.
- The posterior part of the joint capsule is now well exposed (Fig. 1.94C); incise it from distal to proximal along the line of the femoral neck to the rim of the acetabulum.
- Detach the distal part of the capsule from the femur.
- Flex the thigh and knee 90 degrees, internally rotate the thigh, and dislocate the hip posteriorly (Fig. 1.94D).

MEDIAL APPROACH TO THE HIP

The medial approach to the hip, first described by Ludloff in 1908, was developed to permit surgery on a congenitally dislocated hip with the hip flexed, abducted, and externally rotated. With the hip in this position, the distance from the skin to the medial aspect of the femoral head and lesser trochanter is about half that present when the hip is in the neutral position.

The muscular interval for the Ludloff approach is believed to be between the sartorius and the adductor longus with the deeper interval being between the iliopsoas and pectineus, although Ludloff did not precisely define the interval in his original German articles. A review by Mallon and Fitch clarifies the anatomic intervals for the various medial approaches.

MEDIAL APPROACH TO THE HIP

Ferguson and Hoppenfeld and deBoer described a medial approach based on Ludloff's approach with the superficial muscular interval between the gracilis and adductor longus and the deep interval between the adductor brevis and adductor magnus (Fig. 1.95).

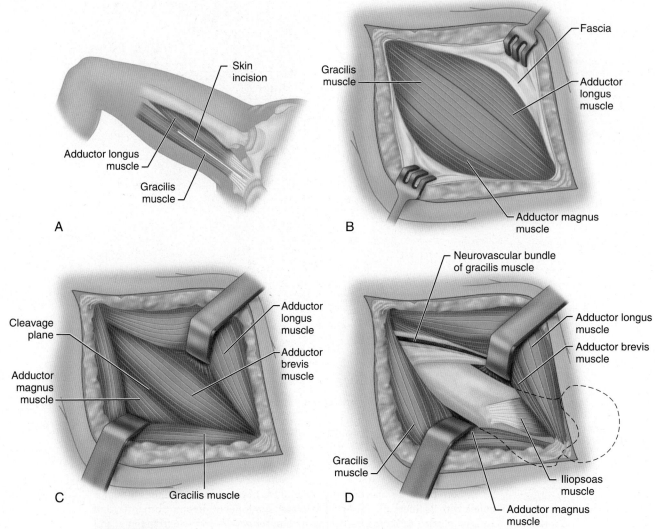

FIGURE 1.95 Ferguson; Hoppenfeld and deBoer medial approach to hip joint. **A,** Skin incision. **B,** Plane between adductor longus and gracilis is to be developed. **C,** Adductor longus has been retracted anteriorly, and gracilis and adductor magnus have been retracted posteriorly. **D,** Lesser trochanter has been exposed. **SEE TECHNIQUE 1.75.**

TECHNIQUE 1.75   *Figure 1.95*

(FERGUSON; HOPPENFELD AND DEBOER)

- Make a longitudinal incision on the medial aspect of the thigh, beginning about 2.5 cm distal to the pubic tubercle and over the interval between the gracilis and the adductor longus muscles.
- Develop the plane between the adductor longus and brevis muscles anteriorly and the gracilis and adductor magnus muscles posteriorly.
- Expose and protect the posterior branch of the obturator nerve and the neurovascular bundle of the gracilis muscle. The lesser trochanter and the capsule of the hip joint are located in the floor of the wound.

Using a modified medial approach, Cavaignac et al. repaired a femoral head fracture. The approach interval in this technique is between the lateral part of the adductor longus

muscle belly and the adductor longus aponeurosis. The lesser trochanter is exposed by blunt dissection. The inferior joint capsule is exposed by retracting the iliopsoas tendon in a lateral direction.

ACETABULUM AND PELVIS

Computed tomography and three-dimensional image reconstruction have aided greatly in characterizing fracture configurations and in preoperative planning for reduction of acetabular and pelvic fractures. Modifications of more traditional approaches have been developed for anterior, posterior, and lateral acetabular fractures. Extensile approaches have been developed for more complex fractures involving the anterior and posterior columns of the acetabulum and pelvis. The procedure for open reduction and internal fixation of acetabular fractures is detailed in other chapter. Complications associated with these more extensile approaches have led to the development of indirect reduction and percutaneous fixation techniques for acetabular fractures using only portions of these approaches if possible. Many of these approaches can be adapted for difficult primary or revision total hip arthroplasty.

STOPPA APPROACH

The modified Stoppa approach can be used for many fractures that were previously treated through the ilioinguinal approach. It is performed through a Pfannenstiel skin incision with a vertical split in the rectus abdominis though the linea alba. The rectus on the involved side is elevated off the superior surface of the pubis, and any anastomoses between the obturator vessels and the external iliac or inferior epigastric vessels (the corona mortis) are ligated to expose the internal surface of the anterior column and the quadrilateral surface. Using the lateral window of the ilioinguinal approach, this approach avoids dissection of the middle window and exposure of the femoral vein and artery, nerve and lymphatics. Combining the complete

ilioinguinal and Stoppa approaches can improve access and fixation of the quadrilateral surface in comminuted anterior fracture patterns. Traditionally most surgeons have preferred to use skeletal traction on a radiolucent fracture table, but some surgeons prefer to drape the limb free to allow positioning of the limb to facilitate exposure.

TECHNIQUE 1.76

(AO FOUNDATION)
- Make a Pfannenstiel incision or alternatively a midline skin incision, starting 1 cm inferior to the symphysis and ending 2 cm to 3 cm inferior to the umbilicus (Fig. 1.96A).
- Divide the subcutaneous tissues in line with the skin incision to expose the fascia overlying both rectus muscles of the abdomen.
- Incise the rectus fascia longitudinally along the linea alba and gently retract both bellies of the rectus abdominis muscle laterally (Fig. 1.96B).

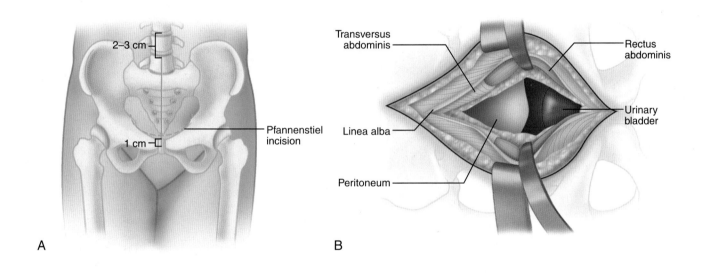

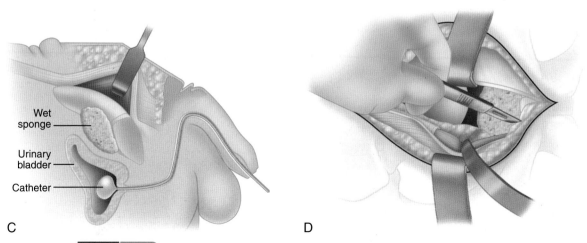

FIGURE 1.96 Stoppa approach for open reduction and internal fixation of acetabular fracture. **A,** Incision. **B,** Retraction of rectus abdominis muscle. **C,** Wet sponge packed into retropubic space to protect the urinary bladder. **D,** Dissection of periosteum from the superior pubic bone.

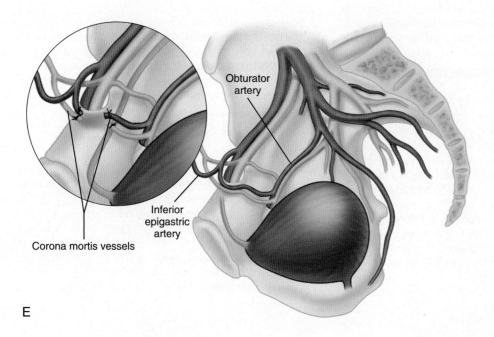

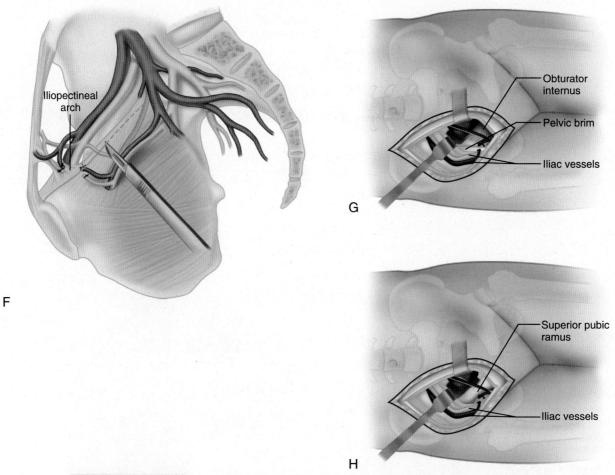

FIGURE 1.96, Cont'd   **E,** Identification of the corona mortis vessels. **F,** Dissection of the iliopectineal arch from the bone. **G,** Elevation of the periosteum and obturator internus to expose the quadrilateral surface. **H,** Placement of Hohmann retractors to expose acetabulum. (A through D, From AO Surgery Reference, **www.aosurgery.org**. Copyright by AO/Spine International, and E through H, Redrawn from AO Foundation, Davos Platz, Switzerland.) **SEE TECHNIQUE 1.76.**

- Identify the fascia between the heads of the rectus muscle. In almost all patients, this fascia has been disrupted by the injury, and the resulting defect can be used as a starting point for blunt dissection.
- In the proximal part of the incision, take care not to incise the peritoneum. The entire approach should stay in the preperitoneal space.
- Loosely pack a wet sponge in the retropubic space to protect the urinary bladder (Fig. 1.96C).
- The medial part of the rectus muscle can be partly detached from the upper and anterior part of the symphysis if necessary.
- Sharply dissect the thick periosteum from the superior pubic bone to allow deeper blunt dissection. At the beginning, dissection should be enlarged also on the anterior part of the symphysis (Fig. 1.96D).
- Identify the upper border of the superior pubic ramus (pectin pubis) and carry the dissection laterally along the pelvic brim. Detach the iliopectineal fascia from the pelvic brim.
- Dissecting carefully along the medial surface of the superior ramus, identify the corona mortis vessels and ligate (or clip) them as necessary (Fig. 1.96E).
- Continue dissection of the periosteum farther laterally, following the upper border of the superior pubic bone to the direction of the pelvic brim, exposing the beginning of the iliopectineal eminence.
- Dissect the beginning of the iliopectineal arch from the bone to allow elevation of the femora vessels and nerve (Fig. 1.96F).
- Continue the dissection subperiosteally more laterally, following the upper border of the pelvic brim. At this point, the entire internal surface of the superior pubic ramus has been exposed adequately for plate fixation.
- At this level, the obturator neurovascular bundle crosses the quadrilateral surface and, in some cases, it should be mobilized. Use a spatula or malleable retractor to protect the obturator neurovascular bundle and pelvic floor.
- With a Cobb elevator, elevate the periosteum and obturator internus to expose the quadrilateral surface (Fig. 1.96G).
- Place a Hohmann retractor in the middle part of the superior pubic ramus and another curved Hohmann retractor on the posterior top of the acetabulum on the iliac part of the pelvic brim. Take care not to injure the external iliac vein, which may be in close proximity to the elevators (Fig. 1.96H).

ANTERIOR APPROACHES TO THE ACETABULUM

ILIOINGUINAL APPROACH TO THE ACETABULUM

Letournel developed the ilioinguinal approach in 1960 as an anterior approach to the acetabulum and pelvis for the operative treatment of anterior wall acetabular and anterior column pelvic fractures. The articular surface of the acetabulum is not exposed, which is a disadvantage. This approach provides exposure of the inner table of the innominate bone from the symphysis pubis to the anterior aspect of the sacroiliac joint, however, including the quadrilateral surface and the superior and inferior pubic rami. The hip abductor musculature is left undisturbed, and rapid postoperative rehabilitation is possible.

A thorough knowledge of the surgical anatomy of this area is necessary to avoid disastrous complications.

TECHNIQUE 1.77

(LETOURNEL AND JUDET, AS DESCRIBED BY MATTA)

- Position the patient supine on a fracture table with skeletal traction applied on the injured side through a distal femoral pin. Traction should not be used in the presence of contralateral superior and inferior pubic rami fractures because deformity of the anterior pelvic ring results from pressure from the perineal post. Apply lateral traction, if necessary, through a traction screw inserted into the greater trochanter and attached to a lateral support on the fracture table.
- Begin an incision 3 cm above the symphysis pubis and carry it laterally across the lower abdomen to the anterior superior iliac spine. Continue it posteriorly along the iliac crest to the junction of the middle and posterior thirds of the crest (Fig. 1.97A).
- Sharply elevate the origins of the abdominal muscles and the iliacus muscle from the iliac crest.
- Elevate the iliacus by subperiosteal dissection from the inner table of the ilium as far as the anterior aspect of the sacroiliac joint. Continue the incision anteriorly through the superficial fascia to the external oblique aponeurosis and the external fascia of the rectus abdominis muscle (Fig. 1.97B).
- Sharply incise the aponeurosis of the external oblique and the external fascia of the rectus abdominis at least 1 cm proximal to the external inguinal ring and in line with the skin incision.
- Open the inguinal canal by elevating and reflecting the distal edge of the external oblique aponeurosis and the adjacent fascia of the rectus abdominis (Fig. 1.97C). Protect the lateral femoral cutaneous nerve, which may be adjacent to the anterior superior iliac spine or 3 cm medial to it.
- Identify the spermatic cord or round ligament and adjacent ilioinguinal nerve. Bluntly free these structures and secure them with a Penrose drain.
- Clean the areolar tissue from the inguinal ligament and incise the ligament along its length carefully with a scalpel, leaving 1 mm of ligament attached to the internal oblique and transversus abdominis muscles and the transversalis fascia (Fig. 1.97D). Exercise extreme caution to avoid damaging the structures beneath the inguinal ligament.
- Having released the common origin of the internal oblique and transversus abdominis from the inguinal ligament, the psoas sheath is entered. Continue to protect the lateral femoral cutaneous nerve beneath the inguinal ligament.
- To gain further exposure medially, retract the spermatic cord or round ligament laterally, exposing the transversalis fascia and conjoined tendon, which form the floor of the inguinal canal.
- Divide the conjoined tendon of the internal oblique and transversus abdominis and the tendon of the rectus abdominis at their insertions on the pubis to open the retropubic space.

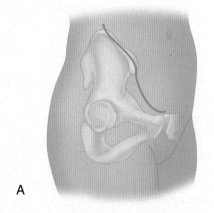

A

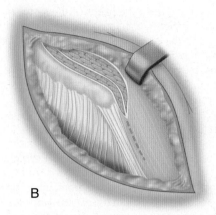

B

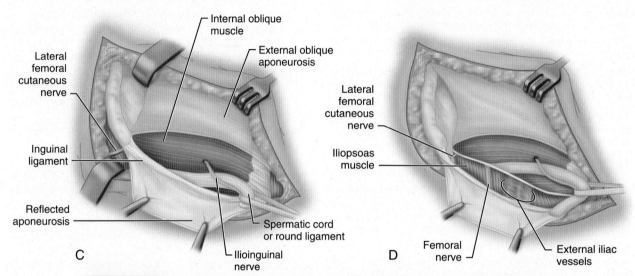

Internal oblique
muscle

External oblique
aponeurosis

Lateral
femoral
cutaneous
nerve

Inguinal
ligament

Reflected
aponeurosis

C

Spermatic cord
or round ligament

Ilioinguinal
nerve

Lateral
femoral
cutaneous
nerve

Iliopsoas
muscle

Femoral
nerve

D

External iliac
vessels

FIGURE 1.97 Letournel and Judet ilioinguinal approach. **A,** Skin incision. **B,** Origins of abdominal and iliacus muscles have been elevated from iliac crest. *Broken line* shows incision through superficial fascia and external oblique aponeurosis. **C,** Lateral femoral cutaneous nerve has been exposed, and aponeurosis of external oblique has been incised. Iliacus has been reflected from inner table of ilium. Inguinal canal has been opened by reflecting incised flap of external oblique aponeurosis distally. Internal oblique, inguinal ligament, and spermatic cord or round ligament have been exposed. **D,** Inguinal ligament has been incised, releasing common origin of internal oblique and transversus abdominis muscles.

- The structures beneath the inguinal ligament lie within two compartments or lacunae. The lacuna musculorum is lateral and contains the iliopsoas muscle, the femoral nerve, and the lateral femoral cutaneous nerve. The lacuna vasorum is medial and contains the external iliac vessels and lymphatics. The iliopectineal fascia, or psoas sheath, separates the two compartments (Fig. 1.97E). Carefully elevate the external iliac vessels and lymphatics from the iliopectineal fascia by blunt dissection and gently retract them medially.
- Elevate the iliopectineal fascia from the underlying iliopsoas and divide it sharply with scissors down to the pectineal eminence (Fig. 1.97F,G); continue the dissection laterally beneath the iliopsoas until the muscle and surrounding fascia are freed from the underlying pelvic brim.

Pass a Penrose drain beneath the iliopsoas, femoral nerve, and lateral femoral cutaneous nerve for use as a retractor.
- Using blunt finger dissection, begin mobilizing the external iliac vessels and lymphatics, working from lateral to medial. Search for the obturator artery and nerve medial and posterior to the vessels. Occasionally, the obturator artery or vein has an anomalous anastomosis with the external iliac or inferior epigastric artery or vein
- This is known as the *corona mortis*, or "crown of death," because if it is accidentally cut hemostasis is difficult to achieve. If the anomalous obturator vessel is present, clamp, ligate, and divide it to avoid an avulsive traction injury. Place a third Penrose drain around the external iliac vessels and lymphatics. Leave the areolar tissue surrounding the vessels and lymphatics intact.

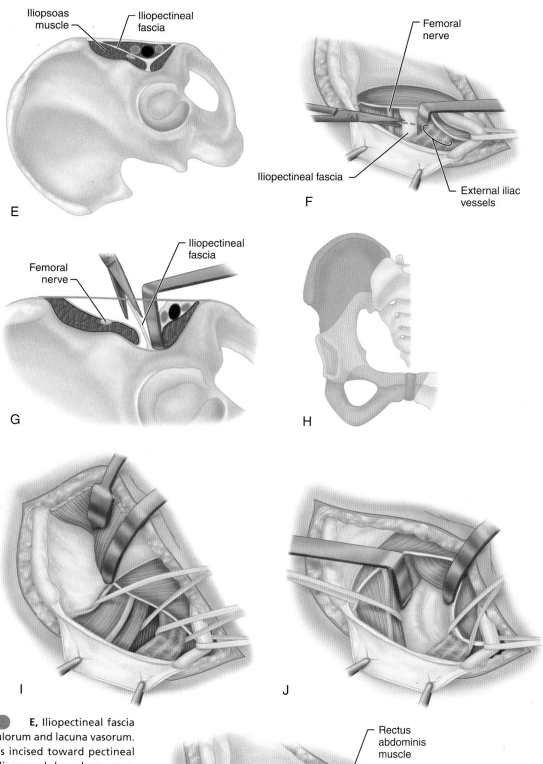

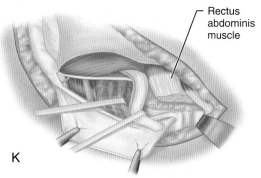

FIGURE 1.97, Cont'd **E,** Iliopectineal fascia separates lacuna musculorum and lacuna vasorum. **F,** Iliopectineal fascia is incised toward pectineal eminence. **G,** Internal iliac vessels have been separated and retracted medially from iliopectineal fascia. **H,** Three regions of pelvis exposed during approach. **I,** Lateral femoral cutaneous nerve, iliopsoas, and femoral nerve have been retracted medially to expose internal iliac fossa. **J,** Pelvic brim and pectineal eminence have been exposed by lateral retraction of iliopsoas and femoral nerve and medial retraction of external iliac vessels. **K,** Medial aspect of superior pubic ramus and pubic symphysis have been exposed by release of rectus abdominis and lateral retraction of external iliac vessels and spermatic cord or round ligament. **SEE TECHNIQUE 1.77.**

- To expose the internal iliac fossa and adjacent pelvic brim, retract the iliopsoas and femoral nerve medially. Continue elevation of the iliacus muscle subperiosteally to the quadrilateral surface of the pelvis as necessary. Avoid injuring the internal iliac and gluteal vessels as the dissection is continued proximally along the quadrilateral space (Fig. 1.97H,I). To increase the exposure of the superior pubic ramus, retract the iliac vessels laterally and release the origin of the pectineus muscle.
- To obtain access to the entire pelvic brim distally to the lateral aspect of the superior pubic ramus, the anterior wall of the acetabulum, the quadrilateral surface, and the superior aspect of the obturator foramen, retract the iliopsoas and femoral nerve laterally and the external iliac vessels medially (Fig. 1.97J). To gain access to the superior aspect of the obturator foramen and the superior pubic ramus, retract the external iliac vessels laterally and the spermatic cord or round ligament medially. During retraction of the external iliac vessels in either direction, check the pulse of the internal iliac artery frequently and lessen the traction force if the pulse is interrupted. To obtain access to the medial aspect of the superior pubic ramus and symphysis pubis, retract the spermatic cord or round ligament laterally (Fig. 1.97K).
- If necessary, release the inguinal ligament and sartorius muscle from the anterior superior iliac spine and elevate the tensor fasciae latae and gluteal muscles from the external surface of the iliac wing.
- In repairing a pelvic fracture, preserve all substantial muscular attachments to the fracture fragments to avoid devitalizing the bone.
- Before wound closure, insert suction drains into the retropubic space and internal iliac fossa overlying the quadrilateral space.
- Reattach the abdominal fascia to the fascia lata on the iliac crest with heavy sutures.
- Reattach the tendon of the rectus abdominis to the periosteum of the pubis.
- Reattach the transversalis fascia and the internal oblique and transversus abdominis muscles to the inguinal ligament.
- Repair the iliopectineal fascia that separates the iliopsoas from the fascia of the rectus abdominis and the aponeurosis of the external oblique.

ILIOFEMORAL APPROACH TO THE ACETABULUM

The Letournel and Judet anterior ilioinguinal approach can be used in a bilateral fashion for extensile exposure of the entire anterior half of the pelvic ring, symphysis pubis, iliac fossae, and the anterior aspects of both sacroiliac joints. The skin incision described in Figure 1.97 is carried across the opposite superior pubic ramus to the anterior superior iliac spine and then posteriorly along the iliac crest (Fig. 1.98). The insertions of both rectus abdominis muscles are released. The remainder of the exposure is developed as described in the unilateral ilioinguinal approach.

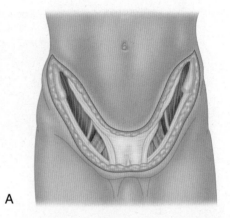

A

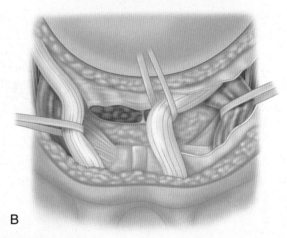

B

FIGURE 1.98 Bilateral ilioinguinal approach. **A,** Skin incision and deep dissection have been performed as described for unilateral ilioinguinal approach (Fig. 1.97). **B,** Insertions of both rectus abdominis muscles have been released, and symphysis and superior pubic rami have been exposed.

Letournel modified and improved the Smith-Petersen, or iliofemoral, approach. The muscles on the inner wall of the ilium are elevated to gain access to the anterior column directly within the pelvis.

TECHNIQUE 1.78

(LETOURNEL AND JUDET)
- Begin the skin incision at the middle of the iliac crest. Carry it anteriorly over the anterior superior iliac spine and distally along the medial border of the sartorius to the middle third of the anterior thigh (Fig. 1.99A).
- Divide the superficial and deep fascia.
- Develop the interval between the tensor fasciae latae laterally and the sartorius medially, exposing the rectus femoris.
- Divide the sartorius at its attachment to the anterior superior iliac spine.
- Divide the external branch of the lateral femoral cutaneous nerve.
- Incise the anterior abdominal musculature from the iliac crest and reflect it medially.

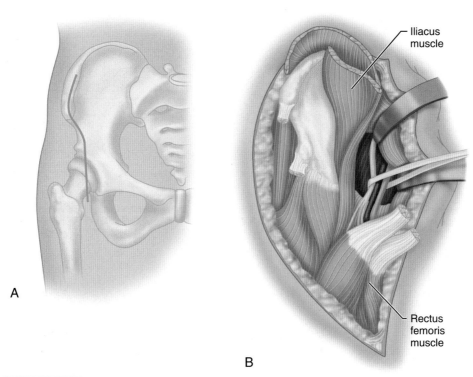

Iliacus muscle

Rectus femoris muscle

A

B

FIGURE 1.99　Letournel and Judet iliofemoral approach. **A,** Skin incision. **B,** Anterior aspect of hip joint and anterior column are exposed by releasing sartorius and rectus femoris and reflecting iliacus medially. **SEE TECHNIQUE 1.78.**

- Expose the iliac fossa by elevating the iliacus muscle (Fig. 1.99B). Carefully protect the femoral nerve and vessels and the remaining branches of the lateral femoral cutaneous nerve that lie just medial to the plane of the dissection.
- Detach both origins of the rectus femoris and reflect the muscle medially to expose the anterior surface of the hip joint capsule and anterior wall of the acetabulum. The iliopsoas tendon can be divided to provide more access to the anterior column. Preserve the musculature on the external surface of the iliac wing in this approach. Further reflection of the iliacus and abdominal musculature posteriorly and medially allows exposure of the inner wall of the ilium to the sacroiliac joint. Anteriorly, the superior pubic ramus can be exposed but the symphysis pubis cannot.

POSTERIOR APPROACHES TO THE ACETABULUM

The combination of the Kocher approach and the Langenbeck approach, described as the Kocher-Langenbeck posterior approach by Letournel and Judet, provides access to the posterior wall and posterior column of the acetabulum.

Gibson modified this approach by moving the superior limb of the incision more anteriorly (see Technique 1.80). Moed further described a modification of the Gibson approach that uses a straight lateral incision and approach that preserve the neurovascular supply to the anterior portion of the gluteus maximus muscle and allow more anterosuperior exposure of the acetabulum and iliac wing. As with the Kocher-Langenbeck technique, this approach is useful for

the treatment of posterior wall, posterior column, and certain transverse and T-type acetabular fractures. For more complex fracture types, it can be performed with the patient prone.

KOCHER-LANGENBECK APPROACH

TECHNIQUE 1.79

(KOCHER-LANGENBECK; LETOURNEL AND JUDET)
- Place the patient in the lateral position with the affected hip uppermost. If a fracture table and a supracondylar femoral traction pin are used, keep the knee joint in at least 45 degrees of flexion to prevent excessive traction on the sciatic nerve.
- Begin the skin incision over the greater trochanter and extend it proximally to within 6 cm of the posterior superior iliac spine (Fig. 1.100A). The incision can be extended distally over the lateral surface of the thigh for approximately 10 cm as necessary.
- Divide the fascia lata in line with the skin incision and bluntly split the gluteus maximus in line with its muscle fibers for a distance of no more than 7 cm (Fig. 1.100B), protecting the branch of the inferior gluteal nerve to the anterosuperior portion of the gluteus maximus to avoid denervating that part of the muscle.
- Identify and protect the sciatic nerve overlying the quadratus femoris (Fig. 1.100C). Incise the short external rotators at their tendinous insertions on the greater

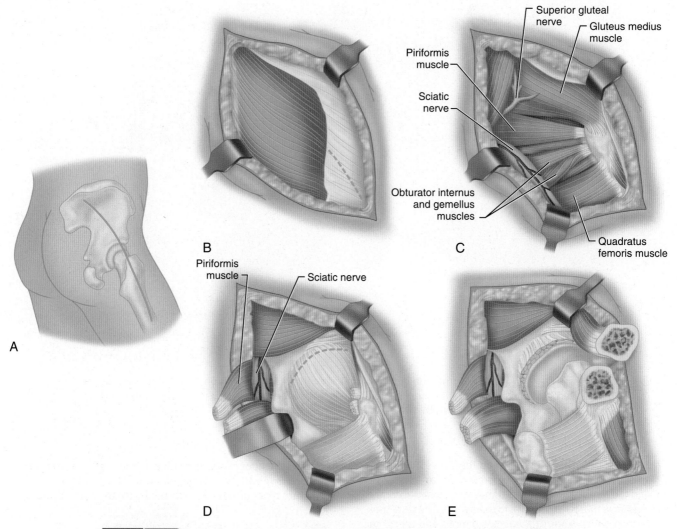

FIGURE **1.100**   Kocher-Langenbeck posterior approach. **A,** Skin incision. **B,** Incision of fascia lata and splitting of gluteus maximus outlined. **C,** Gluteus maximus has been retracted, exposing short external rotators, sciatic nerve, and superior gluteal vessels. Ascending branch of medial circumflex femoral artery underlies obturator externus and quadratus femoris. **D,** Hip joint capsule has been exposed by division and posterior reflection of short external rotators. Quadratus femoris and obturator externus are left intact to protect the ascending branch of the medial circumflex artery. **E,** Osteotomy of greater trochanter and reflection of hamstring origins from ischial tuberosity have enlarged exposure. **SEE TECHNIQUE 1.79.**

trochanter and reflect them medially to protect the sciatic nerve further (Fig. 1.100D). Leave the quadratus femoris and obturator externus intact to protect the underlying ascending branch of the medial circumflex femoral artery. The tendinous insertion of the gluteus maximus on the femur can be incised to increase exposure.

■ Elevate the gluteus medius and minimus subperiosteally from the posterior and lateral ilium. Retraction of these muscles can be maintained by inserting two smooth Steinmann pins into the ilium above the greater sciatic notch. Identify and protect the superior gluteal nerve and vessels as they exit the greater sciatic notch. The entire posterior acetabulum and posterior column are now exposed. Further exposure can be gained by an os-

teotomy of the greater trochanter and reflection of the origins of the hamstrings from the ischial tuberosity (Fig. 1.100E).

■ Reattach the greater trochanter with two 6.5-mm lag screws during wound closure.

MODIFIED GIBSON APPROACH

As with the Kocher-Langenbeck approach, this approach is useful for the treatment of posterior wall, posterior column, and certain transverse and T-type acetabular fractures. For more complex fracture types it can be performed with the patient prone.

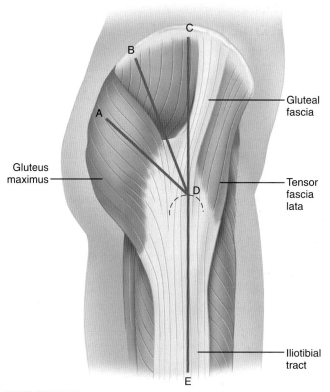

FIGURE 1.101 Modified Kocher approach as described by Gibson. Greater trochanter is dotted line. ADE is the Kocher-Langenbeck incision. BDE is Gibson's original incision. CDE is Moed's modification of the approach. (Redrawn from Moed BR: The modified Gibson posterior surgical approach to the acetabulum, *J Orthop Trauma* 24:315, 2010.) **SEE TECHNIQUE 1.80.**

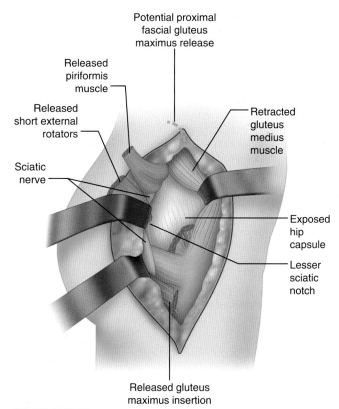

FIGURE 1.102 Deep dissection with gluteus maximus muscle reflected posterior and a retractor in the lesser sciatic notch. Retract the gluteus medius muscle in an anterior direction to expose the hip joint. (Redrawn from Moed BR: The modified Gibson posterior surgical approach to the acetabulum, *J Orthop Trauma* 24:315, 2010.) **SEE TECHNIQUE 1.80.**

TECHNIQUE 1.80

(MODIFIED GIBSON APPROACH, MOED)
- Position the patient in the lateral decubitus position as one would for a Kocher-Langenbeck approach (see Technique 1.79).
- Make a longitudinal incision beginning at the iliac crest, continuing it over the greater trochanter and down the lateral thigh as far as necessary (Fig. 1.101).
- Dissect through the subcutaneous tissue until the iliotibial band and gluteus maximus muscle fascia are reached.
- Identify the anterior border of the gluteus maximus muscle by identifying the branches of the inferior gluteal artery that run in the fascia between the gluteus maximus and gluteus medius muscles. Do not split the gluteus maximus as in the Kocher-Langenbeck approach.
- Release the anterior border of the gluteus maximus, leaving an anterior fascial end for later repair. Release it from the level of the greater trochanter to the level of the iliac crest. Preserve the neurovascular supply to the anterior gluteus maximus.
- Retract the gluteus medius in an anterior direction and the gluteus maximus in a posterior direction. Release the gluteus maximus insertion on the posterior femur if necessary. Release the posterosuperior origin and fascia from the iliac crest as needed.

- Release the piriformis and short external rotators. Leave the obturator externus and quadratus externus intact to protect the medial circumflex femoral artery (Fig. 1.102).

EXTENSILE ACETABULAR APPROACHES
Because complete exposure of anterior and posterior columns of the acetabulum requires separate anterior and posterior approaches, several surgeons developed extensile approaches to the acetabulum to avoid the problems encountered when using these separate approaches. Included here are the approaches that my colleagues and I have found most useful.

EXTENSILE ILIOFEMORAL APPROACH

Letournel developed an extended iliofemoral approach that provides complete exposure of the inner and outer table of the ilium, acetabulum, and anterior and posterior columns. It requires incision, however, of the origins and insertions of the gluteus minimus and medius from the iliac crest and the greater trochanter. Great care should be taken to avoid damaging the superior gluteal vessels to prevent ischemic necrosis of the hip abductors. In the presence of a fracture through the greater sciatic notch and arteriographic evidence of damage to the superior gluteal vessels, this approach should not be used.

TECHNIQUE 1.81

(LETOURNEL AND JUDET)

- Place the patient in the lateral position on a fracture table if distal femoral traction is necessary. If traction is not necessary, a standard operating table can be used. Keep the knee joint flexed more than 45 degrees to avoid excessive traction on the sciatic nerve.
- Begin the incision at the posterior superior iliac spine and extend it along the iliac crest, over the anterior superior iliac spine, and carry it distally halfway down the anterolateral aspect of the thigh (Fig. 1.103A).
- Elevate the gluteal muscles and the tensor fasciae latae from the outer table of the iliac wing as far anteriorly as the anterior superior iliac spine. Division of some of the posterior branches of the lateral femoral cutaneous nerve is inevitable, but protect the main trunk of the nerve.
- Open the fascia covering the greater trochanter and vastus lateralis longitudinally.
- Isolate, ligate, and divide the lateral femoral circumflex artery (Fig. 1.103B).
- Continue the dissection posteriorly to the greater sciatic notch. Carefully identify and protect the superior gluteal vessels and nerve.
- Divide the tendons of the gluteus minimus and medius, dissect these muscles from the hip joint capsule, and reflect them posteriorly (Fig. 1.30C).
- Divide the tendons of the piriformis and obturator internus at their insertions on the greater trochanter and elevate these muscles from the hip joint capsule. The sciatic nerve exits the greater sciatic foramen beneath the piriformis muscle and must be protected. A retractor can be placed in the greater sciatic notch; gentle retraction exposes the posterior column (Fig. 1.103D). Avoid a traction injury to the sciatic nerve in this exposure. Leave the quadratus femoris muscle intact to protect the ascending branch of the medial circumflex femoral artery.
- Open the hip joint by a capsulotomy around the rim of the acetabulum.
- Exposure of the internal surface of the ilium and anterior column proceeds as in a routine iliofemoral approach.
- Elevate the abdominal muscles and iliacus from the iliac crest of the ilium and divide the attachments of the sartorius and inguinal ligament subperiosteally from the anterior superior iliac spine. Divide the origins of the direct and reflected heads of the rectus femoris to expose the anterior portion of the hip joint capsule (Fig. 1.103E).
- During wound closure, reattach the rectus femoris, sartorius, fascial layers of the hip abductor musculature, and tensor fasciae latae to the iliac wing with sutures passed through the bone.
- Repair the gluteus minimus and medius tendons anatomically.
- Reattach the tendons of the piriformis and obturator internus to the greater trochanter also with transosseous sutures.

EXTENSILE ILIOFEMORAL APPROACH

Reinert et al. developed a modification of the Letournel and Judet extended iliofemoral approach designed to allow later reconstructive procedures. It provides exposure for repair of complex and both-column acetabular fractures. The skin incision is positioned more laterally. Also, the hip abductors are mobilized by osteotomies of their origins and insertions. Rigid bone-to-bone reattachment of these muscles permits early rehabilitation with less risk of failure than when the abductors are reattached through soft tissue. As with the extended iliofemoral approach, the patency of the superior gluteal artery is necessary to avoid necrosis of the hip abductors. In the presence of a displaced fracture at the sciatic notch, a preoperative arteriogram is recommended. If a later reconstructive procedure is required, the same operative site can be approached using part or all of the same skin incision as necessary.

TECHNIQUE 1.82

(REINERT ET AL.)

- Place the patient in the lateral position. Drape the lower extremity free on the side of the pelvic injury.
- Begin the skin incision 2 cm posterior to the anterior superior iliac spine and carry it posteriorly along the iliac crest for 8 to 12 cm. Make the vertical limb of the T-shaped incision by incising from the midportion of the iliac crest incision in a curvilinear fashion down the lateral aspect of the thigh to a point 15 cm distal to the greater trochanter (Fig. 1.104A).
- Develop the anterior flap by dissecting the subcutaneous tissue from the deep fascia until the anterior superior iliac spine and the interval between the sartorius and tensor fasciae latae muscles are reached. Protect the lateral femoral cutaneous nerve. Develop the posterior flap in the same fashion.
- Flex the hip to 45 degrees and abduct it. Incise the fascia lata longitudinally from the center of the greater trochanter distally to a point 2 cm distal to the insertion of the tensor fasciae latae muscle.
- Incise the gluteal fascia and bluntly split the gluteus maximus in line with its fibers until the inferior gluteal nerve and vessels are encountered.
- Divide the anterior portion of the fascia lata transversely 2 cm distal to the insertion of the tensor fasciae latae muscle. Release the proximal portion of the gluteus maximus insertion on the femur.
- Bluntly develop the interval between the tensor fasciae latae and the sartorius.
- Continue the deep dissection anterior and posterior to the tensor fasciae latae, separating it from the sartorius and the rectus femoris.
- Carefully identify, ligate, and divide the ascending branch of the lateral femoral circumflex artery in the proximal part of the dissection. Microvascular reanastomosis of this artery can be used as a substitute to restore collateral circulation to the hip abductors should the superior gluteal artery be severely damaged during the procedure.

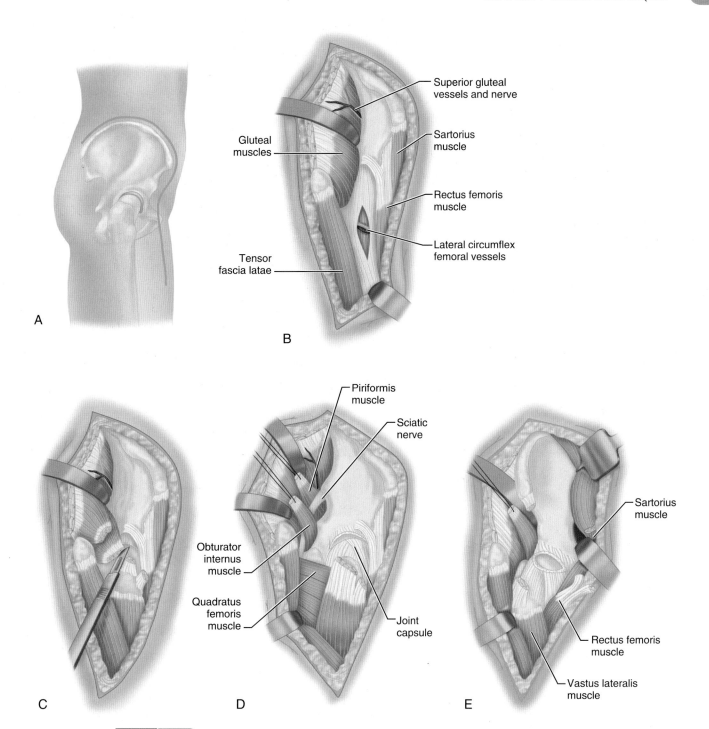

FIGURE 1.103 Letournel and Judet extended iliofemoral approach. **A,** Skin incision. **B,** Gluteal muscles and tensor fasciae latae have been partially elevated and retracted posteriorly. Lateral femoral circumflex vessels have been isolated. **C,** Tendon of gluteus minimus has been completely severed from anterior aspect of greater trochanter. Gluteus medius tendon has been partially incised. **D,** Reflection of piriformis, obturator internus, and gluteal muscles has exposed external surface of innominate bone. **E,** Internal surface of ilium and anterior acetabulum and hip joint have been exposed by reflection of iliacus, sartorius, and rectus femoris (see text). **SEE TECHNIQUE 1.81.**

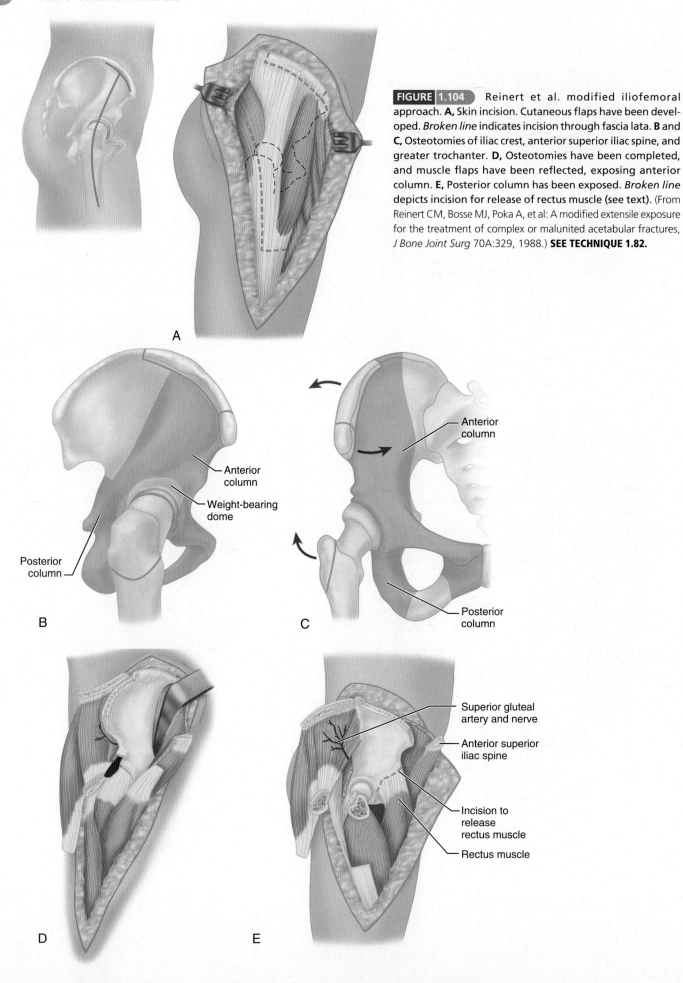

FIGURE 1.104 Reinert et al. modified iliofemoral approach. **A,** Skin incision. Cutaneous flaps have been developed. *Broken line* indicates incision through fascia lata. **B** and **C,** Osteotomies of iliac crest, anterior superior iliac spine, and greater trochanter. **D,** Osteotomies have been completed, and muscle flaps have been reflected, exposing anterior column. **E,** Posterior column has been exposed. *Broken line* depicts incision for release of rectus muscle (see text). (From Reinert CM, Bosse MJ, Poka A, et al: A modified extensile exposure for the treatment of complex or malunited acetabular fractures, *J Bone Joint Surg* 70A:329, 1988.) **SEE TECHNIQUE 1.82.**

- Elevate the abdominal and iliacus muscles from the iliac crest subperiosteally. Extend the dissection posteriorly to expose the anterior aspect of the sacroiliac joint and sciatic notch as necessary.
- Perform an osteotomy of the anterior superior iliac spine and reflect the attached sartorius and inguinal ligament medially, along with the abdominal and iliacus muscles.
- With an osteotome or 90-degree power cutting tool, perform an osteotomy of the tricortical portion of the iliac crest beginning along the inner table and producing a fragment 10 to 12 cm long and 1.5 cm wide (Fig. 1.104B,C). Leave the hip abductor muscles attached to the fragment, and reflect this musculo-osseous flap laterally.
- Elevate the abductors subperiosteally from the outer table of the ilium during this reflection. Carefully preserve the superior gluteal nerve and vessels.
- Perform a standard trochanteric osteotomy and release the abductors from the hip joint capsule.
- Carefully reflect the abductors and attached greater trochanter posteriorly (Fig. 1.104D,E). Release the short external rotators from the greater trochanter. The quadratus femoris is preserved, protecting the ascending branch of the medial circumflex femoral artery.
- Identify and protect the sciatic nerve. Further avoid traction injury to the sciatic nerve by maintaining the hip extended and the knee flexed to at least 45 degrees.
- If further anterior exposure is needed, release the direct and reflected heads of the rectus femoris (Fig. 1.104E). Incise the hip joint capsule circumferentially at the acetabular labrum.
- During closure, reattach the origins of the rectus femoris with heavy sutures through holes drilled in the anterior inferior iliac spine.
- Repair all osteotomies with lag-screw fixation.
- Repair the fascia lata and reattach the iliacus and abdominal muscles to the iliac crest with heavy sutures.

TRIRADIATE EXTENSILE APPROACH TO THE ACETABULUM

Mears and Rubash modified Charnley's initial total hip arthroplasty approach and developed an extensile acetabular approach providing access to the acetabulum, the anterior and posterior columns, the inner iliac wall, the anterior aspect of the sacroiliac joint, and the outer aspect of the innominate bone. This triradiate approach was developed for reduction and repair of complex acetabular fractures. It avoids the potential complication of massive ischemic necrosis of the hip abductors caused by injury to the superior gluteal vessels, which is a possibility when the extended iliofemoral approach is used.

TECHNIQUE 1.83

(MEARS AND RUBASH)
- Place the patient in the lateral position on a conventional operating table. A fracture table can be used if skeletal traction is necessary. Keep the knee joint in at least 45 degrees of flexion to avoid excessive traction on the sciatic nerve.
- Begin the longitudinal portion of the triradiate incision at the tip of the greater trochanter and carry it distally 6 to 8 cm. Carry the anterosuperior limb from the tip of the greater trochanter across the anterior superior iliac spine. Begin the posterosuperior limb of the incision at the tip of the greater trochanter as well, and carry it to the posterior superior iliac spine, forming an angle of approximately 120 degrees (Fig. 1.105A).
- Divide the fascia lata in line with its fibers in the longitudinal limb of the incision.
- Incise the fascia lata and fascial covering of the tensor fasciae latae in line with the anterosuperior limb of the incision (Fig. 1.105B).
- Dissect the anterior border of the tensor fasciae latae from its overlying fascia and elevate the origin of the muscle from the iliac crest. Elevate subperiosteally from the iliac crest the origins of the gluteus medius and minimus from anterior to posterior and distally to the hip joint capsule.
- Incise the fascia of the gluteus maximus in line with the posterosuperior limb of the incision and split the muscle in line with its fibers (Fig. 1.105C).
- Perform an osteotomy of the greater trochanter and reflect the trochanter with the attached insertions of the gluteus medius and minimus proximally.
- Sharply elevate the gluteus medius and minimus from the capsule of the hip joint, preserving the capsule during the dissection. Continue the dissection to the greater sciatic notch and identify and protect the superior gluteal vessels (Fig. 1.105D).
- Divide the insertions of the short external rotators on the proximal femur, including the upper third of the quadratus femoris. Leave intact the remainder of this muscle and the underlying ascending branch of the medial circumflex femoral artery.
- Reflect the divided short external rotators posteriorly to expose the posterior aspect of the hip joint capsule and the posterior column.
- Maintain the exposure of the posterior column by carefully inserting blunt Hohmann retractors into the greater and lesser sciatic notches.
- Secure the abductor muscles superiorly by inserting two Steinmann pins into the ilium 2.5 cm and 5 cm above the greater sciatic notch (Fig. 1.105E).
- Sharply incise the origins of the hamstrings to expose the ischial tuberosity.
- To expose the anterior column and inner table of the ilium, extend the anterosuperior limb of the skin incision 6 to 8 cm medial to the anterior superior iliac crest.
- Incise the abdominal musculature from the anterior iliac crest and elevate subperiosteally the iliacus muscle from the inner table of the ilium. Continue the dissection posteriorly to expose the anterior aspect of the sacroiliac joint (Fig. 1.105F).
- To increase the exposure further, divide the origin of the sartorius from the anterior superior iliac spine and the origins of the direct and reflected heads of the rectus femoris from the anterior inferior iliac spine and hip joint capsule.

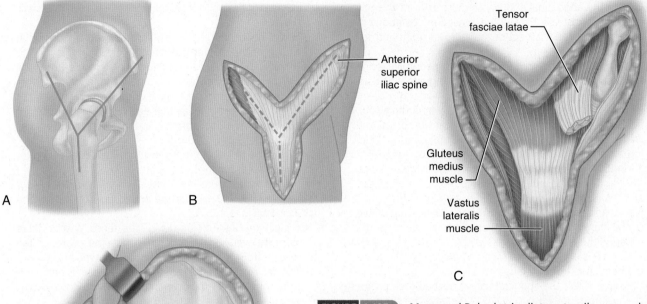

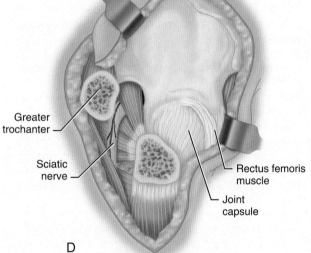

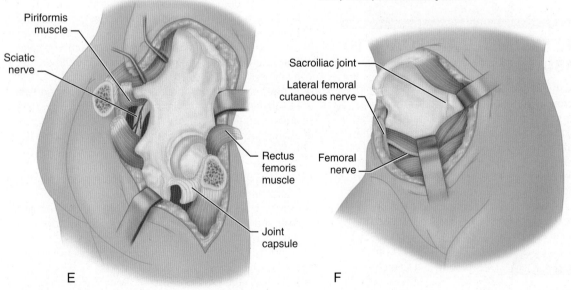

FIGURE **1.105** Mears and Rubash triradiate extensile approach. **A,** Skin incision. **B,** Superficial fascial incision. **C,** Origin of tensor fasciae latae has been elevated from anterior iliac crest. Gluteus maximus has been split in line with its fibers up to inferior gluteal nerve and vessels. **D,** Greater trochanter has been osteotomized and reflected posteriorly exposing sciatic nerve and short external rotators. Gluteal and tensor fasciae latae muscles have been elevated from outer table of ilium and hip joint capsule and reflected posteriorly. **E,** Short external rotators have been severed from greater trochanter and reflected posteriorly. Quadratus femoris remains intact. Gluteal and tensor fasciae latae muscles have been retracted superiorly and held with Steinmann pins to expose posterior column. Joint capsule has been severed circumferentially from acetabulum. **F,** Abdominal muscles have been incised and iliacus muscle elevated subperiosteally from ilium and reflected medially to expose inner table of ilium (see text and also Fig. 1.103). (Modified from Mears DC, Rubash HE: Pelvic and acetabular fractures, Thorofare, NJ, Slack, 1986.) **SEE TECHNIQUE 1.83.**

- Incise the aponeurosis of the external oblique muscle 1 cm proximal to the external inguinal ring and in line with the inguinal ligament as described for the ilioinguinal approach (see Technique 1.77).
- Carefully develop the interval between the external iliac vessels medially and the psoas muscle laterally. Next, develop the interval between the external iliac vessels and the spermatic cord or round ligament (Fig. 1.105B-F).
- Use the longitudinal intervals developed and expose subperiosteally the superior pubic ramus and quadrilateral surface of the pelvis.
- Incise the joint capsule of the hip circumferentially at the edge of the acetabulum as far anteriorly and posteriorly as necessary, but leave the acetabular labrum intact.
- During closure, reattach the abdominal fascia to the fascia lata along the iliac crest with heavy sutures.
- Reattach the gluteal muscle origins and the tensor fasciae latae to the iliac crest.
- Drill small holes in the ilium and use heavy sutures to reattach the origins of the rectus femoris and sartorius muscles.
- Repair the trochanteric osteotomy with two long 6.5-mm cancellous screws with washers.
- Close the three fascial limbs of the triradiate incision, beginning with a single apical suture.
- Complete the closure of each limb of the incision.

EXTENSILE APPROACH TO THE ACETABULUM

Carnesale combined Henry's reflection of the gluteus maximus with several other approaches to the hip joint to form an extensile approach for open reduction of complex acetabular fractures. The posterior or anterior part of the approach may be used alone as indicated in the given instance; the entire approach is rarely required.

TECHNIQUE 1.84

(CARNESALE)
- Secure the patient on the uninjured side on a standard operating table so that the table may be tilted to either side.
- Prepare the skin from the middle of the rib cage to below the knee.
- Drape to allow free manipulation of the extremity.
- Start the skin incision at the posterior superior iliac spine, extend it anteriorly parallel to the iliac crest, and end it just proximal to the anterior superior iliac spine (Fig. 1.106A). If the anterior part of the approach is to be used, extend the incision into the groin crease (see Fig. 1.106G). Perpendicular to this transverse incision, incise the skin distally in the lateral midline of the thigh, cross the center of the greater trochanter, and at the gluteal fold turn the incision 90 degrees posteriorly and extend it to the posterior midline of the thigh; if necessary, extend it distally in the posterior midline of the thigh for 4 or 5 cm.
- Raise appropriate flaps of skin, investing fascia anteriorly and posteriorly (Fig. 1.106B).

- Reflect the gluteus maximus, leaving it attached medially at its pelvic origin as described by Henry as follows:
- In the distal part of the incision, locate the posterior cutaneous nerve of the thigh just beneath the deep fascia. Open this fascia and trace the nerve to the distal edge of the gluteus maximus; the nerve will be freed from the muscle later.
- Free the femoral side of the gluteus maximus by longitudinally splitting the part of the iliotibial band that slides on the femoral shaft and greater trochanter.
- Extend the incision in the iliotibial band slightly proximally; at this point, insert a finger, locate the superior border of the gluteus maximus where it joins the iliotibial band, and, with the scissors, free this border of the muscle proximal to the iliac crest (Fig. 1.106C,D).
- Raise the distal edge of the gluteus maximus and the posterior cutaneous nerve of the thigh, and divide the thick insertion of the muscle from the femur. Control the constant vessel found at this insertion.
- Detach the posterior cutaneous nerve of the thigh from the deep surface of the gluteus maximus and gently reflect the muscle medially, hinged on its pelvic attachment (Fig. 1.106E).
- Detach the short external rotators from the greater trochanter, reflect them medially, and strip them subperiosteally from the ilium sufficiently to expose the posterior acetabular wall. If more superior exposure of the acetabulum is required, osteotomize the greater trochanter, and with it reflect the hip abductors proximally (Fig. 1.106F).
- In fractures of the anterior aspect of the acetabulum, continue the skin incision anteriorly to the groin crease as already described (Fig. 1.106G).
- Locate the lateral femoral cutaneous nerve and preserve it (Fig. 1.106H).
- Detach the inguinal ligament, sartorius, and rectus femoris from the pelvis, but leave the tensor fasciae latae intact (Fig. 1.106I).
- Strip subperiosteally the iliacus and, if necessary, the obturator internus from the medial pelvic wall, exposing the anterior aspect of the acetabulum (Fig. 1.106J).

ILIUM

APPROACH TO THE ILIUM
TECHNIQUE 1.85

- Incise the skin along the iliac crest from the anterior superior spine to the posterior superior spine.
- Reflect the attachments of the gluteal muscles subperiosteally, proximally to distally, as far as the superior rim of the acetabulum, and expose the lateral surface of the ilium.
- Reflect subperiosteally the attachment of the abdominal muscles from the iliac crest, or osteotomize the crest, leaving the abdominal muscles attached to the superior fragment. In children, make the osteotomy of the crest inferior to the epiphyseal plate. Reflect subperiosteally the iliacus muscle from the medial surface of the ilium. Also, divide at their origins the structures attached to the

anterior superior spine and the anterior border of the ilium. Most of the ilium can be denuded.

- In this procedure, a nutrient artery on the lateral surface of the ilium 5 cm inferior to the crest and near the juncture of the anterior and middle thirds is divided. Because ligating it is impossible, control the bleeding with the point of a small hemostat or, if necessary, with bone wax.

SYMPHYSIS PUBIS

APPROACH TO THE SYMPHYSIS PUBIS

TECHNIQUE 1.86

(PFANNENSTIEL)
- Place the patient supine and insert a Foley catheter for intraoperative identification of the base of the bladder and the urethra.

- Make a curvilinear transverse incision 2 cm cephalad to the superior pubic ramus (Fig. 1.107A).
- Incise the external oblique aponeurosis parallel to the inguinal ligament.
- Identify the spermatic cords or round ligaments and adjacent ilioinguinal nerves. Release the aponeurotic insertion of both heads of the rectus abdominis from the superior pubic ramus (Fig. 1.107B).
- Expose subperiosteally the superior, anterior, and posterior surfaces of both rami laterally for 4 to 5 cm as necessary (Fig. 1.107C). During this dissection, identify the urethra and base of the bladder by manual palpation of the Foley catheter.
- During wound closure, insert a suction drain into the retropubic space and repair the rectus abdominis with heavy interrupted sutures.
- Carefully repair the external oblique aponeurosis to prevent an inguinal hernia.

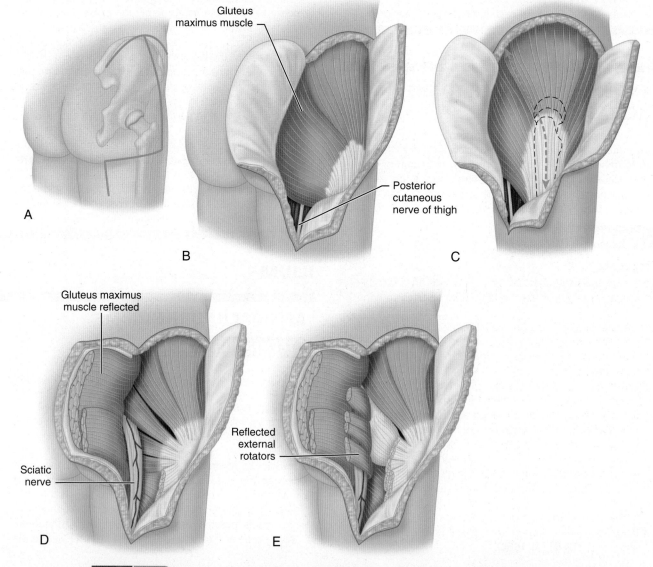

FIGURE 1.106 **A-J,** Carnesale extensile exposure of acetabulum (see text). **SEE TECHNIQUE 1.84.**

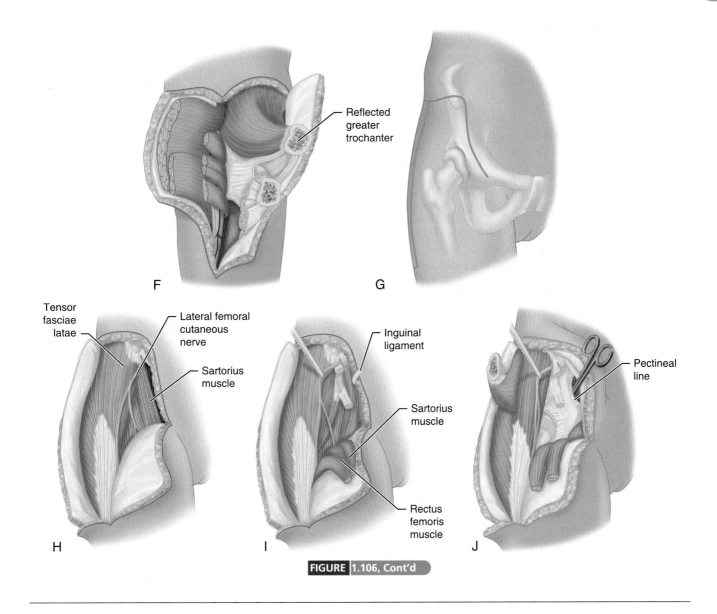

Reflected greater trochanter

F

G

Tensor fasciae latae

Lateral femoral cutaneous nerve

Sartorius muscle

H

Inguinal ligament

Sartorius muscle

Rectus femoris muscle

I

Pectineal line

J

FIGURE 1.106, Cont'd

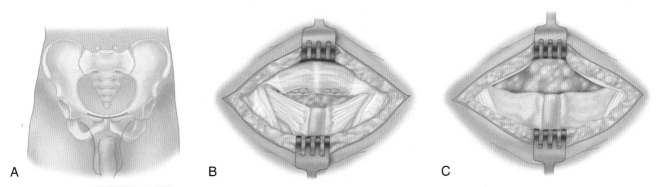

A

B

C

FIGURE 1.107 Pfannenstiel transverse approach to pubic symphysis. **A,** Skin incision. **B,** Rectus abdominis insertions have been released. **C,** Entire pubic symphysis has been exposed. **SEE TECHNIQUE 1.86.**

SACROILIAC JOINT

POSTERIOR APPROACH TO THE SACROILIAC JOINT

TECHNIQUE 1.87

- Make an incision along the lateral lip of the posterior third of the iliac crest to the posterior superior spine (Fig. 1.108A).
- Deepen the dissection down to the crest, separate the lumbodorsal fascia from it, detach and reflect medially the aponeurosis of the sacrospinalis muscle together with the periosteum, and expose the posterior margin of the sacroiliac joint. This exposure is ample for extraarticular fusion.
- To expose the articular surfaces of the joint for drainage or intraarticular fusion, continue the skin incision laterally and distally 5 to 8 cm from the posterior superior spine. Split the gluteus maximus muscle in line with its fibers, or incise its origin on the iliac crest, the aponeurosis of the sacrospinalis, and the sacrum, and reflect it laterally and distally to expose the posterior aspect of the ilium (Fig. 1.108B). Branches of the inferior gluteal nerve and artery may be present.
- To expose more of the ilium, reflect the gluteus medius anterolaterally. The gluteus medius cannot be reflected very far anteriorly because of the presence of the superior gluteal nerve and artery.
- With an osteotome, remove a full-thickness section of the ilium 1.5 to 2 cm wide, beginning at its posterior border between the posterior superior and posterior inferior spines and proceeding laterally and slightly cephalad

for 4 to 5 cm. The inferior border of this section roughly parallels the superior border of the greater sciatic notch.
- Exposure of the joint is limited by the size of the section removed.

ANTERIOR APPROACH TO THE SACROILIAC JOINT

Sometimes primary suppurative arthritis of the sacroiliac joint may localize anteriorly; Avila approaches this region by an intrapelvic route. This approach also is useful for open reduction and plating of sacroiliac joint dislocation.

TECHNIQUE 1.88

(AVILA)

- With the patient supine, make a 10- to 12-cm incision 1.5 cm proximal to and parallel with the iliac crest, beginning at the anterior superior iliac spine (Fig. 1.109).
- Dissect distally to the iliac crest and detach the abdominal muscles from it without disturbing the origin of the gluteal muscles.
- Incise the periosteum and strip the iliacus muscle subperiosteally, following the medial surface of the ilium medially and slightly distally.
- Retract the iliacus medially and complete the stripping by hand with the gloved finger covered with gauze. Proceed as far as the lateral attachments of the anterior sacroiliac ligament; detach them and palpate the joint.
- To expose the anterior aspect of the joint, extend the incision farther posteriorly in the intermuscular plane along the iliac crest.

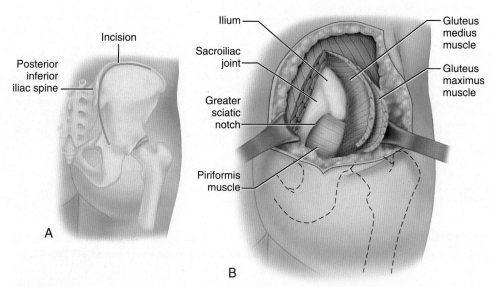

FIGURE 1.108 Posterior approach to the sacroiliac joint. **A,** Incision for the posterior approach to the sacroiliac joint is vertical from just above the posterior superior iliac spine distally about 1.0 cm. **B,** Deeper dissection involves incising the gluteus maximus fascia and subperiosteally elevating the maximus off of the ilium just lateral to the posterior superior iliac spine. **SEE TECHNIQUE 1.87.**

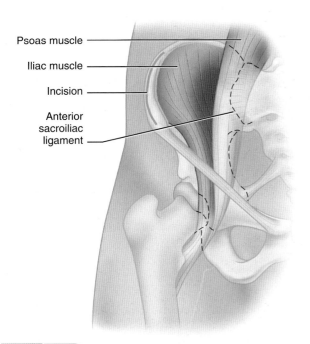

Psoas muscle

Iliac muscle

Incision

Anterior
sacroiliac
ligament

FIGURE 1.109 Anterior approach to the sacroiliac joint. **SEE TECHNIQUE 1.88.**

APPROACH TO BOTH SACROILIAC JOINTS OR SACRUM

When bilateral, unstable sacroiliac disruptions or comminuted vertical fractures of the sacrum occur as part of a pelvic ring disruption, Mears and Rubash approach these through a transverse incision made across the midportion of the sacrum. These injuries can be stabilized with a contoured reconstruction plate through this approach.

TECHNIQUE 1.89

(MODIFIED FROM MEARS AND RUBASH)

- With the patient prone, make a transverse straight incision across the midportion of the sacrum 1 cm inferior to the posterior superior iliac spines (Fig. 1.110A). If one or both of the sciatic nerves are to be explored, curve the ends of the incision distally to allow exposure of the sciatic nerves from the sacrum to the greater sciatic notch.
- Extend the incision through the deep fascia to expose the superior portions of the origins of both gluteus maximus muscles on the posterior superior iliac spines (Fig. 1.110B).
- Elevate the paraspinous muscles from the posterior superior iliac spine and perform an osteotomy of each spine

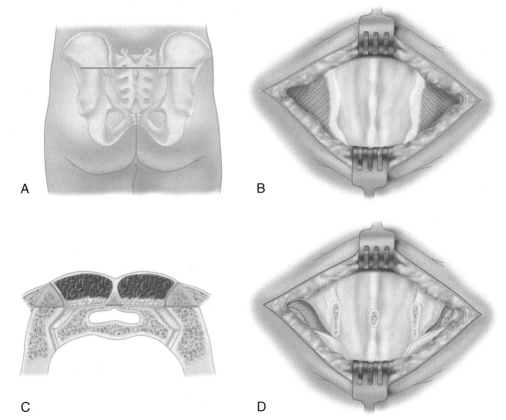

A

B

C

D

FIGURE 1.110 Exposure of both sacroiliac joints or sacrum. **A,** Skin incision. **B,** Posterior iliac crests, gluteus maximus muscles, and paraspinous muscles have been exposed. **C,** Outline of osteotomies of posterior superior iliac spines for application of plate and screws. **D,** Osteotomies have been performed, and gluteus maximus muscles have been reflected laterally. **SEE TECHNIQUE 1.89.**

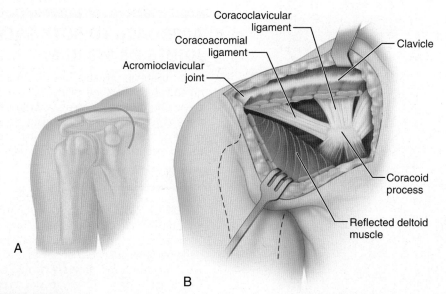

Coracoclavicular
ligament

Coracoacromial
ligament

Acromioclavicular
joint

Clavicle

Coracoid
process

Reflected deltoid
muscle

A

B

FIGURE 1.111 Roberts exposure of acromioclavicular joint and coracoid process of scapula. **A,** Skin incision. **B,** Deltoid muscle detached from clavicle and acromion, exposing acromioclavicular joint, and retracted distally for exposure of coracoid process. **SEE TECHNIQUE 1.91.**

posterior to the sacrum, from medial to lateral, leaving the origins of the gluteus maximus muscles intact (Fig. 1.110C,D). This provides a flat surface for application of a plate.

- Elevate the paraspinous muscles subperiosteally from the sacrum and adjacent posterosuperior iliac spines to provide a tunnel for application of a plate.
- Remove the tips of the spinous processes of the sacrum as necessary.
- If further exposure is necessary for drainage of a sacroiliac joint or intraarticular fusion, split the gluteus maximus muscle on that side or incise its origin from the posterior superior iliac spine, and reflect it laterally to expose the posterior aspect of the ilium.
- Perform a larger osteotomy of the posterior ilium as described for the standard posterior approach to the sacroiliac joint (see Technique 1.87).

SPINE

Surgical approaches to the spine are discussed in other chapter.

STERNOCLAVICULAR JOINT

Contrast computed tomography scans of mediastinal structures have shown that the brachiocephalic vein is the most frequent structure at risk for injury deep to the sternoclavicular joint. If a posterior dislocation is to be reduced or drill holes made in the sternum or medial clavicle during reconstructive procedures, consultation with a cardiothoracic surgeon is recommended.

APPROACH TO THE STERNOCLAVICULAR JOINT

TECHNIQUE 1.90

- Make an incision along the medial 4 cm of the clavicle and over the sternoclavicular joint to the midline of the sternum. Incise the fascia and periosteum.
- Reflect subperiosteally the origins of the sternocleidomastoid and pectoralis major muscles, the first superiorly and the second inferiorly; and expose the sternoclavicular joint.
- When the deep surface of the joint must be exposed, avoid puncturing the pleura or damaging an intrathoracic vessel.

ACROMIOCLAVICULAR JOINT AND CORACOID PROCESS

APPROACH TO THE ACROMIOCLAVICULAR JOINT AND CORACOID PROCESS

TECHNIQUE 1.91   *Figure 1.111*

(ROBERTS)
- Make a curved incision along the anterosuperior margin of the acromion and the lateral one fourth of the clavicle.

- Expose the origin of the deltoid, free it from the clavicle and the anterior margin of the acromion, and expose the capsule of the acromioclavicular joint. (By retracting the deltoid distally, the coracoid process also may be exposed.) To expose the acromioclavicular joint alone, use the lateral third of the incision.

SHOULDER
ANTEROMEDIAL APPROACHES TO THE SHOULDER

Any part of the approaches to the shoulder described can be used for operations on more limited regions around the shoulder.

ANTEROMEDIAL APPROACH TO THE SHOULDER

TECHNIQUE 1.92

(THOMPSON; HENRY)
- Begin the incision over the anterior aspect of the acromioclavicular joint, passing it medially along the anterior margin of the lateral one third of the clavicle and distally along the anterior margin of the deltoid muscle to a point two thirds the distance between its origin and insertion (Fig. 1.112A).
- Expose the anterior margin of the deltoid. The cephalic vein and the deltoid branches of the thoracoacromial artery lie in the interval between the deltoid and pectoralis major muscles (the deltopectoral groove), and although the cephalic vein may be retracted medially along with a few fibers of the deltoid muscle, it may be damaged during the operation. Ligating this vein proximally and distally as soon as it is reached may be indicated.
- Define the origin of the deltoid muscle on the clavicle; detach it by dividing it near the bone or at the bone together with the adjacent periosteum or by removing part of the bone intact with it (Fig. 1.112B). We prefer the first method, leaving enough soft tissue attached to the clavicle to allow suturing the deltoid to its origin later.
- Laterally reflect the anterior part of the deltoid muscle to expose the structures around the coracoid process and the anterior part of the joint capsule.
- To expose the deep aspects of the shoulder joint more easily, including the anterior margin of the glenoid, osteotomize the tip of the coracoid process. First, incise the periosteum of the superior aspect of the coracoid; next, cut through the bone and reflect medially and distally the tip of the bone along with the attached origins of the coracobrachialis, the pectoralis minor, and the short head of the biceps. Predrill the coracoid process.
- For wider exposure, divide the subscapularis at its musculotendinous junction about 2.5 cm medial to its insertion into the lesser humeral tuberosity; separate the tendon medially from the underlying capsule and expose the glenoid labrum.
- When closing the wound, replace the tip of the coracoid and secure with a screw.
- Suture the deltoid in place and close the wound in the usual way.
- If an extensile exposure is unnecessary, the skin incisions and deeper dissection may be limited to the deltopectoral

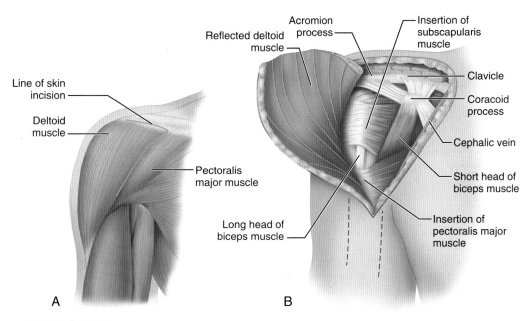

Line of skin incision
Deltoid muscle
Pectoralis major muscle
Long head of biceps muscle

Acromion process
Reflected deltoid muscle
Insertion of subscapularis muscle
Clavicle
Coracoid process
Cephalic vein
Short head of biceps muscle
Insertion of pectoralis major muscle

A   B

FIGURE 1.112   Anteromedial approach to shoulder joint. **A,** Skin incision. Transverse part of incision has been made along anterior border of clavicle and longitudinal part was made along interval between deltoid and pectoralis major. **B,** Deltoid has been detached from clavicle and reflected laterally to expose anterior aspect of joint. **SEE TECHNIQUE 1.92.**

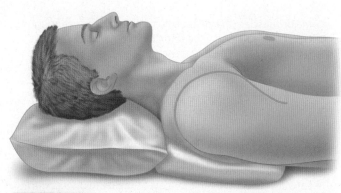

FIGURE 1.113   Henry shoulder strap or suspender incision. **SEE TECHNIQUE 1.92.**

portion of the approach. The anterior deltoid muscle need not be detached from the clavicle. Approach the joint anteriorly without an osteotomy of the coracoid process by retracting the short head of the biceps muscle in a medial direction. Take care to avoid a traction injury to the musculocutaneous nerve lying beneath the short head of the biceps in the distal part of this wound.

- Instead of this curved anteromedial approach, Henry later used an incision that arches like a shoulder strap over the shoulder from anterior to posterior (Fig. 1.113). The anterior part of this incision is similar to the deltopectoral part of his original approach, but at its superior end, it proceeds directly over the superior aspect of the shoulder and distally toward the spine of the scapula. Mobilize a lateral flap by dissecting between the subcutaneous tissues and the deep fascia, and expose the lateral and posterior margins of the acromion and adjacent spine of the scapula. Detach as much of the deltoid as needed to reach the deeper structures sought.

ANTEROMEDIAL/POSTEROMEDIAL APPROACH TO THE SHOULDER

If a wider field is needed, the anteromedial approach may be extended as Cubbins et al. suggest.

TECHNIQUE 1.93

(CUBBINS, CALLAHAN, AND SCUDERI)

- Make the anterior limb of the Cubbins incision similar to that in the anteromedial approach. Extend the incision laterally around the acromion and medially along the lateral half of the spine of the scapula (Fig. 1.114A).
- Detach the origin of the deltoid from the acromion and from the exposed part of the spine of the scapula and reflect the deltoid inferiorly and laterally to expose the anterior, superior, and posterior parts of the joint capsule.
- Reach the joint anteriorly or posteriorly by a corresponding incision of the capsule (Fig. 1.114B). To expose the articular surface of the humerus and the glenoid, incise the capsule continuously from anterior to posterior over

the head of the humerus (Fig. 1.114C); take care not to sever the tendon of the long head of the biceps. In this approach, the fibers of the deltoid are not divided and the axillary nerve that supplies the deltoid is not disturbed.

ANTERIOR AXILLARY APPROACH TO THE SHOULDER

ANTERIOR AXILLARY APPROACH TO THE SHOULDER

The anterior axillary approach as described by Leslie and Ryan is indicated when cosmesis is a factor. This approach can be used with most of the anterior procedures described in this chapter. Placement of the skin incision over the anterior axillary fold is quite satisfactory, and the scar is not noticeable when the arm is at the side. This is not a direct axillary approach to the glenohumeral joint but simply a placement of the skin incision. The remainder of the approach is through the deltopectoral interval.

TECHNIQUE 1.94

(LESLIE AND RYAN)

- Make a straight vertical 3- to 4-cm incision over the anterior axillary fold (Fig. 1.115A).
- Undermine the skin and subcutaneous tissue so they can be retracted anteriorly and superiorly (Fig. 1.115B).
- If needed, both the coracoid process and subscapularis tendon can be easily detached and reattached at closure.
- Close the wound with a continuous subcuticular suture (Fig. 1.115C).

ANTEROLATERAL APPROACHES TO THE SHOULDER

ANTEROLATERAL LIMITED DELTOID-SPLITTING APPROACH TO THE SHOULDER

The limited deltoid-splitting approach is appropriate for limited operations that need only to expose the tendons inserting on the greater tuberosity of the humerus and to reach the subdeltoid bursa.

TECHNIQUE 1.95

- Begin the incision at the anterolateral tip of the acromion and carry it distally over the deltoid muscle about 5 cm.
- Define the avascular raphe 4 to 5 cm long between the anterior and middle thirds of the deltoid; splitting the muscle here provides a fairly avascular approach to underlying structures.
- For maximal exposure, split the deltoid up to the margin of the acromion, but do not split it distally more than 3.8 cm from its origin to avoid damaging the axillary nerve

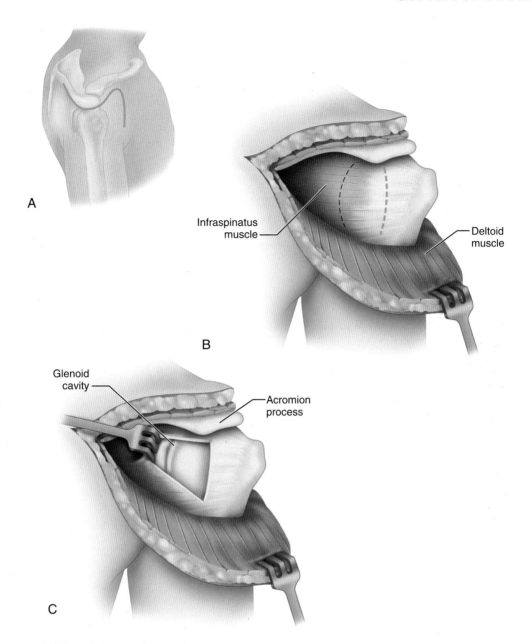

A

B

C

Infraspinatus
muscle

Deltoid
muscle

Glenoid
cavity

Acromion
process

FIGURE **1.114**   Cubbins et al. approach to anterior, superior, and posterior aspects of shoulder joint. **A,** Skin incision. **B,** Origin of deltoid reflected from clavicle, acromion, and spine of scapula; posterior capsule incised vertically. **C,** Capsule retracted, exposing posterior portion of glenoid and humerus. **SEE TECHNIQUE 1.93.**

and paralyzing the anterior part of the deltoid (Fig. 1.116). (The axillary nerve courses transversely just proximal to the midpoint between the lateral margin of the acromion and the insertion of the deltoid.)

- Incise the thin wall of the subdeltoid bursa and explore the rotator cuff as desired by rotating and abducting the arm to bring different parts of it into view in the floor of the wound.

- A transverse skin incision about 6.5 cm long may be used instead of the longitudinal one to leave a less conspicuous scar (Fig. 1.117). Place it about 2.5 cm distal to the inferior border of the acromion, dissect the skin flaps from the

underlying deltoid muscle, and split the muscle in the line of its fibers. The rest of the approach is the same as that just described.

- To approach a more posterior aspect, place the skin incision more laterally and split the deltoid just beneath it. To maintain a dry field, cauterize the intramuscular vessels encountered.

In a cadaver study, Traver et al. demonstrated that irreversible changes in axillary nerve length and strain caused microscopic damage to neuronal structures with prolonged retraction during a deltoid-splitting approach.

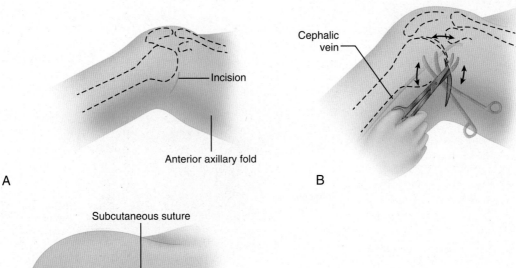

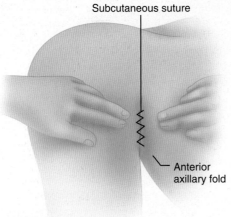

FIGURE 1.115 Anterior axillary incision to approach shoulder joint. **A,** Incision. **B,** Skin and subcutaneous tissue are being undermined all around incision. **C,** Incision closed by continuous subcuticular wire suture. **SEE TECHNIQUE 1.94.**

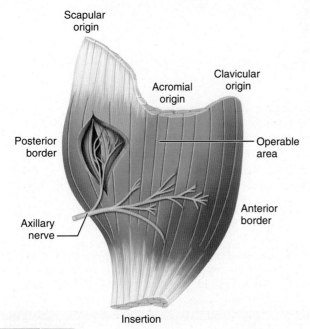

FIGURE 1.116 Deep surface of left deltoid showing location of axillary nerve. Nerve courses transversely at level about 5 cm distal to origin of muscle. One branch of nerve has been exposed fully to show that incision that splits muscle, even in the *operable area,* damages smaller branches of nerve. **SEE TECHNIQUE 1.95.**

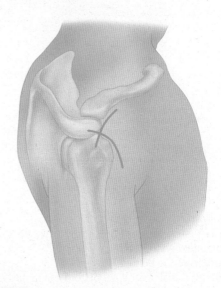

FIGURE 1.117 Incision options for a limited anterolateral deltoid-splitting approach to the anterior rotator cuff. **SEE TECHNIQUE 1.95.**

EXTENSILE ANTEROLATERAL APPROACH TO THE SHOULDER

Gardener et al. demonstrated that the limited deltoid-splitting approach could be successfully extended by isolating the axillary nerve and posterior circumflex artery. This extensile anterolateral approach is very useful for plate fixation of proximal humeral fractures (Fig. 1.118). Chou et al. demonstrated that this approach is also useful for fracture management with hemiarthroplasty.

TECHNIQUE 1.96　　*Figure 1.118*

(GARDNER ET AL.)
- Make an incision beginning at the anterolateral tip of the acromion and carry it distally for 8 to 10 cm.
- By blunt dissection, identify the avascular raphe between the anterior and middle third of the deltoid muscle.
- Make a 2-cm incision in the deltoid raphe beginning at its attachment on the acromion.
- Spread this incision bluntly and insert a finger laterally beneath the raphe. Sweep the undersurface of the deltoid from the proximal humerus. Palpate the cord-like axillary nerve on its undersurface.
- Carefully further incise the raphe and identify the axillary nerve and posterior humeral circumflex artery. Isolate them and tag them with a vessel loop. Thoroughly elevate these structures medially and laterally to free up the deltoid to allow easy passage of a plate.

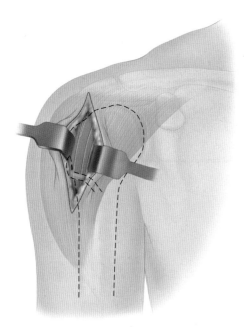

FIGURE 1.118 Extended anterolateral deltoid-splitting approach. The axillary nerve lies approximately 3.5 cm distal to the lateral prominence of the greater tuberosity. The nerve is then identified and protected. **SEE TECHNIQUE 1.96.**

TRANSACROMIAL APPROACH TO THE SHOULDER

The transacromial approach is excellent for surgery of the musculotendinous cuff and for fracture-dislocations of the shoulder.

TECHNIQUE 1.97

(DARRACH; MCLAUGHLIN)
- Incise the skin just lateral to the acromioclavicular joint from the posterior aspect of the acromion superiorly like a shoulder strap and anteriorly to a point 5 cm distal to the anterior edge of the acromion (Fig. 1.119A).
- Deepen the anterior limb through the deltoid muscle, detach the deltoid from its acromial origin, and divide the coracoacromial ligament (Fig. 1.119B-D).
- To repair the rotator cuff, an oblique osteotomy of the acromion (Fig. 1.120A) gives enough exposure, and the cosmetic result is satisfactory; to expose the joint completely, McLaughlin advised using the osteotomy technique shown in Figure 1.120B. In either instance, excise the detached segment of the acromion. Armstrong advised complete acromionectomy (Fig. 1.120C) if subacromial impingement of the rotator cuff would be a problem.
- To expose the joint, split any of the tendons of the cuff in the line of their fibers or separate two of them; the best way is to approach between the subscapularis and supraspinatus tendons through the coracohumeral ligament.
- Close the cuff by side-to-side suture, bevel the stump of the acromion, and suture the edge of the deltoid to the fascia on the stump.

　Kuz et al. recommended a coronal transacromial osteotomy just anterior to the spine of the scapula and parallel to it for hemiarthroplasty and total shoulder arthroplasty. The osteotomy is repaired with two large, absorbable, 1-0, figure-of-eight sutures passed through drill holes. Kuz et al. reported an 87% union rate using this osteotomy, with the remaining patients having a stable, painless, fibrous union.

POSTERIOR APPROACHES TO THE SHOULDER

Similar posterior approaches to the shoulder joint have been described by Kocher, McWhorter, Bennett, Rowe and Yee, Harmon, and others. For any such approach to be done safely, a thorough knowledge of the anatomy of the posterior aspect of the shoulder is essential (Fig. 1.121).

POSTERIOR DELTOID-SPLITTING APPROACH TO THE SHOULDER

Wirth et al. described a posterior deltoid-splitting approach (Fig. 1.122). As with more anterior approaches, it is limited by the location of the axillary nerve and posterior circumflex artery. Karachalios et al. used this approach to successfully reduce a neglected posterior dislocation of the shoulder.

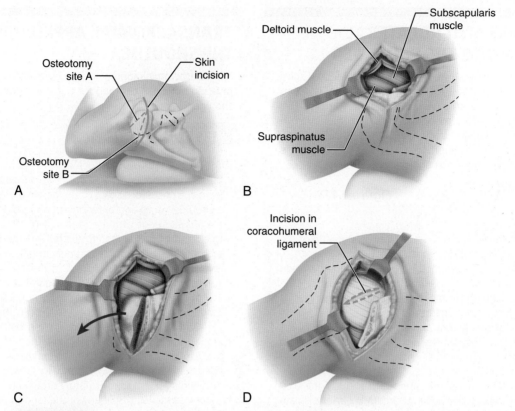

FIGURE 1.119 Transacromial approach to shoulder joint. **A,** Skin incision. **B,** Fibers of deltoid separated. **C,** Osteotomy of acromion. **D,** Line of incision through coracohumeral ligament. Detached segment of acromion is usually discarded. **SEE TECHNIQUE 1.97.**

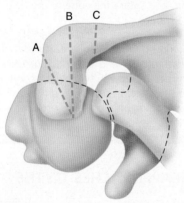

FIGURE 1.120 Lines of osteotomy of acromion. Oblique osteotomy *(A)* is adequate for repair of ordinary shoulder cuff lesion. Resection of acromion at *B* is preferable when complete exposure of shoulder joint is required. Line of osteotomy for complete acromionectomy *(C).* **SEE TECHNIQUE 1.97.**

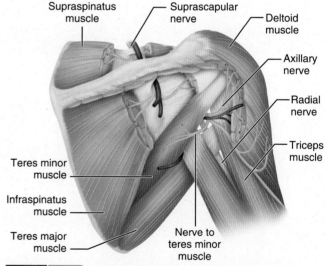

FIGURE 1.121 Anatomy of posterior aspect of shoulder joint.

TECHNIQUE 1.98

(WIRTH ET AL.)
- Place the patient in the lateral decubitus position.
- Make a 10-cm straight incision beginning at the posterior aspect of the acromioclavicular joint and carry it toward the posterior axillary fold (Fig. 1.122).
- Raise sufficient subcutaneous flaps and identify the fibrous septum between the middle and posterior third of

the deltoid muscle. The muscle split should be no longer than two thirds of the length of the muscle to avoid damage to the axillary nerve and posterior circumflex humeral artery (see Fig. 1.126).
- Identify the insertion of the two heads of the infraspinatus muscle and separate them in a medial direction, exposing the posterior capsule of the glenohumeral joint.

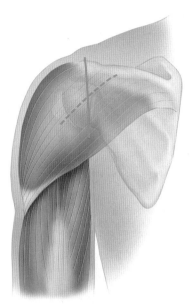

FIGURE **1.122** Posterior deltoid-splitting approach. *Dashed line* represents the deltoid split. **SEE TECHNIQUE 1.98.**

POSTERIOR APPROACH TO THE SHOULDER

One of the most practical posterior approaches to the shoulder joint and inferior scapula is the posterior (Judet) approach. The interval between the infraspinatus (suprascapular nerve innervated) and teres minor (axillary nerve innervated) muscles can be extended medially exposing a large portion of the inferior half of the scapula. One extensive cadaver study showed that the medial branch of the supraclavicular nerve was on average 2.7 cm lateral to the sternoclavicular joint and the lateral branch was on average 1.9 cm medial to the acromioclavicular joint. Between these two points, there is wide variability in nerve branch location and increased risk for injury without meticulous dissection along the shaft of the clavicle.

TECHNIQUE 1.99

(MODIFIED JUDET)
- Begin the skin incision just lateral to the tip of the acromion, pass it medially and posteriorly along the border of the acromion, curve it slightly distal to the spine of the scapula, and end it at the base of the spine of the scapula (Fig. 1.123A, *inset*).
- Reflect the skin and fascia and expose the origin of the deltoid muscle from the spine of the scapula (Fig. 1.123A). Detach this part of the deltoid from the bone by subperiosteal dissection, and reflect it distally and laterally, taking care to avoid injury to the axillary nerve and vessels as they emerge from the quadrangular space and enter the muscle (Fig. 1.123B). As a precaution against injuring this nerve, do not retract the deltoid distal to the teres minor muscle, and to avoid injuring the suprascapular nerve, do not enter the infraspinatus muscle.

- After reflecting the deltoid, expose the posterior surface of the joint capsule by detaching the inferior two thirds of the infraspinatus tendon near its insertion on the humerus and reflecting the detached part medially.
- Alternatively, the posterior part of the joint can be exposed by an oblique incision between the infraspinatus and teres minor muscles (Fig. 1.123C) and then opening the joint capsule by a longitudinal or a transverse incision or by a combination of both, as needed. The interval between the infraspinatus and teres minor muscles can be extended medially, exposing more of the inferior scapula for fracture fixation. Extend the incision distally along the medial border of the scapula if necessary.

SIMPLIFIED POSTERIOR APPROACH TO THE SHOULDER

Brodsky, Tullos, and Gartsman described a simplified posterior approach to the shoulder introduced to Tullos by J.W. King. It is based on the fact that wide abduction of the arm raises the inferior border of the posterior deltoid to the level of the glenohumeral joint. This approach can be used for a wide variety of procedures and does not require freeing large portions of the posterior deltoid from the scapular spine or splitting the deltoid; postoperative immobilization for healing of the muscle is unnecessary. Rehabilitation of the shoulder can be started as soon as tolerated by the patient if the particular procedure performed does not require immobilization.

TECHNIQUE 1.100

(KING, AS DESCRIBED BY BRODSKY ET AL.)
- Place the patient prone or in the lateral position.
- Drape the arm and shoulder free and abduct the shoulder to 90 degrees, but no farther, avoiding excessive traction on the axillary vessels and brachial plexus.
- Begin a vertical incision at the posterior aspect of the acromion and carry it inferiorly for 10 cm (Fig. 1.124A,B).
- Retract the posterior deltoid superiorly (Fig. 1.124C) and, if necessary, release the medial 2 cm of its origin from the scapular spine.
- Develop the interval between the infraspinatus and teres minor muscles.
- Incise the capsule of the joint in a manner dependent on the procedure to be performed; to prevent injury to the axillary nerve and the posterior humeral circumflex vessels beneath the inferior border of the teres minor, avoid dissecting too far inferiorly (Fig. 1.124D).

POSTERIOR INVERTED-U APPROACH TO THE SHOULDER

The deltoid muscle has three parts—three heads of origin—and two relatively avascular intervals separating the three. The anterior part (which originates on the lateral third of

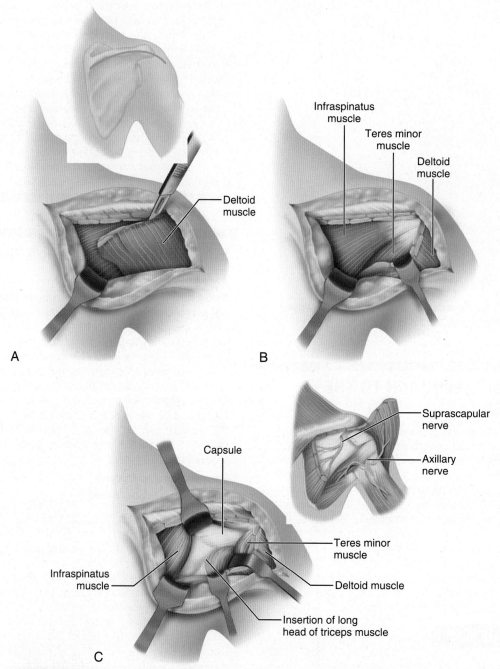

A

B

Capsule

Suprascapular nerve

Axillary nerve

Infraspinatus muscle

Teres minor muscle

Deltoid muscle

Insertion of long head of triceps muscle

C

FIGURE 1.123 Modified Judet posterior approach to shoulder joint. **A,** Deltoid is being detached from spine of scapula and from acromion. *Inset,* Skin incision. **B,** Deltoid has been retracted to expose interval between infraspinatus and teres minor. **C,** Infraspinatus and teres minor have been retracted to expose posterior aspect of joint capsule. *Inset,* Relationships of suprascapular and axillary (circumflex) nerves to operative field. **SEE TECHNIQUE 1.99.**

the clavicle and the anterior border of the acromion) and the posterior part are composed primarily of long parallel muscle fibers extending from the origin to the insertion. The middle part is multipennate, with short fibers inserting obliquely into parallel tendinous bands. The interval between the posterior and middle parts can be found by beginning the dissection at the angle of the acromion and proceeding through the fibrous septum; with care, the division can be extended distally through the proximal two thirds of the muscle without endangering the nerve

supply because the posterior branch of the axillary nerve supplies the posterior part of the muscle and the anterior branch supplies the anterior and middle parts. The interval between the anterior and middle parts is less distinct; it extends distally from the anterior apex of the shoulder formed by the anterolateral tip of the acromion.

In view of this tripartite division, Abbott and Lucas described inverted-U-shaped approaches to reach the anterior, lateral, and posterior aspects of the shoulder joint, dissecting the deltoid distally at the two intervals described

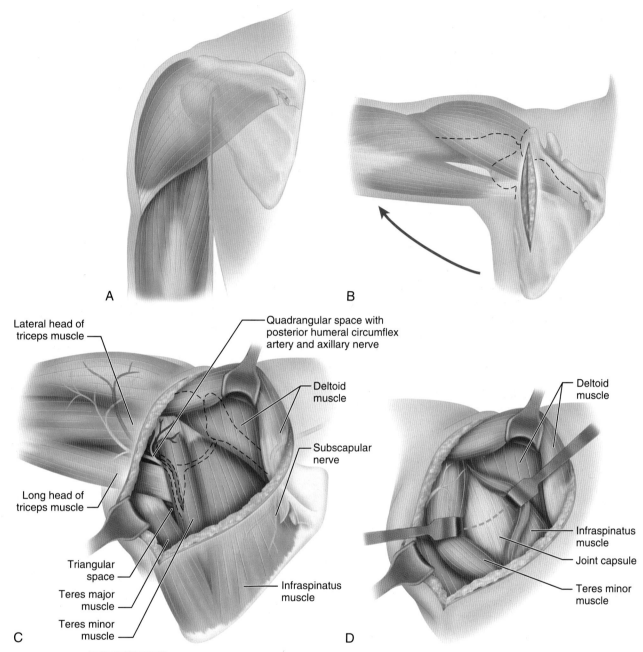

A

B

Lateral head of
triceps muscle

Quadrangular space with
posterior humeral circumflex
artery and axillary nerve

Deltoid
muscle

Deltoid
muscle

Subscapular
nerve

Long head of
triceps muscle

Infraspinatus
muscle

Joint capsule

Triangular
space

Teres major
muscle

Teres minor
muscle

Infraspinatus
muscle

Teres minor
muscle

C

D

FIGURE 1.124 King simplified posterior approach. **A,** Skin incision. **B,** Posterior deltoid muscle has been elevated to level of joint by abduction of arm to 90 degrees. **C,** Deltoid has been retracted superiorly exposing muscles of rotator cuff. **D,** Capsule has been exposed. (Modified from Brodsky JW, Tullos HS, Gartsman GM: Simplified posterior approach to the shoulder joint: a technical note, *J Bone Joint Surg* 71A:407, 1989.) **SEE TECHNIQUE 1.100.**

and detaching the appropriate third of the muscle from its origin. They, too, warn that to separate the anterior and middle thirds distally more than 4 to 5 cm endangers the trunk of the axillary nerve (Fig. 1.125).

TECHNIQUE 1.101

(ABBOTT AND LUCAS)

- Begin the skin incision 5 cm distal to the spine of the scapula at the junction of its middle and medial thirds, and

extend it superiorly over the spine and laterally to the angle of the acromion. Curve the incision distally for about 7.5 cm over the tendinous interval between the posterior and middle thirds of the deltoid muscle (Fig. 1.126A).

- Free the deltoid subperiosteally from the spine of the scapula, split it distally in the interval, and turn the resulting flap of skin and muscle distally for 5 cm to expose the infraspinatus and teres minor muscles and the quadrangular space (Fig. 1.126B). The posterior humeral circumflex artery and the axillary nerve each divide into anterior and

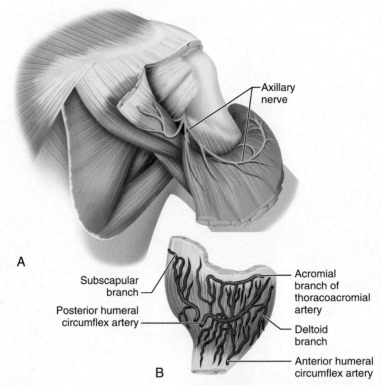

FIGURE 1.125 Nerve and blood supply of deltoid muscle. **A,** Anterior and posterior divisions of axillary nerve to deltoid muscle. **B,** Blood supply of deltoid muscle from posterior humeral circumflex artery and anastomotic branches from adjacent arteries. **SEE TECHNIQUE 1.101.**

posterior branches, so the splitting of the deltoid between its posterior and middle thirds does not injure them.
- Carry this division of the deltoid to its insertion to give full access to the quadrangular space if desired.
- To expose the glenohumeral joint, incise the shoulder cuff in its tendinous part and retract the muscles; then divide the capsule (Fig. 1.126C).
- If exposure of both the posterior and anterior shoulder is needed, bring the lateral portion of the incision around the acromion laterally then medially along the anterior clavicle (see Fig. 1.117).

HUMERUS

Almost all major approaches to the humerus involve isolating or potentially damaging the radial nerve. The radial nerve course and relationships to other structures must be kept in mind with most approaches. Hasan et al. described the "zone of vulnerability" for injury to the radial nerve with a study of 33 cadaver arms. They found the proximal aspect of the triceps tendon to be a reliable landmark being approximately 2.3 cm below the radial nerve at the posterior midline of the humerus. The "zone of vulnerability" was found to be 2.1 cm (average) of radial nerve that lies directly on the lateral cortex before piercing the lateral intramuscular septum and the few centimeters of nerve distal to the septum.

ANTEROLATERAL APPROACH TO THE SHAFT OF THE HUMERUS

TECHNIQUE 1.102

(THOMPSON; HENRY)
- Incise the skin in line with the anterior border of the deltoid muscle from a point midway between its origin and insertion, distally to the level of its insertion, and proceed in line with the lateral border of the biceps muscle to within 7.5 cm of the elbow joint (Fig. 1.127).
- Divide the superficial and deep fasciae and ligate the cephalic vein.
- In the proximal part of the wound, retract the deltoid laterally and the biceps medially to expose the shaft of the humerus.
- Distal to the insertion of the deltoid, expose the brachialis muscle, split it longitudinally to the bone, and retract it subperiosteally, the lateral half to the lateral side and the medial half to the medial. Retraction is easier when the tendon of the brachialis is relaxed by flexing the elbow to a right angle. The lateral half of the brachialis muscle protects the radial nerve as it winds around the humeral shaft (Fig. 1.128; see also Fig. 1.127).

If desired, the distal end of this approach may be carried to within 5 cm of the humeral condyles and the proximal

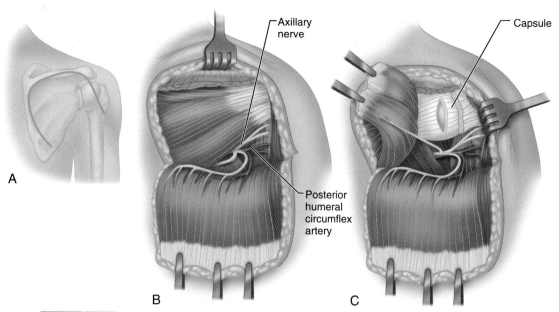

FIGURE 1.126 Abbott and Lucas inverted-U approach to posterior aspect of shoulder. **A,** Skin incision. **B,** Skin and muscle flap turned down, exposing quadrangular space and posterior aspect of rotator cuff and muscles. **C,** Rotator cuff and capsule incised, exposing humeral head. **SEE TECHNIQUES 1.98 AND 1.101.**

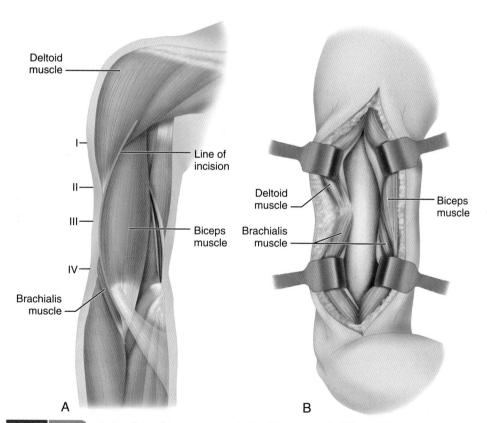

FIGURE 1.127 Anterolateral approach to shaft of humerus. **A,** Skin incision. **B,** Deltoid and biceps muscles retracted; brachialis muscle incised longitudinally, exposing shaft. **SEE TECHNIQUE 1.102.**

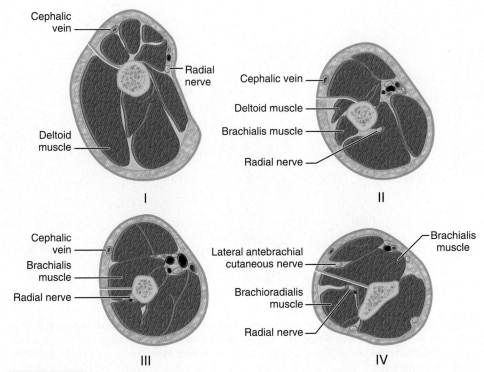

Cephalic vein

Radial nerve

Deltoid muscle

I

Cephalic vein

Deltoid muscle

Brachialis muscle

Radial nerve

II

Cephalic vein

Brachialis muscle

Radial nerve

III

Lateral antebrachial cutaneous nerve

Brachioradialis muscle

Radial nerve

Brachialis muscle

IV

FIGURE 1.128   Cross-sections at various levels in arm (see Fig. 1.127) to show approach through deep structures and relationship to radial nerve. **SEE TECHNIQUES 1.102 AND 1.103.**

end farther proximally, as in the anteromedial approach to the shoulder. The advantages of this approach are that the brachialis muscle usually is innervated by the musculocutaneous and radial nerves and can be split longitudinally without paralysis and that the lateral half of the brachialis muscle protects the radial nerve.

The anterior aspect of the humeral shaft at the junction of its middle and distal thirds also can be approached between the biceps and brachialis muscles medially and the brachioradialis laterally (Fig. 1.128). In a retrospective study, King and Johnston reported that the original anterolateral skin incision as described by Henry (Fig. 1.129; see also Fig. 1.128) frequently transected branches of the lower lateral brachial cutaneous nerve, resulting in painful neuroma formation, numbness, or tingling around the wound scar in 62% of 30 patients. This was confirmed by an anatomic study of seven cadaver arms. King and Johnston recommended a more anteriorly placed incision (Fig. 1.130) in the watershed zone between the lower lateral brachial and the medial brachial cutaneous nerves.

Kuhne and Friess used the anterolateral humeral approach combined with a Kocher lateral elbow approach (Technique 1.112) to expose the lateral humerus from the surgical neck to the lateral condyle. A muscular bridge was maintained to protect the radial nerve during internal fixation.

Using a cadaver study, Phelps et al. described connecting a deltopectoral shoulder approach with an anterolateral humeral approach called an aggregate anterior approach. By adding a lateral elbow approach (extended aggregate anterior approach), the entire humerus could be exposed.

SUBBRACHIAL APPROACH TO THE HUMERUS

The subbrachial approach avoids splitting the brachialis muscle. Both the radial and musculocutaneous nerves are protected, and according to Boschi et al., there is much less brachialis muscle damage as supported by a postoperative electromyoneurography study.

TECHNIQUE 1.103

(BOSCHI ET AL.)
- Flex the elbow taking tension off the biceps brachii muscle. Move the muscle in a medial to lateral direction to define the lateral edge of the muscle.
- Make a longitudinal skin incision 1 cm posterior to the lateral edge of the muscle.
- Develop the interval between the biceps brachii muscle and the brachialis muscle starting in the proximal portion of the wound using blunt dissection.
- Stay on the anterior surface of the brachialis muscle and once over the medial edge bluntly dissect the muscle from the anterior and lateral edge of the humerus (Fig. 1.128, III).

POSTERIOR APPROACH TO THE PROXIMAL HUMERUS

Berger and Buckwalter described a posterior approach to the proximal third of the humeral diaphysis for resection

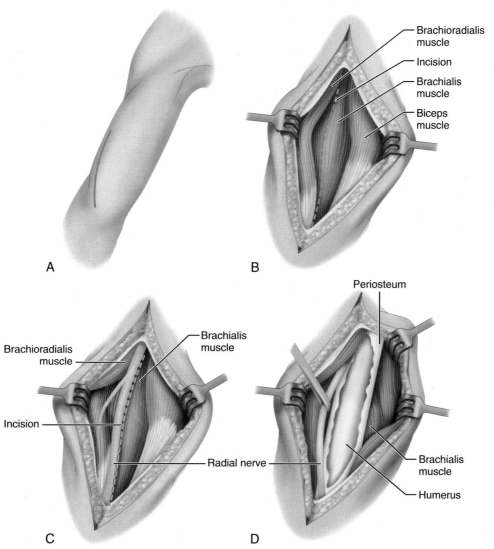

FIGURE 1.129 Exposure of humerus at junction of middle and distal thirds through antero-lateral approach. **A,** Skin incision. **B,** Interval between biceps and brachialis muscles medially and brachioradialis muscle laterally is developed, and muscles are retracted. **C,** Radial nerve identified and retracted. **D,** Nerve is retracted, and brachioradialis and brachialis muscles are separated, exposing humeral shaft. **SEE TECHNIQUE 1.102.**

of an osteoid osteoma. This approach exposes the bone through the interval between the lateral head of the triceps muscle innervated by the radial nerve and the deltoid muscle innervated by the axillary nerve. Approximately 8 cm of the bone can be exposed, with the approach limited proximally by the axillary nerve and posterior circumflex humeral artery and distally by the origin of the triceps muscle from the lateral border of the spiral groove and by the underlying radial nerve.

TECHNIQUE 1.104

(BERGER AND BUCKWALTER)

- Place the patient in the lateral position with the extremity draped free and positioned across the patient's chest. Beginning 5 cm distal to the posterior aspect of the acromion, make a straight incision over the interval between

the deltoid and triceps muscles and extend it distally to the level of the deltoid tuberosity.
- Bluntly develop the interval between the lateral head of the triceps and the deltoid (Fig. 1.131).
- Expose the periosteum of the humerus and incise it longitudinally.
- Elevate the periosteum medially and retract it and the lateral head of the triceps medially.
- Continue the subperiosteal elevation of the triceps proximally until its origin from the proximal humerus is reached. Retract the triceps medially with care to avoid injury to the radial nerve as it comes in contact with the periosteum about 3 cm proximal to the level of the deltoid tuberosity.
- Elevate the periosteum laterally, and retract it and the deltoid laterally.
- To extend the exposure proximally, carefully continue the subperiosteal dissection to the proximal origin of the lateral

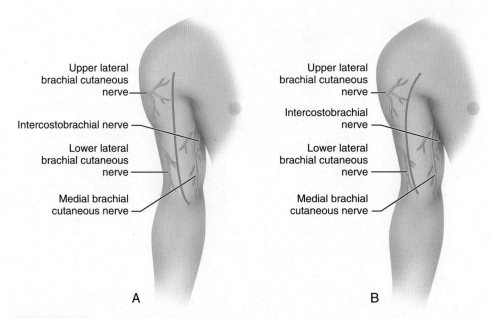

FIGURE 1.130 **A,** Relationship of lower lateral brachial cutaneous nerve and anterior midline skin incision. **B,** Relationship of lower lateral brachial cutaneous nerve and standard Henry anterolateral skin incision. (From King A, Johnston GH: A modification of Henry's anterior approach to the humerus, *J Shoulder Elbow Surg* 7:210, 1998.) **SEE TECHNIQUE 1.102.**

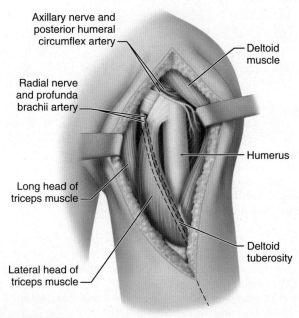

FIGURE 1.131 Berger and Buckwalter posterior approach to proximal humeral diaphysis. *Broken line* indicates course of radial nerve beneath lateral head of triceps muscle (see text). (Modified from Berger RA, Buckwalter JA: A posterior surgical approach to the proximal part of the humerus, *J Bone Joint Surg* 71A:407, 1989.) **SEE TECHNIQUE 1.104.**

head of the triceps. Protect the axillary nerve and posterior circumflex artery at the proximal edge of this exposure.
- To extend the exposure distally, partially release the insertion of the deltoid muscle carefully, avoiding the radial nerve that is beneath the lateral border of the triceps (see Fig. 1.131).

APPROACHES TO THE DISTAL HUMERAL SHAFT

Henry described a posterior approach that splits the triceps to expose the posterior humeral shaft in its middle two thirds. This approach is sometimes valuable when excising tumors that cannot be reached by the anterolateral approach. Medially the humeral shaft can be approached posterior to the intermuscular septum along a line extending proximally from the medial epicondyle. The ulnar nerve is freed from the triceps muscle and retracted medially; the triceps is then separated from the posterior surface of the medial intermuscular septum and the adjacent humeral shaft. If this approach is extended proximally to the inferior margin of the deltoid muscle, one must keep the radial nerve in mind and avoid its path.

POSTEROLATERAL APPROACH TO THE DISTAL HUMERAL SHAFT

Moran described a modified lateral approach to the distal humeral shaft for fracture fixation. This approach uses the interval between the triceps and brachioradialis muscles and does not involve splitting the triceps tendon or muscle.

TECHNIQUE 1.105

(MORAN)
- Place the patient prone or in the lateral decubitus position.
- Make a longitudinal skin incision 15 to 18 cm in length over the posterolateral aspect of the arm (Fig. 1.132A). Extend the incision distally midway between the lateral epicondyle of the humerus and the tip of the olecranon 4 cm distal to the elbow joint. The proximal portion of the

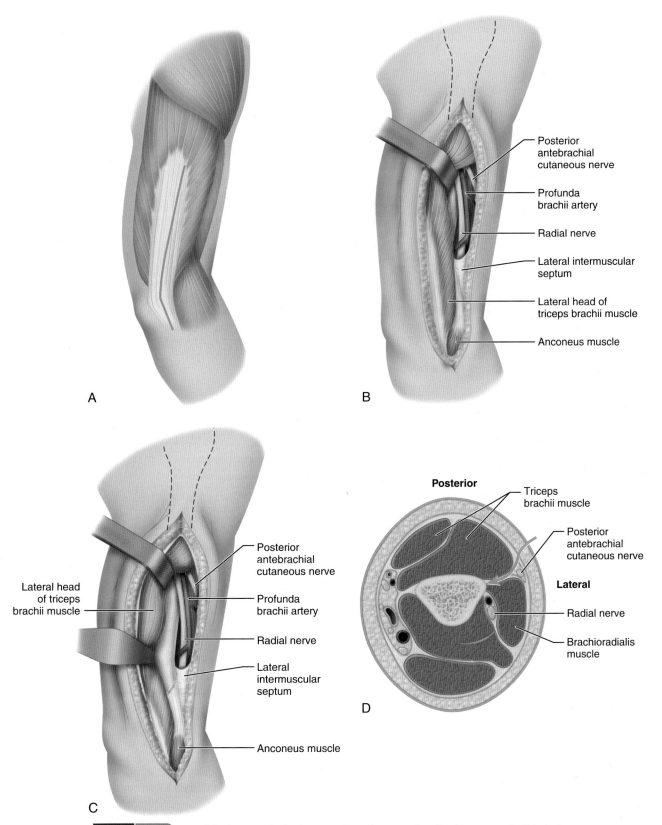

A

B
- Posterior antebrachial cutaneous nerve
- Profunda brachii artery
- Radial nerve
- Lateral intermuscular septum
- Lateral head of triceps brachii muscle
- Anconeus muscle

C
- Lateral head of triceps brachii muscle
- Posterior antebrachial cutaneous nerve
- Profunda brachii artery
- Radial nerve
- Lateral intermuscular septum
- Anconeus muscle

D
- **Posterior**
- Triceps brachii muscle
- Posterior antebrachial cutaneous nerve
- **Lateral**
- Radial nerve
- Brachioradialis muscle

FIGURE 1.132 Modified posterolateral approach to the posterior distal humerus. **A,** Skin incision. **B,** Interval between lateral head of triceps and lateral intermuscular septum is developed. **C,** Medial retraction of triceps exposes the posterior aspect of the humerus. **D,** Cross-section of upper arm at midpoint of skin incision. **SEE TECHNIQUE 1.105.**

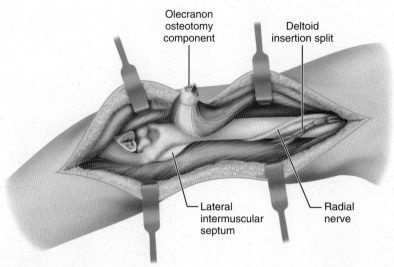

Olecranon osteotomy component

Deltoid insertion split

Lateral intermuscular septum

Radial nerve

FIGURE 1.133 The COLD approach, described by Lewicky, Sheppard, and Ruth, with the patient in the lateral decubitus position *(right arm depicted)*. The olecranon osteotomy component is reflected proximally while dissection proceeds along the lateral intermuscular septum. The radial nerve is seen obliquely crossing the humerus distal to the deltoid insertion split. (Modified from Lewicky YM, Sheppard JE, Ruth JT: The combined olecranon osteotomy, lateral para tricipital sparing, deltoid insertion splitting approach for concomitant distal intra-articular and humeral shaft fractures, *J Orthop Trauma* 21:135, 2007.) **SEE TECHNIQUE 1.106.**

incision is located 4 cm posterior to the lateral intermuscular septum.

- From the midpoint of the wound, dissect laterally until the lateral intermuscular septum is reached.
- Incise the triceps fascia longitudinally a few millimeters posterior to the intermuscular septum and carefully separate the triceps muscle from the intermuscular septum working distally to proximally.
- Distally, incise the fascia at the lateral edge of the anconeus and carry this 4 cm distal to the lateral epicondyle.
- Retract the anconeus muscle and fascia in continuity with the triceps.
- Identify and protect the posterior antebrachial cutaneous nerve as it leaves the posterior compartment at the lateral intermuscular septum (Fig. 1.132B,D).
- Retract the radial nerve anteriorly. The radial nerve passes through the lateral intermuscular septum at the junction of the middle and distal thirds of the humerus (Fig. 1.132B).
- Retract the triceps muscle medially to expose the posterior humeral shaft (Fig. 1.132C). If more proximal exposure is needed, carefully follow the radial nerve proximally and bluntly dissect it from the region of the spiral groove.
- To close the wound, allow the triceps muscle to fall anteriorly into its bed, and loosely close the fascia with interrupted sutures.

POSTEROLATERAL EXTENSILE (COLD) APPROACH TO THE DISTAL HUMERUS

Lewicky et al. described how the posterolateral approach can be extended proximally and distally to expose most of the posterior humeral shaft and elbow joint for complex fracture treatment. They described an extensile approach combining an olecranon osteotomy, lateral triceps sparing, and deltoid insertion splitting (COLD).

TECHNIQUE 1.106

(LEWICKY, SHEPPARD, AND RUTH)

- Carry the distal limb of the incision distally over the subcutaneous border of the ulna far enough to allow an olecranon osteotomy and anterior transposition of the ulnar nerves.
- Extend the proximal limb of the incision to allow further mobilization of the lateral head of the triceps muscle and exposure of the deltoid muscle insertion on the proximal humerus. Dissection can be extended as far proximally as the level of the posterior branch of the axillary nerve in its subdeltoid position.
- Pay careful attention to isolate and protect the radial nerve and profunda brachii artery (Fig. 1.133).

ELBOW

There has been a marked increase in information pertaining to surgery of the elbow. Table 1.9 provides a summary of surgical approaches to the elbow and proximal forearm. Only the more commonly used of these approaches are described here.

POSTERIOR APPROACHES TO THE ELBOW

POSTEROLATERAL APPROACH TO THE ELBOW

Campbell used a posterolateral approach to the elbow for extensive operations such as treatment of old posterior

TABLE 1.9

Summary of Surgical Approaches to the Elbow and Proximal Forearm

AUTHOR	TISSUE PLANE
POSTERIOR APPROACHES	
Campbell	Midline triceps split
Campbell	Triceps aponeurosis tongue
Extended Kocher/ Ewald	ECU and anconeus/triceps
Wadsworth	Triceps aponeurosis tongue and full-thickness deep head
Bryan, Morrey	Elevate triceps mechanism from medial olecranon and reflect laterally
Boyd	Lateral border of triceps/ulna and anconeus/ECU
Muller, MacAusland	Olecranon osteotomy—transverse or chevron
LATERAL APPROACHES	
Kocher	Between ECU and anconeus
Cadenat	Between ECRB and ECRL
Kaplan	Between ECRB and ECU
Key, Conwell	Between BR and ECRL
MEDIAL APPROACH	
Hotchkiss	Between FCU and PL/FCR; brachialis resected laterally with PL/FCR/PT
Molesworth	Medial epicondyle osteotomy
GLOBAL APPROACH	
Patterson, Bain, Mehta	Kocher interval; ±± lateral epicondyle osteotomy; ± Kaplan interval; ± Hotchkiss interval; ± Taylor interval
ANTERIOR APPROACH	
Henry	Between mobile wad and biceps tendon; elevate supinator from radius

BR, Brachioradialis; *ECRB,* extensor carpi radialis brevis; *ECRL,* extensor carpi radialis longus; *ECU,* extensor carpi ulnaris; *FCR,* flexor carpi radialis; *FCU,* flexor carpi ulnaris; *FDP,* flexor digitorum profundus; *PL,* palmaris longus; *PT,* pronator teres.
From Mehta JA, Bain GI: Surgical approaches to the elbow, *Hand Clin* 20:375, 2004.

dislocations, fractures of the distal humerus involving the joint, and arthroplasties.

TECHNIQUE 1.107

(CAMPBELL)
- Begin the skin incision 10 cm proximal to the elbow on the posterolateral aspect of the arm and continue it distally for 13 cm (Fig. 1.134A).
- Deepen the dissection through the fascia and expose the aponeurosis of the triceps as far distally as its insertion on the olecranon.
- When the triceps muscle has been contracted by fixed extension of the elbow, free the aponeurosis proximally

to distally in a tongue-shaped flap and retract it distally to its insertion (Fig. 1.134B); incise the remaining muscle fibers to the bone in the midline.
- If the triceps muscle has not been contracted, divide the muscle and aponeurosis longitudinally in the midline and continue the dissection through the periosteum of the humerus, through the joint capsule, and along the lateral border of the olecranon (Fig. 1.134C).
- Elevate the periosteum together with the triceps muscle from the posterior surface of the distal humerus for 5 cm.
- For wider exposure, continue the subperiosteal stripping on each side, releasing the muscular and capsular attachments to the condyles and exposing the anterior surface, taking care not to injure the ulnar nerve.
- Strip the periosteum from the bone as conservatively as possible because serious damage to the blood supply of the bone causes osteonecrosis. The head of the radius lies in the distal end of the wound.
- When the elbow has been fixed in complete extension with a contracted triceps muscle, it should be flexed to a right angle for closure of the wound. Fill the distal part of the defect in the triceps tendon with the inverted-V-shaped part of the triceps fascia and close the proximal part by suturing the remaining two margins of the triceps.

EXTENSILE POSTEROLATERAL APPROACH TO THE ELBOW

To achieve the maximum safe exposure of the elbow and proximal radioulnar joints, Wadsworth modified the known posterolateral approaches. His extensile approach is useful for displaced distal humeral articular fractures, synovectomy, total elbow arthroplasty, and other procedures requiring extensive exposure.

TECHNIQUE 1.108

(WADSWORTH)
- With the patient prone and the elbow flexed 90 degrees over a support and the forearm dependent, begin a curved skin incision over the center of the posterior surface of the arm at the proximal limit of the triceps tendon and extend it distally to the posterior aspect of the lateral epicondyle and farther distally and medially to the posterior border of the ulna, 4 cm distal to the tip of the olecranon (Fig. 1.135A).
- Dissect the medial skin flap far enough medially to expose the medial epicondyle, and gently elevate the lateral skin flap a short distance; keep both skin flaps retracted with a single suture in each.
- Identify the ulnar nerve proximally and release it from its tunnel by dividing the arcuate ligament that passes between the two heads of the flexor carpi ulnaris muscle; gently retract it with a rubber sling.
- To fashion a tongue of triceps tendon with its base attached to the olecranon, leaving a peripheral tendinous rim attached to the triceps for later repair, begin sharp dissection at the medial surface of the proximal part of

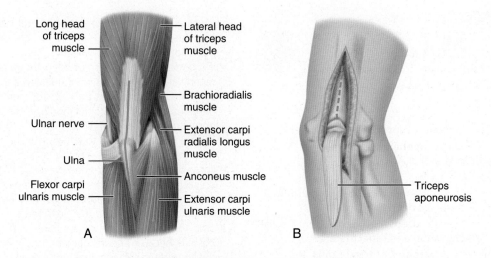

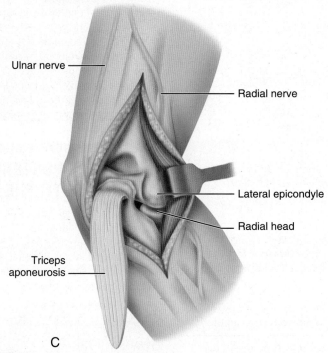

FIGURE 1.134 Campbell posterolateral approach to elbow joint in contracture of triceps. **A,** Skin incision. **B,** Tongue of triceps aponeurosis has been freed and reflected distally. **C,** Elbow joint has been exposed by subperiosteal dissection. Ulnar nerve has been identified and protected. **SEE TECHNIQUE 1.107.**

the olecranon, extend it proximally along the triceps tendon, across laterally, and distally through the tendon to the posterior aspect of the lateral epicondyle. From this point, deviate the incision distally and medially through the triceps aponeurosis to separate the anconeus from the extensor carpi ulnaris (Fig. 1.135B).
- Divide the posterior capsule in the same line.
- Reflect the triceps tendon distally, dividing the muscle tissue with care in an oblique manner for minimal damage to the deep part of the muscle; stay well clear of the radial nerve.

- Reflect the anconeus and underlying capsule medially.
- Behind the lateral epicondyle, the incision lies between the anconeus muscle and the common tendinous origin of the forearm extensor muscles. To increase exposure, partially reflect from the humerus the common extensor origin, the lateral collateral ligament, and the adjacent capsule.
- Excellent exposure is easily achieved (Fig. 1.135C); increase the exposure by putting a varus strain on the elbow joint.
- During closure, repair the triceps tendon, posterior capsule, and triceps aponeurosis with strong interrupted sutures.

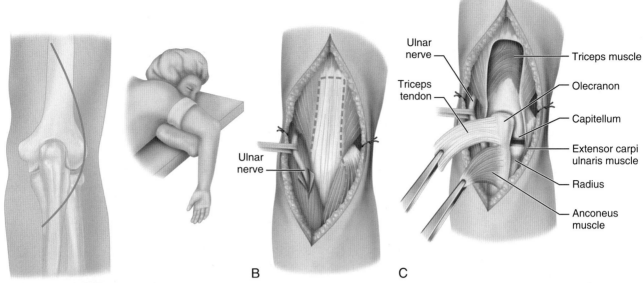

A   B   C

FIGURE 1.135 Wadsworth extensile posterolateral approach to elbow. **A,** Skin incision. *Right,* Patient is prone with elbow flexed 90 degrees and arm supported as shown. **B,** Distally based tongue of triceps tendon with intact peripheral rim is fashioned. Ulnar nerve is protected. **C,** Exposure is complete (see text). (Redrawn from Wadsworth TG: A modified posterolateral approach to the elbow and proximal radioulnar joints, *Clin Orthop Relat Res* 144:151, 1979.) **SEE TECHNIQUE 1.108.**

POSTERIOR APPROACH TO THE ELBOW BY OLECRANON OSTEOTOMY

In a comparative anatomic study, Wilkinson and Stanley showed that an olecranon osteotomy exposed significantly more articular surface of the distal humerus than a triceps-reflecting approach.

TECHNIQUE 1.109

(MACAUSLAND AND MÜLLER)

- Expose the elbow posteriorly through an incision beginning 5 cm distal to the tip of the olecranon and extending proximally medial to the midline of the arm to 10 to 12 cm above the olecranon tip.
- Reflect the skin and subcutaneous tissue to either side carefully to expose the olecranon and triceps tendon.
- Expose the distal humerus through a transolecranon approach.
- Isolate the ulnar nerve and gently retract it from its bed with a Penrose drain or a moist tape.
- Drill a hole from the tip of the olecranon down the medullary canal; then tap the hole with the tap to match a large (6.5-mm) AO cancellous screw 8 to 10 cm in length (Fig. 1.136A).
- Divide three fourths of the olecranon transversely with an osteotome or thin oscillating saw approximately 2 cm from its tip. Fracture the last fourth of the osteotomy (Fig. 1.136B,C).
- Reflect the olecranon and the attached triceps proximally to give excellent exposure of the posterior aspect of the lower end of the humerus.

- Alternatively, the osteotomy may be done in a chevron fashion to increase bone surface area for healing and to control rotation.
- At wound closure, reduce the proximal fragment and insert a cancellous screw using the previously drilled and tapped hole in the medullary canal.
- Drill a transverse hole in the ulna distal to the osteotomy site, pass a No. 20 wire through this hole around the screw neck, and tighten it in a figure-of-eight manner (Fig. 1.136D). In our experience, posterior plate and screw fixation of the osteotomy yields a higher union rate but the hardware often has to be removed after union because of its subcutaneous location.

EXTENSILE POSTERIOR APPROACH TO THE ELBOW

Bryan and Morrey developed a modified posterior approach to the elbow joint that provides excellent exposure and preserves the continuity of the triceps mechanism, which allows easy repair and rapid rehabilitation.

TECHNIQUE 1.110

(BRYAN AND MORREY)

- Place the patient in the lateral decubitus position or tilted 45 to 60 degrees with sandbags placed under the back and hip. Place the limb across the chest.
- Make a straight posterior incision in the midline of the limb, extending from 7 cm distal to the tip of the olecranon to 9 cm proximal to it.

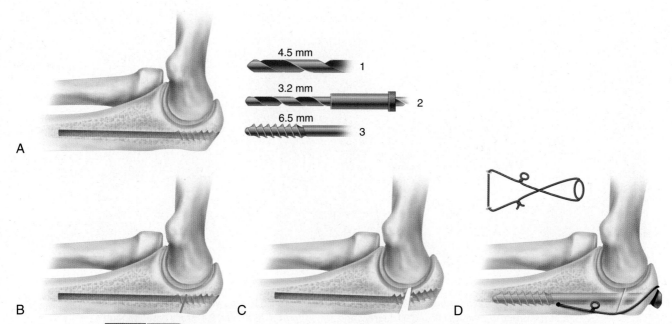

FIGURE 1.136 Osteotomy of olecranon. **A,** Preparation of hole for 6.5-mm cancellous screw. **B,** Incomplete osteotomy made with thin saw or osteotome. **C,** Osteotomy completed by fracturing bone. **D,** Lag screw (6.5 mm) and tension band wire fixation. This technique also is useful for internal fixation of olecranon fractures. **SEE TECHNIQUE 1.109.**

- Identify the ulnar nerve proximally at the medial border of the medial head of the triceps and dissect it free from its tunnel distally to its first motor branch (Fig. 1.137A).
- In total joint arthroplasty, transplant the nerve anteriorly into the subcutaneous tissue (Fig. 1.137B).
- Elevate the medial aspect of the triceps from the humerus, along the intermuscular septum, to the level of the posterior capsule.
- Incise the superficial fascia of the forearm distally for about 6 cm to the periosteum of the medial aspect of the olecranon.
- Carefully reflect as a single unit the periosteum and fascia medially to laterally (Fig. 1.137C). The medial part of the junction between the triceps insertion and the superficial fascia and the periosteum of the ulna is the weakest portion of the reflected tissue. Take care to maintain continuity of the triceps mechanism at this point; carefully dissect the triceps tendon from the olecranon when the elbow is extended to 20 to 30 degrees to relieve tension on the tissues, and then reflect the remaining portion of the triceps mechanism.
- To expose the radial head, reflect the anconeus subperiosteally from the proximal ulna; the entire joint is now widely exposed (Fig. 1.137D).
- The posterior capsule usually is reflected with the triceps mechanism, and the tip of the olecranon may be resected to expose the trochlea clearly (see Fig. 1.137D).
- To attain joint retraction in total joint arthroplasty, release the MCL from the humerus if necessary.
- During closure, carefully repair the MCL when its release has been necessary.

- Return the triceps to its anatomic position and suture it directly to the bone through holes drilled in the proximal aspect of the ulna.
- Suture the periosteum to the superficial forearm fascia, as far as the margin of the flexor carpi ulnaris (Fig. 1.137E).
- Close the wound in layers and leave a drain in the wound. In total joint arthroplasty, dress the elbow with the joint flexed about 60 degrees to avoid direct pressure on the wound by the olecranon tip.

LATERAL APPROACHES

LATERAL APPROACH TO THE ELBOW

The lateral approach is an excellent approach to a fracture of the lateral condyle because the common origin of the extensor muscles is attached to the condylar fragment and need not be disturbed.

TECHNIQUE 1.111   *Figure 1.138*

- Begin the incision approximately 5 cm proximal to the lateral epicondyle of the humerus and carry it distally to the epicondyle and along the anterolateral surface of the forearm for approximately 5 cm.
- To expose the lateral border of the humerus, develop distally to proximally the interval between the triceps posteriorly and the origins of the extensor carpi radialis longus and brachioradialis anteriorly. In the proximal angle of the wound, avoid the radial nerve where it enters the interval between the brachialis and brachioradialis muscles.

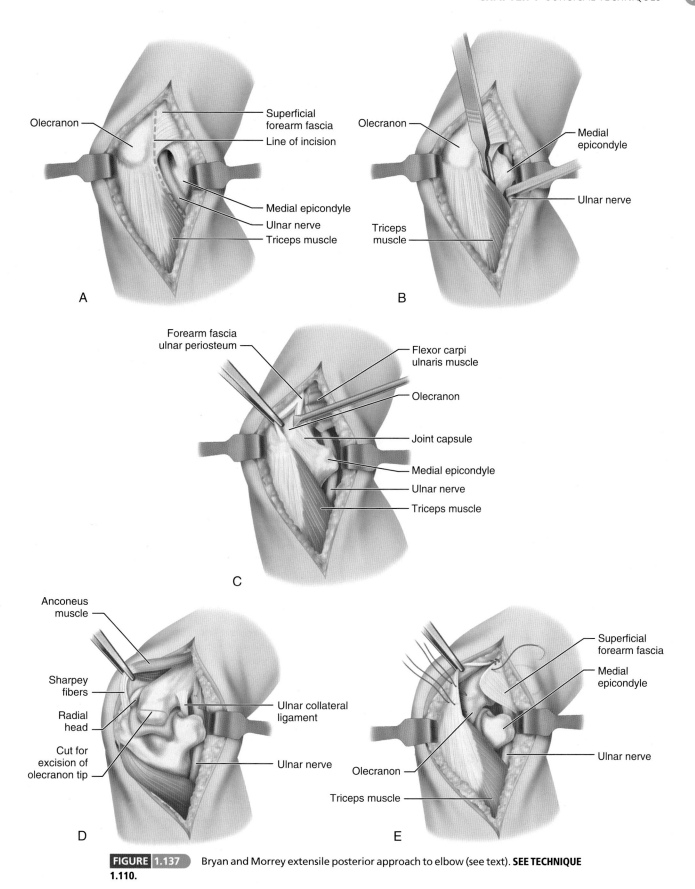

FIGURE 1.137 Bryan and Morrey extensile posterior approach to elbow (see text). **SEE TECHNIQUE 1.110.**

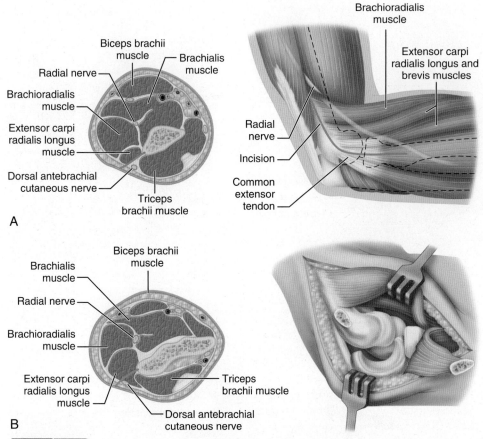

FIGURE 1.138 Lateral approach to elbow joint. **A,** Cross-section shows approach at level of proximal part of incision; *right,* skin incision and its relation to deep structures. **B,** Cross-section shows approach at level just proximal to humeral condyles; *right,* approach has been completed. **SEE TECHNIQUE 1.111.**

- With a small osteotome, separate the common origin of the extensor muscles from the lateral epicondyle together with a thin flake of bone, or divide this origin just distal to the lateral epicondyle.
- Reflect the common origin distally and expose the radio-humeral joint. Protect the deep branch of the radial nerve as it enters the supinator muscle.
- Elevate subperiosteally the origins of the brachioradialis and extensor carpi radialis longus muscles and incise the capsule to expose the lateral aspect of the elbow joint.

LATERAL J-SHAPED APPROACH TO THE ELBOW

TECHNIQUE 1.112

(KOCHER)
- Begin the incision 5 cm proximal to the elbow over the lateral supracondylar ridge of the humerus, extend it distally along this ridge, continue it 5 cm distal to the radial head, and curve it medially and posteriorly to end at the posterior border of the ulna (Fig. 1.139A).

- Dissect between the triceps muscle posteriorly and the brachioradialis and extensor carpi radialis longus muscles anteriorly to expose the lateral condyle and the capsule over the lateral surface of the radial head.
- Distal to the head, separate the extensor carpi ulnaris from the anconeus and divide the distal fibers of the anconeus in line with the curved and transverse parts of the distal skin incision. Reflect the periosteum from the anterior and posterior surfaces of the distal humerus.
- Reflect anteriorly the common origin of the extensor muscles from the lateral epicondyle by subperiosteal dissection or by detachment of the epicondyle.
- Incise the joint capsule longitudinally.
- Reflect the anconeus subperiosteally from the proximal ulna to dislocate and examine the joint under direct vision (Fig. 1.139B).

MEDIAL APPROACH WITH OSTEOTOMY OF THE MEDIAL EPICONDYLE

The medial approach with osteotomy of the medial epicondyle was developed by Molesworth and Campbell,

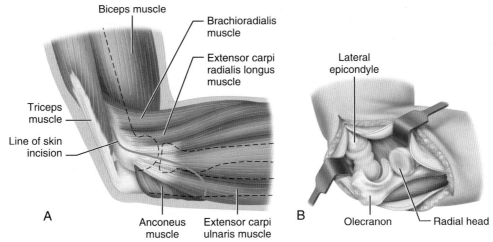

Biceps muscle
Brachioradialis muscle
Extensor carpi radialis longus muscle
Triceps muscle
Line of skin incision
Lateral epicondyle

A
Anconeus muscle
Extensor carpi ulnaris muscle

B
Olecranon
Radial head

FIGURE 1.139 Kocher lateral J approach to elbow joint. **A,** Skin incision. **B,** Approach has been completed, and elbow joint has been dislocated. **SEE TECHNIQUE 1.112.**

working independently of each other. Each needed to treat a fracture of the medial humeral epicondyle. In Campbell's patient, the fragment had been displaced distally and laterally and was incarcerated in the joint cavity. During surgery, Campbell found the radius and ulna could be dislocated on the humerus so that all parts of the joint, including all the articular surfaces, could be inspected.

TECHNIQUE 1.113 *Figure 1.140*

(MOLESWORTH; CAMPBELL)
- With the elbow flexed to a right angle, make a medial incision over the tip of the medial epicondyle from 5 cm distal to the joint to about 5 cm proximal to it.
- Isolate the ulnar nerve in its groove posterior to the epicondyle, free it, and retract it posteriorly.
- Dissect all the soft tissues from the epicondyle except the common origin of the flexor muscles, detach the epicondyle with a small osteotome, and reflect it distally together with its undisturbed tendinous attachments.
- By blunt dissection, continue distally, reflecting the muscles that originate from the medial epicondyle. Protect the branches of the median nerve that supply these muscles, entering along their lateral margins.
- Free the medial aspect of the coronoid process, incise the capsule, and strip the periosteum and capsule anteriorly and posteriorly from the humerus as far proximally as necessary. Avoid injuring the median nerve, which passes over the anterior aspect of the joint.
- With the lateral capsule acting as a hinge, dislocate the joint.

MEDIAL AND LATERAL APPROACH TO THE ELBOW

TECHNIQUE 1.114

- When extensive exposure is not needed, an incision 5 to 7 cm long can be made on either or both sides of the

joint just anterior to the condyles and parallel with the epicondylar ridges of the humerus. The flexion crease of the elbow is proximal to the joint line (Fig. 1.141). On the medial side, carefully avoid the ulnar nerve.
- Incise the capsule from proximal to distal on each side.

GLOBAL APPROACH TO THE ELBOW

The "global" approach allows circumferential exposure of the elbow. The collateral ligaments, coronoid process, and anterior joint capsule can be reached through this approach.

TECHNIQUE 1.115

(PATTERSON, BAIN, AND MEHTA)
- Make a straight posterior midline incision.
- Sharply dissect down through the deep fascia to the triceps tendon and subcutaneous border of the ulna.
- If the medial aspect of the elbow is to be exposed, open the cubital tunnel, isolate the ulnar nerve, and transpose it anteriorly. Protect it throughout the procedure with a Penrose drain (Fig. 1.142A).
- Develop full-thickness medial or lateral fasciocutaneous flaps, depending on the procedure to be performed.

Posterolateral Approach
- Develop the Kocher interval between the anconeus and extensor carpi ulnaris muscle to expose the elbow capsule and lateral epicondyle.
- To expose the olecranon fossa and posterior aspect of the distal humerus, reflect the anconeus and triceps medially.
- To expose the radial head, elevate the common extensor origin anteriorly from the underlying capsule, lateral ulnar collateral ligament, and lateral epicondyle (Fig. 1.142B).
- Make an arthrotomy along the anterior border of the lateral ulnar collateral ligament and carry it distally, dividing the annular ligament.

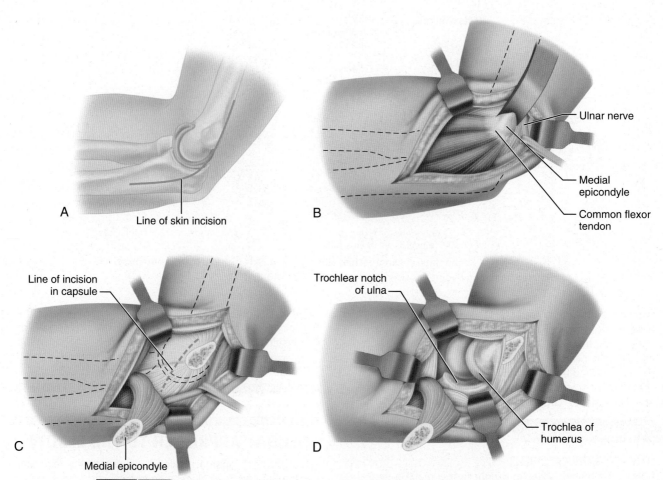

A — Line of skin incision

B — Ulnar nerve
— Medial epicondyle
— Common flexor tendon

Line of incision in capsule —
C — Medial epicondyle

Trochlear notch of ulna —
D — Trochlea of humerus

FIGURE 1.140   Campbell medial approach to elbow joint. **A,** Skin incision. **B,** Ulnar nerve has been retracted posteriorly, and medial epicondyle is being freed. **C,** Epicondyle and attached common origin of flexor muscles have been reflected distally. Joint capsule is to be incised longitudinally. **D,** Approach has been completed, and elbow joint has been dislocated. **SEE TECHNIQUE 1.113.**

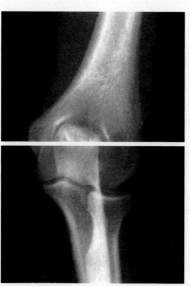

FIGURE 1.141   Kirschner wire has been taped along flexion crease of elbow. Note relation of wire to joint line. **SEE TECHNIQUE 1.114.**

- If additional exposure of the radial head is needed, perform a chevron osteotomy of the lateral epicondyle (Fig. 1.142C).
- Predrill and tap holes to accept one or two 4-mm cancellous or 3.5-mm cortical screws. Use a small sagittal saw or osteotome to perform the cut.
- Elevate the muscles from the supracondylar ridge subperiosteally, keeping them in continuity with the lateral epicondyle and the common extensor origin.
- Develop the interval between the extensor digitorum communis and extensor carpi radialis longus and brevis to the level of the deep radial (posterior interosseous) nerve where it enters the supinator at the arcade of Fröhse. This allows reflection of the common extensor origin, lateral ulnar collateral ligament, and attached lateral epicondyle in an anterior and distal direction.
- If additional exposure of the radial head, neck, and proximal shaft is needed, pronate the forearm to translate the posterior interosseous nerve anteriorly (Fig. 1.142D) and divide the annular ligament 5 mm from the edge of the lesser sigmoid notch (see Fig. 1.142C). Elevate a posterior capsular flap if needed. This violates the lateral ulnar collateral ligament, which must be repaired at closing.

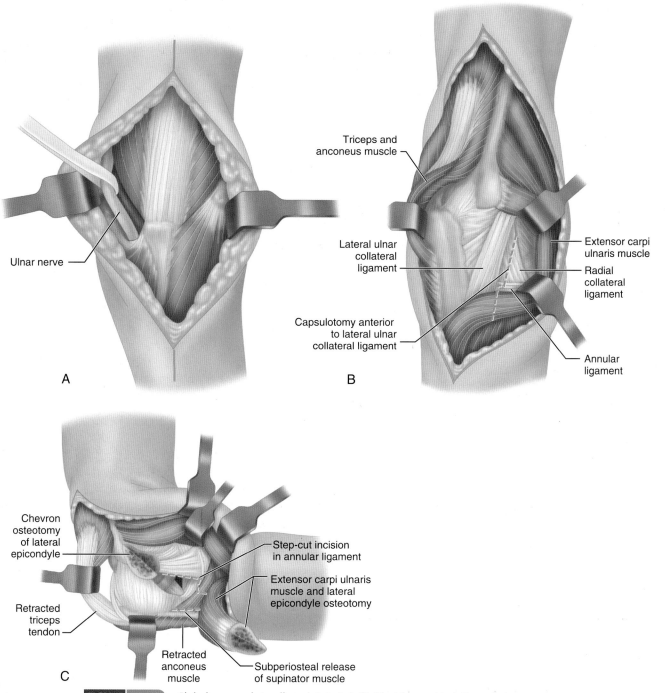

Ulnar nerve

Triceps and
anconeus muscle

Lateral ulnar
collateral
ligament

Capsulotomy anterior
to lateral ulnar
collateral ligament

Extensor carpi
ulnaris muscle

Radial
collateral
ligament

Annular
ligament

A

B

Chevron
osteotomy
of lateral
epicondyle

Retracted
triceps
tendon

Retracted
anconeus
muscle

Step-cut incision
in annular ligament

Extensor carpi ulnaris
muscle and lateral
epicondyle osteotomy

Subperiosteal release
of supinator muscle

C

FIGURE 1.142 Global approach to elbow joint. **A,** Initial incision and isolation of ulnar nerve. **B,** Lateral component. **C,** Chevron osteotomy of lateral epicondyle.

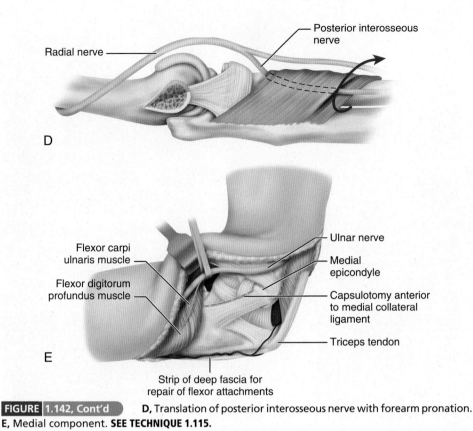

FIGURE **1.142, Cont'd** **D,** Translation of posterior interosseous nerve with forearm pronation. **E,** Medial component. **SEE TECHNIQUE 1.115.**

- Release the supinator muscle from the supinator crest of the ulna and retract it along with the posterior interosseous nerve to expose the proximal radius.

Posteromedial Approach

- To extend the approach medially, release the flexor carpi ulnaris and flexor digitorum profundus muscles subperiosteally from their ulnar origins.
- Retract anteriorly to expose the coronoid process, the anterior bundle of the medial ligament complex, and anterior joint capsule (Fig. 1.142E).

RADIUS

POSTEROLATERAL APPROACH TO THE RADIAL HEAD AND NECK

A posterolateral oblique approach safely exposes the radial head and neck; it corresponds to the distal limb of the lateral-J approach of Kocher to the elbow. It is the best approach for excising the radial head because it is not only extensile proximally and distally without danger to major vessels or nerves, but it also preserves the nerve supply to the anconeus. It is safer than an approach that separates the extensor carpi ulnaris from the extensor digitorum communis or one that separates the latter muscle from the radial extensors because both of these endanger the

posterior interosseous nerve. After experimental work on cadavers, Strachan and Ellis recommended a position of full pronation of the forearm for maximal protection of the nerve during this procedure (see Fig. 1.142D).

TECHNIQUE 1.116

- Begin an oblique incision over the posterior surface of the lateral humeral condyle and continue it obliquely distally and medially to a point over the posterior border of the ulna 3 to 5 cm distal to the tip of the olecranon (Fig. 1.143).
- Divide the subcutaneous tissue and deep fascia along the line of the incision and develop the fascial plane between the extensor carpi ulnaris and the anconeus muscles. This plane can be found more easily in the distal than in the proximal part of the incision because in the proximal part the two muscles blend at their origin.
- Retract the anconeus toward the ulnar side and the extensor carpi ulnaris toward the radial side, exposing the joint capsule in the depth of the proximal part of the wound.
- Note that the fibers of the supinator cross at a right angle to the wound, near its center and deep (anterior) to the extensor carpi ulnaris; retract the proximal fibers of the supinator distally.
- Locate the joint capsule in the depth of the wound, incise it, and expose the head and neck of the radius (Fig. 1.143). The deep branch of the radial nerve that lies between the two planes of the supinator remains undisturbed.

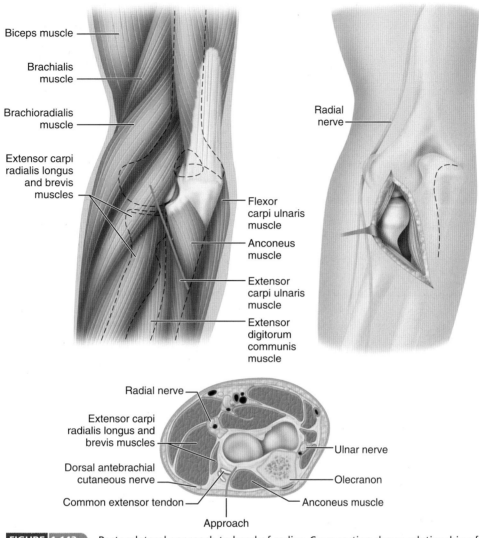

Biceps muscle

Brachialis muscle

Brachioradialis muscle

Extensor carpi radialis longus and brevis muscles

Radial nerve

Flexor carpi ulnaris muscle

Anconeus muscle

Extensor carpi ulnaris muscle

Extensor digitorum communis muscle

Radial nerve

Extensor carpi radialis longus and brevis muscles

Dorsal antebrachial cutaneous nerve

Common extensor tendon

Ulnar nerve

Olecranon

Anconeus muscle

Approach

FIGURE 1.143 Posterolateral approach to head of radius. Cross-section shows relationship of surgical dissection to adjacent anatomy. **SEE TECHNIQUE 1.116.**

APPROACH TO THE PROXIMAL AND MIDDLE THIRDS OF THE POSTERIOR SURFACE OF THE RADIUS

Exposing the proximal third of the radius is difficult because the deep branch of the radial nerve (posterior interosseous) traverses it within the supinator muscle; one must keep this nerve constantly in mind and take care to protect it from injury.

TECHNIQUE 1.117

(THOMPSON)

- Make the skin incision over the proximal and middle thirds of the radius along a line drawn from the center of the dorsum of the wrist to a point 1.5 cm anterior to the lateral humeral epicondyle (Fig. 1.144A); when the forearm is pronated, this line is nearly straight.
- Expose the lateral (radial) border of the extensor digitorum communis muscle in the distal part of the incision.

- Develop the interval between this muscle and the extensor carpi radialis brevis and retract these structures to the ulnar and radial sides.
- The abductor pollicis longus muscle is visible; retract it distally and toward the ulna to expose part of the posterior surface of the radius.
- Continue the dissection proximally between the extensor digitorum communis and the extensors carpi radialis brevis and longus to the lateral humeral epicondyle.
- Reflect the extensor digitorum communis toward the ulna to expose the supinator muscle, or for a wider view, detach the extensor digitorum from its origin on the lateral epicondyle and retract it further medially (Fig. 1.144B).
- Expose the part of the radius covered by the supinator by one of two means. Either divide the muscle fibers down to the deep branch of the radial nerve and carefully retract the nerve or free the muscle from the bone subperiosteally and reflect it proximally or distally along with the nerve; the latter is the better method if the exposure is wide enough (Fig. 1.144C).

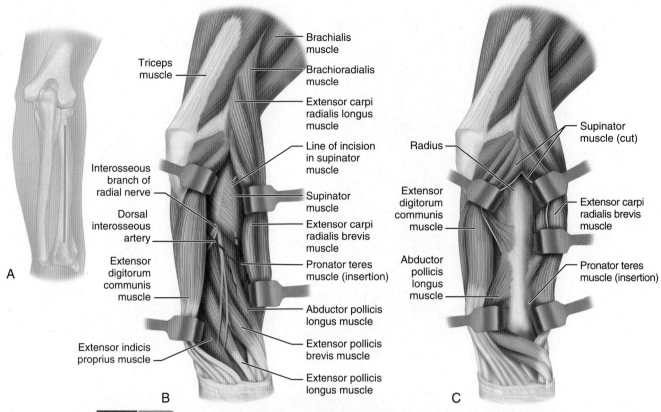

Triceps muscle

Interosseous branch of radial nerve

Dorsal interosseous artery

Extensor digitorum communis muscle

Extensor indicis proprius muscle

A

B

Brachialis muscle

Brachioradialis muscle

Extensor carpi radialis longus muscle

Line of incision in supinator muscle

Supinator muscle

Extensor carpi radialis brevis muscle

Pronator teres muscle (insertion)

Abductor pollicis longus muscle

Extensor pollicis brevis muscle

Extensor pollicis longus muscle

Radius

Extensor digitorum communis muscle

Abductor pollicis longus muscle

Supinator muscle (cut)

Extensor carpi radialis brevis muscle

Pronator teres muscle (insertion)

C

FIGURE 1.144 Thompson approach to proximal and middle thirds of posterior surface of radius. **A,** Skin incision. **B,** Relationships of supinator and deep branch of radial nerve to proximal third of radius. **C,** Approach has been completed. **SEE TECHNIQUE 1.117.**

ANTEROLATERAL APPROACH TO THE PROXIMAL SHAFT AND ELBOW JOINT

TECHNIQUE 1.118

(HENRY)
- With the forearm supinated, begin a serpentine longitudinal incision at a point just lateral and proximal to the biceps tendon and extend it distally in the forearm along the medial border of the brachioradialis and, if necessary, as far as the radial styloid (Fig. 1.145A).
- Expose the biceps tendon by incising the deep fascia on its lateral side; divide the deep fascia of the forearm in line with the skin incision, taking care to protect the radial vessels (Fig. 1.145B,C).
- Isolate and ligate the recurrent radial artery and vein immediately; otherwise, the cut ends may retract, resulting in a hematoma that may cause ischemic (Volkmann) contracture of the forearm flexor muscles. Flex the elbow to a right angle to allow more complete retraction of the brachioradialis and the radial carpal extensor muscles to expose the supinator.
- Incise the bicipital bursa, which lies in the angle between the lateral margin of the biceps tendon and the radius, and from this point distally, strip the supinator subperiosteally

from the radius and reflect it laterally; it carries with it and protects the deep branch of the radial nerve (Fig. 1.145D,E).
- Pronate the forearm and expose the radius by subperiosteal dissection.

ANTERIOR APPROACH TO THE DISTAL HALF OF THE RADIUS

The volar (anterior) surface of the distal half of the radius is broad, flat, and smooth and provides a more satisfactory bed for a plate or a graft than does the dorsal (posterior) convex surface.

TECHNIQUE 1.119

(HENRY)
- With the forearm in supination, make a 15- to 20-cm longitudinal incision over the interval between the brachioradialis and the flexor carpi radialis muscles (Fig. 1.146A-C); this interval, as Kocher stated, "lies in the frontier line between the structures innervated by the different nerves."
- Identify and protect the sensory branch of the radial nerve, which lies beneath the brachioradialis muscle. Carefully mobilize and retract medially the flexor carpi

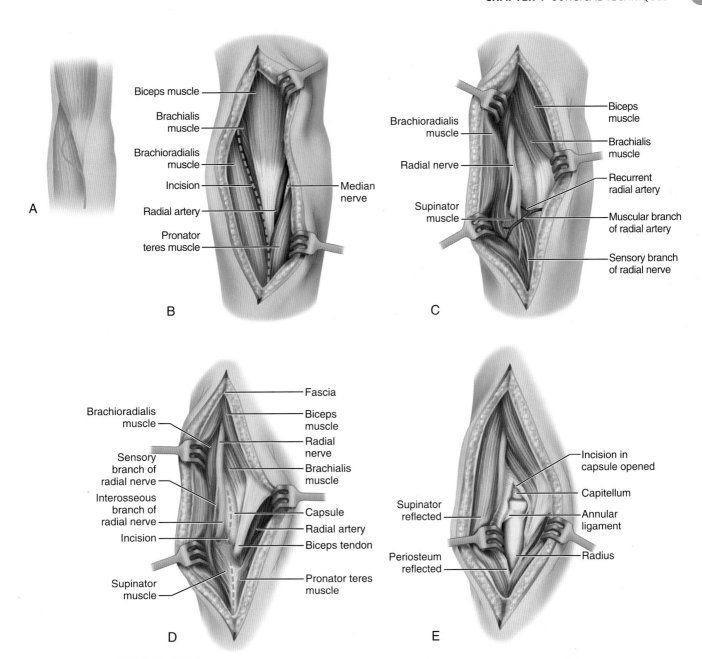

FIGURE 1.145 Modified Henry anterolateral approach to elbow joint. **A,** Incision. **B,** Fascia has been incised to expose brachioradialis laterally and biceps and brachialis medially. Lacertus fibrosus has been divided to permit dissection to be deepened between biceps tendon and pronator teres medially and brachioradialis laterally. **C,** Dissection has been deepened to expose radial nerve. Nerve and its sensory branch are protected, and recurrent radial artery is ligated and divided. **D,** *Broken line* represents incision to be made through joint capsule and along medial border of supinator to expose capitellum and proximal radius. **E,** Forearm has been supinated, and approach has been completed by reflecting supinator. Radial nerve, which courses in supinator, is protected. **SEE TECHNIQUE 1.118.**

radialis tendon and the radial artery and vein. The flexor digitorum sublimis, flexor pollicis longus, and pronator quadratus muscles are now exposed.

- Beginning at the anterolateral edge of the radius, elevate subperiosteally the flexor pollicis longus and the pronator quadratus muscles (Fig. 1.146D-F) and strip them medially (toward the ulna).

ANTERIOR APPROACH TO THE CORONOID PROCESS OF THE PROXIMAL ULNA

Yang et al. described an anterior approach to the proximal ulna for repair of coronoid fractures. This uses the interval between the brachial artery and the median nerve.

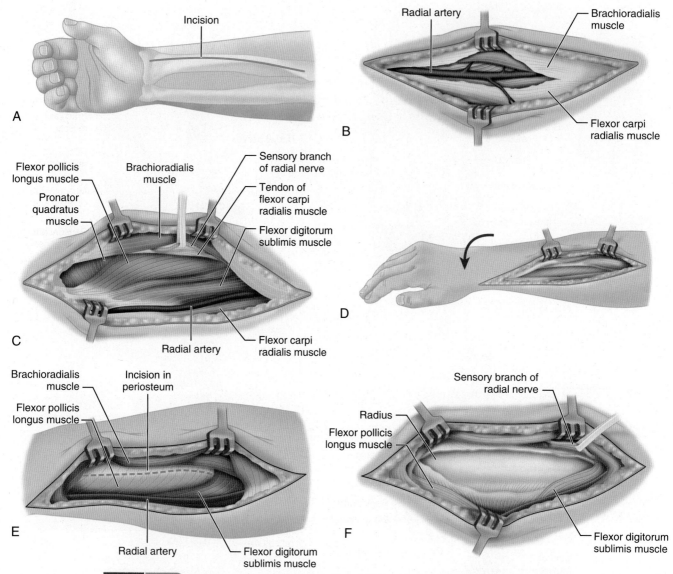

FIGURE 1.146 Henry anterior approach to distal half of radius. **A,** Skin incision. **B,** Fascia has been incised, and brachioradialis has been retracted laterally and flexor carpi radialis medially. Radial artery and sensory branch of radial nerve must be protected because they course deep to brachioradialis. **C,** Radial vessels and flexor carpi radialis tendon have been retracted medially to expose long flexor muscles of thumb and fingers and pronator quadratus. **D,** Forearm has been pronated to expose radius lateral to pronator quadratus and flexor pollicis longus. **E,** *Broken line* indicates incision to be made through periosteum. **F,** Periosteum has been incised, and flexor pollicis longus and pronator quadratus have been elevated subperiosteally from anterior surface of radius. **SEE TECHNIQUE 1.119.**

TECHNIQUE 1.120

(YANG ET AL.)

- Make an S-shaped incision from the ulnar side of the elbow to the radial side (Fig. 1.147A).
- Expose the biceps tendon, the bicipital aponeurosis, and the neurovascular bundle (Fig. 1.147B).
- Incise the biceps aponeurosis transversely exposing the biceps, pronator teres, brachial artery, and median nerve (Fig. 1.147C)

- Incise the space between the brachial artery and median nerve. Laterally retract the brachial artery, biceps, and brachioradialis; retract the median nerve and pronator teres medially. Incise the brachialis muscle and tendon longitudinally (Fig. 1.147D)
- Incise and retract the capsule exposing the coronoid process (Fig. 1.147E).

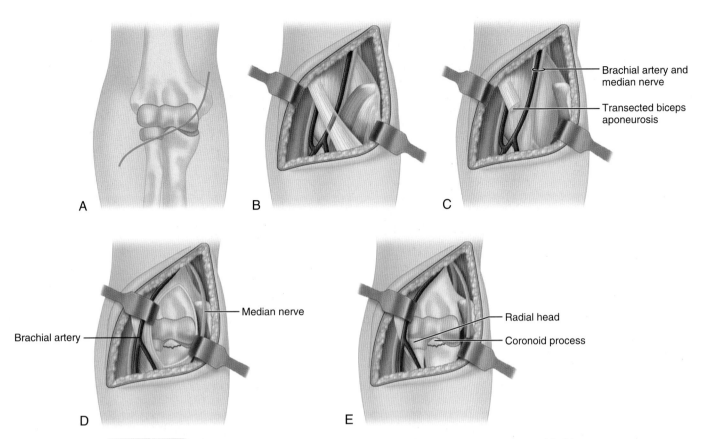

FIGURE 1.147 Anterior approach to the coronoid process. **A,** S-shaped incision in antecubital fossa. **B,** Expose the biceps, biceps aponeurosis, and neurovascular bundle. **C,** Expose the interval between the brachial artery and median nerve. **D,** Retract the brachial artery, biceps, and brachioradialis laterally and median nerve and pronator teres medially. **E,** Open the joint capsule and expose the coronoid process. **SEE TECHNIQUE 2.120.**

ULNA

APPROACH TO THE PROXIMAL THIRD OF THE ULNA AND THE PROXIMAL FOURTH OF THE RADIUS

Because part of the posterior surface of the ulna throughout its length lies just under the skin, any part of the bone can be approached by incising the skin, fascia, and periosteum along this surface.

The following approach is especially useful when treating fractures of the proximal third of the ulna associated with dislocation of the radial head. It also can be used to expose the proximal fourth of the radius alone, with less danger to the deep branch of the radial nerve than with other approaches.

TECHNIQUE 1.121

(BOYD)
- Begin the incision about 2.5 cm proximal to the elbow joint just lateral to the triceps tendon, continue it distally over the lateral side of the tip of the olecranon and along the subcutaneous border of the ulna, and end it at the junction of the proximal and middle thirds of the ulna (Fig. 1.148A).
- Develop the interval between the ulna on the medial side and the anconeus and extensor carpi ulnaris on the lateral side.
- Strip the anconeus from the bone subperiosteally in the proximal part of the incision; to expose the radial head, reflect the anconeus radially.
- Distal to the radial head, deepen the dissection to the interosseous membrane after reflecting the part of the supinator that arises from the ulna subperiosteally.
- Peel the supinator from the proximal fourth of the radius and reflect radially the entire muscle mass, including this muscle, the anconeus, and the proximal part of the extensor carpi ulnaris (Fig. 1.148B). This amply exposes the lateral surface of the ulna and the proximal fourth of the radius. The substance of the reflected supinator protects the deep branch of the radial nerve (Fig. 1.148C,D).
- In the proximal part of the wound, divide the recurrent interosseous artery but not the dorsal interosseous artery.

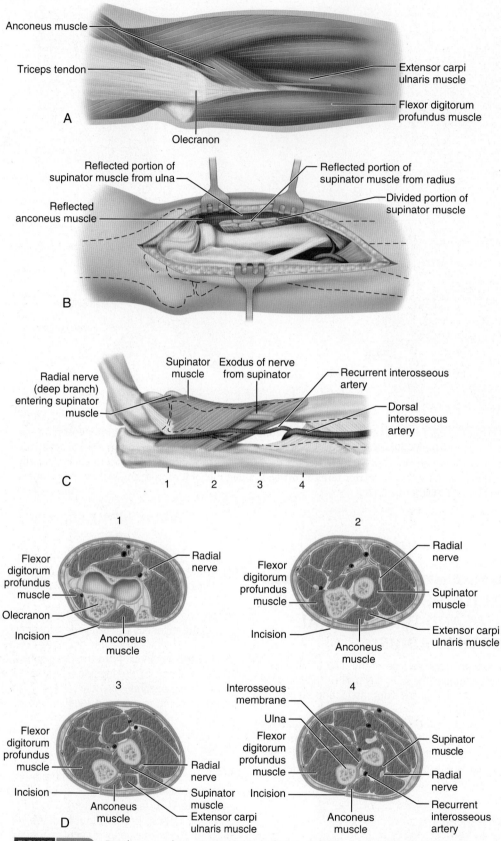

FIGURE 1.148 Boyd approach to proximal third of ulna and fourth of radius. **A,** Skin incision. **B,** Approach has been completed. **C** and **D,** Relationship of deep branch of radial nerve to superficial and deep parts of supinator. **C,** Numbers 1, 2, 3, and 4 correspond to levels of cross-sections in **D** with same numbers. **SEE TECHNIQUE 1.121.**

WRIST

DORSAL APPROACH TO THE WRIST

TECHNIQUE 1.122

- Through a 10-cm dorsal curvilinear incision centered over the Lister tubercle (Fig. 1.149A), expose the dorsal carpal ligament and define the fibrous partitions separating the tendon sheaths on the dorsum of the radius and ulna.
- Divide this ligament and the underlying periosteum over the tubercle, taking care not to injure the tendon of the extensor pollicis longus; dissect between the extensor tendons of the thumb and fingers.

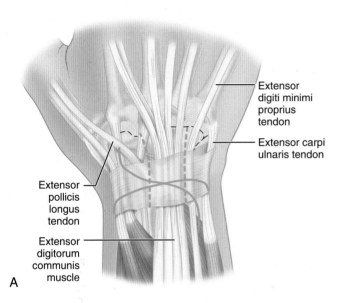

Extensor digiti minimi proprius tendon

Extensor carpi ulnaris tendon

Extensor pollicis longus tendon

Extensor digitorum communis muscle

A

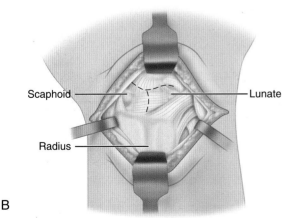

Scaphoid

Lunate

Radius

B

FIGURE 1.149 Dorsal approaches to wrist. **A,** *Solid lines* represent curved longitudinal and transverse skin incisions. *Broken lines* represent incisions through dorsal carpal ligament (see text). **B,** Scaphoid, lunate, and distal radius have been exposed through curved transverse skin incision and through incision in dorsal carpal ligament centered over Lister tubercle. **SEE TECHNIQUES 1.122 AND 1.123.**

- Elevate the periosteum of the distal inch of the radius, but preserve as much as possible of the extensor tendon sheaths.
- Retract the extensor tendons of the fingers medially (toward the ulna) to expose the dorsum of the wrist joint and to allow transverse incision of the capsule (Fig. 1.149B).

DORSAL APPROACH TO THE WRIST

TECHNIQUE 1.123

- Begin a transverse curved skin incision on the medial side of the head of the ulna, and extend it across the dorsum of the wrist to a point 1.5 cm proximal and posterior to the radial styloid (Fig. 1.149A).
- Retract the skin and the superficial and deep fasciae and retract the tendons as described in the first technique, exposing the radial side of the dorsum of the wrist.
- To expose the ulnar side, make a longitudinal incision through the dorsal carpal ligament between the extensor digiti quinti proprius and the common extensor tendons. Retract the common extensor tendons to the radial side and the tendons of the extensor digiti quinti proprius and extensor carpi ulnaris to the ulnar side and incise the capsule transversely.
- By combining these deeper incisions and alternately retracting the tendons of the common extensors of the fingers to the radial or ulnar side, one may reach the entire dorsal aspect of the joint.

VOLAR APPROACH TO THE WRIST

The volar approach often is used to remove or to reduce a dislocated lunate.

TECHNIQUE 1.124

- Make a transverse incision across the volar aspect of the wrist in the distal flexor crease (Fig. 1.150). (A curved longitudinal incision has been used but is less desirable because crossing the flexor creases produces a scar that may cause a flexion contracture.)
- Incise and retract the superficial and deep fasciae.
- Identify the palmaris longus tendon. Find and isolate the median nerve; it is usually deep to the palmaris longus tendon and slightly to its radial side. In patients with congenital absence of the palmaris longus tendon, the median nerve is the most superficial longitudinal structure on the volar aspect of the wrist. Gently retract the palmaris longus tendon (if present) and the flexor pollicis longus tendon to the radial side. Retract the flexor digitorum sublimis and profundus tendons to the ulnar side (Fig. 1.150A, *inset*).
- Incise the joint capsule, exposing the distal end of the radius and the lunate (Fig. 1.150B).

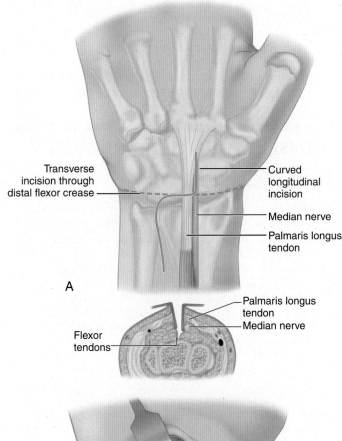

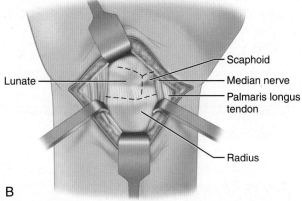

FIGURE 1.150 Volar approach to wrist. **A,** Optional transverse or curved longitudinal skin incisions. **B,** Flexor tendons and median nerve retracted as in cross-section, exposing lunate bone and distal end of radius. **SEE TECHNIQUE 1.124.**

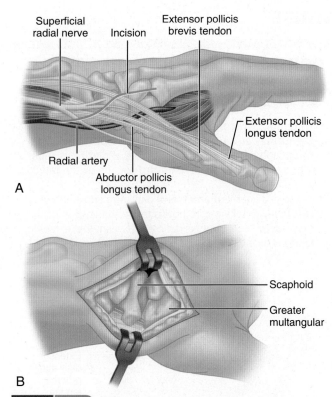

FIGURE 1.151 Lateral approach to wrist joint. **A,** Skin incision. **B,** Approach has been completed. **SEE TECHNIQUE 1.125.**

the radial artery, and the lateral terminal branch of the superficial branch of the radial nerve; retract the extensor pollicis longus tendon dorsally. This retraction exposes the tubercle of the scaphoid (Fig. 1.151B).

■ Longitudinally divide the radial collateral ligament and capsule to expose the lateral aspect of the wrist joint. Take care to protect the radial artery, which passes between the abductor pollicis longus and the extensor pollicis brevis tendons laterally and the radial collateral ligament medially, and the superficial branches of the radial nerve, which supply the skin on the dorsum of the thumb.

MEDIAL APPROACH TO THE WRIST

The medial approach may be used for arthrodesis of the wrist when tendon transfers around the dorsum of the wrist are contemplated. Historically, Smith-Petersen used it for arthrodesis of the wrist when the distal radioulnar joint was diseased or deranged; in his technique, the distal 2.5 cm of the ulna is resected.

TECHNIQUE 1.126   *Figure 1.152*

■ Make a medial curvilinear incision centered over the ulnar styloid. Its proximal limb is parallel to the ulna; at the level of the ulnar styloid, it curves dorsally and toward the palm toward the proximal end of the fifth metacarpal, and its distal limb parallels the fifth metacarpal for about 2.5 cm.

LATERAL APPROACH TO THE WRIST

TECHNIQUE 1.125

■ Make a 7.5-cm lateral curvilinear skin incision shaped like a bayonet on the radial side of the wrist (Fig. 1.151A).
■ Retract to the volar side of the wrist, the extensor pollicis brevis tendon, the abductor tendons of the thumb,

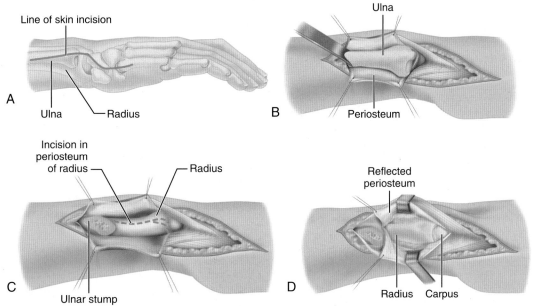

FIGURE 1.152 Smith-Petersen medial approach to wrist. **A,** Medial curvilinear incision. **B,** Ulna osteotomized obliquely 2.5 cm proximal to styloid process. **C,** Distal ulna resected and periosteum of radius incised. **D,** Radiocarpal joint exposed by reflection of capsule and ligaments from carpus and distal end of radius. **SEE TECHNIQUE 1.126.**

While incising the skin and subcutaneous tissue, carefully avoid injuring the dorsal branch of the ulnar nerve, which winds around the dorsum of the wrist immediately distal to the head of the ulna and divides into its three cutaneous branches supplying the little finger and the ulnar half of the ring finger.

- Incise the fascia and open the capsule longitudinally. Do not injure the triangular fibrocartilage attached to the ulnar styloid.

HAND

Surgical approaches to the hand are discussed in other chapter.

REFERENCES

SURGICAL TECHNIQUES

Akinyoola AL, Adegbehingbe OO, Odunsi A: Timing of antibiotic prophylaxis in tourniquet surgery, *J Foot Ankle Surg* 50:374–376, 2011.

Al-Ahaideb A: Surgical treatment of chronic acromioclavicular dislocation using the Weaver-Dunn procedure augmented by the TightRope® System, *Eur J Orthop Surg Traumatol* 24:741, 2014.

American Academy of Orthopaedic Surgeons Information Statement: Preventing the transmission of bloodborne pathogens. Available online at www.aaos.org/about/papers/advistmt/1018.asp. Accessed 12 April 2010.

American Academy of Orthopaedic Surgeons: *Preventing the transmission of bloodborne pathogens*, Rosemont, 2008, AAOS, Reviewed 2012: http://www.aaos.org/about/papers/advistmt/1018.asp.

AORN: Recommended practices for the use of the pneumatic tourniquet in the perioperative practice setting. In Blanchard J, Burlingame B, editors: *Perioperative standards and recommended practices: for inpatient and ambulator settings*, Denver, Colorado, 2011, Association of Perioperative Registered Nurses, pp 177–189.

Association of Surgical Technologists: Recommendation standards of practice for safe use of pneumatic tourniquets. Littleton, Colorado, http://www.ast.org////pdf/Standards_of_Practice/RSOP_Pneumatic_Tourniquets.pdf.

Atesok K, Fu FH, Wolf MR, et al.: Augmentation of tendon-to-bone healing, *J Bone Joint Surg* 96A:513–521, 2014.

Carragee EJ, Chu G, Rohatgi R, et al.: Cancer risk after use of recombinant bone morophogenetic protein-2 for spinal arthrodesis, *J Bone Joint Surg* 95A:1537, 2013.

El Sallakh SA: Evaluation of arthroscopic stabilization of acute acromioclavicular joint dislocation using the TightRope system, *Orthopedics* 35:e18, 2012.

Farber DC, Farber JS: Tourniquet application on the difficult thigh: technique tip, *Foot Ankle Int* 32:735, 2011.

Friesenbichler J, Maurer-Ertl W, Sadoghi P, et al.: Adverse reactions of artificial bone graft substitutes: lessons learned from using tricalcium phosphate geneX®, *Clin Orthop Relat Res* 472:976, 2014.

Gerbert J, Traynor C, Blue K, Kim K: Use of the Mini TightRope® for correction of hallux varus deformity, *J Foot Ankle Surg* 50:245, 2011.

Hernigou P, Pariat J, Queinnec S, et al.: Supercharging irradiated allografts with mesenchymal stem cells improves acetabular bone grafting in revision arthroplasty, *Int Orthop* 38:1913, 2014.

Hidalgo Díaz JJ, Muresan L, Touchal S, et al.: The new digit tourniquet ForgetMeNot®, *Orthop Traumatol Surg Res* 2017.

Jensen G, Katthagen JC, Alvarado LE, et al.: Has the arthroscopically assisted reduction of acute AC joint separations with the double tight-rope technique advantages over the clavicular hook plate fixation? *Knee Surg Sports Traumatol Arthrosc* 22:422, 2014.

Kurien T, Person RG, Scammell BE: Bone graft substitutes currently available in orthopaedic practice. The evidence for their use, *J Bone Joint Surg* 95B:583, 2013.

Lowes R: *Avoid certain bone graft substitutes in children*, FDA warns, January 2015. https://www.medscape.com/viewarticle/838493.

Luo Z-Y, Wang H-Y, Wang D, et al.: Oral vs. intravenous vs topical tranexamic acid in primary hip arthroplasty: a prospective, randomized, double-blind, controlled trial, *J Arthroplasty* 33(3):786, 2018.

Marchand LS, Rothberg DL, Kubiak EN, Higgins TF: Is this autograft worth it?: the blood loss and transfusion rates associated with reamer irrigator aspirator bone graft harvest, *J Orthop Trauma* 31(4):205, 2017.

Mont MA, Beaver WB, Dysart SH, et al.: Local infiltration analgesia with liposomal bupivacaine improves pain scores and reduces opioid use after total knee arthroplasty: results of a randomized controlled trial, 33(1):90, 2018.

Naqvi GA, Shafqat A, Awan N: Tightrope fixation of ankle syndesmosis injuries: clinical outcome, complications and technique modification, *Injury* 43:838, 2012.

Osanai T, Ogino T: Modified digital tourniquet designed to prevent the tourniquet from inadvertently being left in place after the end of surgery, *J Orthop Trauma* 24:387, 2010.

Qvick LM, Ritter CA, Mutty CE, et al.: Donor site morbidity with reamer-irrigator-aspirator (RIA) use for autogenous bone graft harvesting in a single centre 204 case series, *Injury* 44:1263, 2014.

Ramussen LE, Holm HA, Kristense PW, Kjaersgaard-Andersen P: *Tourniquet time in total knee arthroplasty* 2018, https://doi.org10.1016/j.knee.2018.01.002.

Sagi HC, Young ML, Gerstenfeld L, et al.: Qualitative and quantitative differences between bone graft obtained from the medullary canal (with a Reamer/Irrigator/Aspirator) and the iliac crest of the same patient, *J Bone Joint Surg* 94A:2128, 2012.

Taylor BC, French BG, Fowler TT, et al.: Induced membrane technique for reconstruction to manage bone loss, *J Am Acad Orthop Surg* 20:142, 2012.

Thiel E, Mutnal A, Gilot GJ: Surgical outcome following arthroscopic fixation of acromioclavicular joint disruption with the tightrope device, *Orthopedics* 34:e267, 2011.

SURGICAL APPROACHES
KNEE
Chang SM: Selection of surgical approaches to the posterolateral tibial plateau fracture by its combination patterns, *J Orthop Trauma* 25:e32, 2011.

Frosch KH, Balcarek P, Walde T, Stürmer KM: A new posterolateral approach without fibula osteotomy for the treatment of tibial plateau fractures, *J Orthop Trauma* 24:515, 2010.

He X, Ye P, Hu Y, et al.: A posterior inverted L-shaped approach for the treatment of posterior bicondylar tibial plateau fractures, *Arch Orthop Trauma Surg* 133:23, 2013.

Johnson EE, Timon S, Osuji C: Tscherne-Johnson extensile approach for tibial plateau fractures, *Clin Orthop Relat Res* 471:2760, 2013.

Kandemir U, Maclean J: Surgical approaches for tibial plateau fractures, *J Knee Surg* 27:21, 2014.

Keshmiri A, Dotzauer F, Baier C, et al.: Stability of capsule closure and postoperative anterior knee pain after medial parapatellar approach in TKA, *Arch Orthop Trauma Surg* 137:1019, 2017.

Lobenhoffer P: Posterolateral transfibular approach to tibial plateau fractures, *J Orthop Trauma* 25:e31, 2011.

Satish BRJ, Ganesan JC, Chandran P, et al.: Efficacy and mid term results of lateral parapatellar approach without tibial tubercle osteotomy for primary total knee arthroplasty with fixed valgus knees, *J Arthroplasty* 28:1751, 2013.

Solomon LB, Stevenson AW, Baird RPV, Pohl AP: Posterolateral transfibular approach to tibial plateau fractures; technique, results, and rationale, *J Orthop Trauma* 24:505, 2010.

Sun DH, Zhao Y, Zhang JT, et al.: Anterolateral tibial plateau osteotomy as a new approach for the treatment of posterolateral tibial plateau fracture. A case report, *Medicine* 97(3):e9669, 2018.

Yoon YC, Sim JA, Kim DH, Lee BK: Combined lateral femoral epicondylar osteotomy and a submeniscal approach for the treatment of a tibial plateau fracture involving the posterolateral quadrant, Injury, *Int J Care Injured* 46:422, 2015.

Yu B, Han K, Zhan C, et al.: Fibular head osteotomy: a new approach for the treatment of lateral or posterolateral tibial plateau fractures, *Knee* 17:313, 2010.

ACETABULUM AND PELVIS
Guy P: Evolution of the anterior intrapelvic (Stoppa) approach for acetabular fracture surgery, *J Orthop Trauma* 29(2):S1, 2015.

Moed BB: The modified Gibson posterior surgical approach to the acetabulum, *J Orthop Trauma* 24:315, 2010.

HIP
Cavaignac E, Laumond G, Regis P, et al.: Fixation of a fractured femoral head through a medial hip approach: an original approach to the femoral head, *Hip Int* 25(5):488, 2015.

Ishimatsu T, Kinoshita K, Nishio J, et al.: Motor-evoked potential analysis of femoral nerve status during the direct anterior approach for total hip arthroplasty, *J Bone Joint Surg Am* 100:572, 2018.

Mednick RE, Alvi HM, Morgan CE, et al.: Femoral vein blood flow during a total hip arthroplasty using a modified Heuter approach, *J Arthroplasty* 30:786, 2015.

Ohmori T, Kabata T, Maeda T, et al.: Selection of a surgical approach for total hip arthroplasty according to the depth to the surgical site, *Hip Int* 27(3):273, 2017.

York PJ, Smarck CT, Judet T, Mauffrey C: Total hip arthroplasty via the anterior approach: tips and tricks for primary and revision surgery, *Int Orthop* 40:2041, 2016.

FOOT AND ANKLE
Choi JY, Kim JH, Ko HT, Suh JS: Single oblique posterolateral approach for open reduction and internal fixation of posterior malleolar fractures with an associated lateral malleolar fracture, *J Foot Ankle Surg* 54:559, 2015.

Kesemenli CC, Memisogu K, Atmaca H: A minimally invasive technique for the reduction of calcaneal fractures using the Endobutton®, *J Foot Ankle Surg* 52:215, 2013.

Knupp M, Zwicky L, Lang TH, et al.: Medial approach to the subtalar joint. Anatomy, indications, technique tips, *Foot Ankle Clin N Am* 20:311, 2015.

Park J, Che JH: The sinus tarsi approach in displaced intra-articular calcaneal fractures, *Arch Orthop Trauma Surg* 137:1055, 2017.

Schepers T, Den Hartog D, Vogels LMM, Van Lieshout EMM: Extended lateral approach for intra-articular calcaneal fractures: an inverse relationship between surgeon experience and wound complications, *J Foot Ankle Surg* 52:167, 2013.

HUMERUS
Boschi V, Pogorelic Z, Gulan G, et al.: Subbrachial approach to humeral shaft fractures: new surgical technique and retrospective case series study, *Can J Surg* 56:27, 2013.

Kuhne MA, Friess D: Supine extensile approach to the anterolateral humerus, *Orthopedics* 39(1):193, 2016.

Phelps KD, Harmer LS, Crickard CV, et al.: A preoperative planning tool: aggregate anterior approach to the humerus with quantitative comparisons, *J Orthop Trauma* 32:e229, 2018.

Traver JL, Guzman MA, Cannada LK, Kaar SG: Is the axillary nerve at risk during a deltoid-splitting approach for proximal humerus fractures? *J Orthop Trauma* 30:240, 2016.

SHOULDER
Chou YC, Tseng IC, Chiang CW, Wu CC: Shoulder hemiarthroplasty for proximal humeral fractures; comparisons between the deltopectoral and anterolateral deltoid-splitting approaches, *J Shoulder Elbow Surg* 22:e1, 2013.

Nathe T, Tseng S, Yoo B: The anatomy of the supraclavicular nerve during surgical approach to the clavicular shaft, *Clin Orthop Relat Res* 469:890, 2011.

Ponce BA, Kundukulam JA, Pflugner R, et al.: Sternoclavicular joint surgery: how far does danger lurk below? *J Shoulder Elbow Surg* 22:993, 2013.

ELBOW
Hasan SA, Rauls RB, Cordell CL, et al.: "Zone of vulnerability" for radial nerve injury: anatomic study, *J Surg Orthop Adv* 23:105, 2014.

FOREARM
Yang X, Chang W, Chen W, et al.: A novel anterior approach for the fixation of ulnar coronoid process fractures, *Orthop Traumaol Surg Res* 103:899, 2017.

The complete list of references is available online at Expert Consult.com.

CHAPTER 2

ADVANCED IMAGING IN ORTHOPAEDICS

Dexter H. Witte III

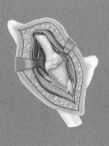

Although routine radiography currently remains the primary imaging modality in orthopaedics, more advanced imaging techniques are now an integral part of the modern orthopaedic practice. Modalities such as magnetic resonance imaging (MRI), computed tomography (CT), and ultrasonography (US) are valuable diagnostic tools and are fundamental components of image-guided interventional procedures. The scope of these advanced imaging techniques across the field of orthopaedics is far too broad to address in a single chapter. Therefore, this chapter provides a brief synopsis of the use of MRI and CT in orthopaedics. Musculoskeletal US is reviewed in various chapters as appropriate.

MAGNETIC RESONANCE IMAGING

Aside from routine radiography, no imaging modality has as great an impact on the current practice of orthopaedics as MRI. MRI provides unsurpassed soft-tissue contrast and multiplanar capability with spatial resolution that approaches that of CT. Consequently, MRI has superseded older imaging methods such as myelography, arthrography, and even angiography. In the past 40 years, MRI has matured to become a critical component of the modern orthopaedic practice.

Unlike radiography or CT, the MR image is generated without the use of potentially harmful ionizing radiation. MR images are created by placing the patient in a strong magnetic field (tens of thousands of times stronger than the earth's magnetic field). The magnetic force affects the nuclei within the field, specifically the nuclei of elements with odd numbers of protons or neutrons. The most abundant element satisfying this criterion is hydrogen, which is plentiful in water and fat. These nuclei, which are essentially protons, possess a quantum spin. When the patient's tissues are subjected to

this strong magnetic field, protons align themselves with respect to the field. Because all imaging is performed within this constant magnetic force, this becomes the steady state, or equilibrium. In this steady state, a radiofrequency (RF) pulse is applied, which excites the magnetized protons in the field and perturbs the steady state. After application of this pulse, a receiver coil or antenna listens for an emitted RF signal that is generated as these excited protons relax or return to equilibrium. This emitted signal is then used to create the MR image.

MRI TECHNOLOGY AND TECHNIQUE

A wide variety of MR imaging systems are commercially available. Scanners can be grouped roughly by field strength. High-field scanners possess superconducting magnets considered to have field strengths greater than 1.0 Tesla (T). Low-field scanners operate at field strengths of 0.3 to 0.7 T. Ultra low-field scanners operate below 0.1 T but are generally limited to studying the appendicular anatomy. The strength of the magnetic field directly correlates with the signal available to create the MR image. High-field scanners generate higher signal-to-noise images, allowing shorter scanning times, thinner scan slices, and smaller fields of view. At lower field strengths, scan field of view or slice thickness must be increased or imaging time lengthened to compensate for lower signal. In the past, lower field strength scanners presented the advantage of an "open" bore, which helped minimize claustrophobia and allow for more comfortable patient positioning when imaging off-axis structures such as elbows and wrists. However, current-generation high-field scanners have bores of larger diameter and shorter length, thus eliminating this low-field advantage.

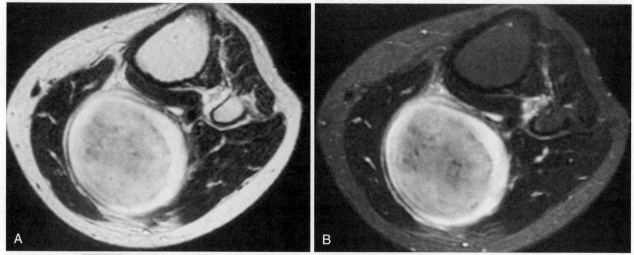

FIGURE 2.1   Chemical shift fat-suppression technique. **A,** Axial fast spin-echo, T2-weighted image of large soft-tissue mass in calf. Hyperintense fat blends with anterior and posterior margins of lesion. **B,** Addition of fat suppression allows for better delineation of tumor margins.

Powerful 3 T scanners have become commercially available in the past several years. Although high-quality musculoskeletal imaging can be performed at 1.5 T, these 3.0 T scanners may be valuable when evaluating small body parts and may provide better image quality in larger patients. At present, the clinical applications of 7 T scanners are being studied at many research centers.

Although an image can be acquired in the main coil (the hollow tube in which the patient lies during the study), almost all MR images are acquired with a separate receiving coil. For evaluation of smaller articular structures, such as the menisci of the knee or the rotator cuff, specialized surface coils are mandatory. Several types of surface coils are available, including coils tailored for specific body parts such as the spine, shoulder, wrist, and temporomandibular joints, as well as versatile flexible coils and circumferential extremity coils. These coils serve as antennae placed close to the joint or limb, markedly improving signal and resolution but also limiting the volume of tissue that can be imaged. Thus, larger surface coils have been developed with phased-array technology, providing the improved signal that is seen in smaller coils with an expanded coverage area. These phased-array coils are available for the knee, shoulder, and torso and are now standard on most state-of-the-art scanners. Optimal coil selection is mandatory for high-quality imaging of joints or small parts.

Although all studies involve magnetization and RF signals, the method and timing of excitation and acquisition of the signal can be varied to affect the signal intensity of the various tissues in the volume. Musculoskeletal MRI examinations primarily use spin-echo technique, which produces T1-weighted, proton (spin) density, and T2-weighted images. T1 and T2 are tissue-specific characteristics. These values reflect measurements of the rate of relaxation to the steady state. By varying the timing of the application of RF pulses (TR, or repetition time) and the timing of acquisition of the returning signal (TE, or echo time), an imaging sequence can accentuate T1 or T2 tissue characteristics. In most cases, fat has a high signal (bright) on T1-weighted images and fluid has a high signal on T2-weighted images. Structures with little water or fat, such as cortical bone, tendons, and ligaments, are

hypointense (dark) in all types of sequences. Improvements in MR techniques have allowed for much faster imaging. Shorter imaging sequences are better tolerated by patients and allow for less motion artifact. One such improvement, fast spin-echo technique, reduces the length of T2-weighted sequences by two thirds or more. Fat signal in fast spin-echo images remains fairly intense, a problem that can be eliminated by chemical-shift fat-suppression techniques (Fig. 2.1). Fat suppression also can be achieved by using a short-tau inversion recovery (STIR) sequence. These fat-suppression techniques can be useful in the detection of edema in both bone marrow and soft tissue and therefore play an important role in the imaging of trauma and neoplasms. For simplicity, imaging series, whether acquired with chemical shift or inversion recovery fat-suppression techniques, are often referred to as "fluid-sensitive" sequences. Another fast imaging method, gradient-echo technique, is more widely used in nonorthopaedic imaging such as MR angiography. The short echo times available with this technique are helpful in minimizing cerebrospinal fluid flow artifacts in cervical spine studies. Gradient echo imaging can be used to generate isovolumetric images that permit multiplanar image reconstruction. These reconstructed images can be used to more accurately assess glenoid bone loss following shoulder dislocation or to evaluate acetabular or femoral head morphology in patients with dysplasia or impingement. Most musculoskeletal MR studies are composed of a number of imaging sequences or series, tailored to detect and define a certain pathologic process. Because the imaging planes (axial, sagittal, coronal, oblique) and the sequence type (T1, T2, gradient-echo) are chosen at the outset, advanced understanding of the clinical problem is required to perform high-quality imaging.

CONTRAINDICATIONS

Some patients are not candidates for MRI. Absolute contraindications to MRI include intracerebral aneurysm clips, automatic defibrillators, internal hearing aids, and metallic orbital foreign bodies. Older cardiac pacemakers generally are not approved for MR imaging; however, a new generation

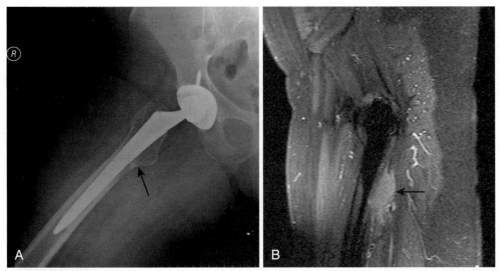

FIGURE 2.2 Magnetic resonance imaging with orthopaedic hardware in a patient with metastatic lung disease. **A,** Lateral radiograph of the proximal femur shows a subtle lesion in the posterior cortex adjacent to the femoral component of a titanium total hip prosthesis *(arrow)*. **B,** Fat-suppressed inversion recovery image displays a metastasis immediately adjacent to the hardware *(arrow)*. Note that minimal artifact is generated by the titanium stem.

of MRI-compatible pacemakers has been developed. Cardiac valve prostheses can be safely scanned. Relative contraindications include first-trimester pregnancy and recently placed intravascular stents. Generally, internal orthopaedic hardware and orthopaedic prostheses are safe to scan, although ferrous metals can create local artifact that can obscure adjacent tissues. Severity of metal artifact depends on hardware bulk, orientation, and material. For example, titanium prostheses generate much less artifact than stainless steel (Fig. 2.2). Certain adjustments to the scan parameters may reduce, but not eliminate, metal artifact. In fact, newly developed imaging sequences are proving useful for detection of periprosthetic bone resorption and soft-tissue masses. Metal prostheses may also become warm during the examination, although this is rarely noticed by the patient and almost never requires termination of the study. Patients with metal external fixation devices should not be scanned. If there is a question regarding the MR compatibility of an implantable device (e.g., pain stimulator, infusion pump), the manufacturer should be consulted.

CONTRAST AGENTS IN MRI

As elsewhere in the body, the administration of gadolinium contrast material can be of great value in evaluating certain musculoskeletal conditions. MR contrast agents are composed of gadolinium ions that are tightly bound to complex macromolecules. These agents can be administered intravenously or intraarticularly with high degree of safety. Normally MR contrast is rapidly filtered and excreted by the kidneys. As opposed to iodinated contrast material used in CT, gadolinium contrast agents are not nephrotoxic. In patients with significantly impaired renal function, however, delayed excretion of gadolinium has been associated with a rare connective tissue disease, nephrogenic systemic fibrosis. The incidence of this complication actually varies with the type of gadolinium macromolecule utilized, and these agents should be administered with caution in patients with acute or chronic kidney disease (stage 4 or 5).

FOOT AND ANKLE

One of the more complex anatomic regions in the human body is the foot and ankle. The complexity of midfoot and hindfoot articulations and the variety of pathologic conditions in the tendons and ligaments make evaluation difficult from a clinical and imaging perspective. Most examinations of the foot and ankle are performed to evaluate tendinopathy, articular disorders, and osseous pathologic conditions, often after trauma. MRI can be quite useful when the examination is directed at solving a certain clinical problem, but its value as a screening study for nonspecific pain is more limited. Given the small size of structures to be examined, optimal imaging is achieved on a high field strength magnet, and the use of a surface coil, typically an extremity coil, is mandatory. Ideally, the clinical presentation will allow the examination to be directed at either the forefoot or ankle/hindfoot. This arbitrary division allows for a sufficiently small field of view (10 to 12 cm) to generate high-resolution images. Images can be prescribed in orthogonal or oblique planes, with combinations of T1-weighted, T2-weighted, and fat-suppressed sequences. The examination should be tailored to best define the clinically suspected problem.

TENDON INJURIES

MRI excels in the evaluation of pathologic conditions in the numerous tendons about the ankle joint. Most commonly affected are the calcaneal and posterior tibial tendons. In chronic tendinitis, the calcaneal tendon thickens and becomes oval or circular in cross-section. The pathologically enlarged tendon maintains low signal on all sequences. When partially torn, the tendon demonstrates focal or fusiform thickening with interspersed areas of edema or hemorrhage that brighten on T2-weighted series (Fig. 2.3). With complete rupture, there is discontinuity of the tendon fibers. Similarly, abnormalities of the posterior tibial tendon can be confidently diagnosed with MRI. Increased fluid in the sheath of the tendon indicates tenosynovitis. Insufficient or ruptured tendons

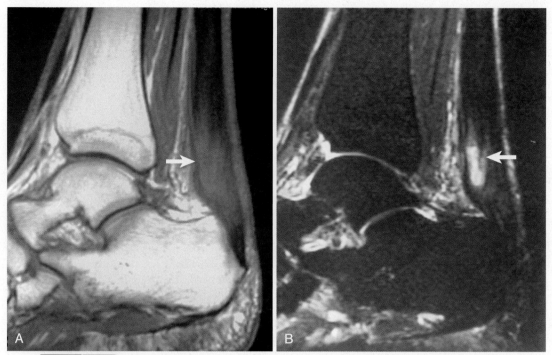

FIGURE 2.3   Partial tear of calcaneal tendon. **A,** Sagittal T1-weighted image demonstrates markedly thickened calcaneal tendon containing areas of intermediate signal *(arrow).* **B,** Sagittal fat-suppressed, T2-weighted image exhibits fluid within tendon substance, indicating partial tear *(arrow).*

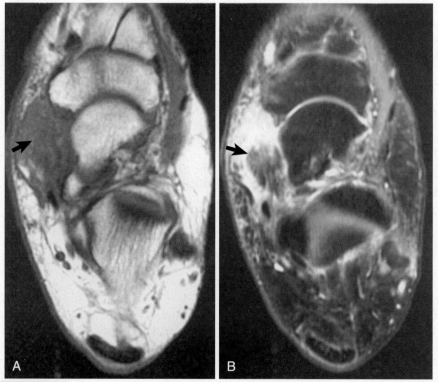

FIGURE 2.4   Posterior tibial tendon tear. **A,** Axial T1-weighted image reveals swollen, ill-defined region of intermediate signal intensity, representing fluid and abnormal tendon *(arrow).* **B,** Axial fat-suppressed, T2-weighted image shows thickened tendon *(arrow)* surrounded by hyper-intense fluid.

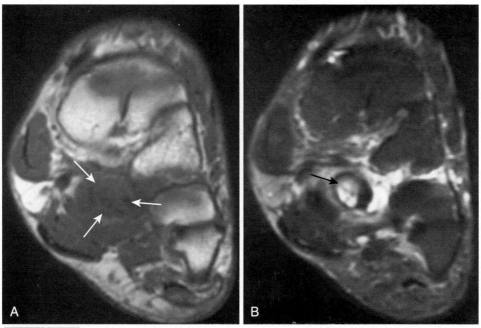

FIGURE 2.5   Peroneus longus tendon rupture. **A,** Coronal T1-weighted image through midfoot shows increased diameter of peroneus longus tendon *(arrows)*. **B,** Coronal fat-suppressed, T2-weighted image reveals fluid signal within ruptured tendon *(arrow)*.

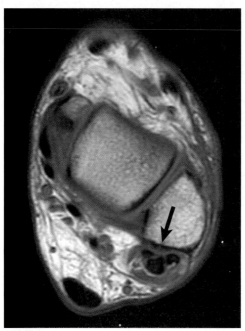

FIGURE 2.6   Longitudinal split tear of the peroneus brevis tendon. T1-weighted axial image at the level of the ankle joint shows a longitudinal split of the peroneus brevis tendon *(arrow)* between the lateral malleolus anteriorly and the peroneus longus tendon posteriorly.

can appear thickened, attenuated, or even discontinuous (Fig. 2.4). Similar abnormalities are often seen in the flexor tendons or peroneus tendons (Fig. 2.5). Longitudinal splitting of the peroneus tendon is usually quite well displayed on axial MRI images (Fig. 2.6).

LIGAMENT INJURIES

The medial and lateral stabilizing ligaments of the tibiotalar and talocalcaneal joints and the distal tibiofibular ligaments are well-visualized with proper positioning of the foot. Although ligamentous injuries about the ankle are common, MRI has a limited role in the evaluation of acute injury. In the acute setting, the MRI examination is helpful in detecting associated occult osteochondral injury. In patients with chronic instability, MRI can provide useful information of the integrity of the lateral ligamentous complex, tibiofibular ligaments, and tibiofibular syndesmosis. Additionally, MRI has proven useful in evaluating the lateral recess of the ankle joint in patients with impingement. Regions of fibrosis associated with anterolateral impingement are identified in the lateral gutter, especially when fluid is present in the ankle joint.

OSSEOUS INJURIES

As with the rest of the skeleton, MRI is especially well-suited for evaluating occult bone pathology in the foot and ankle. MRI is often used to evaluate patients with heel pain, where the differential diagnosis includes both stress fracture and plantar fasciitis. Stress fractures are depicted as areas of marrow edema well before radiographic changes are apparent (Fig. 2.7). MRI is as sensitive as bone scintigraphy while providing greater anatomic detail and specificity. The multiplanar capability of MRI is useful in assessing the ankle and subtalar joints. With high-quality imaging, excellent characterization of osteochondral lesions of the talus can be useful in surgical planning. Hepple et al. developed a classification of osteochondral lesions of the talus based on the MRI appearance. Lesion stability can be inferred by inspection of the overlying articular cartilage and the underlying osseous interface (Fig. 2.8). CT plays a complementary role to MRI if osseous avulsions or tiny intraarticular calcifications are suspected.

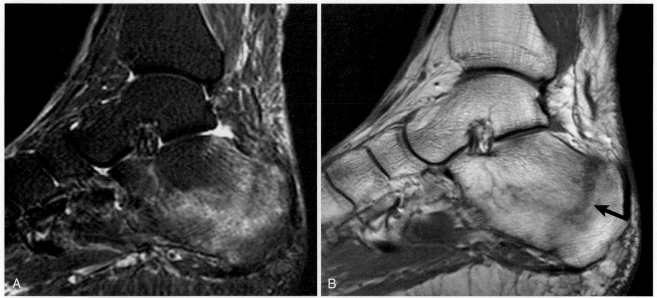

FIGURE 2.7 Calcaneal stress fracture. **A,** Sagittal fat-suppressed T2-weighted image through the hindfoot shows hyperintense marrow edema in the calcaneal tuberosity. **B,** Sagittal T1-weighted image at the same location clearly demonstrates a linear hypointense fracture line *(arrow).*

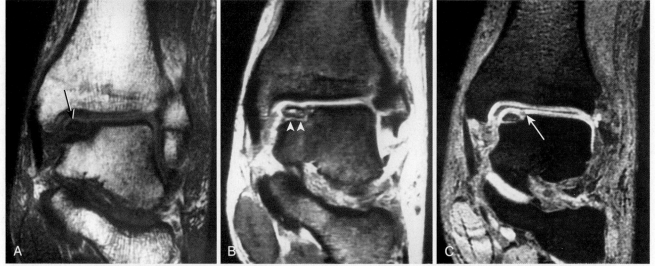

FIGURE 2.8 Osteochondritis dissecans of talus in college football player. **A,** Coronal T1-weighted image shows osteochondral fragment in medial talar dome. Loss of fat signal suggests sclerosis or fibrosis *(arrow).* **B,** Coronal fat-suppressed, T2-weighted image demonstrates fluid signal between lesion and host bone *(arrowheads),* indicating unstable fragment. **C,** Coronal fat-suppressed, spoiled gradient-echo technique reveals abnormal decreased signal *(arrow)* in overlying articular cartilage, indicating defect confirmed by arthroscopy.

Other pathologic marrow processes such as osteonecrosis and tumors can be evaluated as well.

OTHER DISORDERS OF FOOT AND ANKLE

MRI has become an increasingly useful tool in the workup of forefoot pathology. Studies can be designed specifically to evaluate the metatarsals and phalanges and adjacent joints. Focused imaging of the metatarsophalangeal joints can detect sesamoid pathology and plantar plate injuries. MRI is a fundamental tool in the workup of a patient with a soft-tissue or bone tumor. The excellent multiplanar anatomic information provided by MRI allows detection and definition of masses in the foot. Interdigital or Morton neuroma is most frequently found in the distal third metatarsal interspace. Unlike most other tumors, this lesion lacks increased signal on T2-weighted sequences. Another common foot mass, plantar fibroma or plantar fibromatosis, usually is quite easily confirmed by the presence of signal-poor mass arising from the plantar fascia. The MRI evaluation of other neoplasms is discussed later in this chapter.

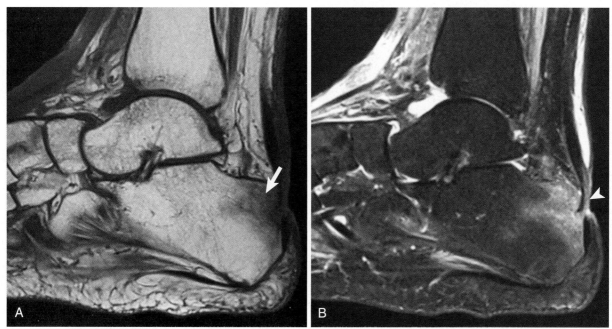

FIGURE 2.9 Osteomyelitis of calcaneus. **A,** Sagittal T1-weighted image shows abnormal hypointense marrow signal throughout the posterior calcaneus *(arrow)*. **B,** Sagittal fat-suppressed T2-weighted image shows subcortical marrow edema consistent with osteomyelitis. Note the overlying soft-tissue ulcer *(arrowhead)*.

MRI also is a valuable imaging modality in the evaluation of patients with suspected bone or soft-tissue infection. Because of the excellent depiction of bone marrow, osteomyelitis can be detected quite early, certainly well before radiographic abnormalities are visible (Fig. 2.9). The anatomic information provided by MRI can assist in surgical planning by defining the extent of bone involvement. Certain fat-suppressed sequences are so sensitive that reactive marrow edema (osteitis) can be seen even before frank osteomyelitis. Although the sensitivity of MRI for osteomyelitis approaches 100%, the reported specificity is less. Some authors have suggested relying on T1-weighted marrow replacement rather than T2-weighted signal abnormality (edema) to increase specificity. In neuropathic patients, the specificity of MR signal abnormalities is reduced; therefore the current workup of osteomyelitis in the diabetic foot often involves a combination of scintigraphy, MRI, laboratory data, and especially physical examination. In almost all cases of pedal osteomyelitis, osseous involvement is secondary to spread from adjacent soft-tissue infection and ulceration. Conversely, the presence of bone marrow signal abnormalities in the absence of a regional soft-tissue wound strongly favors neuropathic disease rather than osteomyelitis. For the evaluation of surrounding soft-tissue infection, MRI is the modality of choice. The addition of contrast-enhanced sequences is helpful in defining nonenhancing fluid collections/abscesses and devascularized or gangrenous tissue. Although the diabetic foot can be a diagnostic challenge, normal MRI marrow signal confidently excludes osteomyelitis.

KNEE

The knee is the most frequently studied region of the appendicular skeleton. Standard extremity coils allow high-resolution images of the commonly injured internal structures of the joint. The routine MRI examination of the knee consists of spin-echo sequences obtained in sagittal, coronal, and usually axial planes. Most examiners prefer to evaluate the menisci on sagittal proton (spin) density–weighted images. The sagittal images are prescribed in a plane parallel to the course of the anterior cruciate ligament (ACL), approximately 15 degrees internally rotated to the true sagittal plane. Coronal images are useful in evaluating medial and lateral supporting structures. The patellofemoral joint is best studied in the axial plane.

PATHOLOGIC CONDITIONS OF MENISCI

A large percentage of knee pain or disability is caused by pathologic conditions of the menisci. The menisci are composed of fibrocartilage and appear as low-signal structures on all pulse sequences. The menisci are best studied in the sagittal and coronal planes. On sagittal images, the menisci appear as dark triangles in the central portion of the joint and assume a "bow tie" configuration at the periphery of the joint. Regions of increased signal can often be seen within the normally dark fibrocartilage of the menisci. Areas of abnormal hyperintense signal may or may not communicate with a meniscal articular surface. Noncommunicating signal changes correspond to areas of mucoid degeneration that are not visible arthroscopically. Conversely, abnormalities that extend to the meniscal articular surface represent tears (Figs. 2.10 to 2.12). Although it has been suggested that noncommunicating signal or mucoid changes progress to meniscal tears, follow-up examinations have not confirmed this progression. Generally, communicating signal abnormalities that are seen on only one image should not be considered tears unless there is associated anatomic distortion of the meniscus. Meniscal tears should be defined as to location (anterior horn, body, posterior horn, free edge, or periphery) and orientation (horizontal, vertical/longitudinal, radial, complex).

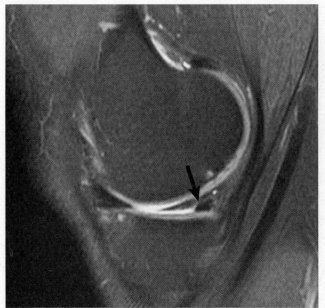

FIGURE 2.10   Meniscal tear. Sagittal fat-suppressed proton density–weighted image demonstrates linear increased signal traversing posterior horn of medial meniscus, indicating horizontal oblique tear *(arrow)*.

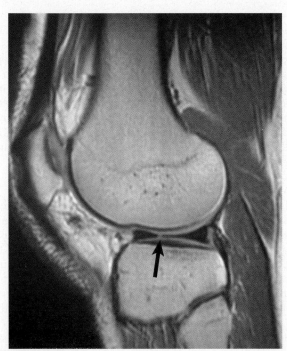

FIGURE 2.11   Meniscal tear. Sagittal proton density–weighted image reveals small defect in free edge of body of lateral meniscus, indicating radial tear *(arrow)*.

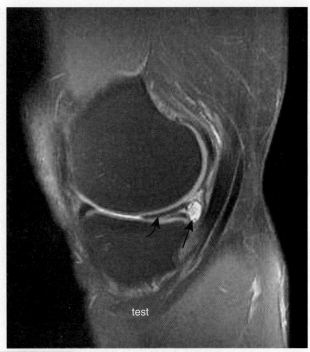

test

FIGURE 2.12   Meniscal cyst. Sagittal fat-suppressed, proton density–weighted image of knee shows a hyperintense meniscal cyst *(straight arrow)* adjacent to medial meniscus. Associated tear is present in inferior articular surface of meniscus *(curved arrow)*.

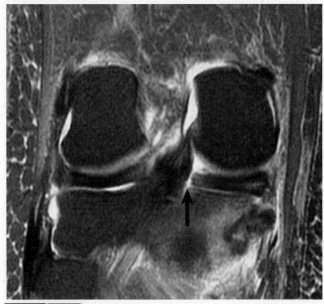

FIGURE 2.13   Root ligament tear of the posterior horn of the medial meniscus. Coronal fat-suppressed proton density-weighted image demonstrates a fluid-filled defect *(arrow)* in the posterior horn of the medial meniscus at the root ligament.

Relatively common and particularly debilitating in elderly patients, radial tears of the posterior horn or posterior root ligament of the medial meniscus are best seen on far posterior coronal images (Fig. 2.13). These root ligament injuries allow for peripheral meniscal displacement and frequently are associated with subchondral stress or insufficiency fractures of the medial compartment. Complications of tears, such as displaced fragments (bucket-handle tears, inferiorly

displaced medial fragment), should be suspected when the orthotopic portion of the meniscus is small or truncated. Careful examination of the joint, often in the coronal plane, will reveal the displaced, hypointense meniscal fragment (Figs. 2.14 and 2.15). The sensitivity and specificity of MRI in detecting meniscal tears routinely exceed 90%.

Studies have shown that many factors affect the accuracy of MRI with respect to meniscal evaluation, including the

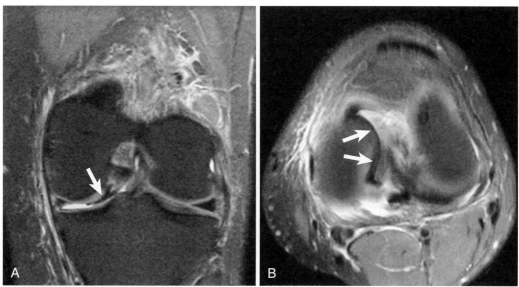

FIGURE 2.14 Bucket handle tear of medial meniscus. Coronal **(A)** and axial **(B)** fat-suppressed, proton density-weighted images demonstrate centrally displaced portion of medial meniscus *(arrows)*.

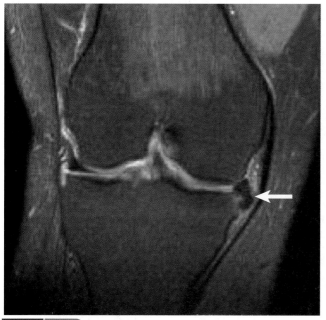

FIGURE 2.15 Inferiorly displaced medial meniscal fragment. Fat-suppressed, proton density–weighted image demonstrates portion of medial meniscus displaced inferiorly and deep to medial collateral ligament *(arrow)*.

experience of both the radiologist in interpreting studies as well as the orthopaedist performing the correlating arthroscopy. Many pitfalls in interpretation exist. When studying the central portions of the menisci, the meniscofemoral ligaments and transverse meniscal ligament can create problems. Recognition of the hiatus for the popliteus tendon will prevent the false diagnosis of a tear in the posterior horn of the lateral meniscus. Meniscocapsular separation is often difficult to detect in the absence of a complete detachment and resulting free-floating meniscus. Elderly patients often exhibit a greatly increased intrameniscal signal that can be mistaken

for a tear. The specificity of MRI for meniscal tear is reduced in patients who have undergone prior meniscal surgery. Most examiners, however, continue to rely on MRI in such patients, using caution with menisci that have greater degrees of surgical resection. Awareness of any history of prior meniscal debridement or repair may affect the interpretation of the examination, and such history should be provided to the interpreting physician. If possible, correlation of the postoperative examination with preoperative MR images is quite helpful in identifying the presence of a new tear. Rarely, the intraarticular injection of gadolinium (MR arthrography) can help differentiate healed or repaired tears from reinjury.

Other morphologic abnormalities of the menisci and adjacent structures are nicely shown with MRI. The abnormally thick or flat discoid meniscus is seen more commonly on the lateral side. Although visualization of the "bow tie" configuration of the lateral meniscus in the sagittal plane on more than three adjacent images indicates a discoid meniscus, the abnormal cross-section usually is quite apparent on the coronal images (Fig. 2.16). Meniscal cysts, which usually are associated with and adjacent to meniscal tears, frequently can be easily seen as discrete T2-weighted hyperintense fluid collections located medially or laterally (see Fig. 2.12).

CRUCIATE LIGAMENT INJURY

MRI is the only noninvasive means of imaging the cruciate ligaments. As described earlier, the sagittal imaging plane of the knee examination is prescribed to approximate the plane of the ACL. The normal ACL appears as a linear band of hypointense fibers interspersed with areas of intermediate signal. The ACL courses from its femoral attachment on the lateral condyle at the posterior extent of the intercondylar notch to the anterior aspect of the tibial eminence. High-resolution images often will define discreet anteromedial and posterolateral bands. On the sagittal images, the orientation of the normal ACL is parallel to the roof of the intercondylar notch. Reliable signs of ACL rupture include an abnormal horizontal course, a wavy or irregular appearance, or fluid-filled gaps in

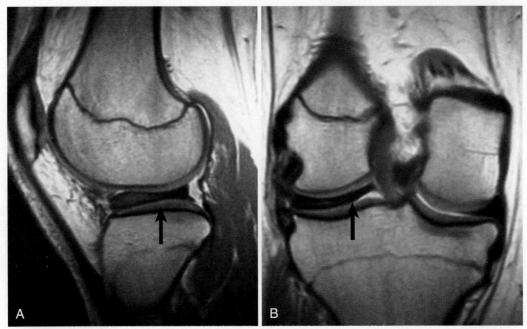

FIGURE 2.16 Discoid meniscus in 3-year-old boy. **A,** Sagittal proton density–weighted image reveals abnormally thick lateral meniscus *(arrow)*. **B,** Coronal fat-suppressed, proton density–weighted image demonstrates extension of discoid meniscus centrally *(arrow)* into weight-bearing portion of lateral compartment.

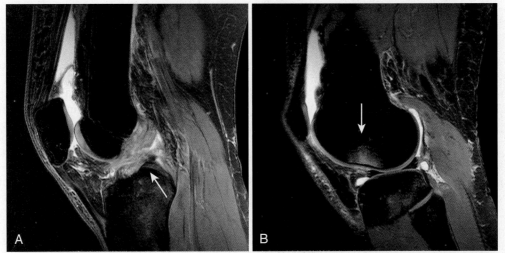

FIGURE 2.17 Acute anterior cruciate ligament tear. **A,** Fat-suppressed, proton density–weighted sagittal image shows edema throughout abnormally oriented anterior cruciate ligament fibers *(arrow)*. **B,** Fat-suppressed proton density–weighted image demonstrates typical associated bone contusion in the lateral femoral condyle *(arrow)*.

a discontinuous ligament (Fig. 2.17). Chronic tears can reveal either ligamentous thickening without edema or, more often, complete atrophy. Several secondary signs of ACL rupture exist. In acute injuries, bone contusions are manifested as regions of edema in the subchondral marrow, typically in the lateral compartment. The overlying articular cartilage should be closely inspected for signs of injury. These bone contusions usually resolve within 6 to 12 weeks of injury. Anterior translocation of the tibia with respect to the femur, the MRI equivalent of the drawer sign, is highly specific for acute or chronic tears. Buckling of the posterior cruciate ligament often is present, but this sign is more subjective. Although usually best evaluated in the sagittal plane, the ACL can and should be seen in coronal and axial planes as well. In large series correlated with arthroscopic data, MRI has achieved an accuracy rate of 95% in the assessment of ACL pathologic conditions. Unfortunately, as is frequently the case with the physical examination, the imaging distinction between partial and complete ACL tears is more challenging. Even when the diagnosis of an ACL tear is a clinical certainty, MRI is valuable in assessing associated meniscal and ligament tears and posterolateral corner injuries. MRI can accurately depict the reconstructed ACL within the intercondylar notch and define the position of intraosseous tunnels. A redundant graft

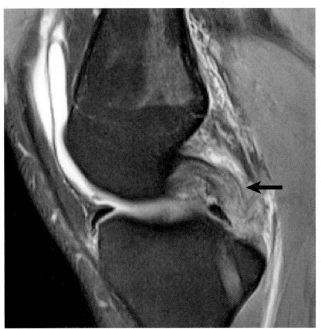

FIGURE 2.18 Posterior cruciate ligament tear. Sagittal fat-suppressed proton density-weighted image shows abnormal increased signal *(arrow)* within the disorganized fibers of the distal posterior cruciate ligament.

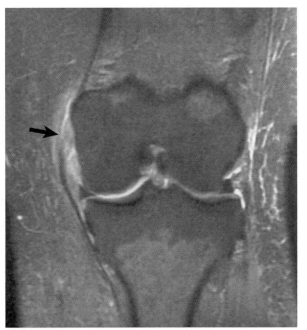

FIGURE 2.19 Medial collateral ligament tear. Complete disruption of proximal medial collateral ligament *(arrow)* is demonstrated in coronal fat-suppressed, proton density–weighted image; this appearance suggests grade 3 medial collateral ligament injury.

or absence of the graft on MRI suggests graft failure. Because the normal revascularization process may result in areas of increased signal within and around the graft, edematous changes in the early postoperative period should be interpreted with caution.

In extension, the posterior cruciate ligament is a gently curving band of fibrous tissue, appearing as a homogeneously hypointense structure of uniform thickness on sagittal MRI series. Discontinuity of the ligament or fluid signal within its substance indicates a tear (Fig. 2.18). In the coronal imaging plane, the medial collateral ligament (MCL) appears as a thin dark band of tissue closely applied to the periphery of the medial meniscus. Mild injuries result in edema about the otherwise normal ligament. Severe strain or rupture causes ligamentous thickening or frank discontinuity (Fig. 2.19). Although mild degrees of MCL injury correlate nicely with MRI appearance, imaging is less accurate in grading more severe injuries. Injuries of the lateral supporting structures, including the lateral collateral ligament, iliotibial band, biceps femoris, and popliteus tendon, also are depicted with MRI.

OTHER KNEE PROBLEMS

Severe injuries to the extensor mechanism of the knee are usually clinically obvious, but when partial tears of the patellar or quadriceps tendon are suspected, MRI can confirm the diagnosis. Discontinuity of tendinous fibers and fluid in a gap within the tendon are seen with complete tears. Incomplete tears show thickening of the tendon with interspersed edema. Generally, tendinitis demonstrates tendon thickening, although normal low signal is maintained. Posteriorly, popliteal, or Baker, cysts are noted in the medial aspect of the popliteal fossa. These cysts can rupture distally into the calf, mimicking thrombophlebitis. In this situation, MRI will demonstrate fluid dissecting inferiorly along the medial

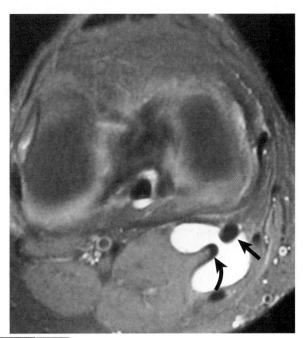

FIGURE 2.20 Popliteal fossa cyst. Axial proton density–weighted image demonstrates hyperintense fluid extending from knee joint into popliteal fossa between semimembranosus tendon *(straight arrow),* and medial gastrocnemius tendon *(curved arrow).*

gastrocnemius muscle belly. Caution should be used when evaluating T2-weighted hyperintense popliteal fossa structures because other lesions, such as popliteal artery aneurysms and tumors, are common in this location. Demonstration of the neck of a popliteal cyst at its communication with the joint between the medial gastrocnemius and the semimembranosus tendon will avoid potential misdiagnosis (Fig. 2.20).

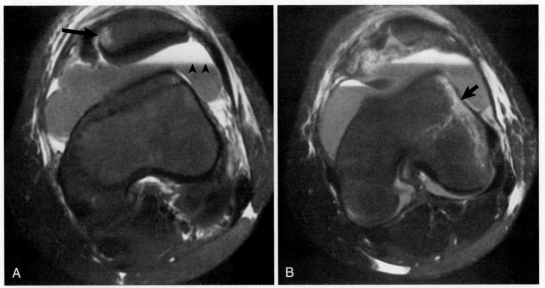

FIGURE 2.21   Patellar dislocation. **A** and **B,** Axial fat-suppressed, proton density–weighted images through patellofemoral joint show regions of increased signal, representing marrow edema beneath medial facet of patella *(long arrow)* and in lateral aspect of lateral femoral condyle *(thick arrow).* This pattern of osseous contusion indicates recent lateral patellar dislocation. Note hematocrit level in joint effusion *(arrowheads).*

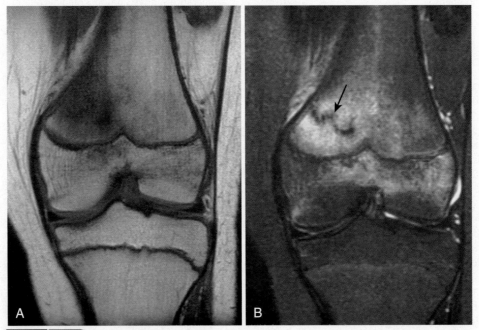

FIGURE 2.22   Occult Salter II fracture of distal femur in 14-year-old boy. **A,** Coronal T1-weighted image reveals ill-defined reduced signal in medial distal femoral metaphysis. **B,** Fat-suppressed, T2-weighted image demonstrates irregular hypointense fracture *(arrow)* surrounded by hyperintense marrow edema. Edema continues along lateral physis, indicating extension of fracture.

Other potential problems about the knee for which MRI is well-suited include osteonecrosis, synovial pathologic conditions, osseous contusions (Fig. 2.21), and occult fractures (Fig. 2.22). Direct coronal and sagittal MRI is helpful in assessing complications of physeal injuries in children (Fig. 2.23) and in demonstrating osteochondritis dissecans. T2-weighted or gradient-echo sequences can show fluid surrounding an unstable osteochondral fragment. MRI is also helpful in

determining the integrity of the overlying cartilage (Fig. 2.24). The fat-suppressed proton density–weighted sequence is most commonly used in the assessment of hyaline cartilage in the routine knee examination. Fat-suppressed, fast spin-echo, proton density–weighted, or gradient-echo sequences obtained with volumetric technique are helpful in the evaluation of articular cartilage in the knee and many other joints (Figs. 2.8, 2.24, and 2.25). Loose bodies are best seen in the

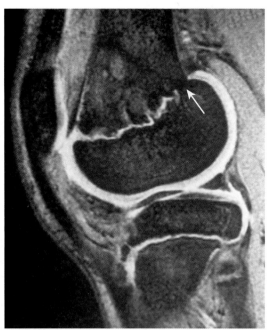

FIGURE 2.23   Physeal bar in 12-year-old boy. Gradient-echo sagittal image of knee demonstrates interruption of posterior extent of distal femoral physis *(arrow)*. Osseous bridge has resulted in posterior angulation of articular surface of distal femur. Articular and physeal cartilage exhibits increased signal with most gradient-echo techniques.

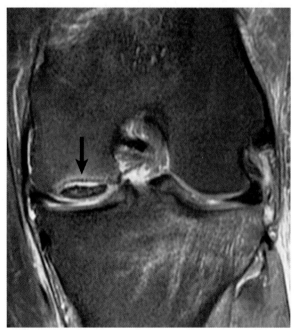

FIGURE 2.24   Osteochondritis dissecans. Coronal fat-suppressed proton density-weighted image of the knee demonstrates hyperintense fluid signal *(arrow)* surrounding an unstable osteochondral fragment.

presence of joint effusion with conventional radiographs as a reference. Specialized cartilage imaging techniques such as T1rho and T2 mapping, and delayed gadolinium-enhanced magnetic resonance imaging of cartilage (D-GEMRIC) require additional scan time or contrast injection. Presently,

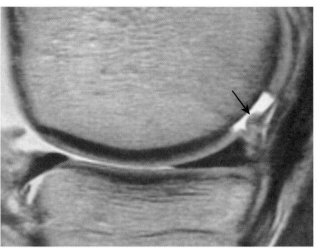

FIGURE 2.25   Chondral lesion. Fat-suppressed proton density weighted sagittal image of knee reveals a small, well-defined fluid filled full-thickness defect in the articular cartilage of the postero-medial femoral condyle *(arrow)*.

these advanced cartilage imaging techniques are used primarily in the research setting or for clinically difficult cases.

HIP

MRI is an extremely useful tool in the evaluation of the hip and pelvis. With the unsurpassed ability to image marrow in the proximal femur, MRI can detect a spectrum of pathologic conditions of the hip. When evaluating patients for processes that may be bilateral, such as osteonecrosis, or conditions that might involve the sacrum or sacroiliac joints, the examination should include both hips and the entire pelvis. A surface coil such as a torso or large wrap coil with phased-array design combines improved signal for high-resolution images coupled with large field-of-view coverage. For patients with suspected unilateral conditions, such as femoral stress fractures, suspected occult trauma, or labral injury, a unilateral study with a smaller field of view is desirable and surface coils are indispensable. Spin-echo sequences are usually performed in axial and coronal planes. Sagittal images are quite useful when investigating osteonecrosis.

OSTEONECROSIS

One of the most frequent indications for hip imaging is evaluation of osteonecrosis because early diagnosis is desirable whether nonoperative or operative treatment is considered. Although initial radiographs are often normal, either scintigraphy or MRI may confirm the diagnosis. Of the two techniques, MRI is the more sensitive in detecting early osteonecrosis and better delineates the extent of marrow necrosis. The percentage of involvement of the weight-bearing cortex of the femoral head as defined by MRI, as well as the presence of perilesional marrow edema and joint effusion, may be helpful in predicting prognosis and the value of surgical intervention. On T1-weighted images, the classic MRI appearance of osteonecrosis is that of a geographic region of abnormal marrow signal within the normally bright fat of the femoral head (Fig. 2.26). This area of abnormal signal, often circumscribed by a low-signal band, represents ischemic bone. The T2-weighted images reveal a margin of bright signal, and the resulting appearance has been termed

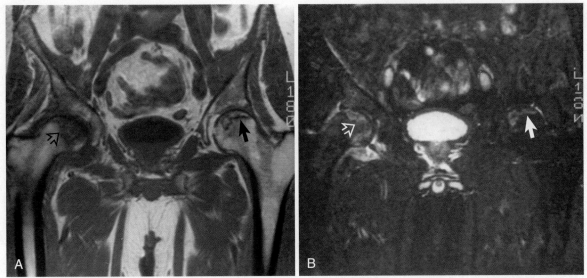

FIGURE 2.26   Corticosteroid-induced bilateral osteonecrosis of femoral head. **A** and **B,** Coronal T1-weighted and inversion recovery images through both hips reveals geographic focus of marrow replacement in weight-bearing aspect of left femoral head, indicating osteonecrosis *(solid arrows)*. More advanced disease is seen in right femoral head with collapse of articular surface, adjacent marrow edema *(open arrows),* and effusion.

the "double line" sign. This sign essentially is diagnostic of osteonecrosis. Initially appearing in the anterosuperior sub-chondral marrow, the central area of necrotic bone can demonstrate various signal patterns throughout the course of the disease, depending on the degree of hemorrhage, fat, edema, or fibrosis. Subchondral fracture, articular surface collapse, cartilage loss, reactive marrow edema, and effusion are seen in more advanced cases of osteonecrosis.

TRANSIENT OSTEOPOROSIS

A second condition also well depicted with MRI is transient osteoporosis of the hip. This unilateral process, initially described in pregnant women in their third trimester, is most commonly seen in middle-aged men. Transient osteoporosis is a self-limited process of uncertain etiology, although ischemic, hormonal, or stress-related etiologies have been proposed. Many patients have later involvement of nearby joints, such as the opposite hip, hence the association with regional migratory osteoporosis. Initial radiographs may be normal or may reveal diffuse osteopenia of the femoral head, with preservation of the joint space. The MRI appearance is that of diffuse edema in the femoral head, extending into the intertrochanteric region. Focal MRI signal abnormalities, as seen in osteonecrosis, generally are not present in transient osteoporosis. Occasionally, a tiny focal, often linear lesion in the subcortical marrow in the weight-bearing portion of the femoral head indicates an insufficiency fracture in the demineralized bone. T1-weighted sequences depict diffuse edema as relative low signal in contrast to background fatty marrow. The edema becomes hyperintense on T2-weighted series and is accentuated when fat-suppression techniques are used (Fig. 2.27). This marrow appearance has been termed a "bone marrow edema pattern." Rare case reports have documented this pattern presenting as the earliest phase of osteonecrosis. For this reason, if initial radiographs are normal, repeat films 6 to 8 weeks after the onset of symptoms should demonstrate osteopenia of the femoral head, confirming the diagnosis of

transient osteoporosis. Transient osteoporosis of the hip generally resolves without treatment within 6 months, and the radiographs and MRI appearance return to normal.

TRAUMA

Frequently, MRI can be helpful in evaluation of the hip after trauma. Radiographs are often negative or equivocal for fracture of the proximal femur in elderly individuals. Although bone scintigraphy has been used to confirm or exclude fracture, this study can be falsely negative in elderly patients in the first 48 hours after injury. The MRI abnormalities are immediately apparent, with linear areas of low signal easily seen in the fatty marrow on T1-weighted images and surrounding edema seen with T2-weighted images (Fig. 2.28). In addition, the anatomic information provided can assist in determining the type of fixation required. In fact, many radiographically occult fractures subsequently discovered by MRI are confined to the greater trochanter or incompletely traverse the femoral neck and, in certain patients, may be treated conservatively.

A great deal of effort has been directed at the imaging evaluation of femoroacetabular impingement and the acetabular labrum. Original reviews of the accuracy of conventional MRI in the assessment of labral pathologic conditions were disappointing because of large field of view images that lacked adequate resolution. The advent of MRI arthrography performed with surface coil or phased-array technique has greatly improved visualization of the cartilaginous labrum. Unfortunately, the geometry of the labrum of the hip displays a wide range of normal variation, even in asymptomatic individuals. As the vast majority of labral tears are found in the anterior or anterolateral labrum, these labral segments should be closely evaluated for the presence of deep or irregular intralabral clefts suggestive of a labral tear (Fig. 2.29). Adjacent regions of acetabular cartilage delamination often are present. In patients with mechanical hip symptoms or possible femoroacetabular impingement, the addition of an anesthetic injection at the time of arthrography may be useful in confirming

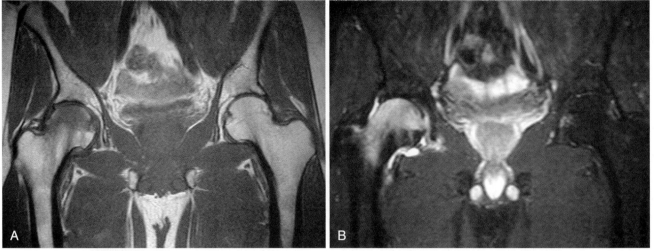

FIGURE 2.27 Transient osteoporosis of hip in 30-year-old man. **A,** Coronal T1-weighted image reveals diminished signal intensity within right femoral head and neck. **B,** Coronal inversion recovery sequence demonstrated hyperintense bone marrow edema in more diffuse pattern than seen in osteonecrosis.

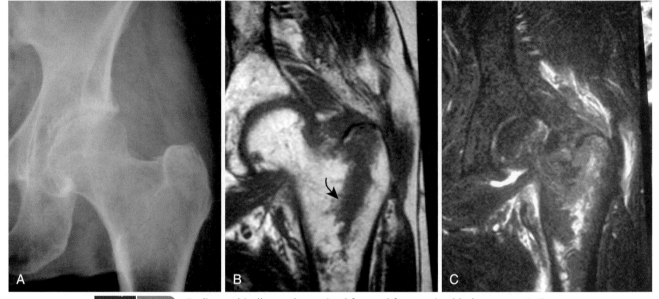

FIGURE 2.28 Radiographically occult proximal femoral fracture in elderly woman. **A,** Questionable cortical disruption is noted on radiograph of left hip obtained after fall. **B,** Coronal T1-weighted image confirms greater trochanter fracture manifested as vertically oriented band of reduced signal *(curved arrow)* within normal bright fat signal of femoral neck. **C,** Coronal inversion recovery sequence shows edema at fracture.

an intraarticular origin of pain. The improved resolution provided by 3 T MRI studies has allowed labral assessment without the need for intraarticular contrast. Nonarthrographic examinations for the workup of hip impingement and labral pathology should be specifically ordered with such history to ensure the necessary sequence selection and small field of view required to appropriately evaluate the labrum.

SPINE

MRI of the spine accounts for a large percentage of examinations at most centers. MRI allows a noninvasive evaluation of the spine and spinal canal, including the spinal cord.

The anatomy of the spine, cord, nerve roots, and spinal ligaments is complex. Because the spine is anatomically divided into three sections—cervical, thoracic, and lumbar—each is evaluated with coils specifically designed for spine imaging. Spinal examinations include series obtained in both axial and sagittal planes. Coronal images may be helpful in patients with significant scoliosis. There is no one correct imaging construct, and the makeup of the study depends on many factors, including the type and field strength of the magnet, the availability of hardware (coils) and software, and the preferences of the examiner. However, all studies should produce images that can detect and define pathologic conditions of the cord, thecal sac, vertebral bodies, and intervertebral discs.

INTERVERTEBRAL DISC DISEASE

The most common indication for MRI of the spine is evaluation of intervertebral disc disease. After routine radiography, MRI is the procedure of choice for screening patients with low back or sciatic pain. In the lumbar and thoracic spine, MRI has supplanted CT myelography because it is noninvasive and less expensive. The combination of high soft-tissue contrast and high resolution allows ideal evaluation of the intervertebral discs, nerve roots, posterior longitudinal ligament, and intervertebral foramen. Additionally, MRI provides excellent assessment of the spinal cord. Because of bony structures, such as osteophytes and bone fragments, CT myelography is invasive and more costly and is therefore reserved for patients who have contraindications to MRI or who have equivocal MRI examinations. Regardless of the region of the spine being evaluated, sagittal images provide an initial evaluation of the intervertebral discs and posterior longitudinal ligament. Because of its high water content, a normal disc exhibits signal hyperintensity on T2-weighted images. The aging process results in a gradual desiccation of the disc material and therefore loss of this signal. Disc herniations or extrusions appear as convex or polypoid masses extending posteriorly into the ventral epidural space, frequently maintaining a signal intensity similar to that of the disc of origin (Fig. 2.30). Sagittal T2-weighted or gradient-echo images create a "myelographic" effect and are useful in evaluating compromise of the subarachnoid space. However, sagittal T1-weighted images should be closely examined to identify narrowing of the neuroforamina. The normal T1-weighted hyperintense perineural fat in the foramina provides excellent contrast to darker displaced disc material. Far lateral disc herniations are best seen on selected axial images that are localized through disc levels. Free disc fragments appear discontinuous with the intervertebral disc, usually of intermediate T1-weighted signal in contrast to the hypointense cerebrospinal fluid. Of great significance in the cervical and thoracic spine is the ability of MRI to detect significant spinal cord compromise. Edema within the cord is readily demonstrated as hyperintensity with T2 weighting.

The terminology of pathologic conditions of the intervertebral disc is confusing. In an effort to standardize terminology, Jensen et al. proposed the following terms: a *bulge* is a circumferential, symmetric extension of the disc beyond the interspace around the endplates; a *protrusion* is a focal or asymmetric extension of the disc beyond the interspace, with the base against the disc of origin broader than any other dimension of the protrusion; an *extrusion* is a more extreme extension of the disc beyond the interspace, with the base against the disc of origin narrower than the diameter of the extruding material itself or with no connection between the material and the disc of origin; and, finally, a *sequestration* specifically refers to a disc fragment that has completely separated from the disc of origin.

POSTOPERATIVE BACK PAIN

In a patient with persistent postoperative back pain, residual disc, epidural hematoma or abscess, and discitis must

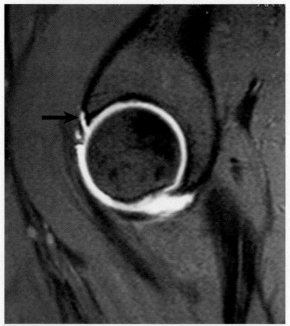

FIGURE 2.29   Anterior labral tear of the hip. Postarthrogram sagittal fat-suppressed T1-weighted image shows contrast opacifying a tear of the anterior labrum of the hip *(arrow)*.

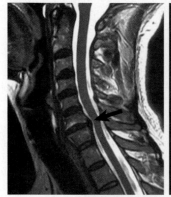 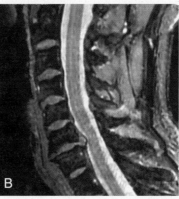 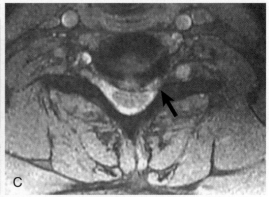

FIGURE 2.30   Cervical disc extrusion (herniation). **A,** T2-weighted sagittal image of the cervical spine reveals extruded C6-C7 disc *(arrow)*. **B,** Gradient-echo sagittal image demonstrates displaced disc material isointense to nucleus pulposus. Note the absence of cerebrospinal fluid pulsation artifact seen on the T2-weighted image. **C,** Gradient-echo axial image shows left eccentric extrusion compressing the cervical cord and filling the left neuroforamen *(arrow)*.

be considered. Distinguishing between recurrent or resid-ual disc material and scar tissue often is impossible with CT myelography or unenhanced MRI, and the administration of intravenous gadolinium is extremely useful in MRI of the postoperative spine. After contrast administration, repeat T1-weighted images typically demonstrate enhancement of scar or fibrosis (Fig. 2.31). Beyond the immediate postopera-tive period, disc material (in the absence of infection) will not enhance. For this reason, examinations performed on patients with a history of disc surgery are usually done with and with-out intravenous contrast. Epidural hematomas and abscesses appear as collections within the spinal canal, demonstrating peripheral enhancement with gadolinium on T1-weighted images. Gadolinium contrast agents are also helpful in post-operative evaluation of the spine for discitis. Signal changes in the disc space and adjacent vertebral endplates frequently are seen after surgery on the spine even when complica-tions do not occur, but the triad of vertebral body endplate enhancement, disc space enhancement, and enhancement of the posterior longitudinal ligament is highly suggestive of postoperative discitis. Correlation with the erythrocyte sedi-mentation rate, C-reactive protein, gallium or tagged white blood cell radionuclide imaging, and percutaneous aspiration is often necessary.

Although diagnosis of disc space infection in a patient who has not undergone surgery generally is more straightfor-ward, the MRI appearance of degenerative disc disease is var-ied and can be confusing. Although vertebral endplate edema and even enhancement do occur in the absence of infec-tion, the presence of disc space enhancement strongly sug-gests infection (Fig. 2.32). Pyogenic and fungal/tuberculous infection is frequently associated with epidural and paraspi-nal abscesses. In the lumbar spine, extension into the adja-cent psoas muscles is best demonstrated on axial T2-weighted sequences because hyperintense fluid and edema invade the normal hypointense musculature. Subligamentous spread of

infection with relative sparing of the intervertebral disc should raise the suspicion of tuberculous spondylitis. Both pyogenic and tuberculous infections demonstrate abnormal enhance-ment with gadolinium administration. Abscesses, given the lack of central perfusion, enhance only at the periphery.

SPINAL TUMORS

Although tumor imaging in general is discussed later in this text, MRI has proven valuable in the assessment of spi-nal neoplasms. Excellent delineation of vertebral body mar-row allows detection of both primary and metastatic disease with high sensitivity on T1-weighted sequences. Normally, T1-weighted vertebral body marrow signal progressively increases with age, a reflection of a gradually higher percent-age of fatty marrow. Diseases such as chronic anemia result in a higher percentage of hematopoietic marrow, thus dif-fusely diminishing this T1-weighted signal. Malignant osse-ous tumor foci appear as discrete areas of diminished T1 signal. As is typical with tumors, these lesions become hyper-intense to surrounding marrow on T2-weighted studies and enhance with contrast. These aggressive lesions can be distin-guished from benign bony hemangiomas, which usually are hyperintense on T1-weighted images because of their inter-nal fat content. Neoplastic processes that diffusely involve vertebral marrow, such as leukemia and occasionally multi-ple myeloma, may be more problematic because differentia-tion from diffusely prominent hematopoietic marrow can be challenging.

SPINAL TRAUMA

CT remains the most useful advanced imaging technique for spinal trauma. The inherent contrast provided by bone and unmatched spatial resolution makes CT the preferred initial examination in trauma patients. MRI is helpful in patients with suspected spinal cord injury, epidural hematoma, or trau-matic disc herniation. Soft-tissue injuries, such as ligamentous

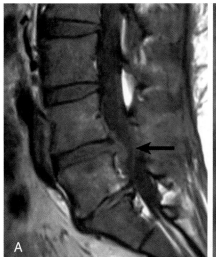
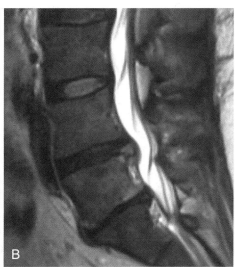
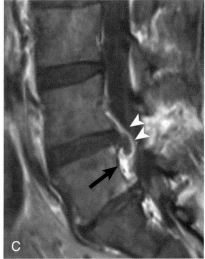

FIGURE 2.31 Recurrent lumbar disc extrusion (herniation). **A,** Sagittal T1-weighted image demonstrates intermediate signal intensity in L4-L5 disc material *(arrow)* surrounded by hypoin-tense cerebrospinal fluid. **B,** Sagittal T2-weighted image shows displaced disc material contiguous with intervertebral disc. Hyperintense cerebrospinal fluid provides improved contrast. **C,** Sagittal T1-weighted image after gadolinium administration demonstrates enhancement of epidural venous plexus *(arrow)* and overlying granulation tissue but no enhancement of disc material.

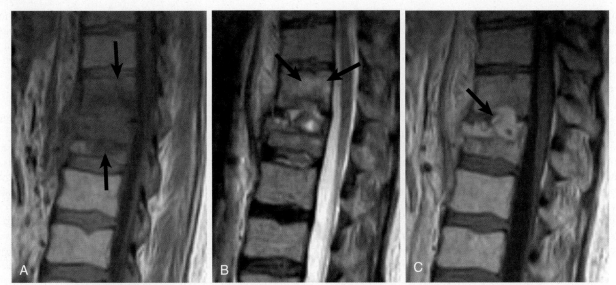

FIGURE 2.32 Thoracic discitis. **A,** Sagittal T1-weighted image exhibits reduced marrow signal *(arrows)* adjacent to the irregular and collapsed lower thoracic interspace. **B,** Sagittal T2-weighted image reveals corresponding hyperintense areas of marrow edema *(arrows).* **C,** After administration of gadolinium, sagittal T1-weighted image exhibits enhancement of the intervertebral disc *(arrow).*

tears, can be identified in the acute stage. Discontinuity of normally hypointense ligaments, hemorrhage, and edema can be seen on sagittal T2-weighted images. In the setting of trauma, MRI usually is reserved for neurologically impaired patients whose CT examinations are negative or for patients in whom spinal fracture reduction is planned and associated disc pathology must be excluded. The role of MRI in evaluating nontraumatic compressed vertebrae and in the exclusion of any underlying pathologic condition is critical. Preservation of normal marrow signal in a portion of the compressed vertebral body, especially with a linear pattern of signal abnormality, is suggestive of a fracture caused by a benign process, such as osteoporosis. Complete marrow replacement or the presence of additional focal abnormal marrow signal at other levels should prompt consideration of biopsy. The association of an irregular or asymmetric soft-tissue mass or broad convexity of the dorsal vertebral cortex is also suggestive of underlying neoplasm. In questionable cases, a follow-up MRI at 6 to 8 weeks may demonstrate at least partial reconstitution of normal marrow signal around osteoporotic fractures. The identification of edema within a compressed vertebra can confirm a fracture as either acute or subacute because normal marrow signal is typically restored in chronic compression fractures.

SHOULDER

The major indications for MRI evaluation of the shoulder include three interrelated problems: rotator cuff tear, impingement, and instability. The complex anatomy of the shoulder requires oblique imaging planes and surface coil technique. The typical MRI shoulder examination includes axial spin-echo or gradient-echo sequences to evaluate the labrum. Oblique coronal images prescribed in the plane of the supraspinatus tendon best detect pathologic conditions of the rotator cuff. Oblique sagittal images confirm abnormalities of the cuff tendons and evaluate rotator cuff muscles in cross-section. Both conventional arthrography and MRI can detect complete tears of the rotator cuff. However, although arthrography shows full-thickness tears and partial tears along the articular (inferior) surface, noninvasive MRI also detects partial-thickness intrasubstance and bursal surface tears and can reliably determine the size of full-thickness defects.

PATHOLOGIC CONDITIONS OF THE ROTATOR CUFF

Oblique coronal spin-echo imaging with T2 weighting optimally detects most pathologic conditions of the rotator cuff. With the humerus in neutral to external rotation, the oblique coronal plane is chosen parallel to the supraspinatus tendon. As is the case with all other tendons, the tendons of the supraspinatus, infraspinatus, and teres minor muscles normally maintain low signal on all pulse sequences. Rotator cuff tears appear as areas of increased T2-weighted signal, representing fluid within the tendon substance. This signal may traverse the entire tendon substance, indicating a full-thickness tear (Fig. 2.33). Alternatively, intact cuff fibers may persist along the articular surface, bursal surface, or both, as seen in partial-thickness tears. Fluid may be identified in the subacromial-subdeltoid bursa. In patients with large or chronic tears, the cuff may be so atrophied that its identification is impossible. In these cases, fluid freely communicates between the glenohumeral joint and the subacromial bursa and the humeral head often migrates superiorly. Excessive retraction of the cuff tendons and atrophy of the cuff musculature portend a poor surgical result.

Most examiners have used the terms *tendinosis* or *tendinopathy* to describe focal signal abnormalities within the cuff that do not achieve the signal intensity of fluid on T2-weighted images. Because artifacts frequently occur within tendons on T1-weighted and gradient-echo images, the diagnosis of rotator cuff tear should not be made in the absence of discrete foci of T2-weighted fluid signal abnormalities or complete absence of the tendon. Typically, areas of normal fluid can be appreciated elsewhere in the glenohumeral joint for reference. Diffuse or focal signal abnormalities less intense than fluid should be

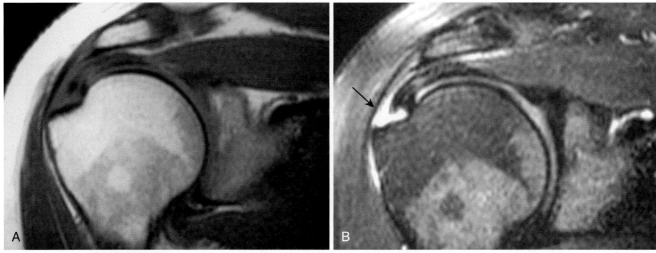

FIGURE 2.33 Full-thickness rotator cuff tear. **A,** Oblique coronal T1-weighted image poorly differentiates normal tendon from pathologic condition. **B,** At same location, oblique coronal fat-suppressed, T2-weighted image clearly shows fluid-filled, full-thickness tear *(arrow)* in supraspinatus tendon.

considered tendinosis. MRI has shown greater than 90% sensitivity in detecting full-thickness rotator cuff tears. For the assessment of partial tears, the sensitivity is greater than 85%. The addition of fat suppression to T2-weighted images has been shown to improve detection of partial-thickness tears. MRI assessment of the repaired rotator cuff should be done with caution. Often irregular foci of increased T2-weighted signal normally can be seen with an intact healing tendon, likely representing areas of granulation tissue. For this reason, the diagnosis of partial-thickness tears in the postoperative shoulder should be avoided. However, larger, fluid-filled, full-thickness defects and tendon retraction correlate well with failed repairs or re-tears. MR arthrography is often helpful in the evaluation of the postoperative rotator cuff.

IMPINGEMENT SYNDROMES

Although impingement can be suggested by an imaging technique, it remains a clinical diagnosis. MRI can be helpful in confirming the clinical impression or providing additional information. Imaging findings that suggest the possibility of impingement include narrowing of the subacromial space by spurs or osteophytes, a curved or hooked acromial morphology, and signal abnormalities in the cuff indicating tendinosis or tendinopathy.

PATHOLOGIC CONDITIONS OF LABRUM

Much study has been directed at MRI evaluation of the labroligamentous complex of the shoulder. The cross-sectional anatomy of the normal labrum is quite variable, and the adjacent glenohumeral ligaments create many potential diagnostic pitfalls (Fig. 2.34). For these reasons, early conventional MRI evaluation of the glenohumeral joint for instability achieved mixed results. With modern scanner and coil technology, however, the labrum often is quite well depicted in routine shoulder MRI. Nevertheless, many investigators still believe that the distension of the joint achieved by the injection of intraarticular fluid improves evaluation of the labrum, biceps tendon origin, and joint capsule. MR arthrography most often uses dilute gadolinium as a contrast agent and subsequent T1-weighted sequences in the axial, oblique sagittal,

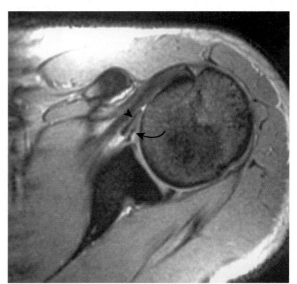

FIGURE 2.34 Anterior labral tear. Axial gradient-echo image through glenohumeral joint shows anterior displacement of avulsed anterior labral fragment *(curved arrow)*. Hypointense middle glenohumeral ligament *(arrowhead)* lies between labral fragment and subscapularis tendon and should not be mistaken for portion of labrum.

and oblique coronal planes performed in a standard position with the arm at the patient's side (Fig. 2.35A). Additional imaging can be performed with the humerus in abduction and external rotation (ABER) position for assessment of the inferior glenohumeral ligament and its labral attachment (Fig. 2.35B). Anterior labral injuries are best seen in the axial plane, whereas superior labral abnormalities or SLAP (superior labral anterior posterior) lesions are best depicted in the axial or coronal images (Fig. 2.36). Using MR arthrography, a sensitivity of 91% and a specificity of 93% have been reported in the detection of pathologic labral conditions. The accuracy of MRI in evaluation of SLAP lesions is somewhat less. Some investigators have proposed indirect arthrography as an alternative method of joint opacification. In this technique,

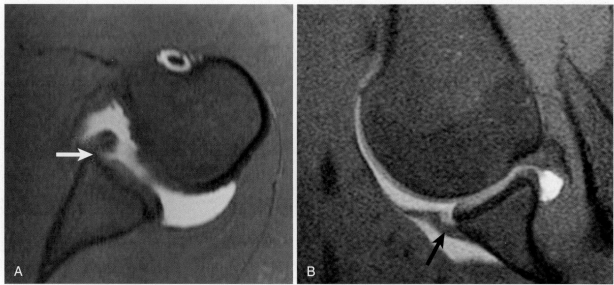

FIGURE 2.35 Anterior labral tear. **A,** Postarthrogram fat-suppressed T1-weighted axial image of the shoulder shows a small defect in the anteroinferior labrum *(arrow)*. **B,** Oblique axial imaging in abduction/external rotation places tension on the inferior glenohumeral ligament, better demonstrating the tear *(arrow)*.

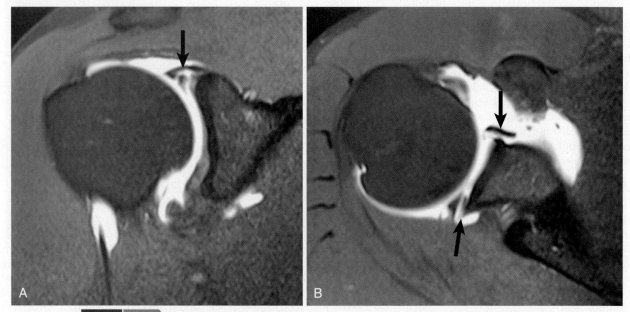

FIGURE 2.36 Superior labral anterior posterior tear. **A,** Fat-suppressed T1-weighted oblique coronal image from MR arthrogram shows contrast opacifying a defect in the long head biceps anchor *(arrow)*. **B,** Fat-suppressed T1-weighted axial image shows extension of the tear into the anterior and posterior labrum *(arrows)*.

delayed intraarticular enhancement is achieved by exercising the joint after intravenous administration of gadolinium. Although this is a less invasive technique, the degree of distention is less than that achieved with direct arthrography.

OTHER CAUSES OF SHOULDER PAIN

MRI also can demonstrate additional causes of shoulder pain, such as occult fractures or osteonecrosis (Fig. 2.37). Pathologic conditions of the tendon of the long head of the biceps, including rupture, dislocation, or tendinitis, should be detected on routine MRI examination. A less frequent cause

of shoulder pain, suprascapular nerve entrapment, is a ganglion cyst of the spinoglenoid notch. Like ganglia elsewhere, these lesions appear as lobular, multiseptate, hyperintense collections on T2-weighted or gradient-echo sequences (Fig. 2.38). The presence of these ganglia may be associated with infraspinatus atrophy and should trigger a careful search for an associated labral injury. Of note, neither the pectoralis muscle/tendon nor the brachial plexus is imaged on the routine shoulder MRI examination, and if a pathologic condition of these structures is suspected, a study dedicated to this anatomic region should be performed.

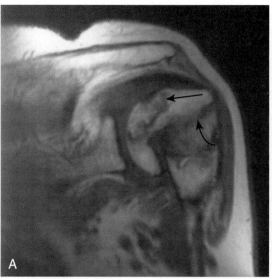
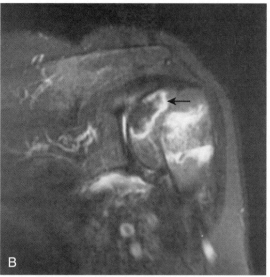

FIGURE 2.37 Osteonecrosis complicating comminuted fracture of proximal humerus. **A,** Oblique coronal T1-weighted image demonstrates displaced fracture through neck of proximal humerus *(curved arrow)*. Geographic region of abnormal marrow within articular fragment is characteristic of osteonecrosis *(long arrow)*. **B,** Oblique coronal fat-suppressed, T2-weighted image shows hyperintense rim of reactive tissue *(arrow)* surrounding now hypointense fatty avascular marrow.

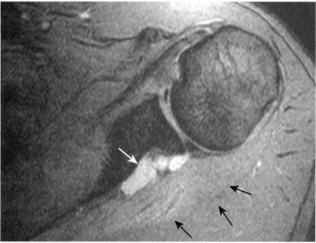

FIGURE 2.38 Soft-tissue ganglion in painful shoulder. Gradient-echo axial image of right shoulder reveals lobulated homogeneous hyperintense lesion in spinoglenoid notch *(white arrow)*. Ganglia and other masses in this location can be associated with suprascapular nerve entrapment. Note subtle hyperintensity indicating edema in the infraspinatus muscle along the posterior scapula related to denervation *(black arrows)*.

WRIST AND ELBOW

MRI has an expanding role in the evaluation of pathologic conditions of the elbow and wrist. Successful study of both articulations requires high-resolution images that are best obtained with surface coil technique and high field system. Often these joints are examined in the extremity coil, requiring extension of the arm overhead within the center of the magnet field. This position is difficult to maintain in elderly patients. The larger-diameter bore current generation of high-field scanners can allow for off-axis imaging with the arm at the side. Dedicated wrist coils, when available, or coupled surface coils also are designed for imaging of this articulation at the patient's side. Again, the MRI examination should be directed at solving a specific clinical problem or question.

CARPAL LIGAMENT DISRUPTIONS

In the wrist, a common indication for MRI is evaluation of the intrinsic carpal ligaments. With proper technique, injuries to the triangular fibrocartilage complex (TFCC) can be demonstrated with MRI. The TFCC is composed of signal-poor fibrocartilage, and perforations in the TFCC appear as linear defects or gaps filled with hyperintense fluid on coronal gradient-echo or T2-weighted pulse sequences (Fig. 2.39). Although evaluation of the scapholunate and lunotriquetral ligaments is more challenging, with optimal technique and equipment the integrity of these structures can be consistently assessed. The addition of arthrographic contrast improves the visualization of these ligaments on MR images. The extrinsic carpal ligaments can be identified with three-dimensional volumetric scanning and subsequent reconstruction; however, at present, the MRI assessment of these ligaments has less impact on treatment.

OTHER PATHOLOGIC CONDITIONS OF HAND AND WRIST

MRI has gained a greater role in the evaluation of acute wrist trauma. Not infrequently, bone marrow edema may reveal fractures of the carpal bones or distal radius that are radiographically occult. MRI is useful in detecting additional marrow abnormalities in osteonecrosis, as seen in the lunate in Kienböck disease (Fig. 2.40) or in the scaphoid after fracture. Asymmetry of marrow signal in proximal and distal fragments of a fractured scaphoid is suggestive of proximal pole ischemia (Fig. 2.41). MRI currently has a limited role in the evaluation of carpal tunnel syndrome. Although this remains a clinical diagnosis, axial imaging with T2 weighting can clearly display masses within the confines of the carpal

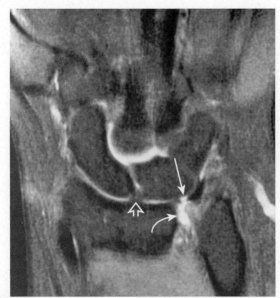

FIGURE 2.39 Triangular fibrocartilage complex (TFCC) perforation. Coronal fat-suppressed, proton density–weighted image of wrist demonstrates central perforation of TFCC *(long arrow)*. Note fluid in distal radioulnar joint *(curved arrow)*. Scapholunate ligament *(open arrow)* is intact in this wrist.

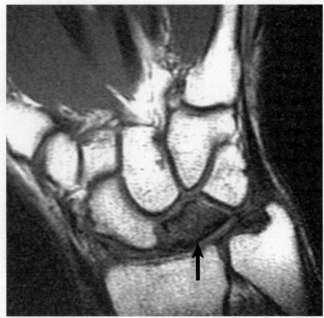

FIGURE 2.40 Osteonecrosis of lunate (Kienböck disease). Coronal T1-weighted image of wrist shows loss of normal high-signal fat in lunate *(arrow)*, indicating osteonecrosis.

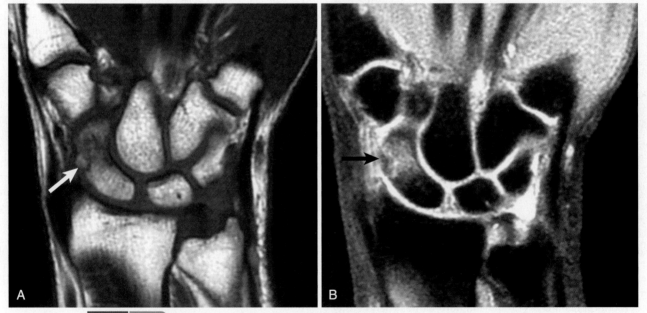

FIGURE 2.41 Early osteonecrosis of scaphoid following fracture. **A,** T1-weighted coronal image of the wrist shows a transverse fracture of the mid-scaphoid *(arrow)*. **B,** Fat-suppressed T2-weighted coronal image reveals marrow edema in the distal pole fragment only *(arrow)*, suggesting proximal pole ischemia.

tunnel, as well as edema and swelling of the median nerve. As in the ankle, tenosynovitis and tendon injuries in the wrist and hand can be assessed (Fig. 2.42). Additionally, MRI has an expanding role in the evaluation of inflammatory arthritis. Numerous studies have shown that MRI provides earlier detection of synovitis and erosive bone changes associated with rheumatoid arthritis than do radiographs.

ELBOW

In the elbow, MRI is useful in assessment of the biceps and triceps tendons. Although complete tears of these tendons are frequently clinically apparent, MRI can assist in surgical planning (Figs. 2.43 and 2.44). MRI can detect partial tears as well. Conventional MRI and MR arthrography have a critical role in the evaluation of medial instability and the study of the ulnar collateral ligament. The ulnar collateral ligament is a complex structure, and its anterior band is normally visible as a linear hypointense structure along the medial aspect of the joint on all sequences. When injured, fluid is seen within and around the disrupted ligament. In a throwing athlete, MR arthrography may be helpful especially in assessment of partial-thickness ligament tears (Fig. 2.45). Conventional MRI is also valuable for detection of occult elbow fractures in adults as well as in children in whom unossified epiphyses are radiographically problematic.

TUMOR IMAGING

Perhaps nowhere in orthopaedics has MRI had as profound an impact as in the field of surgical oncology. Exquisite soft-tissue contrast combined with detailed anatomy and

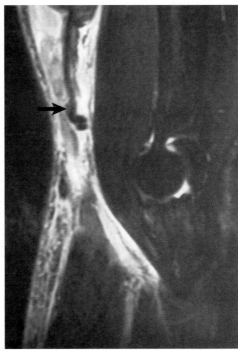

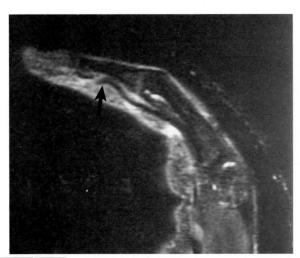

FIGURE 2.42 Image of rupture of flexor digitorum profundus tendon in long finger made 2 weeks after repair. Sagittal inversion recovery image demonstrates abrupt discontinuity of flexor tendon *(arrow)* with laxity of more proximal tendon segment.

FIGURE 2.43 Rupture of distal biceps tendon. Sagittal inversion recovery image of elbow demonstrates ruptured distal biceps tendon. Proximal tendon *(arrow)* has retracted several centimeters, and edema is present in tissues anterior to brachialis muscle.

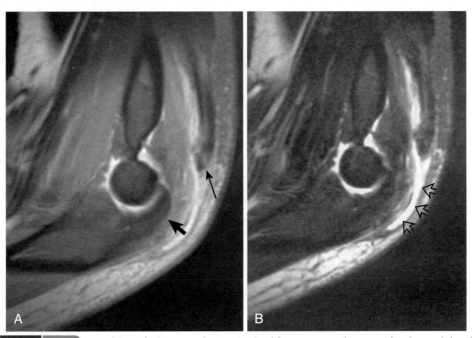

FIGURE 2.44 Avulsion of triceps tendon. **A,** Sagittal fat-suppressed, proton density–weighted image of elbow shows avulsed triceps tendon *(long arrow)* retracted proximally from olecranon *(thick arrow).* **B,** Sagittal fat-suppressed, T2-weighted image demonstrates hyperintense fluid *(arrows)* in gap between bone and detached tendon.

multiplanar capability place MRI at the forefront of musculoskeletal tumor imaging methods. Excellent bone marrow delineation is most helpful in defining tumor extent and planning surgical and radiation therapy. MRI is frequently helpful in defining aggressive versus indolent processes; however, the contribution of routine radiographs cannot be overemphasized. In tumor imaging, interpreting MRI studies without radiographs is risky.

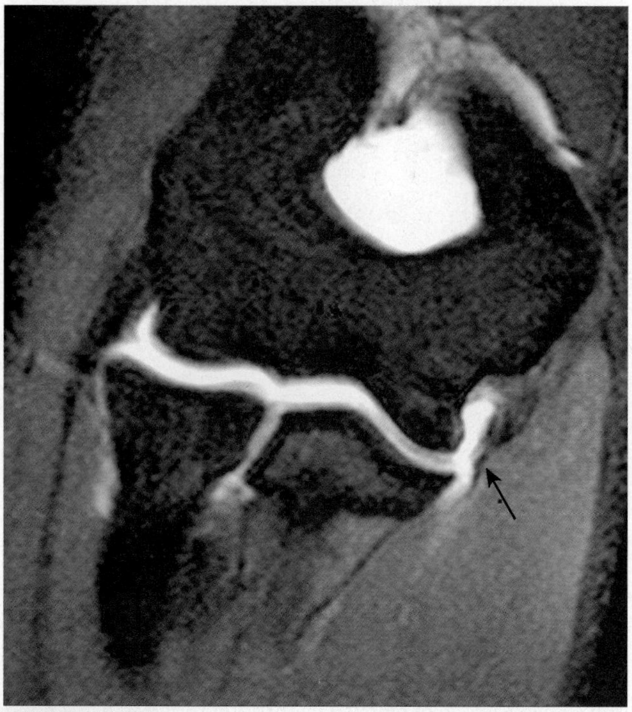

Most oncologic MRI examinations are performed after radiographic detection of a bone lesion or discovery of a clinically palpable soft-tissue mass. Whether imaging bone or soft-tissue neoplasms, the basic concepts are similar. If the lesion is sufficiently small (<20 cm), surface coil technique is preferred. Larger masses or lesions in the pelvis or thigh are usually best imaged in the body coil or with a phased-array torso coil. Imaging should be performed in at least two planes, one of which should be axial (or transverse). This plane is most helpful in defining the relationship of lesions to nearby muscles and neurovascular structures and best demonstrates extraosseous extension of bone tumors. Compartmental anatomy is also best demonstrated in this imaging plane. The sagittal or coronal images define the proximal and distal extents of bone or soft-tissue involvement. T1-weighted images are useful in identifying areas of marrow replacement of edema. T2-weighted sequences delineate soft-tissue extension because most neoplasms become hyperintense in contrast to surrounding muscle and fat (Figs. 2.46 and 2.47). The addition of fat-suppression techniques, when available, can prove invaluable in defining subtle foci of tumor or edema. The role of intravenous gadolinium in the study of musculoskeletal oncology is expanding. In the evaluation of soft-tissue masses, contrast-enhanced, T1-weighted images can differentiate solid from cystic lesions and may assist in biopsy planning by distinguishing active from necrotic tumors. Unfortunately, because active tumor, tumor edema, and granulation tissue all demonstrate enhancement, this enhancement cannot separate tumor from surrounding reactive changes. Dynamic contrast enhancement has shown promise in distinguishing tumor from surrounding edema based on relative enhancement rates, but this technique is not widely available. Currently, routine use of intravenous gadolinium in the initial evaluation of neoplasm is probably not necessary.

FIGURE 2.45 Partial ulnar collateral ligament tear at MR arthrography of elbow. Coronal fat-suppressed, T1-weighted image reveals contrast tracking deep to ulnar attachment of ulnar collateral ligament *(arrow)*.

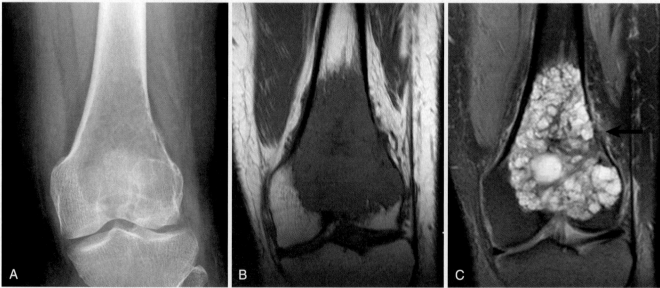

FIGURE 2.46 Giant cell tumor of distal femur. **A,** Radiograph shows lytic lesion in the distal femoral metaphysis and epiphysis. **B,** T1-weighted coronal image confirms a well-demarcated intermediate-signal lesion replacing the normal hyperintense fatty marrow of the distal femur. **C,** Fat-suppressed proton density-weighted coronal image shows heterogeneous hyperintense tumor in a similar distribution. There is subtle cortical destruction of the lateral metaphyseal cortex *(arrow)*.

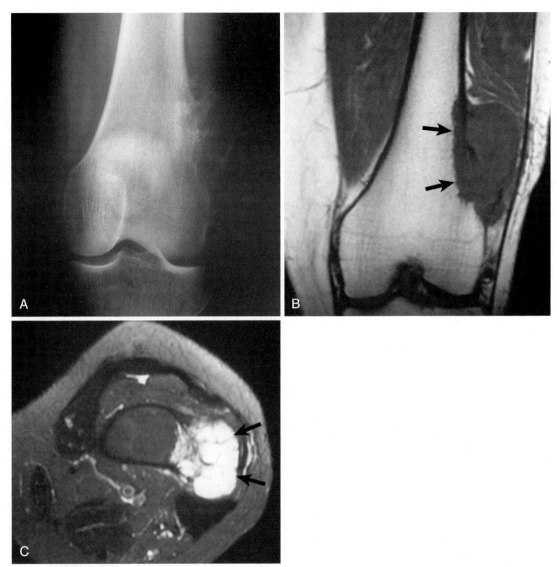

FIGURE 2.47 Chondrosarcoma arising in osteochondroma. **A,** Radiograph reveals irregular ossification throughout exostosis of distal femur. **B,** T1-weighted coronal image shows hypointense marrow signal within lesion and extension of this abnormal signal into medullary canal of femur *(arrows)*. **C,** Axial fat-suppressed, T2-weighted image demonstrates typical hyperintensity of neoplastic tissue *(arrows)*, in contrast to surrounding normal tissues.

Conversely, in a patient who has undergone surgery, the presence of nodular areas of contrast enhancement in the surgical bed is suggestive of recurrent or residual neoplasm, and the use of intravenous gadolinium is advised in these patients. Preoperative MR angiography with gadolinium enhancement can provide important information regarding the blood supply of very vascular lesions.

The differential diagnosis of most bone tumors is derived from routine radiographs, and the role of MRI is to define the extent of disease. With the exception of densely sclerotic lesions, such as osteoid osteoma, MRI has replaced CT for the assessment of skeletal tumors.

The detection of soft-tissue masses is more dependent on the history and physical examination, given the infrequency of radiographic abnormalities. Most soft-tissue lesions present a nonspecific MRI appearance, typically isointense to muscle on T1-weighted images and hyperintense to muscle and fat on T2-weighted images (Fig. 2.48).

Certain lesions do exhibit signal patterns that allow a tissue-specific diagnosis. For example, soft-tissue lipomas reveal homogeneous fat signal intensity on all sequences (Fig. 2.49). In fact, subcutaneous lipomas are notoriously difficult to image because of the lack of contrast with the surrounding subcutaneous fat. Certain subtypes of liposarcoma exhibit regions of fat and nonfat signal. Therefore, the diagnosis of lipoma should be restricted to those lesions that contain only fat and almost imperceptible fibrous septae. As do their intraosseous counterparts, soft-tissue hemangiomas show areas of bright signal on both T1- and T2-weighted studies (Fig. 2.50). These signal characteristics result from the presence of fat and large amounts of slow-flowing blood within the lesion. Situated within or around joints, pigmented villonodular synovitis reveals marked T2-weighted hypointensity because of the presence of hemosiderin (Fig. 2.51). In general, malignant soft-tissue masses are well defined, subfascial, large

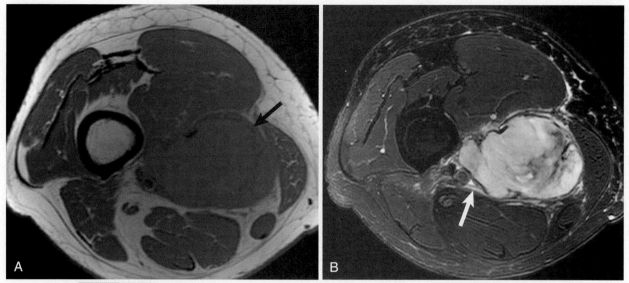

FIGURE 2.48 Synovial sarcoma of the thigh. **A,** T1-weighted axial image reveals a large, well-defined mass *(arrow)* in isointense surrounding muscle in the deep posterior compartment of the mid-thigh. **B,** Fat-suppressed T2-weighted axial image shows a well-defined hyperintense lesion abutting the neurovascular structured *(arrow)*.

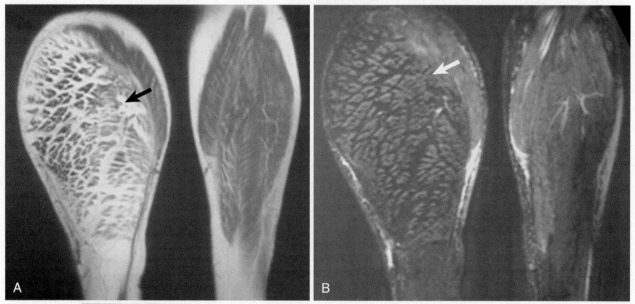

FIGURE 2.49 Intramuscular lipoma of soleus muscle. **A,** Coronal T1-weighted image through calf shows marked fatty infiltration of soleus muscle *(arrow)*. **B,** Coronal inversion recovery image shows complete suppression of fat signal within mass. Muscle fibers exhibit slightly more signal than dark fat *(arrow)*.

(>5 cm), and heterogeneous. Exceptions to these rules are plentiful, and the distinction between benign and malignant disease must be made with caution.

COMPUTED TOMOGRAPHY

CT is a valuable problem-solving tool for orthopaedic conditions too numerous to list in entirety. CT is frequently used and often invaluable in evaluation and treatment planning in patients with acute complex fractures. The modality can be quite helpful in defining post-traumatic, developmental, or congenital osseous deformity. Preoperative CT imaging

can assist with planning for arthroplasty and arthrodesis in patients with advanced degenerative arthropathy. CT may occasionally be of value in tumor evaluation and is certainly often used for image-guided aspirations, injections, or biopsies. Often, CT becomes the default imaging modality of choice in patients who have a contraindication to MR, such as a pacemaker or intracranial clips, or who are claustrophobic.

CT TECHNOLOGY AND TECHNIQUE

Computed x-ray tomography is an advanced radiographic technique that uses a rotating x-ray beam to generate a cross-sectional image. Although the CT also is used in single

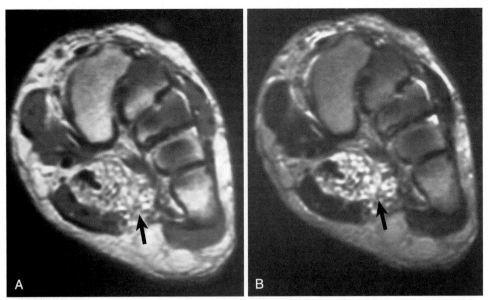

FIGURE 2.50 Soft-tissue hemangioma of foot. **A,** Coronal T1-weighted image of midfoot shows infiltrating mass of heterogeneous increased signal *(arrow)*. **B,** Corresponding fat-suppressed, T2-weighted image demonstrates markedly increased signal within mass *(arrow)*. Morphology and signal characteristics of this lesion (hyperintense T1- and T2-weighted signal) are typical of hemangiomas.

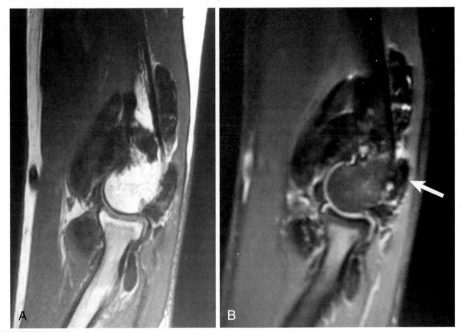

FIGURE 2.51 Pigmented villonodular synovitis. **A,** Sagittal T1-weighted image of the elbow shows lobulated intermediate to hypointense soft tissue distributed diffusely throughout the synovium. **B,** T2-weighted imaging reveals the typical dramatic decrease in signal throughout these masses *(arrow)* due to the presence of hemosiderin.

photon emission computed tomography (SPECT) or positron emission tomography (PET), in this chapter, CT refers to computed x-ray tomography. Current CT scanners use high-heat capacity x-ray tubes and slip-ring technology, which allows image acquisition with a helical or spiral technique. Rather than acquiring individual slices in a stepwise fashion, helical scanners generate imaged volumes as the patient continuously moves through the scanner. The acquired or "raw"

data is then manipulated to generate cross-sectional images for interpretation. Two-dimensional images can be created in orthogonal or oblique planes. Additionally, three-dimensional images can be generated with various post-processing techniques. The acquisition and storage of this raw data allow much greater post-processing flexibility than MR.

Current CT scanners also use multichannel technology, with multiple rows or banks of rotating detectors that capture

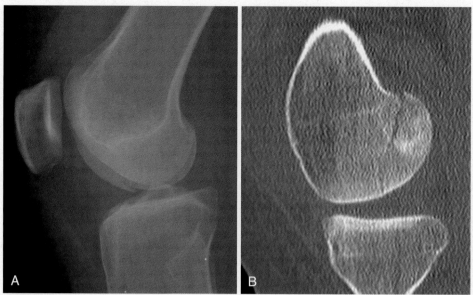

FIGURE 2.52 Medial femoral condyle fracture. **A,** Lateral radiograph of the knee shows very subtle deformity of the articular surface **B,** Sagittal reformatted CT image more clearly shows a coronally oriented intraarticular fracture (Hoffa fracture) of the medial femoral condyle.

the x-rays after they pass through the patient. Analysis of the data acquired in these detector rows individually or in combination affects the reconstructed image collimation or slice thickness. Most modern scanners allow slice thickness of less than 0.5 mm. Therefore, spatial resolution of CT is significantly better than MR. CT is a powerful tool when used to evaluate high-contrast structures such as bone but is of less value is studying soft-tissue structures where MR excels. Additionally, the presence of potentially harmful ionizing radiation associated with the generation of CT images should always be considered, especially in younger patients. Technologists should appropriately reduce doses when performing examinations on younger or smaller patients. Additionally, radiation dose can be easily minimized by limiting the extent of the studied volume. For example, the study of a single-level lumbar pars defect can be localized to the level of concern rather than the entire lumbar spine, reducing exposure by at least two thirds. Dose reduction technology such as iterative reconstruction should be used when available. In certain clinical situations, similar diagnostic information can be obtained with MR or US, avoiding radiation exposure entirely.

TRAUMA

CT can be extremely useful is the setting of trauma. For example, in an acutely injured patient, CT may detect radiographically occult fractures in the spine and appendicular skeleton. In some studies, conventional radiography missed up to 70% of cervical spine fractures. Trauma radiographs often are compromised by body habitus or osteopenia. Many trauma patients require cranial or body scanning, and the addition of spinal CT can be done with little or no additional scan time and dose. In the lumbar spine, CT can better assess compression fractures and can frequently distinguish acute from chronic deformities. Certainly, CT is the modality of choice in assessing bony canal compromise in patients with vertebral burst fractures. CT also is critical in assessing radiographically occult or obvious pelvic fractures. CT can detect

occult fractures of the appendicular skeleton as well, particularly those involving the elbow, hip, and knee. It should be noted that in almost all situations, the sensitivity of MR exceeds CT in detection of occult fracture; however, because of the excellent spatial resolution of CT, this modality better demonstrates small fracture fragments such as avulsions involving the scapular glenoid or metatarsal bases.

In many situations, CT is requested to further assess a radiographically known fracture. In most cases, the severity of fracture displacement is better appreciated with CT. Because this displacement is especially critical when fractures involve an articular surface, CT imaging is commonly requested for intraarticular fractures of the proximal humerus, wrist, proximal tibia, or calcaneus. Image reconstruction in planes orthogonal to the articular surface is needed to best appreciate displacement of the subchondral bone (Fig. 2.52). With severe displacement or bony deformity, three-dimensional shaded surface rendering is also valuable (Fig. 2.53).

CT is also the modality of choice to assess for fracture healing. Bony bridging of the fracture site is visible with CT before it becomes radiographically apparent. If local implants are present, scan technique should be optimized to minimize artifact. Current generation scanners use metal artifact reduction software (MARS technique), which can be valuable when imaging in the vicinity of implants such as joint prostheses or bulky plates. Again, images must be reconstructed in planes orthogonal to the fracture. In the setting of malunion, CT imaging may assist in quantifying bony displacement or angulation and especially rotational deformity. In adolescents, CT analysis of lumbar spondylosis can often distinguish immature from chronic fractures.

DEVELOPMENTAL SKELETAL PATHOLOGY

Development skeletal abnormalities can be accurately characterized with CT imaging. Vertebral anomalies such as butterfly or hemivertebrae are clearly displayed on three-dimensional CT images, assisting in operative planning. Developmental

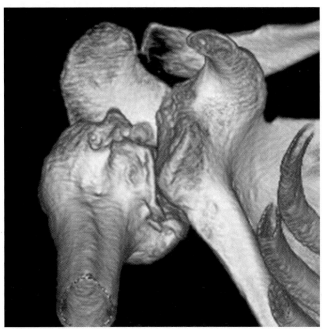

FIGURE 2.53 Posterior shoulder dislocation. Three-dimensional shaded surface rendering clearly demonstrates posterior dislocation of the humerus with respect to the glenoid.

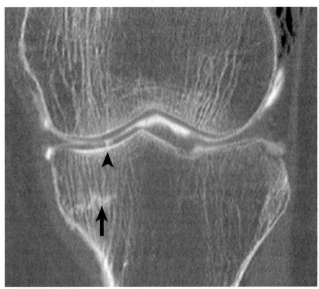

FIGURE 2.55 CT arthrogram knee. Coronal CT image obtained after intraarticular injection of iodinated contrast demonstrates normal menisci with focal fissuring of medial tibial articular cartilage *(arrowhead)*. A transverse band of sclerosis in the medial tibial plateau *(arrow)* represents stress fracture.

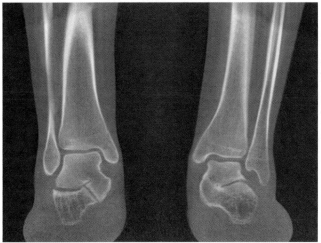

FIGURE 2.54 Talocalcaneal coalition. A coronal reformatted CT image of both feet reveals bilateral middle facet subtalar coalitions, fibrous on the patient right and osseous on patient left.

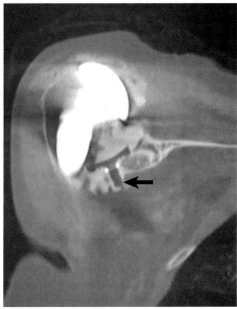

FIGURE 2.56 Displaced glenoid prosthesis. A coronal reformatted CT arthrogram image of the glenohumeral joint in a patient with a total shoulder prosthesis reveals displaced low-density glenoid component *(arrow)* surrounded by radiodense intraarticular contrast.

rotational deformities of the long bones, particularly the femur and tibia, can be precisely quantified. Synostosis or osseous coalition also is nicely displayed with CT (Fig. 2.54).

ARTHROPATHY

In general, CT has a limited role in the evaluation of arthropathy. When MR imaging is contraindicated because of clinical factors or technical reasons, CT arthrography of the shoulder and knee may be a reasonable next-best option (Fig. 2.55). In patients with advanced glenohumeral osteoarthritis, CT is often used to assess glenoid morphology before arthroplasty. Similarly, custom prostheses are often templated based on preoperative CT data. In painful post-arthroplasty patients,

MR imaging can be a challenge due to ferromagnetic artifact. Often, CT is helpful in detecting and defining the extent of periarticular osteolysis and prosthesis displacement when planning revision arthroplasty (Fig. 2.56). Finally, newer techniques using dual energy techniques can produce images that specifically highlight monosodium urate crystals in patients with gout.

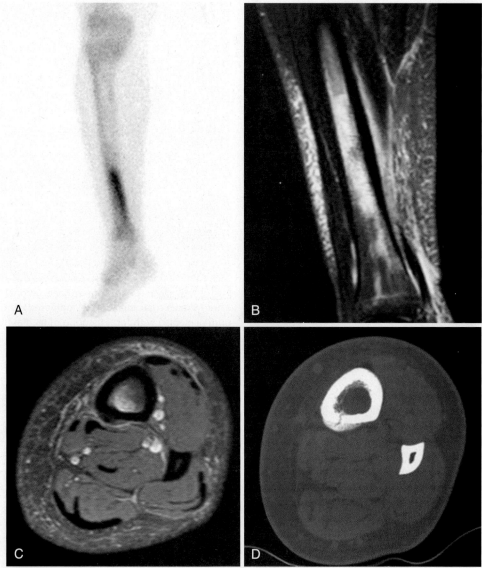

FIGURE 2.57 Longitudinal stress fracture of tibia. **A,** Delayed bone scan demonstrates longitudinally oriented activity in the distal tibia. **B** and **C,** Fluid sensitive longitudinal and axial MR images reveal nonspecific ill-defined marrow edema. **D,** Axial CT image shows clearly defined longitudinally orient fracture in the posterior tibial cortex.

TUMOR EVALUATION

Although radiography and MRI are the primary imaging modalities used in bone and soft-tissue tumor evaluation, there are certain situations in which CT imaging is valuable. Occasionally, MRI detects marrow or cortical signal abnormalities that are indeterminate for fracture or tumor. CT images may reveal a cortical fracture not previously appreciated, essentially excluding tumor (Fig. 2.57). The nidus of an osteoid osteoma is often better visualized with CT than with MRI (Fig. 2.58). In almost all cases, MRI is preferred to CT is evaluation of soft-tissue masses. One exception involves myositis ossificans, in which the calcified margin of the post-traumatic lesion is much better appreciated with CT (Fig. 2.59). In patients with known osseous metastatic disease, the cross-sectional capability of CT is often of value in evaluating cortical integrity when assessing for risk of pathologic fracture. Finally, CT guidance is quite frequently used

for percutaneous biopsy or treatment of bone and soft-tissue lesions (see Fig. 2.58D).

CONCLUSION

As the growing field of musculoskeletal imaging is far broader than can be covered in this text, innumerable clinical situations in which MRI and CT can be used have not been discussed. Ongoing research is continually defining new indications for advanced imaging in orthopaedic patients. The MRI and CT techniques described in this chapter are widely available with most commercial imaging systems. Optimal image quality can be obtained only when meticulous attention is paid to imaging technique by both the radiologist and the technician. Greater interaction between orthopaedists and radiologists will ensure that studies are performed appropriately to solve the specific clinical problem.

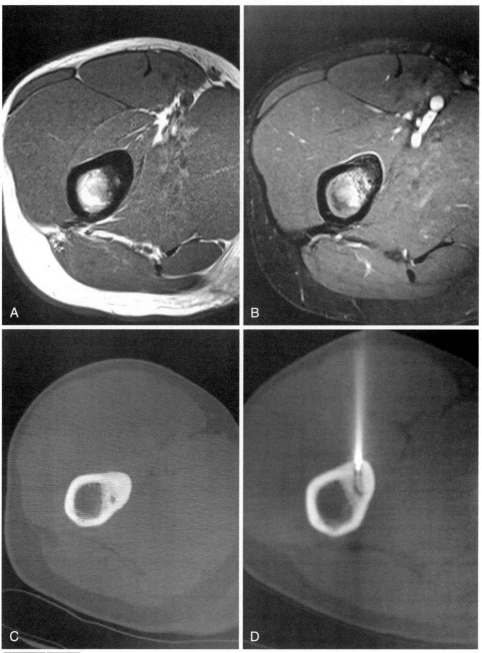

FIGURE 2.58   Osteoid osteoma. **A,** T1-weighted axial MR image shows medial femoral cortical thickening. **B,** Fluid sensitive axial MR image demonstrates bone marrow edema without a discrete lesion. **C,** Axial CT image reveals a radiolucent nidus within the thickened cortical bone consistent with osteoid osteoma. **D,** Axial CT image acquired during radiofrequency ablation confirms coaxial placement of the RF probe into the nidus.

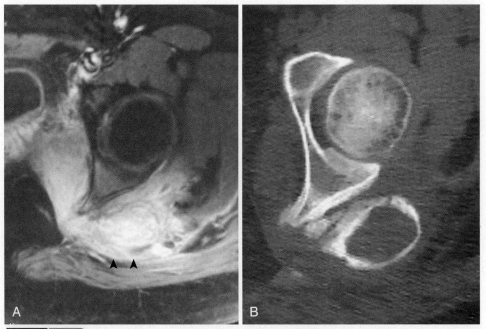

FIGURE 2.59 Myositis ossificans. **A,** Fluid sensitive axial image reveals a nonspecific increased signal intensity soft tissue mass posterior to the hip (*arrowheads*). **B,** Axial CT image shows a peripherally calcified mass confirming the diagnosis of myositis ossificans.

REFERENCES

GENERAL

Kijowski R, Gold GE: Routine 3D magnetic resonance imaging of joints, *J Magn Reson Imaging* 33:758, 2011.

FOOT AND ANKLE

Boonthathip M, Chen L, Trudell DJ, Resnick DL: Tibiofibular syndesmotic ligaments: MR arthrography in cadavers with anatomic correlation, *Radiology* 254:827, 2010.

Chhabra A, Soldatos TR, Challan M, et al.: 3-Tesla magnetic resonance imaging evaluation of posterior tibial tendon dysfunction with relevance to clinical staging, *J Foot Ankle Surg* 50:320, 2011.

Ferkel RD, Tyorkin M, Applegate GR, Heinen GT: MRI evaluation of anterolateral soft tissue impingement of the ankle, *Foot Ankle Int* 31:655, 2010.

Ford GM, Genuario J, Kinkartz J, et al.: Return-to-play outcomes in professional baseball players after medial ulnar collateral ligament injuries: comparison of operative versus nonoperative treatment based on magnetic resonance imaging findings, *Am J Sports Med* 44:723, 2016.

Gonzalez FM, Morrison WB: Magnetic resonance imaging of sports injuries involving the ankle, *Top Magn Reson Imaging* 24:205, 2015.

Hembree WC, Wittstein JR, Vinson EN, et al.: Magnetic resonance imaging features of osteochondral lesions of the talus, *Foot Ankle Int* 33:591, 2012.

Ikoma K, Ohashi S, Maki M, et al.: Diagnostic characteristics of standard radiographs and magnetic resonance imaging of ruptures of the tibialis posterior tendon, *J Foot Ankle Surg* 55:542, 2016.

Joshy S, Abdulkadir U, Chaganti S, et al.: Accuracy of MRI scan in the diagnosis of ligamentous and chondral pathology in the ankle, *Foot Ankle Surg* 16:78, 2010.

Jung HG, Kim NR, Kim TH, et al.: Magnetic resonance imaging and stress radiography in chronic lateral ankle instability, *Foot Ankle Int* 38:621, 2017.

Kanamoto T, Shiozaki Y, Tanaka Y, et al.: The use of MRI in pre-operative evaluation of anterior talofibular ligament in chronic ankle instability, *Bone Joint Res* 3:241, 2014.

Kraeutler MJ, Purcell JM, Hunt KJ: Chronic Achilles tendon ruptures, *Foot Ankle Int* 38:921, 2017.

Kwon DG, Sung KH, Chung CY, et al.: Associations between MRI findings and symptoms in patients with chronic ankle sprain, *J Foot Ankle Surg* 53:411, 2014.

Nazarenko A, Beltran LS, Bencardino JT: Imaging evaluation of traumatic ligamentous injuries of the ankle and foot, *Radiol Clin North Am* 51:455, 2013.

Petersen B, Fitzgerald J, Schreibman K: Musculotendinous magnetic resonance imaging of the ankle, *Semin Roentgenol* 45:250, 2010.

Porrino JA, Pettis CR, Lewis G, et al.: CT and MR imaging of the postoperative ankle and foot, *Radiographics* 36:1828, 2016.

Sofka CM: Technical considerations: best practices for MR imaging of the foot and ankle, *Magn Reson Imaging Clin N Am* 25(1), 2017.

Sung W, Weil Jr L, Weil LS, Rolfes RJ: Diagnosis of plantar plate injury by magnetic resonance imaging with reference to intraoperative findings, *J Foot Ankle Surg* 51:570, 2012.

KNEE

Cho HW, Suh JS, Park JO, et al.: Three-dimensional fast spin-echo imaging without fat suppression of the knee: diagnostic accuracy comparison to fat-suppressed imaging on 1.5T MRI, *Yonsei Med J* 58:1186, 2017.

Choi JY, Chang EY, Cunha GM, et al.: Posterior medial meniscus root ligament lesions: MRI classification and associated findings, *AJR Am J Roentgenol* 203:1286, 2014.

Choi SH, Bae S, Ji SK, Chang MJ: The MRI findings of meniscal root tear of the medial meniscus: emphasis on coronal, sagittal, and axial images, *Knee Surg Sports Traumatol Arthrosc* 20:2098, 2012.

Davis KW, Rosas HG, Graf BK: Magnetic resonance imaging and arthroscopic appearance of the menisci of the knee, *Clin Sports Med* 32:449, 2013.

Derby E, Imrecke J, Henckel J, et al.: How sensitive and specific is 1.5 Tesla MRI for diagnosing injuries in patients with knee dislocation? *Knee Surg Sports Traumatol Arthrosc* 25:517, 2017.

Dufka FL, Lansdown DA, Zhang AL, et al.: Accuracy of MRI evaluation of meniscus tears in the setting of ACL injuries, *Knee* 23:460, 2016.

Gnannt R, Chhabra A, Theodoropoulos JS, et al.: MR imaging of the postoperative knee, *J Magn Reson Imaging* 34:1007, 2011.

Hash TW: Magnetic resonance imaging of the knee, *Sports Health* 5:78, 2013.

Kijowski R, Rosas H, Williams A, et al.: MRI characteristics of torn and untorn post-operative menisci, *Skeletal Radiol* 46:1353, 2017.

Kosy JD, Eyres KD, Toms AD: The value of magnetic resonance imaging in investigating a painful total knee arthroplasty, *J Arthroplasty* 26:977, 2011.

Lance V, Heilmeier UR, Joseph GB, et al.: MR imaging characteristics and clinical symptoms related to displaced meniscal flap tears, *Skeletal Radiol* 44:375, 2015.

Lin E: Magnetic resonance imaging of the knee: clinical significance of common findings, *Curr Probl Diagn Radiol* 39:152, 2010.

Mohankumar R, White LM, Naraghi A: Pitfalls and pearls in MRI of the knee, *AJR Am J Roentgenol* 203:516, 2014.

Nacey NC, Geeslin MG, Miller GW, et al.: Magnetic resonance imaging of the knee: an overview and update of conventional and state of the art imaging, *J Magn Reson Imaging* 45:1257, 2017.

Naraghi AM, White LM: Imaging of athletic injuries of knee ligaments and menisci: sports imaging series, *Radiology* 281(23), 2016.

Naraghi A, White LM: MR imaging of cruciate ligaments, *Magn Reson Imaging Clin N Am* 22:557, 2014.

Nicandri GT, Slaney SL, Neradilek MB, et al.: Can magnetic resonance imaging predict posterior drawer laxity at the time of surgery in patients with knee dislocation or multiple-ligament knee injury? *Am J Sports Med* 39:1053, 2011.

Quatman CE, Hettrich CM, Schmitt LC, Spindler KP: The clinical utility and diagnostic performance of magnetic resonance imaging for identification of early and advanced knee osteoarthritis: a systematic review, *Am J Sports Med* 39:1557, 2011.

Rosas HG: Magnetic resonance imaging of the meniscus, *Magn Reson Imaging Clin N Am* 22:493, 2014.

Slattery T, Major N: Magnetic resonance imaging pitfalls and normal variations: the knee, *Magn Reson Imaging Clin North Am* 18:675, 2010.

Smith C, McGarvey C, Harb Z, et al.: Diagnostic efficacy of 3-T MRI for knee injuries using arthroscopy as a reference standard: a meta-analysis, *AJR Am J Roentgenol* 207:369, 2016.

Subhas N, Patel SH, Obuchowski NA, Jones MH: Value of knee MRI in the diagnosis and management of knee disorders, *Orthopedics* 37:e109, 2014.

Tyler P, Datir A, Saifuddin A: Magnetic resonance imaging of anatomical variations in the knee: part 1. Ligamentous and musculotendinous, *Skeletal Radiol* 39:1161, 2010.

Tyler P, Datir A, Saifuddin A: Magnetic resonance imaging of anatomical variations in the knee: part 2. Miscellaneous, *Skeletal Radiol* 39:1175, 2010.

Van Dyck P, Vanhoenacker FM, Gielen JL, et al.: Three Tesla magnetic resonance imaging of the anterior cruciate ligament of the knee: can we differentiate complete from partial tears? *Skeletal Radiol* 40:701, 2011.

Zheng L, Shi H, Feng Y, et al.: Injury patterns of medial patellofemoral ligament and correlation analysis with articular cartilage lesions of the lateral femoral condyle after acute lateral patellar dislocation in children and adolescents: an MRI evaluation, *Injury* 46:1137, 2015.

HIP

Albers CE, Wambeek N, Hanke MS, et al.: Imaging of femoroacetabular impingement—current concepts, *J Hip Preserv Surg* 3:245, 2016.

Annabell L, Master V, Rhodes A, et al.: Hip pathology: the diagnostic accuracy of magnetic resonance imaging, *J Orthop Surg Res* 13:127, 2018.

Berkowitz JL, Potter HG: Advanced MRI techniques for the hip joint: focus on the postoperative hip, *AJR Am J Roentgenol* 209:534, 2017.

Carstensen SE, McCrum EC, Pierce JL, et al.: Magnetic resonance imaging (MRI) and hip arthroscopy correlations, *Sports Med Arthrosc Rev* 25:199, 2017.

Chopra A, Grainger AJ, Dube B, et al.: Comparative reliability and diagnostic performance of conventional 3T magnetic resonance imaging and 1.5T magnetic resonance arthrography for the evaluation of internal derangement of the hip, *Eur Radiol* 28:963, 2018.

Coker DJ, Zoga AC: The role of magnetic resonance imaging in athletic pubalgia and core muscle injury, *Top Magn Reson Imaging* 24:183, 2015.

Crema MD, Watts GJ, Guermazi A, et al.: A narrative overview of the current status of MRI of the hip and its relevance for osteoarthritis research—what we know, what has changed and where are we going? *Osteoarthritis Cartilage* 25(1), 2017.

Crespo-Rodriguez AM, De Lucas-Villarrubia JC, Pastrana-Ledesma M, et al.: The diagnostic performance of non-contrast 3-Tesla magnetic resonance imaging (3-T) MRI) vrsus 1.5-Tesla magnetic resonance arthrography (1.5T MRA) in femoro-acetabular impingement, *Eur J Radiol* 88:109, 2017.

Di Pietto F, Chianca V, Zappia M, et al.: Articular and peri-articular hip lesions in soccer players. The importance of imaging in deciding which lesions will need surgery and which can be treated conservatively? *Eur J Radiol* 105:227, 2018.

Friedman T, Chen T, Chang A: MRI diagnosis of recurrent pigmented villonodular synovitis following total joint arthroplasty, *HSS J* 9:100, 2013.

Gold SL, Burge AJ, Potter HG: MRI of hip cartilage: joint morphology, structure, and composition, *Clin Orthop Relat Res* 470:3321, 2012.

Hayter CL, Potter HG, Su EP: Imaging of metal-on-metal hip resurfacing, *Orthop Clin North Am* 42:195, 2011.

Haubro M, Stougaard C, Torfing T, Overgaard S: Sensitivity and specific of CT- and MRI-scanning in evaluation of occult fracture of the proximal femur, *Injury* 46:1557, 2015.

Jayakar R, Merz A, Plotkin B, et al.: Magnetic resonance arthrography and the prevalence of acetabular labral tears in patients 50 years of age and older, *Skeletal Radiol* 45:1061, 2016.

Jazrawi LM, Alaia MJ, Chang G, et al.: Advances in magnetic resonance imaging of articular cartilage, *J Am Acad Orthop Surg* 19:420, 2011.

Kavanagh EC, Read P, Carty F, et al.: Three-dimensional magnetic resonance imaging analysis of hip morphology in the assessment of femoral acetabular impingement, *Clin Radiol* 66:742, 2011.

Kim HT, Oh MH, Lee JS: MR imaging as a supplement to traditional decision-making in the treatment of LCP disease, *J Pediatr Orthop* 31:246, 2011.

Linda DD, Naraghi A, Murnaghan L, et al.: Accuracy of non-arthrographic 3T MR imaging in evaluation of intra-articular pathology of the hip in femoroacetabular impingement, *Skeletal Radiol* 46:299, 2017.

Matharu GS, Mansour R, Dada O, et al: Which imaging modality is most effective for identifying pseudotumours in metal-on-metal hip resurfacings requiring revision: ultrasound or MARS-MRI or both?

Nachtrab O, Cassar-Pullicino VN, Lalam R, et al.: Role of MRI in hip fractures, including stress fractures, occult fractures, avulsion fractures, *Eur J Radiol* 81:3813, 2012.

Naraghi A, White LM: MRI of labral and chondral lesions of the hip, *AJR Am J Roentgenol* 205:479, 2015.

Newman JS, Newberg AH: MRI of the painful hip in athletes, *Clin Sports Med* 25:613, 2006.

Park JH, Shon HC, Chang JS, et al.: How can MRI change the treatment strategy in apparently isolated greater trochanteric fracture? *Injury* 49:824, 2018.

Petchprapa CN, Rosenberg ZS, Sconfienza LM, et al.: MR imaging of entrapment neuropathies of the lower extremity: part 1. The pelvis and hip, *Radiographics* 30:983, 2010.

Potter HG, Schachar J: High resolution noncontrast MRI of the hip, *J Magn Reson Imaging* 31:268, 2010.

Rakhra KS: Magnetic resonance imaging of acetabular tears, *J Bone Joint Surg* 93A(Suppl 2):28, 2011.

Rehman H, Clement RG, Perks F, et al.: Imaging of occult hip fractures: CT or MRI? *Injury* 47:1297, 2016.

Riley GM, McWalter EJ, Stevens KJ, et al.: MRI of the hip for the evaluation of femoroacetabular impingement: past, present, and future, *J Magn Reson Imaging* 41:558, 2015.

Robinson P: Conventional 3-T MRI and 1.5-T MR arthrography of femoroacetabular impingement, *AJR Am J Roentgenol* 199:509, 2012.

Sutter R, Zubler V, Hoffman A, et al.: Hip MRI: how useful is intraarticular contrast material for evaluating surgically proven lesions of the labrum and articular cartilage? *AJR Am J Roentgenol* 202:160, 2014.

Tannast M, Pleus F, Bonel H, et al.: Magnetic resonance imaging in traumatic posterior hip dislocation, *J Orthop Trauma* 24:723, 2010.

Tosum O, Algin O, Yalcin N, et al.: Ischiofemoral impingement: evaluation with new MRI parameters and assessment of their reliability, *Skeletal Radiol* 41:575, 2012.

Tsifountoudis I, Kraniotis P, Karantanas AH: Hip and pelvic: MRI of muscu-lotendinous trauma and mimickers, *Semin Musculoskelet Radiol* 27:218, 2017.

Walsh CP, Hubbard JC, Nessler JP, et al.: MRI findings associated with recalled modular femoral neck Rejuvenate and ABG implants, *J Arthroplasty* 30:2021, 2015.

Zoga AC, Hegazi TM, Roedl JB: Algorithm for imaging the hip in adoles-cents and young adults, *Radiol Clin North A* 54:913, 2016.

SPINE

Bozzo A, Marcoux J, Radhakrishna M, et al.: The role of magnetic resonance imaging in the management of acute spinal cord injury, *J Neurotrauma* 28:1401, 2011.

Como JJ: The role of MRI in the clearance of the cervical spine in the obtunded blunt trauma patient, *J Trauma* 68:1269, 2010.

D'Aprile P, Nasuto M, Tarantino A, et al.: Magnetic resonance imaging in degenerative disease of the lumbar spine: fat saturation technique and contrast medium, *Acta Biomed* 89:208, 2018.

Diab M, Landman Z, Lubicky J, et al.: Use and outcome of MRI in the surgi-cal treatment of adolescent idiopathic scoliosis, *Spine* 36:667, 2011.

Durand DJ, Huisman TA, Carrino JA: MR imaging features of common vari-ant spinal anatomy, *Magn Reson Imaging Clin N Am* 18:717, 2010.

Dutoit JC, Vanderkerken MA, Verstraete KL: Value of whole body MRI and dynamic contrast enhanced MRI in the diagnosis, follow-up and evalu-ation of disease activity and extent in multiple myeloma, *Eur J Radiol* 82:1444, 2013.

Fehlings MG, Arvin B: Magnetic resonance imaging and outcome, *J Neurosurg Spine* 12:56, 2010.

Ganiyusufoglu AK, Onat L, Karatoprak O, et al.: Diagnostic accuracy of mag-netic resonance imaging versus computed tomography in stress fractures of the lumbar spine, *Clin Radiol* 65:902, 2010.

Goldberg AL, Kershah SM: Advances in imaging of vertebral and spinal cord injury, *J Spinal Cord Med* 33:105, 2010.

Hanrahan CJ, Shah LM: MRI of spinal bone marrow: part 2, T1-weighted imaging-based differential diagnosis, *AJR Am J Roentgenol* 197:1309, 2011.

Khanna P, Chau C, Dublin A, et al.: The value of cervical magnetic resonance imaging in the evaluation of the obtunded or comatose patient with cer-vical trauma, no other abnormal neurological findings, and a normal cer-vical computed tomography, *J Trauma* 72:699, 2012.

Kumar Y, Hayashi D: Role of magnetic resonance imaging in acute spinal trauma: a pictorial review, *BMC Muculoskelet Disord* 17:310, 2016.

Land N, Su MY, Yu HJ, et al.: Differentiation of myeloma and metastatic cancer in the spine using dynamic contrast-enhanced MRI, *Magn Reson Imaging* 31:1285, 2013.

Lattig F, Fekete TF, Grob D, et al.: Lumbar facet joint effusion in MRI: a sign of instability in degenerative spondylolisthesis? *Eur Spine J* 21:276, 2012.

Lee S, Lee JW, Yeom JS, et al.: A practical MRI grading system for lumbar foraminal stenosis, *AJR Am J Roentgenol* 194:1095, 2010.

Machino M, Yukawa Y, Ito K, et al.: Can magnetic resonance imaging reflect the prognosis in patients of cervical spinal cord injury without radio-graphic abnormality? *Spine* 36:E1568, 2011.

Malhorta A, Wu X, Kalra VB, et al.: Utility of MRI for cervical spine clearance after blunt traumatic injury: a meta-analysis, *Eur Radiol* 27:1148, 2017.

Merhemic Z, Stosic-Opincal T, Thurnher MM: Neuroimaging of spinal tumors, *Magn Reson Imaging Clin N Am* 24:563, 2016.

Murphy JM, Park P, Patel RD: Cost-effectiveness of MRI to assess for post-traumatic ligamentous cervical spine injury, *Orthopedics* 37:e148, 2014.

Nouri A, Martin AR, Mikulis D, et al.: Magnetic resonance imaging assess-ment of degenerative cervical myelopathy: a review of structural changes and measurement techniques, *Neurosurg Focus* 40:(E5), 2016.

Ostergaard M, Poggenborg RP, Axelsen MB, Pedersen SJ: Magnetic reso-nance imaging in spondyloarthritis—how to quantify findings and mea-sure response, *Best Pract Res Clin Rheumatol* 24:637, 2010.

Ozturk C, Karadereler S, Orneck I, et al.: The role of routine magnetic reso-nance imaging in the preoperative evaluation of adolescent idiopathic scoliosis, *Int Orthop* 34:543, 2010.

Park HJ, Kim SS, Chung EC, et al.: Clinical correlation of a new practical MRI method for assessing cervical spinal canal compression, *AJR Am J Roentgenol* 199:W197, 2012.

Pizones J, Castillo E: Assessment of acute thoracolumbar fractures: chal-lenges in multidetector computed tomography and added value of emer-gency MRI, *Semin Musculoskelet Radiol* 17:389, 2013.

Pizones J, Izwuierdo E, Alvarez P, et al.: Impact of magnetic resonance imag-ing on decision making for thoracolumbar traumatic fracture diagnosis and treatment, *Eur Spine J* 20(Suppl 3):390, 2011.

Rihn JA, Yang N, Fisher C, et al.: Using magnetic resonance imaging to accu-rately assess injury to the posterior ligamentous complex of the spine: a prospective comparison of the surgeon and radiologist, *J Neurosurg Spine* 12:391, 2010.

Roudarsi B, Jarvik JG: Lumbar spine MRI for low back pain: indications and yield, *AJR Am J Roentgenol* 195:550, 2010.

Savvopoulou V, Martis TG, Koureas A, et al.: Degenerative endplate changes of the lumbosacral spine: dynamic contrast-enhanced MRI profiles related to age, sex, and spinal level, *J Magn Reson Imaging* 33:382, 2011.

Schoenfeld AJ, Bono CM, McGuide KJ, et al.: Computed tomography alone versus computed tomography and magnetic resonance imaging in the identification of occult injuries to the cervical spine: a meta-analysis, *J Trauma* 68:109, 2010.

Shah LM, Hanrahan CJ: MRI of spinal bone marrow: part 1, techniques and normal age-related appearances, *AJR Am J Roentgenol* 197:1298, 2011.

Sheehan NJ: Magnetic resonance imaging for low back pain: indications and limitations, *Ann Rheum Dis* 69:(7), 2010.

Soult MC, Weireter LJ, Britt RC, et al.: MRI as an adjunct to cervical spine clearance: a utility analysis, *Am Surg* 78:741, 2012.

Weber U, Maksymowych WP: Sensitivity and specificity of magnetic reso-nance imaging for axial spondyloarthritis, *Am J Med Sci* 341:272, 2011.

SHOULDER

Ajuied A, McGarvey CP, Harb Z, et al.: Diagnosis of glenoid labral tears using 3-tesla MRI vs. 3-tesla MRA: a systematic review and meta-analysis, *Arch Orthop Trauma Surg* 138:699, 2018.

Beltran LS, Bencardino JT, Steinbach LS: Postoperative MRI of the shoul-der, *J Magn Reson Imaging* 40:1280, 2014.

Chang IY, Polster JM: Pathomechanics and magnetic resonance imaging of the thrower's shoulder, *Radiol Clin North Am* 54:801, 2016.

Cook TS, Stein JM, Simonson S, Kim W: Normal and variant anatomy of the shoulder on MRI, *Magn Reson Imaging Clin North Am* 19:581, 2011.

Fitzpatrick D, Walz DM: Shoulder MR imaging normal variants and imaging artifacts, *Magn Reson Imaging Clin North Am* 18:615, 2010.

Garwood ER, Mitti GS, Alaia M, et al.: Use of shoulder imaging in the out-patient setting: a pilot study, *Curr Probl Diagn Radiol* pii: S0363-0188 (17):30260–30268, 2017, https://doi.org/10.1067/j.cpradiol.2017.10.011, [Epub ahead of print].

Gazzola S, Bleakney RR: Current imaging of the rotator cuff, *Sports Med Arthrosc* 19:300, 2011.

Giles JW, Owens BD, Athwal GS: Estimating glenoid width for instability-related bone loss: a CT evaluation of an MRI formula, *Am J Sports Med* 43:1726, 2015.

Gottsegen CJ, Merkle AN, Bencardino JT, et al.: Advanced MRI techniques of the shoulder joint: current applications in clinical practice, *AJR Am J Roentgenol* 209:544, 2017.

Gyftopoulos S, Strauss EJ: MRI-arthroscopy correlation for shoulder anat-omy and pathology: a teaching guide, *AJR Am J Roentgenol* 204:W684, 2015.

Gyftopoulos S, Yemin A, Beltran L, et al.: Engaging Hill-Sachs lesion: is there an association between this lesion and findings on MRI? *AJR Am J Roentgenol* 201:W633, 2013.

Houtz CG, Schwartzberg RS, Barry JS, et al.: Shoulder MRI accuracy in the community setting, *J Shoulder Elbow Surg* 20:537, 2011.

Knapik DM, Voos JE: Magnetic resonance imaging and arthroscopic correla-tion in shoulder instability, *Sports Med Arthrosc Rev* 25:172, 2017.

Lee SC, Williams D, Endo Y: The repaired rotator cuff: MRI and ultrasound evaluation, *Curr Rev Musculoskelet Med* 11:92, 2018.

Lin DJ, Wong TT, Kazam JK: Shoulder injuries in the overhead-throwing athlete: epidemiology, mechanisms of injury, and imaging findings, *Radiology* 286:370, 2018.

Llopis E, Montesinos P, Guedez MT, et al.: Normal shoulder MRI and MR arthrography: anatomy and technique, *Semin Musculoskelet Radiol* 19:212, 2015.

Major NM, Browne J, Domzalski T, et al.: Evaluation of the glenoid labrum with 3-T MRI: is intraarticular contrast necessary? *AJR Am J Roentgenol* 196:1139, 2011.

Park S, Lee DH, Yoon SH, et al.: Evaluation of adhesive capsulitis of the shoulder with fat-suppressed T2-weighted MRI: association between clinical feature and MRI findings, *AJR Am J Roentgenol* 207:135, 2016.

Petchprapa CN, Beltran LS, Jazrawi LM, et al.: The rotator interval: a review of anatomy, function, and normal and abnormal MRI appearance, *AJR Am J Roentgenol* 195:567, 2010.

Roy EA, Cheyne I, Andrews G, et al.: Beyond the cuff: MR imaging of labroligamentous injuries in the athletic shoulder, *Radiology* 278:316, 2016.

Shin YK, Ryu KN, Prk JS, et al.: Predictive factors of retear in patients with repaired rotator cuff tear on shoulder MRI, *AJR Am J Roentgenol* 210:134, 2018.

Stillwater L, Koenig J, Maycher B, et al.: 3D-MR vs. 3D-CT of the shoulder in patients with glenohumeral instability, *Skeletal Radiol* 46:325, 2017.

Suh CH, Yun S, Jin W, et al.: Systematic review and meta-analysis of magnetic resonance imaging features for diagnosis of adhesive capsulitis of the shoulder, *Eur Radiol* 2018, https://doi.org/10.1007/s00330-018-5604-y, [Epub ahead of print].

Veen EJD, Donders CM, Westerbeek RE, et al.: Predictive findings on magnetic resonance imaging in patients with asymptomatic aromioclavicular osteoarthritis, *J Shoulder Elbow Surg* 27:e252, 2018.

Welton KL, Bartley JH, Major NM, et al.: MRI to arthroscopy correlations in SLAP lesions and long head biceps pathology, *Sports Med Arthrosc Rev* 25:179, 2017.

ELBOW, WRIST, AND HAND

Awan H, Goitz R: MRI correlation of radial head fractures and forearm injuries, *Hand (N Y)* 12:145, 2017.

Bergh TH, Steen K, Lindau T, et al.: Costs analysis and comparison of usefulness of acute MRI and 2 weeks of case immobilization for clinically suspected scaphoid fractures, *Acta Orthop* 86:303, 2015.

Datis A: MRI of the hand and fingers, *Top Magn Reson Imaging* 24:109, 2015.

Ersoy H, Pomeranz SJ: Palmer classification and magnetic resonance imaging findings of ulnocarpal impingement, *J Surg Orthop Adv* 24:257, 2015.

Festa A, Mulieri PJ, Newman JS, et al.: Effectiveness of magnetic resonance imaging in detecting partial and complete distal biceps tendon rupture, *J Hand Surg [Am]* 35:77, 2010.

Gupta P, Lenchik L, Wuertzer SD, Pacholke DA: High-resolution 3-T MRI of the fingers: review of anatomy and common tendon and ligament injuries, *AJR Am J Roentgenol* 204:W314, 2015.

Haillotte G, Bachy M, Delpont M, et al.: The use of magnetic resonance imaging in management of minimally displaced or nondisplaced lateral humeral condyle fractures in children, *Pediatr Emerg Care* 33:21, 2017.

Joyner PW, Bruce J, Hess R, et al.: Magnetic resonance imaging-based classification for ulnar collateral ligament injuries of the elbow, *J Shoulder Elbow Surg* 25:1710, 2016.

Krabben A, Stomp W, van Nies JA, et al.: MRI-detected subclinical joint inflammation is associated with radiographic progression, *Ann Rheum Dis* 73:2034, 2014.

Magee T: Accuracy of 3-T MR arthrography versus conventional 3-T MRI of elbow tendons and ligaments compared with surgery, *AJR Am J Roentgenol* 204:W70, 2015.

Mahmood A, Fountain J, Vasireddy N, Waseem M: Wrist MRI arthrogram v wrist arthroscopy: what are we finding? *Open Orthop J* 6:194, 2012.

Mallee W, Doornberg JN, Ring D, et al.: Comparison of CT and MRI for diagnosis of suspected scaphoid fractures, *J Bone Joint Surg Am* 93:20, 2011.

Malone WJ, Snowden R, Alvi F, Klena JC: Pitfalls of wrist MR imaging, *Magn Reson Imaging Clin N Am* 18:643, 2010.

Mete BD, Gursoy M, Resnick D: A rare cause of posterolateral elbow pain: radiohumeral plica syndrome with typical MRI findings, *JBR-BTR* 97:371, 2014.

Onen MR, Kayalara AE, Ilbas EN, et al.: The role of wrist magnetic resonance imaging in the differential diagnosis of the carpal tunnel syndrome, *Turk Neurosurg* 25:701, 2015.

Ringler MD: MRI of wrist ligaments, *J Hand Surg [Am]* 38:2034, 2013.

Sampaio ML, Schweitzer ME: Elbow magnetic resonance imaging variants and pitfalls, *Magn Reson Imaging Clin North Am* 18:633, 2010.

Simonson S, Lott K, Major NM: Magnetic resonance imaging of the elbow, *Semin Roentgenol* 45:180, 2010.

Stein JM, Cook TS, Simonson S, Kim W: Normal and variant anatomy of the wrist and hand on MR imaging, *Magn Reson Imaging Clin North Am* 19:595, 2011.

Stevens KJ, McNally EG: Magnetic resonance imaging of the elbow in athletes, *Clin Sports Med* 29:521, 2010.

Taljanovic MS, Malan JJ, Sheppard JE: Normal anatomy of the extrinsic capsular wrist ligaments by 3-T MRI and high-resolution ultrasonography, *Semin Musculoskelet Radiol* 16:104, 2012.

Thorkelson M, Augustyn R, Barnes CE: Pediatric elbow fracture diagnosis using 3-D MR imaging, *Radiol Technol* 89:75, 2017.

Tsujimoto Y, Ryoke K, Yamagami N, et al.: Delineation of extensor tendon of the hand by MRI: usefulness of "soap-bubble" mip processing technique, *Hand Surg* 20:93, 2015.

Walton MJ, Mackie K, Fallon M, et al.: The reliability and validity of magnetic resonance imaging in the assessment of chronic lateral epicondylitis, *J Hand Surg [Am]* 36:475, 2011.

TUMORS

Bancroft LW: Postoperative tumor imaging, *Semin Musculoskelet Radiol* 15:425, 2011.

Costa FM, Ferreira EC, Vianna EM: Diffusion-weighted magnetic resonance imaging for the evaluation of musculoskeletal tumors, *Magn Reson Imaging Clin North Am* 19:159, 2011.

D'Ippolito G, Torres LR, Saito Filho CF, Ferreira RM: CT and MRI in monitoring response: state-of-the-art and future developments, *Q J Nucl Med Mol Imaging* 55:603, 2011.

Hansford BG, Stacy GS: From tumor to trauma: etiologically deconstructing a unique differential diagnosis of musculoskeletal entities with high signal intensity on T1-weighted MRI, *AJR Am J Roentgenol* 204:817, 2015.

Padhani AR, Makris A, Gall P, et al.: Therapy monitoring of skeletal metastases with whole-body diffusion MRI, *J Magn Reson Imaging* 39:1049, 2014.

Subhawong TK, Jacobs MA, Fayad LM: Insights into quantitative diffusion-weighted MRI for musculoskeletal tumor imaging, *AJR Am J Roentgenol* 203:560, 2014.

Vandergugten S, Traore SY, Cartiaux O, et al.: MRI evaluation of resection margins in bone tumour surgery, *Sarcoma* 2014:967848, 2014.

COMPUTED TOMOGRAPHY

Barg A, Bailey T, Richter M, et al.: Weightbearing computed tomography of the foot and ankle: emerging technology topical review, *Foot Ankle Int* 39:376, 2018.

Brink M, Steenbakkers A, Holla M, et al.: Single-shot CT after wrist trauma: impact on detection accuracy and treatment of fractures, *Skeletal Radiol*, 2018, https://doi.org/10.1007/s00256-018-3097-z, [Epub ahead of print].

Cahill CW, Radcliff KE, Reitman CA: Enhancing evaluation of the cervical spine: thresholds for normal CT relationships in the subaxial cervical spine, *Int J Spine Surg* 12:510, 2018.

Castiglia MT, Nogueira-Barbosa MH, Messias AMV, et al.: The impact of computed tomography on decision making in tibial plateau fractures, *J Knee Surg* 31:1007, 2018.

Cerquiglini A, Henckel J, Hothi HS, et al.: Computed tomography techniques help understand wear patterns in retrieved total knee arthroplasty, *J Arthroplasty* 33:3030, 2018.

Cheema AN, Niziolek PJ, /Steinberg D, et al.: The effect of computed tomography scans oriented along the longitdinual scaphoid axis on measurements of deformity and displacement in scaphoid fractures, *J Hand*

Surg Am 2018. pii: S0363-5023(18)30628-2, https://doi.org/10.1016/j.jhsa.2018.05.006, [Epub ahead of print].

Figueroa J, Guarachi JP, Matas J, et al.: Is computed tomography an accurate and reliable method for measuring total knee arthroplasty component rotation? *Int Orthop* 40:709, 2016.

Gupta P, Prakash M, Sharma N, et al.: Computed tomography detection of clinically unsuspected skeletal tuberculosis, *Clin Imaging* 39:1056, 2015.

Haubro M, Stougaard C, Torfing T, et al.: Sensitivity and specificity of CT- and MRI-scanning in evaluation of occult fracture of the proximal femur, *Injury* 46:1557, 2015.

Hecht G, Shelton TJ, Saiz Jr AM, et al.: CT-measurement predicts shortening of stable intertrochanteric hip fractures, *J Orthop* 15:952, 2018.

Ho A, Kurdziel MD, Koueiter DM, et al.: Three-dimensional computed tomography measurement of varying Hill-Sachs lesion size, *J Shoulder Elbow Surg* 27:350, 2018.

Imerci A, Aydogan NH, Topsakal FE: The role of computed tomography scans in diaphyseal femur fractures following gunshot injuries: a survey of orthopaedic traumatologists, *Injury* 49:731, 2018.

Jakubietz MG, Mages L, Zahn RK, et al.: The role of CT scan in postoperative evaluation of distal radius fractures: retrospective analysis in regard to complications and revision rates, *J Orthop Sci* 22:434, 2017.

Jaroma A, Suomalainen JSm Niemitukia L, et al.: Imaging of symptomatic total knee arthroplasty with cone beam computed tomography, *Acta Radiol* 59:1500, 2018.

Kozaci N, Avci M, Ararat E, et al.: Comparison of ultrasonography and computed tomography in the determination of traumatic injuries, *Am J Emerg Med* 2018. pii: S0735-6757(18)30637-5, https://doi.org/10.1016/j.ajem.2018.08.002, [Epub ahead of print].

Kumar A, Mishra P, Tandon A, et al.: Effect of CT on management plan in malleolar ankle fractures, *Foot Ankle Int* 39:59, 2018.

Li WY, Lin KC: Three-dimensional computed tomography reduced fixation failure of intramedullary nailing for unstable type of intertrochanteric fracture, *J Orthop Trauma* 32:e381, 2018.

Mansfield C, Ali S, Komperda K, et al.: Optimizing radiation dose in computed tomography of articular fractures, *J Orthop Trauma* 31:401, 2017.

Neubauer J, Benndorf M, Ehritt-Braun C, et al.: Comparison of the diagnostic accuracy of cone beam computed tomography and radiography for scaphoid fractures, *Sci Rep* 8:3906, 2018.

Rajasekaran S, Vaccaro AR, Kanna RM, et al.: The value of CT and MRI in the classification and surgical decision-making among spine surgeons in thoracolumbar spinal injuries, *Eur Spine J* 26:1463, 2017.

Stoltny T, Pasek J, Leksowska-Pawliczek M, et al.: Importance of computed tomography (CT) in talar neck fractures, Case studies, *Ortop Traumatol Rehabil* 20:31, 2018.

Thomas RW, Williams HL, Carpenter EC, et al.: The validity of investigating occult hip fractures using multidetetor CT, *Br J Radiol* 89:20150250, 2016.

Wiewiorski M, Hoechel S, Anderson AE, et al.: Computed tomographic evaluation of joint geometry in patients with end-stage ankle osteoarthritis, *Foot Ankle Int* 37:644, 2016.

Wu XD, Xiang BY, Schotanus MGM, et al.: CT- versus MRI-based patient-specific instrumentation for total knee arthroplasty: a systematic review and meta-analysis, *Surgeon* 15:336, 2017.

The complete list of references is available online at Expert Consult.com.

PART **II**

INFECTIONS

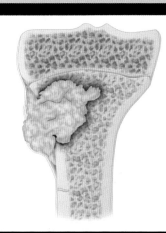

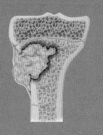

ETIOLOGY

Bone and joint infections pose a formidable challenge to the orthopaedic surgeon. The high success rate obtained with antibiotic therapy in most bacterial diseases has not been obtained in bone and joint infections because of the physiologic and anatomic characteristics of bone. Approximately 80 million surgical cases are performed in the United States yearly, and with the rise in aging population, this will most likely increase. The overall surgical site infection (SSI) rate has been estimated by the U.S. Centers for Disease Control and Prevention (CDC) to be 2.8% in the United States. Approximately 300,000 SSIs occur each year in the United States, with affected patients requiring 6.5 more hospital days on average, which increases the cost of surgery two to five times. Although bacteremia is common (estimated to occur 25% of the time after simple tooth brushings), other etiologic factors must be present for an infection to occur. The mere presence of bacteria in bone, whether from bacteremia or from direct inoculation is insufficient to produce osteomyelitis. Illness, malnutrition, and inadequacy of the immune system can contribute to bone and joint infections. As in other parts of the body, bones and joints produce inflammatory and immune responses to infection. Osteomyelitis occurs when an adequate number of a sufficiently virulent organism overcomes the host's natural defenses (inflammatory and immune responses) and establishes a focus of infection. Local skeletal factors also play a role in the development of infection. For example, the relative absence of phagocytic cells in the metaphysis of bones in children may explain why acute hematogenous osteomyelitis is more common in this location.

The peculiarity of an abscess in bone is that it is contained within a firm structure with little chance of tissue expansion. As infection progresses, purulent material works its way through the Haversian system and Volkmann canals and lifts the periosteum off the surface of bone. The combination of pus in the medullary cavity and in the subperiosteal space causes necrosis of cortical bone. This necrotic cortical bone, known as a sequestrum, can continue to harbor bacteria despite antibiotic treatment. Antibiotics and inflammatory cells cannot adequately access this avascular area, resulting in failure of medical treatment of osteomyelitis.

Recognizing these unique characteristics of bone infections, the best course of action is prevention. The orthopaedic surgeon should evaluate the risk of infection in each patient by considering patient-dependent and surgeon-dependent factors. Patient-dependent factors include nutrition, immunologic status, alcohol abuse, smoking, infection at a remote site, congestive heart failure, depression, and other comorbidities (Table 3.1). Surgeon-dependent factors include prophylactic antibiotics, skin and wound care, operating environment, surgical technique, and treatment of impending infections, such as in open fractures. Duration of hospital stay also has been directly correlated with an increased risk of SSI. Simply stated, it is much easier to prevent an infection than it is to treat it.

PATIENT-DEPENDENT FACTORS

It has been discovered that up to 80% of patients have at least one modifiable risk factor that, if corrected, could decrease the risk of SSI. Alcohol abuse, for instance, doubles the risk, and tobacco use more than triples the risk for infection. These substances should be discontinued 1 month before surgery is recommended. Intra-articular injections also should be discontinued 3 to 6 months before elective surgery, and any poor dentition issues should be treated.

■ NUTRITIONAL STATUS

A patient's nutritional status and immunologic response are important. A body mass index greater than 40 is associated with an eight times greater risk for SSI. Despite their appearance, obese patients are frequently malnourished. In fact, over half of patients are noted to be malnourished. If a patient is malnourished or immunocompromised and cannot mount a response to an infection, the effects of any treatment are diminished. Malnutrition adversely affects humoral and cell-mediated immunity, impairs neutrophil chemotaxis, diminishes bacterial clearance, and depresses neutrophil bactericidal function, the delivery of inflammatory cells to infectious foci, and serum complement components. Basal energy requirements of a traumatized or infected patient increase from 30% to 55% of normal. Fever of just 1°F above normal increases the body's metabolic rate by 13%.

Nutritional status can be determined preoperatively by (1) anthropometric measurements (height, weight, triceps

TABLE. 3.1

Summary of Risk Factors Associated With Development of Surgical Joint Infection/Prosthetic Joint Infection

NONMODIFIABLE HOST FACTORS	MODIFIABLE HOST FACTORS	FACTORS WITH LIMITED EVIDENCE OF ASSOCIATIONS WITH SSI/PJI
Age (≥75 years)—moderate	BMI—strong	Age—(as a continuous exposure)—limited
Male sex—strong	Smoking—strong	Hispanic ethnicity—limited
Black race—strong	High alcohol intake (alcohol abuse)—strong	Native American and Eskimo ethnicity—limited
TKA vs. THA—strong	Low income—strong	Asian race—limited
	Malnutrition (low serum albumin)—strong	History of drug abuse—limited
	History of DM—strong	Rural location vs. nonrural location—limited
	History of CVD—moderate	Underweight—limited
	History of CHF—strong	History of hypertension—limited
	History of cardiac arrhythmia—strong	History of osteoarthritis—limited
	History of peripheral vascular disease—strong	History of posttraumatic arthritis—limited
	Chronic pulmonary disease—strong	Low- or high-risk dental procedures—limited
	Chronic obstructive pulmonary disease	History of urinary tract infection—limited
	History of renal disease—strong	History of dementia—limited
	History of liver disease/cirrhosis—strong	Hypercholesterolemia—limited
	History of RA—strong	Peptic ulcer disease—limited
	History of cancer/malignancy—strong	Valvular disease—limited
	History of osteonecrosis—strong	Metastatic tumor—limited
	History of depression—strong	History of coagulopathy—limited
	History of psychosis—strong	History of venous thromboembolism—limited
	History of HIV/AIDS—strong	Pulmonary circulatory disorders—limited
	Neurologic disease (hemiplegia, paraplegia)—moderate	Hypothyroidism—limited
	History of corticosteroid administration—strong	Hepatitis (B or C)—limited
	History of intra-articular corticosteroid injection—moderate	Electrolyte imbalance—limited
	Previous joint surgery—strong	Autogenous blood transfusion—limited
	Revision arthroplasty—strong	
	Previous joint infection—moderate	
	Frailty—moderate	
	Preoperative anemia—strong	
	American Society of Anesthesiologists grade >2—strong	
	Charlson comorbidity index (high)—strong	
	Preoperative hyperglycemia and high HbA1c—moderate	
	Allogenic blood transfusion—strong	
	Prophylaxis with warfarin or low-molecular weight heparin—moderate	

BMI, Body mass index; *CHF*, congestive heart failure; *CVD*, cardiovascular disease; *DM*, diabetes mellitus; *PJI*, periprosthetic joint infection; *RA*, rheumatoid arthritis; *SSI*, surgical site infection; *THA*, total hip arthroplasty; *TKA*, total knee arthroplasty.
From Zainul-Abidin S, Amanatullah DF, Anderson MB, et al: General assembly, prevention, host related general: proceedings of international consensus on orthopedic infections, *J Arthroplasty* 34(2S):S13–S35, 2019.

skinfold thickness, and arm muscle circumference), (2) measurement of serum proteins or cell types (lymphocytes), and (3) antibody reaction to certain antigens in skin testing.

Nutritional support is recommended before elective surgery for patients with recent weight losses of more than 10 lb, serum albumin levels less than 3.5 g/dL, or lymphocyte counts of less than 1500 cells/mm³, which can be obtained from a routine complete blood cell count and BMP-24. With the use of serum albumin and transferrin levels, the formula that follows can be used to screen for patients who may need nutritional support: [(1.2 × serum albumin) + (0.013 × serum transferrin)] − 6.43. If the sum is 0 or a negative number, the patient is nutritionally depleted and is at high risk for sepsis. If nutritional support is needed, enteral therapy should always be used when the gastrointestinal tract is functional; if not, hyperalimentation must be employed. Vitamin D deficiency also has been linked to an increase in SSIs. Vitamin D levels should be obtained preoperatively, and any deficiencies corrected at that time.

GLUCOSE

Glycemic control is a patient modifiable risk factor that can lead to a decrease in SSI. The optimal hemoglobin A1c (HbA1c) has yet to be determined. Some advocate 7%, whereas others believe 8% is the correct value for risk stratification. Fructosamine levels have been utilized to detect hyperglycemia especially in the 2 to 3 week period before surgery. A level greater than 292 mmol/L has been shown to be a better indicator of deep infection than HbA1c (>7%). Most agree that hyperglycemia, even in nondiabetic patients, is a risk factor for developing SSI. A glucose level greater than 200 mg/dL requires treatment before elective surgery.

RHEUMATOID ARTHRITIS

The incidence of periprosthetic joint infection (PJI) is 1.6 times higher in patients with rheumatoid arthritis than with osteoarthritis. Most believe that this is associated with their use of disease-modifying antirheumatic drugs. To decrease the incidence of SSI in this population, it is recommended that these medications be discontinued according to their half-life and resumed 2 weeks postoperatively.

IMMUNOLOGIC STATUS

To fight infection, the patient must mount inflammatory (white blood cell [WBC] count) and immune (antibody) responses that initially stop the spread of infection and then, ideally, destroy the infecting organisms. The body's main cellular defense mechanisms are (1) neutrophil response, (2) humoral immunity, (3) cell-mediated immunity, and (4) reticuloendothelial cells. A deficiency in production or function of any of these predisposes the host to infection by specific groups of opportunistic pathogens. Deficiencies in the immune system may be acquired or may result from congenital abnormalities. Immunocompromised hosts are not susceptible to all opportunistic pathogens. The susceptibility to a microorganism depends on the specific defect in immunity. Abnormal neutrophils or humoral and cell-mediated immunities have been implicated in infections caused by encapsulated bacteria in infants and elderly patients, in the increased incidence of *Pseudomonas* infections in heroin addicts, and in *Salmonella* and *Pneumococcus* infections in patients with sickle cell anemia.

Diabetes, alcoholism, hematologic malignancy, and cytotoxic therapy are common causes of neutrophil abnormalities. If the neutrophil count decreases to less than 55/mm^3, infections caused by *Staphylococcus aureus,* gram-negative bacilli, *Aspergillus* organisms, and *Candida* organisms become a major threat.

Immunoglobulins and complement factors are two plasma proteins that play crucial roles in humoral immunity. Patients with hypogammaglobulinemia or who have had a splenectomy are at increased risk of infection caused by encapsulated bacteria, such as *Streptococcus pneumoniae, Haemophilus influenzae,* and *Neisseria* organisms. When a defect in a component of the complement cascade is present, *S. aureus* and gram-negative bacillus infections are common. Septic arthritis caused by unusual organisms such as *Mycoplasma pneumoniae* and *Ureaplasma urealyticum* has been reported and should be suspected in patients with hypogammaglobulinemia and culture-negative septic arthritis.

Cell-mediated immunity depends on an interaction between T lymphocytes and macrophages. Primary cell-mediated deficiencies are rare, but secondary cell-mediated deficiencies are common. Corticosteroid therapy, malnutrition, lymphoma, systemic lupus erythematosus, immunodeficiency in elderly patients, and autoimmune deficiency syndrome all can cause a secondary cell-mediated deficiency, which predisposes the host to fungal and mycobacterial infections as well as infection with herpes virus and *Pneumocystis jiroveci.*

Vaccinations also play a role in host response. The hepatitis B vaccine has dramatically reduced the incidence of hepatitis B virus (HBV), and the *H. influenzae* type B vaccine, that is given to children, has all but eliminated musculoskeletal infections caused by *H. influenzae.*

SURGEON-DEPENDENT FACTORS
SKIN PREPARATION

Wound contamination exists whenever the skin barrier is broken, but proper skin preparation decreases the contamination caused by bacteria present on the skin. Skin barriers also may decrease skin contamination during surgery. Although the skin can never be disinfected completely, the number of bacteria present can be reduced markedly before surgery. The skin and hair can be sterilized with alcohol, iodine, hexachlorophene, or chlorhexidine, but it is almost impossible to sterilize the hair follicles and sebaceous glands where bacteria normally reside and reproduce. Skin preparations have a limited effect on sebaceous glands and hair follicles because they do not penetrate an oily environment. Disinfectants that penetrate the oily environment are absorbed by the body and have potentially toxic side effects. Hexachlorophene has better penetration but also has neurotoxic side effects. Very few level I evidence-based studies discuss if preoperative skin antiseptics actually decrease SSI and, if so, the correct method of cleansing. Most agree that the patient should bathe the night before surgery with soap and water. Some advocate adding chlorhexidine wipes. A Cochrane Library systematic review concluded that 4% chlorhexidine in 70% alcohol had the most favorable results in reducing SSI. Most agree that some form of alcohol needs to be employed with whatever skin preparation is used, whether it be chlorhexidine or iodophor. We agree with the CDC guidelines for skin preparation with slight modifications:
1. The size of the area being prepared should be enough to include any additional exposure that may be required.
2. The solution should be applied in concentric circles from the incision site peripherally.
3. A dedicated instrument may be utilized that is removed from the operative field after preparation and before draping (i.e., sponge clamp).
4. Time should be allowed for the alcohol to dry because a fire risk exists.

Hand washing is the single-most important procedure for prevention of nosocomial infections and should be performed before and after each patient encounter. Studies suggest that hand scrubbing for 2 minutes is as effective as traditional hand scrubbing for 5 minutes. The optimal duration of hand scrubbing has yet to be determined. Hand rubbing with an aqueous

TABLE. 3.2

Antimicrobial Activity* and Summary of Properties of Antiseptics Used in Hand Hygiene

ANTISEPTICS	GRAM-POSITIVE BACTERIA	GRAM-NEGATIVE BACTERIA	VIRUSES ENVELOPED	VIRUSES NONENVELOPED	MYCOBACTERIA	FUNGI	SPORES
Alcohols	+++	+++	+++	++	+++	+++	−
Chloroxylenol	+++	+	+	±	+	+	−
Chlorhexidine	+++	++	++	+	+	+	−
Hexachlorophene[†]	+++	+	?	?	+	+	−
Iodophors	+++	+++	++	++	++	++	±[‡]
Triclosan[¶]	+++	++	?	?	±	±[¶]	−
Quaternary ammonium compounds[§]	++	+	+	?	±	±	−

ANTISEPTICS	TYPICAL CONC. IN%	SPEED OF ACTION	RESIDUAL ACTIVITY	USE
Alcohols	60%–70%	Fast	No	HR
Chloroxylenol	0.5%–4%	Slow	Contradictory	HW
Chlorhexidine	0.5%–4%	Intermediate	Yes	HR/HW
Hexachlorophene[†]	3%	Slow	Yes	HW, but not recommended
Iodophors	0.5%–10%	Intermediate	Contradictory	HW
Triclosan[‖]	0.1%–2%	Intermediate	Yes	HW; seldom
Quaternary ammonium compounds[§]		Slow	No	HR, HW; Seldom; +alcohols

Good = +++, moderate = ++, poor = +, variable = ±, none = −
*Activity varies with concentration.
[†]Bacteriostatic.
[‡]In concentrations used in antiseptics, iodophors are not sporicidal.
[‖]Mostly bacteriostatic.
[¶]Activity against *Candida spp.*, but little activity against filamentous fungi.
[§]Bacteriostatic, fungistatic, microbicidal at high concentrations.
HR, Hand rubbing; *HW*, hand washing.
From Pittet D, Allegranzi B, Boyce J, et al: The World Health Organization guidelines on hand hygiene in health care and their consensus recommendations. *Infec Control Hosp Epidemiol* 30:611–622, 2009.

alcohol solution that is preceded by a 1-minute nonantiseptic hand washing for the first case of the day was found by Parienti et al. to be just as effective in prevention of SSI as traditional hand scrubbing with antiseptic soap. The effectiveness of common antiseptics is summarized in Table 3.2.

Hair removal at the operative site is not recommended unless done in the operating room with clippers. Shaving the operative site the night before surgery can cause local trauma that produces a favorable environment for bacterial reproduction.

Prevention of infection transmission between the patient and the surgeon also includes proper surgical attire. Edlich et al. showed that a narrow glove gauntlet (cuff) significantly increased the security of the gown-glove interface. The U.S. Food and Drug Administration accepts there is a 2.5% failure rate of new unused sterile gloves. Glove perforation has been reported to occur in up to 48% of operations. Perforations usually occur approximately 40 minutes into the procedure, and as much as 83% of the time the surgeon is unaware of the perforation. Most frequently, the perforation occurs on the index finger of the nondominant hand. Double gloving reduces the exposure rate by as much as 87%. In addition, double gloving decreases the volume of blood on a solid needle (through a wipe-clean pass mechanism from the outer glove)

as much as 95%. A meta-analysis by Tanner and Parkinson found that double gloving decreased skin contamination, and the use of Biogel indicator gloves (Regent Medical, Norcross, GA) increased the awareness of glove perforation. A darker glove should be worn as the indicator glove. When both gloves were compromised, however, the indicator gloves did not increase the awareness of a perforation. As long as the indicator glove was intact, perforation of the outer glove was promptly detected in 90% of cases. Wearing an outer cloth glove over a latex glove significantly reduced the number of perforations to the innermost latex glove. When a liner glove was used between two latex gloves, the perforation rate of the innermost glove decreased. No reduction in perforations was seen when using an outer steel–weave glove. Double gloving does not provide reduction in perforations when tears occur as a result of geometry configurations such as bone or hollow-core needles. At a minimum, surgical gloves should be changed after draping, before handling implants, and then every 2 hours. No level I evidence exists currently that conclusively proves reduction of SSI with the use of surgical mask, caps, shoe covers, cloth versus disposable gowns, or operating room attire worn outside the hospital; however, experience dictates their usefulness. A very large number of patients will be required to sufficiently power future level I studies.

OPERATING ROOM ENVIRONMENT

Airborne bacteria are another source of wound contamination in the operating room. These bacteria usually are gram positive and originate almost exclusively from humans in the operating room; 5000 to 55,000 particles are shed per minute by each individual in the operating room. Conventional operating room air may contain 10 to 15 bacteria per cubic foot and 250,000 particles per cubic foot. The number of door openings and surgical personnel has been shown to increase the number of airborne particles and, therefore, should be kept to a minimum. Bouffant style hats allow significantly greater microbial shedding than disposable skull caps and perhaps should be avoided. In past research, airborne bacterial concentrations in the operating room were thought to be reduced by at least 80% with laminar-airflow systems and even more with personnel-isolator systems. Wound contamination rates have been reported to be reduced by 80% with the use of these systems, although an increased infection rate has been reported with the use of horizontal laminar flow after total knee arthroplasty, possibly from deposition of bacteria shed by scrubbed personnel who were not wearing personnel-isolator systems. However, most recent studies have shown that the use of laminar flow does not decrease SSI. At this time, laminar flow is no longer required. Ultraviolet light also has been noted to decrease the incidence of wound infection by reducing the number of airborne bacteria; however, the use of ultraviolet light rooms is not recommended by the Hospital Infection Control Practice Advisory Committee or the CDC because of the increased risk to surgical personnel of exposure to ultraviolet light. It can be employed as a method for terminal cleaning of the unoccupied operating room.

No level I evidence exists that forced air warming increases SSI; however, a multicentered pooled data study by Augustine showed a 78% reduction in SSI after discontinuing forced air warming. Normothermia has shown to decrease SSI.

Additional evidence exists for changing the scalpel after the first incision, changing the suction tip every hour, avoiding a back-table splash basin (the dirty pond), keeping operative time to less than 2.5 hours to decrease the occurrence of infection. Of note, low-pressure (bulb) lavage has been demonstrated to be equal to high-pressure (pulse) lavage. The addition of antibiotics to the irrigation fluid had no additional benefit and, therefore, is not recommended. Although little has changed in over 50 years in our use of surgical attire and little clinically based evidence exists for scrub masks, head coverings, iodine-impregnated plastic drapes, and many of our "standard sterile techniques," we believe that the practices listed in Table 3.3 should be adhered to in an effort to minimize the risk of SSI.

PROPHYLACTIC ANTIBIOTIC THERAPY

Many studies have shown the effectiveness of prophylactic antibiotics in reducing infection rates after orthopaedic procedures. During the first 24 hours, infection depends on the number of bacteria present. During the first 2 hours, the host defense mechanism works to decrease the overall number of bacteria. During the next 4 hours, the number of bacteria remains constant, with the bacteria that are multiplying and the bacteria that are being killed by the host defenses being about equal. These first 6 hours are called the "golden period," after which the bacteria multiply exponentially. Antibiotics decrease bacterial growth geometrically and delay the reproduction of the bacteria. The administration of prophylactic antibiotics expands the golden period.

A prophylactic antibiotic should be safe, bactericidal, and effective against the most common organisms causing infections in orthopaedic surgery. Because the patient's skin remains the major source of orthopaedic infection, prophylactic antibiotics should be directed against the organism most commonly found on the skin, which is *S. aureus,* although the frequency of *Staphylococcus epidermidis* is increasing. This increase in *S. epidermidis* is important because this organism has antibiotic resistance and often gives erroneous sensitivity data. *Escherichia coli* and *Proteus* organisms also should be covered by antibiotic prophylaxis. In the United States, first-generation cephalosporins (cefazolin weight adjusted, but a minimum of 2 g for patients weighing more than 70 kg and 3 g for patients weighing over 120 kg) have been favored for many reasons. They are relatively nontoxic, inexpensive, and effective against most potential pathogens in orthopaedic surgery. Cephalosporins are more effective against *S. epidermidis* than are semisynthetic penicillins. Clindamycin can be given if a patient has a history of anaphylaxis to penicillin. Routine use of vancomycin for prophylaxis should be avoided. If a patient has risk factors that predisposes to an infection, then weight-adjusted vancomycin (15 mg/kg, 1 g over 1 hour to avoid red man syndrome) may be added to the preoperative antibiotic protocol.

Antibiotic therapy should begin immediately before surgery (30 to 60 minutes before skin incision). A maximal dose of antibiotic (weight adjusted) should be given and can be repeated every 4 hours intraoperatively or whenever the blood loss exceeds 1000 to 1500 mL. Little is gained by extending antibiotic coverage over 24 hours, and the possibility of side effects, such as thrombophlebitis, allergic reactions, superinfections, or drug fever, is increased. Prophylactic antibiotics should not be extended past 24 hours even if drains and catheters are still in place. The current CDC recommends no additional antibiotics after skin closure. Namias et al. found that antibiotic coverage for longer than 4 days led to increased bacteremia and intravenous line infections in patients in intensive care units. Evidence now shows that 24 hours of antibiotic administration is just as beneficial as 48 to 72 hours. Currently, antibiotic prophylaxis for patients undergoing colonoscopy, upper gastrointestinal endoscopy, or dental procedures (even in patients with total joint arthroplasty) is not recommended. For current prophylaxis please visit www.orthoguidelines.org/auc. If antibiotics are to be used see Table 3.4 for recommended antibiotics and dosing.

Antibiotic irrigation has not found a definite role in orthopaedic surgery. Several studies have shown a decrease in colony counts in wounds and a decrease in infection rates with the use of antibiotic irrigation in general surgical procedures. When a topical antibiotic is used, it should have (1) a wide spectrum of antibacterial activity, (2) the ability to remain in contact with normal tissues without causing significant local irritation, (3) low systemic absorption and toxicity, (4) low allergenicity, (5) minimal potential to induce bacterial resistance, and (6) availability in a topical preparation that can be easily suspended in a physiologic solution. We have employed the recommendations of the CDC as well as the World Health Organization (WHO) in utilizing a dilute (sterile water not tap) povidone-iodine wound soak before closure to decrease SSI. We follow the recommendations of Brown et al., utilizing

---

TABLE. 3.3

Methods for Reducing Surgical Site Infection

PATIENT FACTORS

Diabetes mellitus	Aggressive glucose control; if HgbA1c >7%, recommend delaying elective surgery DMARDs and methotrexate should *NOT* be stopped
Rheumatoid arthritis	Perioperative steroids are generally not required (stress dose steroids) Balance the risks and benefits of stopping anti-TNF at 3–5 half-lives preoperatively, restarting after wound healing and no evidence of infection
Obesity (BMI ≥30 kg/m²)	Dietician input to encourage weight loss over long period before surgery without rapid weight loss preoperatively Adjust perioperative antibiotic doses appropriately In extremely obese, consider bariatric surgery before surgery
Smoking	Consider a smoking cessation program 4–6 weeks preoperatively
Carrier screening	MRSA and MSSA screening based on local guidelines, and decolonize before admission which may include mupirocin ointment to the area for 5 days and chlorhexidine betadine for 5 days
Oral hygiene	Complete any dental treatment before elective surgery

PREOPERATIVE FACTORS

Patient preparation	Shower on day of surgery If shaving required, use electric clippers on day of surgery Avoid oil-based skin moisturizers
Antibiotics	Prophylactic antibiotics should be given within 1 h before incision and continued for 24 h postoperatively (antibiotic type dependent on local guidelines) Administer antibiotics at a minimum of 5 min before tourniquet inflation If cementation is required, should be antibiotic-impregnated
NSAIDs	Those with short half-lives (including ibuprofen) stop a minimum of 48 h prior; those with long half-lives (naproxen) stop within 3–7 days prior

PERIOPERATIVE FACTORS

Theater	Keep theater door opening to a minimum
Personnel	Hand wash with antiseptic surgical solution, using a single-use brush or pic for the nails Before subsequent operations hands should be washed with either an alcoholic hand rub or an antiseptic surgical solution Double glove and change gloves regularly minimum at 2 h; change outer gloves when draping
Skin preparation	Use an alcohol prewash followed by a 2% chlorhexidine-alcohol scrub solution
Anesthetic	Maintain normothermia Maintain normovolemia A higher inspired oxygen concentration perioperatively and for 6 h postoperative may be of benefit
Drapes	Use of iodine-impregnated incise drapes may be of benefit (in patients without allergy)
Blood transfusion	Optimize preoperative hemoglobin If possible, transfusion should be avoided intraoperatively and, if anticipated, should be given more than 48 h before surgery Antifibrinolytics may indirectly reduce SSI by reducing the need for transfusion

POSTOPERATIVE FACTORS

Dental procedures	Insufficient evidence to recommend the use of prophylactic antibiotics for patients undergoing routine dental procedures following joint replacement

BMI, Body mass index; *DMARDs,* disease-modifying antirheumatic drugs; *MRSA,* methicillin-resistant *Staphylococcus aureus*; *MSSA,* methicillin-sensitive *S. aureus*; *NSAIDs,* nonsteroidal antiinflammatory drugs; *SSI,* surgical site infection; *TNF,* tumor necrosis factor.
Modified from Johnson R, Jameson SS, Sanders RD, et al: Reducing surgical site infection in arthroplasty of the lower limb. A multi-disciplinary approach, *Bone Joint Res* 2(3):58–65, 2013.

17.5 mL of 10% povidone-iodine in 500 to 1000 mL sterile normal saline irrigation of the wound for 3 minutes. The wound is then irrigated with normal saline. This has led to a decrease in SSI from 0.97% to 0.15%. Although the numbers may appear small, the overall increase in surgeries (by 2030: TKA increase 673% and THA increase by 174%) will significantly reduce infections in individual patients. This solution should be avoided in patients who are allergic to iodine or when cartilage-sparing procedures are performed (i.e., unicompartmental knee replacements). In addition, when liposomal bupivacaine is used, the povidone-iodine solution should be applied before the bupivacaine because it is toxic to liposomes. We no longer routinely add antibiotics to our irrigation solutions. The use of powdered vancomycin sprinkled locally into the wound remains controversial. Hydrogen peroxide also is no longer recommended for wound irrigation because

TABLE. 3.4
Appropriate Prophylactic Antibiotics and Dosages

SITUATION	AGENT	REGIMEN—SINGLE DOSE 30–60 MIN BEFORE DENTAL PROCEDURES	
		Adults	*Children*
Oral	*Amoxicillin*	2 g	50 mg/kg
Unable to take oral medication	Ampicillin or ceftriaxone	2 g IM or IV* 1 g IM or IV	50 mg/kg IM or IV 50 mg/kg IM or IV
Allergic to oral penicillins or ampicillin	Cephalexin[†,‡] or azithromycin or clarithromycin	2 g 500 mg	50 m/kg 15 mg/kg
Allergic to penicillins or ampicillin and unable to take oral medication	Ceftriaxone,[‡] azithromycin, clarithromycin	1 g IM or IV Equivalent dose 500 mg IV	50 mg/kg IM or IV Equivalent dose

*Intramuscular injections should be avoided in persons receiving anticoagulants.
[†]Or other first-or second-generation oral cephalosporin in equivalent adult or pediatric dosage.
[‡]Cephalosporins should not be used in an individual with a history of anaphylaxis, angioedema, or urticaria with penicillins or ampicillin.
From, American Academy of Orthopaedic Surgeons Board of Directors and the American Dental Association Council on Scientific Affaris: Appropriate use criteria for the management of patients with orthopaedic implants undergoing dental procedures, 2016.

of its associated cytotoxicity, impaired wound healing, and oxygen embolic phenomenon.

The importance of irrigation and debridement in the treatment of open fractures has been well documented. The principles of elimination of devitalized tissue and dead space, evacuation of hematomas, and soft-tissue coverage also can be applied to "clean" orthopaedic cases.

METHICILLIN-RESISTANT STAPHYLOCOCCUS AUREUS

The evolution of *S. aureus* into a multiple-drug–resistant pathogen, methicillin-resistant *S. aureus* (MRSA), has become a major health concern worldwide. Approximately 57% of *S. aureus* bacteria are methicillin resistant, and now vancomycin-resistant strains are being reported. This is probably one of the most worrisome problems in the fight against bacterial infections. Initially, MRSA was seen only in hospital settings and long-term care facilities; however, it is now becoming increasingly prevalent in young, healthy individuals in the community (Table 3.5; At-Risk Groups). It has been estimated that 4% of the population in the United States are carriers of MRSA. It is particularly virulent, with a mortality rate of approximately 20%.

S. aureus infection in orthopaedic hospitalized patients generally is around 3%; however, over half of these patients have MRSA. Osteomyelitis caused by MRSA is an infrequent presentation, but treatment can be especially troublesome, and reports of subperiosteal abscess and necrotizing fasciitis also are increasing. Estimates of MRSA infection after total joint replacement range from 1% to 4%, and infection can occur up to 12 years after surgery. Kim et al. prospectively studied the feasibility of bacterial prescreening before elective orthopaedic surgery. They found that 22.6% of 7019 patients were *S. aureus* carriers and 4.4% were MRSA carriers. MRSA carriers had a statistically significantly higher rate of SSIs than methicillin-sensitive *S. aureus* (MSSA) carriers (0.97% compared with 0.14%; $P = 0.0162$). Although not statistically significant, MSSA carriers, approximately 30% of the United States population, also had higher rates of SSIs. After screening was initiated, the institutional infection rate dropped from 0.45% to 0.19% (P

TABLE. 3.5
At-Risk Groups and Risk Factors for Community-Acquired Methicillin-Resistant *Staphylococcus aureus*

AT-RISK GROUPS	RISK FACTORS
Athletes in contact sports Children in day care Homeless persons Intravenous drug users Homosexual males Military recruits Alaskan natives, Native Americans, and Pacific Islanders Prison inmates	Antibiotic use within the preceding year Close, crowded living conditions Compromised skin integrity Contaminated surfaces Frequent skin-to-skin contact Shared items Suboptimal cleanliness

From Marcotte AL, Trzeciak MA: Community-acquired methicillin-resistant *Staphylococcus aureus:* an emerging pathogen in orthopaedics, *J Am Acad Orthop Surg* 16:98–106, 2008.

= 0.0093). The cost-effectiveness of such screening programs has not been determined, although with the increasing prevalence of MRSA, these costs may be justified.

Approximately 3% of MRSA outbreaks have been attributed to asymptomatic colonized health care workers. Schwarzkopf et al. prospectively studied the prevalence of *S. aureus* colonization in orthopaedic surgeons and their patients and found that among surgeons and residents there was a higher prevalence of MRSA compared with a high-risk group of patients. Junior residents had the same prevalence of MRSA colonization as institutionalized patients, most likely because of the substantial time spent in direct patient care. These researchers recommended hand hygiene for the prevention of MRSA. In addition, universal decolonization of patients with mupirocin was recommended before total joint and spine surgeries, although further study of this practice is indicated. Skramm et al. proved that the *S. aureus* colonies that were isolated from operating personnel were indeed the same strain found at the SSI up to 85% of the time. No true proof exists that decolonization of MRSA carriers decreases SSI incidence. There is no definitive recommendation on screening and preoperative treatment of MRSA carriers. However, some advocate povidone-iodine nasal ointment, which would also ease fears of emerging resistance to mupirocin use.

Because of the prevalence of community-acquired (CA)-MRSA, it is necessary to rapidly identify the organism, determine antibiotic sensitivity, and begin antibiotic therapy (for empirical coverage see Table 22.3). Polymerase chain reaction (PCR) can be used to detect *Staphylococcus* with results within 24 hours as opposed to conventional cultures that can take 3 days before results are available. Vancomycin or teicoplanin should be considered in patients with colonization of MRSA or when screening results before surgery are not available. For invasive infections, intravenous vancomycin is recommended or, alternatively, daptomycin, gentamicin, rifampin, and linezolid can be used. In cases of necrotizing fasciitis, clindamycin, gentamicin, rifampin, trimethoprim-sulfamethoxazole, and vancomycin are effective. Rifampin should never be used alone as the single antibiotic. Until a sensitivity determination can be made, antimicrobial coverage specifically of CA-MRSA is recommended. For deep subperiosteal abscesses or superficial abscesses, irrigation and debridement are necessary to reduce bacterial counts. Overuse of quinolones may be driving the selection of MRSA over MSSA and should be avoided. Obtaining an infectious disease consult is highly recommended.

In summary, despite few direct evidence-based studies, best current efforts at controlling SSI are described in Table 3.3.

DIAGNOSIS

The diagnosis of infection may be obvious or obscure. Signs and symptoms vary with the rate and extent of bone and joint involvement. Characteristic features of fever, chills, nausea, vomiting, malaise, erythema, swelling, and tenderness may or may not be present. The classic triad is fever, swelling, and tenderness (pain). Pain probably is the most common symptom. Fever is not always a consistent finding. Infection may also be as indolent as a progressive backache or a decrease in or loss of function of an extremity. No single test is able to serve as a definitive indicator of the presence of musculoskeletal infection.

LABORATORY STUDIES

A complete blood cell count, including differential and erythrocyte sedimentation rate (ESR) and C-reactive protein (CRP), should be obtained during initial evaluation of bone and joint infections. The WBC count is an unreliable indicator of infection and often is normal, even when infection is present. The differential shows an increase in neutrophils during acute infections. The ESR becomes elevated when infection is present, but this does not occur exclusively in the presence of infection. Fractures or other underlying diseases can cause elevation of the ESR. The ESR also is unreliable in neonates, patients with sickle cell disease, patients taking corticosteroids, and patients whose symptoms have been present for less than 48 hours. Peak elevation of the ESR occurs at 3 to 5 days after infection and returns to

normal approximately 3 weeks after treatment is begun. The ESR should very rarely be used alone in diagnosing infection. CRP synthesized by the liver in response to infection, is a better way to follow the response of infection to treatment. CRP increases within 6 hours of infection, reaches a peak elevation 2 days after infection, and returns to normal within 1 week after adequate treatment has begun. CRP can be misleading, however, in patients with chronic inflammatory conditions, neoplasms, and metabolic disease. D-dimer has been shown to better evaluate a patient for infection than ESR or CRP, with a specificity of 93% and a sensitivity of 89%. D-dimer can return to normal levels after 2 days postoperatively. However, if an infection exists it usually re-spikes at 2 weeks. Interleukin-6 (IL-6) also is a useful marker for infection. It provides a rapid diagnosis and returns to normal level 3 days after surgery. Alpha-defensin is another effective marker for infection. It is unaffected by antibiotic treatment, but it is expensive and has a high false-positive rate. Leukocyte esterase also has been employed as a marker for infection. It is inexpensive and can be measured quickly. Other tests, such as the *S. aureus* surface antigen or antibody test and counterimmunofluorescence studies of the urine, are promising, but their usefulness in clinical situations has not been proved. Material obtained from aspiration of joint fluid can be sent to the laboratory for a cell count and differential to distinguish acute septic arthritis from other causes of arthritis. In septic arthritis, the cell count usually is greater than 80,000/mm³, with more than 75% of the cells being neutrophils (Table 3.6). A Gram stain also should be obtained. Gram stains identify the types of organisms (gram-positive or gram-negative) in about a third of bone and joint aspirates. However, intraoperative Gram stain is not recommended in the face of PJI because it is unreliable. Intraoperative frozen sections also should be obtained in cases in which infection is suspected. A WBC count greater than 10 per high-power field is considered indicative of infection, whereas a count less than five per high-power field all but excludes infection. Combining these test results in a higher sensitivity and specificity. The future of serum biomarkers most likely lies with using genomics and proteomics to identify proteins associated with infections.

IMAGING STUDIES

Radiographic studies are helpful but are not as useful in the diagnosis of acute bone and joint infections as they are in

TABLE. 3.6

Synovial Fluid Analysis

	LEUKOCYTES	NEUTROPHILS (%)
Normal	<200	<25
Traumatic	<5000	<25
Toxic synovitis	5000–15,000	<25
Acute rheumatic fever	10,000–15,000	50
Juvenile rheumatoid arthritis	15,000–80,000	75
Septic arthritis	>80,000	>75

From Morrissy RT: Septic arthritis. In Gustilo RB, Genninger RP, Tsukayama DT, editors: *Orthopaedic infection: diagnosis and treatment*, Philadelphia, 1989, WB Saunders.

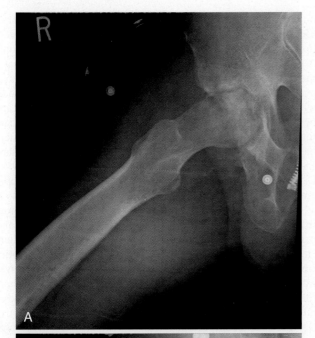

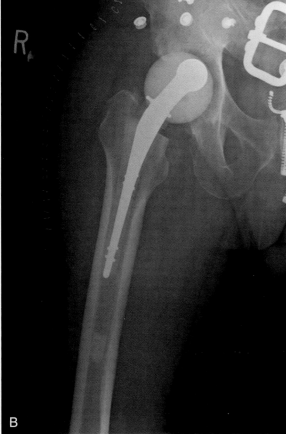

FIGURE 3.1 **A,** Radiographic evidence of acute bone and joint infection. **B,** Treatment with antibiotic cement spacer. (Courtesy Andrew Crenshaw, MD.)

following responses to treatment. Plain radiographs show soft-tissue swelling, joint space narrowing or widening, and bone destruction (Fig. 3.1). Bone destruction is not apparent on radiographs, however, until an infection has been present for 10 to 21 days. In addition, 30% to 50% of the bone matrix

must be lost to show a lytic lesion on radiographs (Fig. 3.2). Wheat found that fewer than 5% of plain radiographs were initially abnormal in bone and joint infections, and fewer than 30% were abnormal at 1 week; however, 90% were abnormal at 3 to 4 weeks. If initial radiographs are normal in the evaluation of bone and joint infections, other imaging methods that show soft-tissue swelling and loss of normal fat planes around the involved bone or joint should be used.

CT is useful in identifying a sequestrum or subchondral bony plate destruction. Arthrography helps document proper aspiration of a suspected septic joint. Dye should be injected only after fluid is obtained from the joint because the bactericidal effect of iodinated contrast material can cause a false-negative culture result. CT can help determine the extent of medullary involvement. Pus within the medullary cavity replaces the marrow fat, causing an increased density on the CT scan. Adjacent soft-tissue abscesses also are seen easily (Fig. 3.3). CT diagnosis of acute osteomyelitis is based on detection of intraosseous gas, osteolysis, soft-tissue masses, abscesses, or foreign bodies. Additionally, increased vascularity after administration of a contrast agent also can aid in the diagnosis. Narrowing of the medullary cavity by granulation tissue and new bone is readily shown during the healing phase of osteomyelitis. CT identifies sequestra in chronic osteomyelitis (Fig. 3.4). It also is helpful in identifying alterations in areas poorly seen on plain films, such as the sternoclavicular joint, sacroiliac joint, and spine. Contrast material can be used to delineate abscesses in necrotic tissue that does not enhance from surrounding hyperemic tissue.

Ultrasonography can also be used to localize an abscess cavity, detect joint effusion, or guide a physician in the proper placement of the needle when obtaining aspirate from a bone or joint.

Radionuclide scanning is a useful imaging adjunct in the diagnosis of osteomyelitis. Although radiography and CT give a structural or anatomic picture, radionuclide scanning gives a more physiologic picture. Bone scintigraphy does not detect the presence of infection but, instead, reflects inflammatory changes or the reaction of bone to the infection. Radionuclide scanning can be used for patients with metallic implants in whom CT and MRI are of limited value because of contraindications and metallic-generated artifact, although metal subtracting software is improving imaging in these patients. The three most commonly used radioisotopes are technetium-99m (^{99m}Tc) phosphate, gallium-67 (^{67}Ga) citrate, and indium-111 (^{111}In)–labeled leukocytes. The most common is ^{99m}Tc phosphate, which can detect osteomyelitis within 48 hours after clinical onset of infection. The uptake of this compound is related primarily to osteoblastic activity, although regional blood flow also plays a role in skeletal uptake. After intravenous injection, the technetium is distributed rapidly throughout the extracellular compartment. Bone uptake is rapid, with more than 50% of the administered dose being delivered to bone within 1 hour. The remainder of the dye is excreted by the kidneys into the urine.

The standard technique of ^{99m}Tc phosphate imaging is to perform a three-phase study. Although this does not increase the sensitivity of the test significantly, it does increase specificity from 74% to 94%. The three-phase bone scan consists of images taken in (1) the flow phase, (2) the immediate or equilibrium phase, and (3) the delayed phase. The flow-phase

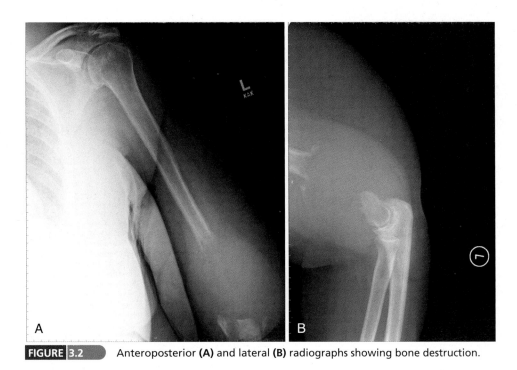

FIGURE 3.2   Anteroposterior **(A)** and lateral **(B)** radiographs showing bone destruction.

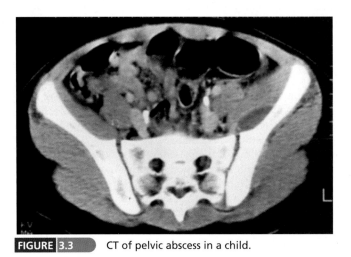

FIGURE 3.3   CT of pelvic abscess in a child.

TABLE. 3.7			
Three-Phase Bone Scan Uptake			
	FLOW	**EQUILIBRIUM**	**DELAYED**
Osteomyelitis	↑	↑	↑
Cellulitis	↑	↑	↔
Osteoarthritis	↔	↔	↑

image is similar to a radionuclide angiogram in that it shows blood flow. The equilibrium or blood pool image shows relative vascular flow and distribution of the radioisotope into the extracellular space. The delayed-phase image is generally obtained 2 to 4 hours after injection, when renal excretion has eliminated most of the isotope except that taken up by osteoblastic activity. This image shows osteoblastic activity and is positive in numerous disease states, including osteomyelitis, tumors, degenerative joint disease, trauma, and postsurgical changes. Usually, a focus of osteomyelitis appears as an area of increased tracer uptake on delayed images. To have a "hot spot" on a bone scan, the vasculature to the involved bone must be intact. If blood flow to the involved area is decreased by subperiosteal pus, necrosis (i.e., sequestrum), joint effusion, vasospasm, or soft-tissue swelling, a "cold" scan may result.

A major disadvantage of three-phase ^{99m}Tc phosphate bone scintigraphy is that the increased uptake caused by osteomyelitis is difficult to distinguish from that caused by degenerative joint disease or posttraumatic or postsurgical changes. The relative activity in each of the three phases may be helpful in differentiating other causes of increased uptake. Cellulitis causes increased activity during the flow and equilibrium phases and a decreased or normal uptake in the delayed phase. Osteomyelitis causes increased uptake in all three phases (Fig. 3.5). Increased uptake in the delayed phase but not in the flow or equilibrium phase suggests degenerative joint disease (Table 3.7). ^{99m}Tc phosphate bone scans are unreliable in neonates (<6 weeks old) and usually are negative in 60% of these patients with bone or joint infections.

^{67}Ga citrate is the oldest tracer and has been used to localize inflammatory lesions as well as malignant tissue. The mechanism of gallium deposition is controversial; it seems to be related to increased endothelial permeability or diffusion by transportation as gallium-transferrin. The specificity of a ^{67}Ga citrate scan alone is poor (82%). ^{67}Ga citrate scanning can be useful in osteomyelitis when it is used in conjunction with ^{99m}Tc phosphate scanning. In purely reactive bone formation (posttraumatic or postsurgical), the intensity on the ^{99m}Tc phosphate scan is proportionally greater than that on the ^{67}Ga citrate scan. In areas of inflammation, however, gallium

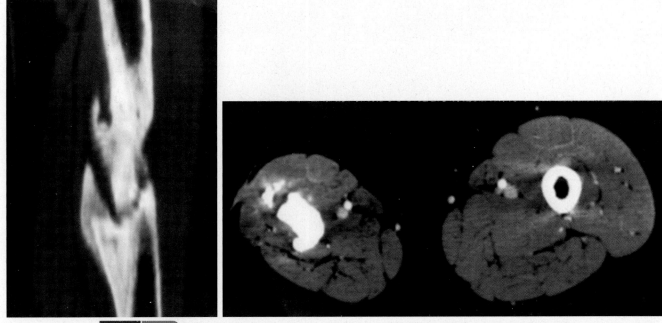

FIGURE 3.4 CT scans showing sequestra. (Courtesy Todd Williams, MD.)

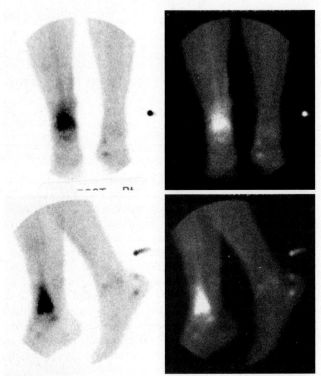

FIGURE 3.5 Three-phase bone scan showing osteomyelitis. (Courtesy Michael Fleming, MD.)

uptake either exceeds that of technetium in relative magnitude or displays a different spatial configuration of activity. A disadvantage of ^{67}Ga citrate imaging is its slow clearance after injection, which requires a delay in imaging ranging from 24 hours after injection for the appendicular skeleton to 72 hours for the axial skeleton. Specificity decreases in ^{67}Ga citrate scintigraphy when the lesion is located peripherally

rather than centrally. With the combination of ^{67}Ga citrate and ^{99m}Tc phosphate scans, sensitivity and specificity are 70% and up to 93%, respectively, for the detection of osteomyelitis.

^{111}In–labeled leukocytes have been utilized for differentiating between osteomyelitis and reactive bone formation. This scan is positive at earlier stages of osteomyelitis than ^{99m}Tc phosphate scintigraphy. The leukocyte scanning technique involves in vitro radionuclide labeling and injection of autologous leukocytes, predominantly polymorphonuclear neutrophilic leukocytes, followed by imaging 24 to 48 hours later. About 50 mL of the patient's venous blood is obtained, separated from the other blood elements in vitro, and labeled with ^{111}In. The labeled leukocytes are reinjected into the patient, and scans are obtained at 24 hours. A scan is positive if focal accumulation of activity exceeds adjacent normal bone activity. Scintigraphy with ^{111}In has been reported to be helpful in the diagnosis of acute osteomyelitis, but there is disagreement about its efficacy in chronic osteomyelitis because the latter is predominantly lymphocytic and may give a negative or "cold" scan. The ^{111}In scan is also unreliable for differentiating between aseptic and septic loosening of a painful arthroplasty. Teller et al. did not recommend the routine use of ^{99m}Tc phosphate with ^{111}In-labeled scans for detecting aseptic or septic loosening of arthroplasty because of the high cost associated with these tests and the low specificity and sensitivity of 78% and 64%, respectively. In a meta-analysis, Prandini et al. found that ^{99m}Tc-labeled white blood cells had a greater sensitivity (89%) and specificity (90.1%) than ^{111}In-labeled white blood cells. Several authors have recommended prolonging the scan time until 24 hours for the ^{99m}Tc-labeled white blood cell scan to improve detection. ^{111}In-labeled monoclonal immunoglobulin is a substitute for ^{111}In-labeled leukocytes. It seems to be as effective as ^{111}In-labeled leukocytes, does not require phlebotomy, and avoids the risk of radiation to white blood cells and the perceived risk of malignant transformation. According to

Hakki et al., compared with ^{111}In-labeled leukocytes and ^{99m}Tc phosphate scintigraphy, monoclonal antibody fragment (LeukoScan, Granuloscint, NeutoSpect) has better sensitivity, specificity, and diagnostic accuracy. In addition, these researchers suggested that ^{99m}Tc-sulesomab (LeukoScan) is a stronger diagnostic tool in patients with a low leukocyte count (i.e., human immunodeficiency virus [HIV] infected patients) and in patients with chronic osteomyelitis. However, meta-analysis studies show that these agents are less accurate than in vitro–labeled white blood cells in most patients, and a risk of allergic reaction (some fatal) does exist, especially when repeated scans are necessary. These agents have limited availability in the United States; however, the quest for a more perfect monoclonal antibody fragment continues.

The detection of chronic osteomyelitis, especially of the central skeleton, can be enhanced with a ^{99m}Tc/ciprofloxacin (infection) scan and fluorine-18 (^{18}F)-fluorodeoxyglucose-labeled positron emission tomography (FDG-PET). FDG-PET is the most accurate test (92%) with the most positive predictive value (94%). It is extremely useful for chronic infections and infections already treated with antibiotics. In addition, it is more advantageous than an ^{111}In bone scan in that it only requires one injection (less exposure to body fluids by personnel and less radiation exposure to the patient) and is completed within hours instead of days. However, it is the most expensive and is not readily available in all health care centers.

MRI has been used for evaluating bone and joint infections. MRI is a complex imaging method that aligns the body's protons along the axis of a powerful external magnetic field and records the motion of the protons as they return to the magnetic field alignment after absorbing energy from a radio-frequency-generating coil. Each type of tissue has its own unique signal characteristics. Two parameters are evaluated. The first is the echo time (TE), which is the time that elapses between the initial radiofrequency pulse and its return back to the radio antenna (akin to a sonar ping). The second is repetition time (TR), which is the time between the applied consecutive radiofrequency pulses to the patient (the frequency of pings). When the TR and TE are short, a T1 image is produced that shows fat as a high, bright signal. When the TR and TE are long, a T2 image is obtained that shows water as a bright signal. An additional signal is obtained by suppressing the fat signal; this is called short tau inversion recovery (STIR). STIR signals have a high negative predictive value for osteomyelitis of almost 100%; however, STIR cannot be used to differentiate fluid collections (e.g., abscesses) from circumscribed soft-tissue edema. The reported abnormal images reflect an increase in water content, resulting from edema in the marrow cavity. Marrow fat is replaced by edema and cellular infiltrates that are lower in signal than fat on T1 images and higher in signal than fat on T2 and STIR images. The classic findings of osteomyelitis on MRI are a decrease in the normally high marrow signal on T1 images and a normal or increased signal on T2 images (Fig. 3.6). According to Boutin et al., MRI is the most appropriate tool to rule out cartilaginous epiphyseal infection. Mazur et al. showed that MRI was superior in sensitivity (97%) and specificity (92%) to ^{99m}Tc phosphate bone scintigraphy for detection of osteomyelitis. MRI detects changes (e.g., lytic areas) much earlier in the course of disease than radiographs because it shows the condition of the intramedullary cavity. The signal changes seen on MRI are nonspecific, and anything that causes edema or hyperemia (e.g.,

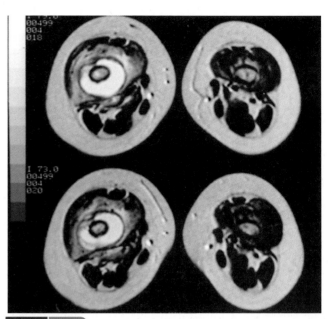

FIGURE 3.6 MRI of abscess *(images on left)*. (Courtesy Amber Turner, MD.)

fractures, tumors, and inflammatory processes) produces signal changes similar to that of osteomyelitis. Although MRI is good for detailing marrow involvement and discitis, it does little to detect early cortical bone involvement.

Gadolinium contrast material can be added to MRI to help distinguish an abscess (bright signal involved abscess with no enhancements of the fluid within the abscess) from coexisting cellulitis. In addition, it enhances granulation tissue surrounding a sinus tract or sequestrum but does not enhance the tract or sequestrum in the bone. Gadolinium contrast does not help in differentiating osteomyelitis from bone marrow edema. The addition of gadolinium to increase detection of CA staphylococcus musculoskeletal infections in patients 0 to 18 months of age has been recommended.

In general, sequestra in sinus tracks, abscesses, and subperiosteal fluid collections are all positive MRI signs that suggest osteomyelitis. MRI should be reserved for patients with inconclusive findings, patients with infections involving the pelvis or spine, and patients who may require surgical intervention. It is extremely useful for detection of acute hematogenous osteomyelitis.

In summary:
1. Patients suspected of having musculoskeletal infection should have plain radiographs of the area in question.
2. CT is useful in detecting bone abnormalities such as sequestra.
3. Ultrasonography helps to establish whether a joint effusion is present and to localize needle aspiration to diagnose septic arthritis.
4. A three-phase bone scan accurately detects osteomyelitis in nonviolated bone. If hardware is in place or if there has been previous trauma to the bone or a Charcot joint, for instance, is present, a three-phase bone scan is only useful as a screening test. A white blood cell–labeled bone scan helps with detection of complicated osteomyelitis and combining this with a colloid scan maximizes accuracy. This is especially useful in total joint infections and diabetic feet, but less so in neuropathic joints. It is not

helpful with spinal osteomyelitis. ^{99m}Tc-HMPAO-labled WBC count can be helpful in detecting chronic recurrent multifocal osteomyelitis (CRMO).

5. MRI shows surrounding tissue and is excellent in detecting osteomyelitis. Adding gallium improves detection of spinal osteomyelitis.
6. FDG-PET also is helpful in the diagnosis of spinal infection and chronic osteomyelitis but is not readily available in all health care institutions. It is generally not recommended because infections can be detected by other less expensive means.
7. The best combination of imaging for osteomyelitis is WBC scintigraphy with single-photon emission computed tomography (SPECT).

CULTURE STUDIES

Although blood tests, radiographic imaging, and clinical signs all give presumptive evidence of an infection, they do not suffice for an actual bacteriologic diagnosis that would allow development of a treatment plan including correct antibiotic selection. The laboratory has the responsibility of isolating and identifying the offending organism and determining antibiotic susceptibility. This process can be easier and more informative when there is proper communication between the orthopaedic surgeon and laboratory personnel. The latter should be informed of patient risk factors, type of antibiotic therapy (which should be stopped 14 days before culture), culture site (three to five different sites are preferred), how the culture was obtained, and what possible organisms are sought.

The timing and selection of the culture are crucial. Most orthopaedic infections are deep seated, and adequate culture specimens are difficult to obtain. Despite this, every effort should be made to obtain a culture specimen before antibiotic therapy is begun. Cultures of superficial wounds or sinus tracks should not be relied on because they are poor indicators of deep infection and usually are polymicrobial. Swab cultures of a sinus track give misleading results unless *S. aureus* coagulase is the predominant isolate or unless a single species is isolated in pure culture. The preferred specimen in most bacterial and yeast infections is aspirated fluid (joint or purulent fluid). A deep wound biopsy or a curetted specimen after cleaning the wound is acceptable. In certain bacterial and fungal infections, a tissue biopsy specimen from the edge of the wound is preferable. Aerobic and anaerobic swabs are more commonly used, but aspirated fluid or a tissue biopsy specimen is preferable. According to Levine and Evans, the use of blood culture vials intraoperatively for placement of aspirated fluid is more sensitive than swab cultures or tissue biopsy; however, others, such as Wilson and Winn, saw no advantage in using blood culture vials or swabs and state that fluid sent to the laboratory in a sterile environment was all that was required. Tissue specimens should be placed in small carbon dioxide–filled containers to reduce exposure to air.

Rapid diagnostic procedures that may aid in initial decision-making are qualitative tests only. A Gram stain determines if gram-negative or gram-positive bacteria are present. Bacterial morphology and some measure of inflammation also can be obtained from a Gram stain. If the Gram stain is negative and infection is strongly suspected because of the presence of many acute inflammatory cells, an acridine orange stain using a fluorescent microscope may aid in the detection of gram-negative bacteria.

When a fungal infection is suspected, a 10% potassium hydroxide wet mount preparation or a fluorescein calcofluor white stain aids in the detection of characteristic fungal morphology. Other special stains, such as acid-fast, rhodamine-auramine, or fluorescein-tagged antibody stains, also can help in making a rapid diagnosis. The development of monoclonal antibodies to specific bacterial antigens has had a major effect, but except for the detection of the bacterial antigens of *H. influenzae, Neisseria meningitidis,* and *S. pneumoniae* in synovial fluid, these tests are useful only in the rapid identification of already isolated bacteria and not for detecting specific bacteria in a clinical specimen.

Several different types of media are available for isolation and identification of bacteria. The initial specimen should be cultured for aerobic and facultative and strict anaerobic organisms. Media for these organisms should include blood agar, chocolate agar for *H. influenzae* and *Neisseria gonorrhoeae,* and a nutrient-enriched broth for fastidious organisms. Selective media should be used when fungi or acid-fast bacteria are suspected. Usually an organism can be identified in 24 to 48 hours, but some isolates can take several days or weeks (i.e., *Cutibacterium acnes*).

After the organism has been isolated and identified, its antimicrobial sensitivity should be determined. The three principal ways to test sensitivity or antimicrobial effectiveness are (1) in vitro susceptibility testing of a bacterial isolate, (2) measurement of the patient's inhibiting or bactericidal serum level against his or her own infectious bacteria, and (3) measurement of actual serum concentration of the antibiotic the patient is receiving.

The National Committee for Clinical Laboratory Standards provides recommendations for standardized tests and suggests the prototype generic antibiotic that can be tested to represent each class of antibiotic when in vitro antimicrobial susceptibilities are performed. The in vitro susceptibility studies are based on (1) serial dilution of the test antibiotic in broth or on a solid agar medium, (2) antibiotic diffusion from a paper disc into a solid agar medium, or (3) antibiotic elution from paper disc into broth. The lowest concentration of an antibiotic that inhibits growth of the patient's isolate is designated the minimal inhibitory concentration (MIC). If the MIC level can be easily achieved in the patient's serum using normal dosage and route of administration, the organism is said to be susceptible or sensitive. After the MIC has been determined, a subculture can be performed to determine the minimal bactericidal concentration, which is the lowest concentration of antimicrobial agent that allows survival of less than 0.1% of the original cultured inoculum.

In the disc diffusion method, the zone of inhibited growth around an antibiotic-impregnated disc is measured and compared with a standard test bacterium. This is reported as sensitive, intermediate, or resistant, depending on the magnitude of the zone of inhibition. Broth disc elution is used for anaerobic bacteria. An antibiotic-impregnated paper disc is placed in an anaerobic broth and incubated along with the bacterium to be tested. Visual results are read as "no growth" (sensitive) or "growth" (resistant).

Measuring the serum bactericidal concentration (SBC) is another way of measuring antimicrobial effectiveness. The SBC measures the activity of the patient's own serum against the infecting organism. The lowest dilution of the patient's serum that kills 99.9% of a standard inoculum is called the

SBC. This requires that the patient's serum be obtained at peak and trough concentrations. This method has gained popularity in the treatment of pediatric septic arthritis and osteomyelitis to test the adequacy of oral antibiotic dosage. The oral dose is adjusted to give a peak SBC of 1:8 or 1:16 and a trough SBC of 1:2 or higher.

Actual antimicrobial concentration in serum also can be measured. This is usually done to determine whether an effective therapeutic level is being obtained and to guide antibiotic dosage to avoid toxic side effects.

Two special tests that can be used in orthopaedic infections are quantitative tissue cultures and in vitro antibiotic synergism versus antagonism susceptibility. Quantitative tissue culture has been helpful in detecting clinically significant infections in burn patients. Its use in orthopaedics has aided in decisions regarding wound closure and antibiotic therapy. After debridement of an open wound, a 1 mL tissue specimen is obtained, and a quantitative Gram stain smear is performed from 0.01 mL of an undiluted homogenate. This is transferred onto a clean glass microscope slide and spread in an area not exceeding 15 mm in diameter. After drying, the slide is Gram stained and the entire smear is examined microscopically at a magnification of 1000×. The presence of a single organism in any field indicates a positive smear, suggesting ongoing infection. The remainder of the tissue homogenate can be serially diluted in nutrient broth for quantitative culture. Cultures containing 10 organisms per gram of tissue have a high probability of remaining infected if closed. The accuracy of quantitative microbiologic techniques has been reported to be 84% for Gram stain and 89% for culture. In vitro antibiotic testing for synergism and antagonism should be considered when a persistent infection is refractory to antibiotic treatment. This test measures the sum effect in vitro of two different antibiotics.

Often, antibiotic therapy is begun before a definitive culture result is obtained, and the selection of an antibiotic is based on the most probable causative bacteria, which varies considerably depending on age and epidemiologic factors. *S. aureus* is most frequently isolated in infectious arthritis. After this, *N. gonorrhoeae* is more common in adults younger than 30 years, and *H. influenzae* type B is more common in children younger than 2 years. These three bacteria, along with various *Streptococcus* species, constitute most known isolates in joint infections. In contrast, PJIs most often are caused by skin flora, such as *S. epidermidis* and other coagulase-negative *Staphylococcus* and gram-negative bacilli that are transient skin colonizers. *Cutibacterium acnes* (*C. acnes*; formerly *Propionibacterium acnes*), a nonspore-forming anaerobic gram-positive bacillus usually found in cutaneous tissue in the respiratory or digestive system, has been recognized to be responsible for severe infections in orthopaedics, particularly in total shoulder replacement and spine surgery. *C. acnes* is challenging to diagnose because it presents late without the usual clinical signs of infection, and laboratory studies may be equivocal. Biological and radiographic signs are usually very discrete. This bacillus requires prolonged culture (>21 days) for diagnosis. Microbiological methods have improved the diagnosis. Sonification of the extracted implant can be helpful as well to identify the infectious organism. *C. acnes* has shown resistance to broad-spectrum antibiotics; however, it is reasonably susceptible to clindamycin, quinolones, rifampin, and beta-lactams. A 2 to 4 week course of intravenous antibiotic or a highly available oral antibiotic followed

by oral treatment for 3 months is recommended. If the infection is found and treated before 4 weeks, only antibiotic medication is required to treat the infection because a biofilm has yet to be created. If, however, it is discovered after 4 weeks, a one- or two-stage replant is warranted along with the antibiotic coverage. Prevention of infection is enhanced by copious irrigation, short operative times, changing the scalpel after skin incision, and avoiding contact of the implant with the skin edge. Consultation with an infectious disease specialist is warranted in these patients.

The etiologic agent for osteomyelitis also depends on age, epidemiologic factors, and whether the osteomyelitis is primary or secondary. *S. aureus* is the most frequent isolate in osteomyelitis, but *Salmonella* organisms have an increased incidence in patients with sickle cell anemia or neonatal osteomyelitis. Postsurgical osteomyelitis also has a predominance of skin flora and hospital flora. This is where an individual hospital statistical survey of infections would be beneficial.

Molecular diagnostic tests for detection of infections are still experimental, expensive, and not readily available. However, next-generation sequencing, such as PCR techniques, aimed at the bacterial 16 S rRNA DNA and sequence, can be performed. This identifies the presence of bacteria but not the specific organism. A high false-positive rate still exists, and improvements are still forthcoming with additional research and development. Moojen et al. have added a reverse line hybridization process that will identify some of the more common orthopaedic pathogens. The clinical usefulness of these molecular diagnostic tests is evident in several areas. They can identify the specific pathogens responsible for musculoskeletal infection, even if pretest antibiotics have already been given, can identify organisms that cause low-grade infections (a small concentration of organisms), and can rapidly recognize infections that usually have long culture times (e.g., tuberculosis).

TREATMENT

Treatment of an orthopaedic infection may require antimicrobial and surgical treatment. Antibiotic treatment alone may be sufficient, but several principles should be followed: (1) the organism should be accurately identified, and its antimicrobial susceptibility should be determined; (2) the correct antibiotic, preferably bactericidal, should be chosen based on the MIC and SBC; (3) the antibiotic must be delivered to the organism in sufficient concentration to destroy it.

Surgery may go hand-in-hand with antibiotic treatment. Surgery can accomplish in 1 hour what the body and antibiotic treatment may require days or weeks to do. The purpose of surgery is augmentation of the host response. Debridement reduces the inoculum and removes necrotic and avascular bone, bacteria, and harmful bacterial products. Surgery is not always necessary, but it is essential when pus is found on aspiration or when radiographic changes of osteomyelitis are seen, indicating pus, necrotic material, and chronic inflammation. If these are not present, a trial of antibiotic treatment is appropriate only after culture material has been obtained. If the patient does not respond to antibiotic treatment in 36 to 48 hours, then it indicates that a wrong antibiotic has been chosen or an abscess has formed. After 48 hours, the sensitivity should have been reported, and a correct organism specific antibiotic can be chosen. If an abscess has formed, surgery is indicated.

Several routes of antibiotic treatment exist. Oral antibiotics are still the most commonly used. Intravenous application may be required for more serious infections that do not respond to oral antibiotics. Local delivery of antibiotics also can be beneficial. Polymethyl methacrylate (PMMA) beads impregnated with heat-stable antibiotics (tobramycin, vancomycin, and gentamicin) have been used since the early 1970s. A 2 to 3 cm area around each bead has a high concentration of antibiotic. With tobramycin and vancomycin, the peak concentration of antibiotic delivered to local tissue occurs on the first day and lasts for only approximately 1 week. This local delivery system avoids systemic toxicity; however, it requires removal (usually surgical) within 4 weeks. A more attractive biodegradable system is the collagen-gentamicin sponge, which obviates the need for surgical removal and delivers higher concentrations of antibiotics than PMMA beads. It has been suggested that antibiotic release by this method may be complete within 4 days. Lactic acid polymerase may be the next step in local biodegradable antibiotic delivery systems. This system delivers a high concentration of quinolines (bactericidals for probable pathogens of chronic osteomyelitis) for 60 days, with a peak release of antibiotics at day 15. An additional method of local antibiotic delivery is that of mixing autogenous iliac crest bone graft with piperacillin or vancomycin. Antibiotics must be chosen carefully. For example, heat-stable antibiotics are required for PMMA applications; quinolones have shown detrimental effects on chondrocytes and fracture healing; and tobramycin at intermediate levels of concentration (400 µg/mL) can decrease cell replication. In general, vancomycin is less toxic to osteoblasts at high local concentrations than other aminoglycosides, and rifampin and quinolones should not be administered when bone regeneration is an issue.

In general, MSSA can be treated with nafcillin/oxacillin, or cefazolin. For *Kingella kingae* infections (best diagnosed with PCR technique) a beta–lactam antibiotic is recommended. For MRSA, clindamycin and vancomycin are recommended. A short course of intravenous antibiotics can be followed with an oral antibiotic regime, which avoids the use of a peripherally inserted central catheter (PICC) line. This treatment has been shown to be equally as effective as long-time intravenous therapy. An infectious disease consult can help guide the appropriate antibiotic in each patient and can be especially useful with the ever-changing microbial picture. Although many surgical techniques have been described for the treatment of osteomyelitis, prevention is still the best course of action, and adherence to the basic principles of treatment of infections will help achieve success.

HUMAN IMMUNODEFICIENCY VIRUS AND HEPATITIS B AND C

The management of patients with HIV infection or acquired immunodeficiency syndrome (AIDS) has reached all fields of medicine. The orthopaedic surgeon may be required to treat HIV-positive patients in the emergency department, clinic, or operating room. Because of this increasing likelihood, the orthopaedist should know the causes, associated diseases affecting the musculoskeletal system, the risks of transmission, and precautions in regard to this infection.

AIDS was diagnosed in 1981 in several patients with disease complexes previously seen only in patients with immunodeficiencies of known causes. After the diagnosis of AIDS, HIV was identified and was found to cause this disease complex. Two strains of HIV have been identified: HIV-1, which is the strain most common in the United States, and HIV-2, which has been reported primarily in Europeans, Africans, and rarely, in the United States.

AIDS is caused by HIV, a human RNA retrovirus. This group of RNA viruses has the ability to produce reverse transcriptase, which converts RNA to DNA and incorporates into the host chromosome. The HIV retrovirus is trophic for the CD4 surface receptors of T lymphocytes. The virus causes deregulation and destruction of these T lymphocytes, ultimately resulting in an immunodeficient state. Initial infection results in stimulation of B cells and an initial increase in the number of suppresser and T killer cells, followed by a progressive decline in the number of circulating CD4 lymphocytes over several years. When the CD4 cell count is less than $200/mm^3$, opportunistic infections occur, and clinical manifestations of AIDS begin.

This progressive destruction of the body's immune function leaves an individual susceptible to a variety of infections, malignancies, and neuropsychiatric abnormalities. *P. jiroveci* pneumonia and malignancies such as Kaposi sarcoma are the most common opportunistic diseases associated with AIDS in the United States.

Four stages of HIV infection have been identified, although not all individuals infected with HIV go through all four stages. The stages are (1) acute primary HIV infection, (2) chronic asymptomatic HIV infection, (3) symptomatic HIV infection, and (4) advanced HIV-associated opportunistic disease or AIDS. Acute primary HIV infection appears clinically similar to infectious mononucleosis and occurs 2 to 6 weeks after viral transmission. Clinical features include pharyngitis, dysphagia, lymphadenopathy, rash, fever, fatigue, hepatosplenomegaly, and leukopenia. This stage is self-limiting, and most patients do not seek medical attention. Within 3 months after viral transmission, most patients develop positive serology, and virtually all patients seroconvert by 6 months, although delayed seroconversion 1 year after infection has been reported. After acute infection, a prolonged period ranging from 5 to more than 15 years of symptomless, chronic infection ensues. In the third stage (AIDS-related complex), the HIV-infected patient is no longer symptom free but has not yet developed AIDS-defining opportunistic infection as defined by the CDC or an absolute CD4 cell count of less than $200/mm^3$. In the final stage, a potentially life-threatening opportunistic disease develops as a result of the severe cell-mediated immunodeficiency.

The epidemiologic data on HIV transmission overwhelmingly indicate that the virus is transmitted through sexual, parenteral, and maternal-infant routes. HIV has been isolated from many organs and tissues. Blood, semen, vaginal secretions, bone, breast milk, and possibly saliva have been implicated in HIV transmission. With current screening of donors and HIV testing techniques, the risk of HIV infection per unit of blood transfused is 1 in 2 million. Although the risk from any single transfusion is low, each transfusion has the potential to be fatal. This potential has increased physician awareness and decreased the elective use of allogeneic blood. When an individual does become infected from a transfusion, the development of AIDS seems to be more rapid than with other forms of transmission. In the United States, two donors were responsible for the transmission of HIV in four musculoskeletal grafts in 1985 and 1988. No further transmissions of HIV through allografts have been reported since 1988. However, the risk of transmission of HIV through allografts is estimated to be 1 in 1.6 million (one to two cases every 2 years), related to the fact that a window period still exists between testing methods and the patient having detectable viral antibodies. Once again this is very rare. Nucleic antibody testing has a window period for HIV and hepatitis C of 7 days and 8 days for hepatitis B. Additionally, there has been one reported case of hepatitis B and two reported cases of hepatitis C, with the most recent occurring in 2002. With better screening techniques including patient history and serologic and nucleic acid testing, rates remain low. Additionally, chemical sterilization techniques have also decreased the opportunity for disease transmission through allografts. The current risk of acquiring an infection from the allograft remains well below the overall perioperative nosocomial risk. Intraoperative culturing of the allograft has a low sensitivity and is generally not recommended. However, it is important that each surgeon knows the specifications of the tissue bank that he or she uses and ensure that it is American Association of Tissue Banks (AATB) accredited (Table 3.8).

DIAGNOSTIC TESTS

Because the serologic tests currently used for the detection of HIV depend on the formation of antibodies by the infected patient, there is a period of time known as the "window period" during which the patient is infectious before the appearance of the HIV antibodies. Most patients (approximately 99%) develop antibodies to HIV within 6 months of the initial infection, but delayed seroconversion (after 1 year) has been reported. Reliance on a single test may give a false sense of security.

The enzyme-linked immunosorbent assay (ELISA) was developed to test antibodies to the retrovirus. Because it is a serologic test, the detection of HIV antibodies by ELISA indicates a past infection. The antibodies usually increase to levels detectable by this test in 1 to 3 months. If the test is reactive, it is repeated; if it remains reactive, a confirmatory test, usually a Western blot, is performed. According to the CDC, the sensitivity of the ELISA is at least 99% when it is performed under optimal laboratory conditions on serum specimens from individuals infected for 3 months or longer. The ELISA was designed to be overly sensitive and is more likely to produce false-positive than false-negative results. The most frequent reason for a false-negative result is that the infected individual had not yet developed antibodies to HIV at the time of testing.

CONFIRMATORY TESTS

The Western blot test is the most common confirmatory test. It is far less likely to produce false results, but they do occur. The probability of obtaining false-positive tests with the ELISA and Western blot testing sequence in a population with a low incidence of infection has been estimated to be 1 in approximately 350,000. Other confirmatory tests are the antigen detection test, in situ hybridization test, indirect immunofluorescence assay, radioimmunoprecipitation assay, and PCR test. The CD4 lymphocyte count is not a diagnostic test but rather a measurement of the degree of immunosuppression.

TABLE. 3.8 Process of Allograft Procurement and Storage	
Donor screening	Precluded by history of autoimmune disease Ingestion or exposure to toxic substances Rheumatoid arthritis Systemic lupus erythematosus Polyarteritis nodosa Sarcoidosis Clinically significant bone disease Blood testing must be negative for antibodies to HIV Nucleic acid test for HIV-1 Hepatitis B surface antigen Total antibody to hepatitis B core antigen Antibodies to hepatitis C virus Nucleic acid test for hepatitis C virus Antibodies to human T-lymphotropic virus Syphilis
Tissue harvest	Within 24 h of death if body cooled Within 15 h of death if body not cooled Aseptic technique Tissue cultured before processing
Disinfection: removal of contaminants	Antibiotic soaks
Secondary sterilization: destruction of all life forms	Ethyl oxide, other chemical sterilants Gamma/electron-beam irradiation Proprietary protocols (i.e., Allowash, BioCleanse, Clearant)
Storage	Fresh allograft (use within 24 days) Fresh-freezing (3–7 years) Cryopreservation (up to 10 years) Lyophilization (3–5 years at room temperature)

Adapted from Azar FM: Tissue processing: role of secondary sterilization techniques, *Clin Sports Med* 28:191–201, 2009.

MUSCULOSKELETAL SYNDROMES IN HUMAN IMMUNODEFICIENCY VIRUS–INFECTED PATIENTS

The most common musculoskeletal syndromes in HIV-infected patients are manifestations of drug toxicity, reactive arthritis, infectious arthritis, myositis, tendinitis, and bursitis. Osteopenia and osteoporosis are increasing in HIV-infected patients being treated with highly active antiretroviral therapy (HAART) and must be as aggressively treated as patients without HIV. General principles to be kept in mind when evaluating an HIV-infected patient with musculoskeletal problems include the following: (1) any musculoskeletal syndrome that occurs in non–HIV-infected patients can occur in HIV-infected patients; (2) HIV infection can alter the clinical presentation, severity, and course of musculoskeletal problems; and (3) early diagnosis of infections is especially important to prevent their spread in an immunocompromised patient (Table 3.9).

TABLE. 3.9

Musculoskeletal Syndromes in Human Immunodeficiency Virus–Infected Patients

CONDITION	COMMENTS
Arthralgias	Causes include systemic bacterial infection, inflammation, drug toxicity
Reactive arthritis (Reiter syndrome)	Possibly more severe in HIV disease
Psoriatic arthritis	Most commonly *Staphylococcus aureus* or *Streptococcus pneumoniae*
Osteomyelitis	Reported in HIV disease as a result of extension of infection from septic joint
MYOSITIS	
Pyomyositis	Focal pain, tenderness
Idiopathic	Focal pain, tenderness
From zidovudine	Usually resolves when zidovudine is discontinued

From Lane N: HIV disease and arthritis: diagnostic and therapeutic dilemmas. In Cohen PT, Sande MA, Volberding PA, editors: *The AIDS knowledge base*, Boston, 1994, Little, Brown.

Reactive arthritis usually occurs in the foot and ankle. Tendinitis involving the Achilles tendon and the anterior and posterior tibial tendons is common. Septic arthritis occurs more commonly in intravenous drug abusers and hemophiliacs who have become infected with HIV. Gram-positive bacteria, such as *S. aureus* and *S. pneumoniae*, commonly found in noninfected patients with septic arthritis and bursitis, are also the most frequently reported organisms causing septic arthritis and bursitis in HIV-infected individuals. Primary osteomyelitis has been reported in HIV-infected patients, but usually it is the result of direct extension from a septic joint. An HIV-infected patient with a total joint prosthesis may be at an increased risk for infection as immunosuppression progresses.

Muscle pain or myositis occurs in up to 75% of HIV-infected patients, including idiopathic polymyositis, polymyositis secondary to zidovudine toxicity, and pyomyositis. Idiopathic polymyositis and zidovudine polymyositis have similar signs and symptoms. Patients complain of muscle weakness and have elevated creatine phosphokinase levels, and muscle biopsy specimens show myofibril necrosis and associated inflammation. Pyomyositis, usually caused by *S. aureus,* can present as a solitary abscess or multiple abscesses within the muscle. The patient has fever, localized muscle pain, swelling, and erythema. Aspiration and systemic antibiotics usually are adequate treatment of pyomyositis, but surgical incision and drainage are occasionally necessary.

RISKS AND PREVENTION

The risk of orthopaedic surgeons contracting HIV infection from patients is unknown at this time. However, no documented seroconversion has ever been reported in orthopaedic surgeons. According to the CDC, only 58 confirmed cases of occupational seroconversion transmission have occurred in health care workers (mostly nurses and technicians). Additionally, from 2000 to 2013, no new documented cases of HIV seroconversion have occurred in any health care worker.

The majority of seroconversions came from a single needle stick. It has been reported that 385,000 sharps-related injuries occur in the United States per year. It is important for health care personnel to continue universal precautions to continue to keep the risk low. The potential for disease transmission still exists. Three factors that must be known to calculate an orthopaedic surgeon's risk of incurring HIV from punctures in the operating room are (1) the frequency of punctures, (2) the percentage of surgical patients who are HIV positive, and (3) the risk of HIV transmission per needle stick from known HIV-positive patients.

At the end of 2013, the WHO estimated that approximately 35 million people worldwide were infected with HIV, and approximately 39 million had died of HIV-related diseases. These numbers are expected to increase as more individuals are living longer with HIV because of antiviral medications. Individuals with new infections worldwide in 2013 numbered 2.1 million. In the United States, approximately 40,000 people are newly diagnosed with HIV infection per year. Approximately 25% of HIV patients will require surgical or anesthetic treatment at some point. At the end of 2008, women accounted for 50% of all adults worldwide with HIV infection. In the United States, it has been estimated that 0.4% of the population is HIV-positive with approximately 21% of positive patients unaware of their HIV infection. The exact prevalence of HIV-infected patients in a specific surgeon's practice is impossible to calculate without prospective testing; however, it has been reported to be 10% with regional and local variations, in that trauma centers have a greater prevalence of HIV-infected patients. According to the CDC in 1986, the overall prevalence of HIV infection was 1% of the U.S. hospital population admitted for reasons other than HIV infection. The CDC reported in 1993 that only 30% of HIV-infected patients were recognized at the time of treatment.

Lemaire and Masson noted that 6% to 50% of operations result in at least one blood contact between patient and health care worker, and 1.3% to 15.4% of procedures involve a sharp injury. Risk decreased with surgical experience but increased with operative time. Fitch et al. found that the greatest risk for occupational transmission of HIV involved parenteral injection of blood through orthopaedic pins or hollow-core needles. No cases of transmission from solid-core needles or exposure of an open wound to blood have been documented. Other potential sites of transmission include mucous membranes and isolated skin exposure, which is extremely rare. Risk increases with increased viral load of the patient, quantity of blood injected, and depth of inoculation (BOX 3.1).

Based on data obtained by the American Board of Orthopaedic Surgeons, the estimated puncture rate for the orthopaedic attending physician is 2.8%, averaging approximately 10 punctures a year. In 1998, the CDC estimated that the percentage of HIV-positive patients averaged 1% to 5.6%, depending on the geographic area and the type of practice. The risk of transmission per needle stick has been estimated by the CDC to be approximately 0.3%. This number has been reduced by the CDC to 0.23%, which means 2.3 of every 1000 contaminated needle sticks would result in seroconversion if the healthcare individual elected to decline postinjury treatment. These figures put the annual risk to the orthopaedic surgeon between 0.025% and 0.5%, a cumulative (>40 years of practice) risk of 0.6%. The risk of transmission of HIV from an infected orthopaedic surgeon to a noninfected patient has not been reported.

BOX 3.1

Risk Factors for Human Immunodeficiency Virus Transmission from a Needle Stick

- Large-gauge (≤18-gauge) hollow-bore needle
- Deep injury
- Visible blood on device
- Procedure involving a needle in an artery or vein
- Emergency procedures
- Terminal illness in source patient

From: Grabowski G, Pilato A, Clark C, et al: HIV in orthopaedic surgery, *J Am Acad Orthop Surg* 25:569–576, 2017.

In the absence of an effective means of prophylaxis, including a vaccine, the chief defense against HIV infection is the prevention of its transmission. Health care workers at risk are those most prone to sustain needle sticks, cuts, and skin tears in the presence of contaminated body fluids and tissues. The cases of HIV transmission through wounds underscore the importance of infection control procedures, especially in the operating room.

During orthopaedic surgical procedures, contact with blood and other body fluids containing blood in gross or microscopic amounts is frequent (3.7%). Lacerations from bone fragments and edges and cuts and needle sticks must be avoided. The estimated risk after a mucocutaneous exposure was reported to be 0.09% based on one seroconversion in six studies. The American Academy of Orthopaedic Surgeons (AAOS) has developed several basic recommendations for procedures in the operating room (BOX 3.2). These precautions involve wearing surgical gowns that offer protection against contact with blood, using no touch techniques for surgery and suturing, not passing sharp instruments from hand to hand (establishing a "hands-free" zone), and proper removal of contaminated gowns and postoperative scrub. Specific recommendations by the AAOS can be found in their information statement Preventing the Transmission of Bloodborne Pathogens (2012).

Chemoprophylaxis for occupational exposure to HIV is controversial. The most effective means of avoiding occupational HIV seroconversion is the employment of universal precautions. The practice of using protective eyewear is advised because projection of blood causes 3% to 5% of contaminations. Standard eyeglasses may provide protection because less than 5% of contamination has been found to be present on the protective side flaps of wraparound eye protectors. Double gloving reduces the risk of blood contact from 29% to 13%; however, the gloves must be changed at least every 2 hours or every hour for trauma cases. Indicator gloves also can be used to alert the surgeon to breaks in glove protection. Kevlar gloves should be used when bone fragments are present, or when saws are used. HIV-positive patients should be placed on HAART protocol before surgery. Elective surgery is contraindicated in untreated patients. The CDC recommends preexposure prophylaxis with daily dosing of tenofovir disoproxil fumarate (TDF)/emtricitabine (FTC) for individuals at high risk of HIV infection.

After exposure of a health care worker to blood, a rapid HIV test should be performed on the source. If it is negative, no chemoprophylaxis should be offered. However, if it is positive, chemoprophylaxis should be offered. The rapid HIV test does have a low false-positive rate; therefore all positive results should be followed with standard enzyme immunoassay and a Western blot assay. The test also will not identify HIV-positive patients if they have been infected less than 3 months. A decrease in seroconversion rates of 81% has been shown with the use of chemoprophylaxis after exposure using zidovudine and lamivudine, chain terminators for reverse transcriptase within 72 hours of exposure. Adding the protease inhibitor, indinavir further decreases antiretroviral activity. These drugs should be started as soon as possible but no later than 72 hours after exposure and generally are recommended for at least a 4-week course. Recommendations from WHO for postexposure prophylaxis (PEP) for HIV are found in Boxes 3.3 and 3.4.

The most current PEP drug regimen can be found at the CDC website www.ncbi.nlm.nih.gov/pubmed/239179 01. Also, questions about PEP can be answered at National Clinicians postexposure prophylaxis hot line (PEPline) at (888) HIV-4911. Most exposures to HIV-infected blood do not cause seroconversion. No confirmed cases of occupational HIV transmission to a health care professional has occurred since 1999, and as of 2013, only 58 documented and 143 possible transmissions have been reported in the United States. Again, there is only a 0.23% chance of seroconversion after exposure to a patient with HIV. Therefore the toxicity of a chemoprophylactic regimen must be considered before the initiation of treatment. If available, consultation with infectious disease expert is recommended.

Additional concern for bloodborne pathogens extends to hepatitis. Approximately 10,000 health care workers become infected with the HBV annually after an occupational exposure. Occupational exposure of health care workers to HBV-infected patients can result in disease transmission up to 30% of the time. The development of a vaccine for HBV has resulted in a decrease of transmission by 98% since 1983 and is recommended for most health care workers. After vaccination it is recommended that the health care worker be tested for anti-HBs to ensure proper antibody response has occurred (titer >10 mIU/mL). If so, lifelong immunity has been acquired. If it has not, a repeat round (three doses) of vaccination is warranted. Retesting should be performed 1 to 2 months after the final injection. Few health care workers remain nonresponders and should be identified. They should be tested for hepatitis B surface antigen (HbsAg). These nonresponders should report any exposures within 7 days so they may receive PEP with hepatitis B immune globulin (HBIg). HBV and HBIg can be administered at the same time but in different arms. The risk of hepatitis C virus (HCV) has continued to increase. It is now the most chronic blood-borne infection in the United States. An estimated 926,000 health care professionals are exposed to HCV per year, resulting in 16,400 new infections worldwide. There is an approximate 2% risk of transmission of HCV after percutaneous exposure. There is no PEP recommendation after contact with HCV. However, effective treatment is available, which can lower the risk of developing chronic HCV infection. The CDC PEP for HBV and HCV is summarized in Table 3.10. Universal precautions should be used to decrease the risk of seroconversion from these pathogens. Seroconversion rates are listed in Table 3.11. In addition to HBV vaccination, it is recommended that all health care personnel be immune to measles, mumps, rubella, varicella, pertussis, and influenza.

Recommended treatments of infectious disease exposure are shown in Boxes 3.5 and 3.6.

Recommendations for Safety During Procedures and Examinations

Hand Hygiene
- Hands should be cleaned with alcohol-based hand rub if not visibly soiled or washed with either plain or antimicrobial soap before and immediately after each patient contact.
- Gloves are not a substitute for hand washing.
- Gloves should be worn during any procedure that may result in contact with blood or body fluids and when handling needles or other sharp instruments (the volume of blood transmitted by a needle stick is reduced by 50% when the needle first passes through a glove). Double gloving is recommended.
- For procedures such as dressing changes or pin removals, gloves, protective eye cover (not just prescription glasses), masks, gowns, and shoe covers should be worn as necessary.

Surgical Garb
- Appropriate footwear such as boots or surgical shoe covers should be worn to prevent skin exposure outside of the surgical field.
- Surgical gown should be worn during all surgical procedures.
- Double gloves should be worn during all surgical procedures and the outer pair changed at least every 2 hours.
- Reinforced gloves should be worn when sharp instruments and devices are used or when bone fragments are likely to be encountered.
- Head covers and facemasks should be worn during surgical procedures with facemasks changed if they become splattered or moist.
- Goggles are better than glasses, but face shields offer the greatest level of protection.

Handling of Sharp Instruments
- Sharp instruments should not be left unattended in surgical field.
- Sharp instruments should not be passed from hand to hand but on intermediate trays, announcing when they are being passed.
- The location of a returned sharp instrument should be announced.

Surgeon Supervision
- Surgeons supervising trainees should take experience into consideration when assigning roles.

- In advance of the procedure, surgeons should inform surgical team of aspects that place them at a higher risk.
- Surgeons should periodically remind surgical team of the importance of caution.

Suturing
- No-touch suturing techniques should be used whenever possible.
- Sutures should not be tied with the suture needle in the surgeon's hand.
- Blunt suture needles are recommended when their use is technically feasible.
- Two surgeons should not suture the same wound simultaneously.

Special Considerations
- Exposed ends of all orthopaedic pins should be securely covered with plastic caps or other appropriate devices.
- The points of pins that have passed through soft tissue or bone should be cut off.
- All power tools should be inspected before and after each use to ensure they are properly maintained.
- When using power tools, appropriate surgical attire should be worn to prevent exposure to blood or aerosols containing blood and to reduce the likelihood of bone chips contacting the surgeon's eyes.

After the Surgical Procedure
- Care should be taken not to contaminate areas outside of the surgical field.
- The outside layer of gloves should be changed before applying the dressing.
- Contaminated drapes should be removed and discarded into a biohazard container.
- Clean, nonsterile gloves should be used to handle operating equipment not grossly contaminated and the gloves discarded thereafter, and hand washing commenced.
- All contaminated clothing should be removed in a manner that avoids contact with blood.
- All contaminated materials from the procedure should be placed in appropriate biohazard bags or containers and discarded.
- Instruments and other reusable equipment should be disinfected and sterilized.

Data from American Academy of Orthopaedic Surgeons Information Statement on Preventing the Transmission of Bloodborne Pathogens, www.aaos.org. Accessed January 2015.

BOX 3.3

Practical Guidance for Assessing Postexposure Prophylaxis Eligibility

- HIV PEP should be offered and initiated as early as possible in all individuals with an exposure that has the potential for HIV transmission, and ideally within 72 h.*
- Eligibility assessment should be based on the HIV status of the source whenever possible and may include consideration of background prevalence and local epidemiologic patterns.†
- Exposures that may warrant HIV PEP include:
  - Bodily fluids: blood, blood-stained saliva, breast milk, genital secretions; cerebrospinal, amniotic, peritoneal, synovial, pericardial, or pleural fluids
  - Mucous membrane: sexual exposure; splashes to eye, nose, or oral cavity
  - Parenteral exposures

- Exposures that do not require HIV PEP include:
  - When the exposed individual is HIV already positive.
  - When the source is established to be HIV negative.
  - Exposures to bodily fluids that do not pose a significant risk, i.e., tears, nonblood-stained saliva, urine, and sweat.

In cases that do not require PEP, the exposed person should be counseled about limiting future exposure risk. Although HIV testing is not required, it may be provided if desired by the exposed person.

*Although PEP is ideally provided within 72 hours of exposure, there may be instances when patients are unable to access services within this timeframe. Providers should consider the range of other essential interventions and referrals that should be offered to clients presenting after the 72-hour period.
†In some settings with high HIV prevalence or where the source is known to be at high risk for HIV infection, all exposures may be considered for PEP without a risk assessment.
HIV, Human immunodeficiency virus; *PEP*, postexposure prophylaxis.
From Ford N, Mayer K: World Health Organization Guidelines on Postexposure Prophylaxis for HIV: Recommendations for a public health approach, *Clin Infect Dis* 60(Suppl 3): S161, 2015.

BOX 3.4

Recommended Regimens for Postexposure Prophylaxis for Adults, Adolescents, and Children

Number of antiretroviral drugs
- A two-drug PEP regimen is effective, but three drugs are preferred. (Conditional recommendation, low quality of evidence).
- Preferred antiretroviral regimen for adults and adolescents:
  - TDF + 3TC (or FTC) is recommended as the preferred backbone regimen for HIV PEP in adults and adolescents. (Strong recommendation, low-to-moderate quality of evidence)
  - LPV/r or ATV/r are suggested as the preferred third drug for HIV PEP in adults and adolescents. Where available, RAL, DRV/r, or EFV can be considered as alternative options. (Conditional recommendation, very low quality of evidence)
Preferred antiretroviral regimen for children ≤10 years:
  - ZDV + 3TC is recommended as the preferred backbone for HIV PEP in children aged ≤10 years. ABC + 3TC or TDF

+ 3TC (or FTC) can be considered as alternative regimens. (Strong recommendation, low quality evidence)
- LPV/r is recommended as the preferred third drug for HIV PEP in children aged ≤10 years. An age-appropriate alternative regimen can be identified among ATV/r, RAL, DRV, EFV, and NVP. (Conditional recommendation, very low quality of evidence).
Prescribing frequency:
- A full 28-day prescription for antiretrovirals should be provided for HIV PEP, following initial risk assessment. (Strong recommendation, very low quality of evidence)
Adherence support:
- Enhanced adherence counseling is suggested for all individuals initiating HIV PEP. (Conditional recommendation, moderate quality of evidence)

3TC, Lamivudine; *ABC*, abacavir; *ATV*, atazanavir; *DRV*, darunavir; *EFV*, efavirenz; *FTC*, emtricitabine; *HIV*, human immunodeficiency virus; *LPV*, lopinavir; *NVP*, nevirapine; *PEP*, postexposure prophylaxis; */r*, boosted with ritonavir; *RAL*, raltegravir; *TDF*, tenofovir; *ZDV*, zidovudine.
From Ford N, Mayer K: World Health Organization Guidelines on Postexposure Prophylaxis for HIV: Recommendations for a public health approach, *Clin Infect Dis* 60[Suppl 3]: S161, 2015.

TABLE. 3.10

Recommended Postexposure Prophylaxis Regimens for Hepatitis B and C

INFECTION	SOURCE PATIENT'S DISEASE STATUS	STATUS OF EXPOSED PERSON	REGIMEN
Hepatitis B virus	Hepatitis B surface antigen positive	Unvaccinated	A single dose of hepatitis B immune globulin, 0.06 mL/kg IM within 24 h of exposure, followed by hepatitis B vaccine series
		Previously vaccinated with documented inadequate response*	A single dose of hepatitis B immune globulin, 0.06 mL/kg IM within 24 h of exposure, followed by hepatitis B vaccine booster
		Previously vaccinated, nonresponder*	A single dose of hepatitis B immune globulin, 0.06 mL/kg IM within 24 h of exposure, followed by hepatitis B vaccine series Or Hepatitis B immune globulin, 0.06 mL/kg IM twice within 24 h of exposure, for individuals who did not respond to two vaccine series
		Previously vaccinated with adequate response†	None
Hepatitis C virus	Anti-hepatitis C virus positive with detectable hepatitis C virus RNA	Hepatitis C seronegative	None available

*Serum levels of hepatitis B surface antigen antibodies <10 MIU/mL.
†Serum levels of hepatitis B surface antigen antibodies ≥10 MIU/mL.
IM, Intramuscularly.
From Bader MS, McKinsey DS: Postexposure prophylaxis for common infectious disease, *Am Fam Physician* 88:25–32, 2013.

BOX 3.5

Methods of Reducing Percutaneous, Mucous Membrane, or Nonintact Skin Exposure to Blood or Potentially Infectious Body Fluids

- Strict adherence to standard precautions including appropriate hand hygiene and use of personal protective equipment (e.g., gloves, gowns, masks, and eye shields)
- Use of safety engineered devices (needles, syringes, scalpels, etc.)
- Use of double gloves during surgical procedures with an increased risk of glove puncture
- Use of blunted surgical needles, when possible
- Work practice controls to reduce risk of injuries, such as elimination of capping needles, using a tray to pass sharp devices, and immediately and appropriately discard used sharp instruments
- Puncture-resistant sharps disposal units
- Precautions should be taken to prevent sharps injuries during procedures and during cleaning/disinfection of instruments
- Mouthpieces, resuscitation bags, or other ventilation devices should be available whenever their need can be anticipated
- Health care personnel who have exudative lesions or weeping dermatitis on exposed body areas (hand/wrist and face/neck) must be excused from providing direct patient care or working patient equipment (OSHA regulation)
- Enhanced education on the proper use of safety engineered device

From Weber DJ, Rutala WA: Occupational health update: Focus on preventing the acquisitions of infections with pre-exposure prophylaxis and postexposure prophylaxis, *Infect Dis Clin N Am* 30:729–757, 2016.

TABLE. 3.11

Risk of Seroconversion After Exposure

Human immunodeficiency virus	0.3%
Hepatitis C virus	1.8%
Hepatitis B virus	30%

BOX 3.6

Management of an Infectious Disease Exposure

- Obtain name, medical record number, and location of source case
- Determine if source case has an infection and is infectious (i.e., capable of transmitting infection)
- Determine if transmission possible (i.e., appropriate exposure without appropriate personal protection)
- Determine if health care provider is susceptible (may require laboratory tests)
- Determine if PEP is available and indicated
- Consider alternative prophylaxis (if available) if health care provider has a contraindication to the prophylaxis of first choice
- Administer prophylaxis with informed consent (healthcare provider may choose not to accept prophylaxis)
- Arrange follow-up
- Document all of the above in the medical record

PEP, Postexposure prophylaxis.
From Weber DJ, Rutala WA: Occupational health update: Focus on preventing the acquisitions of infections with pre-exposure prophylaxis and postexposure prophylaxis, *Infect Dis Clin N Am* 30:729–757, 2016.

REFERENCES

ETIOLOGY AND PROPHYLAXIS

Aalirezaie A, Akkaya M, Barnes CL, et al.: Proceedings of international consensus meeting on orthopedic infections: general assembly, prevention, operating room environment, *J Arthroplasty*, 2018, Article in press.

Aalirezaie A, Anoushiravani A, Cashman J, et al.: General assembly, prevention, host risk mitigation – local factors: proceedings of international consensus on orthopedic infections, *J Arthroplasty*, 2018, Article in press.

Adeli B, Parvizi J: Strategies for the prevention of periprosthetic joint infection, *J Bone Joint Surg* 94B(SA), 2012, 42.

Akesson P, Chen A, Deirmengian GK, et al.: General assembly, prevention, risk mitigation, local factors: proceedings of international consensus on orthopedic infections, *J Arthroplasty* 32(2S):S49, 2019.

Akins GJ, Alberdi MT, Beswick A, et al.: General assembly, prevention, surgical site preparation: proceedings of international consensus on orthopedic infections, *J Arthroplasty* 34(2S):S85, 2019.

Alaee F, Angerame M, Bradbury T, et al.: General assembly, prevention, operating room – surgical technique: proceedings of international consensus on orthopedic infections, *J Arthroplasty* 34(2S):S139, 2019.

Alsadaan M, AlRumaih H, Brown T, et al.: General assembly, prevention, operating room, surgical field: proceedings of international consensus on orthopedic infections, *J Arthroplasty* 34(2S):S127, 2019.

American Academy of Orthopaedic Surgeons: *Information statement. Preventing the transmission of bloodborne pathogens*, Rosemont, IL, 2001, AAOS. revised, 2008, reviewed 2012.

Arciola CR, Montanaro L, Costerton JW: New trends in diagnosis and control strategies for implant infections, *Int J Artif Organs* 34:727, 2011.

Ares O, Arnold WV, Atilla B, et al.: General assembly section, prevention, host related local: proceedings of international consensus on orthopedic infections, *J Arthroplasty*, 2018, Article in press.

Augustine SD: Forced-air warming discontinued: periprosthetic joint infection rates drop, *Orthop Rev (Pavia)* 9(2):6998, 2017.

Autorino CM, Battenberg A, Blom A, et al.: General assembly, prevention, operating room – surgical attire: proceedings of international consensus on orthopedic infections, *J Arthroplasty* 34(2S):S117, 2019.

Baldini A, Blevins K, Del Gaizo D, et al.: General assembly, prevention, operating room – personnel: proceedings of international consensus on orthopedic infections, *J Arthroplasty* 34(2S):S97, 2019.

Berríos-Torres SI, Umscheid CA, Bratzler DW, et al.: Centers for Disease Control and Prevention Guideline for the Prevention of Surgical Site Infection, *JAMA Surg* 152:784, 2017, 2017.

Bhars CH, Marschal M, Weise K, et al.: Acute musculoskeletal infection: comparison of different methods for intraoperative bacterial identification, *Acta Chir Orthop Traumatol Cech* 73:237, 2006.

Bibi S, Shah SA, Qureshi S, et al.: Is chlorhexidine-gluconate superior than povidone-iodine in preventing surgical site infections? A multicenter study, *J Pak Med Assoc* 65(11):1197, 2015.

Bigliardi PL, Alsagoff SAL, El-Kafrawi HY, et al.: Povidone iodine in wound healing: a review of current concepts and practices, *Int J Surg* 44:260, 2017.

Bischoff P, Kubilay NZ, Allegranzi B, et al.: Effect of laminar airflow ventilation on surgical site infections: a systematic review and meta-analysis, *Lancet Infect Dis* 17(5):553, 2017.

Blevins K, Aalirezaie A, Shohat N, Parvizi J: Malnutrition and the development of periprosthetic joint infection in patients undergoing primary elective total joint arthroplasty, *J Arthroplasty* 33:2971, 2018.

Blom A, Cho J, Fleischman A, et al.: General assembly, prevention, antiseptic irrigation solution: proceeding of international consensus on orthopedic infections, *J Arthroplasty*, 2018, Articles in press.

Bondarenko S, Chang CB, Cordero-Ampuero J, et al.: General assembly, prevention, antimicrobials (systemic): proceedings of international consensus on orthopedic infections, *J Arthroplasty*, 2018, Article in press.

Boyle KK, Duquin TR: Antibiotic prophylaxis and prevention of surgical site infection in shoulder and elbow surgery, *Orthop Clin North Am* 49(2):241, 2018.

Bravo T, Budhiparama N, Flynn S, et al.: Hip and knee section, prevention, postoperative issues: proceedings of international consensus on orthopedic infections, *J Arthroplasty*, 2018, Article in press.

Brown NM, Cipriano CA, Moric M, et al.: Dilute betadine lavage before closure for the prevention of acute postoperative deep periprosthetic joint infection, *J Arthroplasty* 27(1):27, 2012.

Cadena J, Thinwa J, Walter EA, Frei CR: Risk factors for the development of active methicillin-resistant Staphylococcus aureus (MRSA) infection in patients colonized with MRSA at hospital admission, *Am J Infect Control* 44:1617, 2016.

Cai Y, Xu K, Hou W, et al.: Preoperative chlorhexidine reduces the incidence of surgical site infections in total knee and hip arthroplasty: a systematic review and meta-analysis, *Int J Surg* 39:221, 2017.

Capriotti K, Pelletier J, Barone S, Capriotti J: Efficacy of dilute povidone-iodine against multi-drug resistant bacterial biofilms, fungal biofilms and fungal spores, *Clin Res Dermatol Open Access* 5(1):1, 2018.

Centers for Disease Control and Prevention, Centers for Disease Control and Prevention: Update: allograft-associated bacterial infections–United States, 2002. Available at http://www.cdc.gov/mmwr/preview/mmwrhtml/mm5110a2.htm. Accessed November 18, 2010.

Centers for Disease Control and Prevention, Hepatitis C: 2010 STD treatment guidelines. Available at http://www.cdc.gov/std/treatment/2010/hepc.htm.

Centers for Disease Control and Prevention: HIV in the United States: at a glance, Available at http://www.cdc.gov/hiv/statistics/basics/ataglance.html. Accessed January 8, 2015.

Centers for Disease Control and Prevention: MDRO Guideline, www.cdc.gov/hicpac/pdf/MDRO/MDROGuideline2006.pdf. Accessed January 5, 2015.

Chou DT, Achan P, Ramachandran M: The World Health Organization '5 moments of hand hygiene, *J Bone Joint Surg* 94B(441), 2012.

Cross MB, Yi PH, Thomas CF, et al.: Evaluation of malnutrition in orthopaedic surgery, *J Am Acad Orthop Surg* 22:193, 2014.

Deuffic-Burban S, Delarocque-Astagneau E, Abiteboul D, et al.: Blood-borne viruses in health care workers: prevention and management, *J Clin Virol* 52(4), 2011.

Cizmic Z, Feng JE, Huang R, et al.: Hip and knee section, prevention, host related: proceedings of international consensus on orthopedic infections, *J Arthroplasty* 34(2S):S255, 2019.

Dumville JC, McFarlane E, Edwards P, et al.: Preoperative skin antiseptics for preventing surgical wound infections after clean surgery (review), *Cochrane Database Syst Rev* 4:CD003949, 2015.

De Vries FE, Wallert ED, Solomkin JS, et al.: A systematic review and meta-analysis including GRADE qualification of the risk of surgical site infections after prophylactic negative pressure wound therapy compared with conventional dressings in clean and contaminated surgery, *Medicine* 95(36):e4673, 2016.

Farach SM, Kelly KN, Farkas RL, et al.: Have recent modifications of operating room attire policies decreased surgical site infections? An American College of Surgeons NSQIP review of 6517 patients, *J Am Coll Surg* 226(5):804, 2018.

Fleischman AN, Restrepo C, Goswami K, Parvizi J: A decade of protocol developments for SSI prevention: intraoperative betadine irrigation prevails, Presentation at 2017 AAHKS Annual Meeting, Dallas, Texas.

Goodman SM, Springer B, Guyatt G, et al.: American College of Rheumatology/American Association of Hip and Knee Surgeons guideline for the perioperative management of antirheumatic medication in patients with rheumatic diseases undergoing elective total hip or total knee arthroplasty, *J Arthroplasty* 32:2628, 2017, 2017.

Goyal N, Miller A, Tripathi M, Parvizi J: Methicillin-resistant Staphylococcus aureus (MRSA), *Bone Joint J* 95B(1):4, 2013.

Guillamet CV, Kollef MH: How to stratify patients at risk for resistant bugs in skin and soft tissue infections, *Curr Opin Infect Dis* 29:116, 2016.

Igbal HJ, Ponniah N, Long S, et al.: Review of MRSA screening and antibiotics prophylaxis in orthopaedic trauma patients; the risk of surgical site infection with inadequate antibiotic prophylaxis in patients colonized with MRSA, *Injury* 48(7):1382, 2017.

Hsu JE, Bumgarner RE, Matsen FA: Propionibacterium in shoulder arthroplasty, *J Bone Joint Surg Am* 98:597, 2016.

Jernigan J, Kallen A, ELC Prevention Collaboratives: Methicillin-resistant Staphylococcus aureus (MRSA) infections, Healthcare-associated infections, *Centers for Disease Control Presentation* January 19, 2010.

Jiranek W, Kigera JWM, Klatt BA, et al.: General assembly, prevention, host risk mitigation – general factors: proceedings of International Consensus on Orthopedic Infections, *J Arthroplasty* 34(2S):S43, 2019.

Johnson R, Jameson SS, Sanders RD, et al.: Reducing surgical site infection in arthroplasty of the lower limb. A multi-disciplinary approach, *Bone Joint Res* 2(3):58, 2013.

Katarincic JA, Fantry A, DePasse JM, Feller R: Local modalities for preventing surgical site infections: an evidence-based review, *J Am Acad Orthop Surg* 26(1):14, 2018.

Kearns KA, Witmer D, Makda J, et al.: Sterility of the personal protection system in total joint arthroplasty, *Clin Orthop Relat Res* 469:3065, 2011.

Kheir MM, Tan TL, Azboy I, et al.: Vancomycin prophylaxis for total joint arthroplasty: incorrectly dosed and has a higher rate of periprosthetic infection than cefazolin, *Clin Orthop Relat Res* 475(7):1767, 2017.

Kim DH, Spencer M, Davidson SM, et al.: Institutional prescreening for detection and eradication of methicillin-resistant *Staphylococcus aureus* in patients undergoing elective orthopaedic surgery, *J Bone Joint Surg* 92A:1820, 2010.

Lu M, Hansen EN: Hydrogen peroxide wound irrigation in orthopaedic surgery, *J Bone Jt Infect* 2(1):3, 2017.

Luedicke C, Slickers P, Ehricht R, Monecke S: Molecular fingerprinting of *Staphylococcus aureus* from bone and joint infections, *Eur J Clin Microbiol Infect Dis* 29:457, 2010.

Marculescu CE, Mabry T, Berbari EF: Prevention of surgical site infections in joint replacement surgery, *Surgical Infections* 17(2):152, 2016.

Marmor S, Kerroumi Y: Patient-specific risk factors for infection in arthroplasty procedure, *Orthop Traumatol Surg Res* 102(Suppl 1):S113, 2016.

Moucha CS, Clyburn T, Evans RP, Prokuski L: Modifiable risk factors for surgical site infection, *J Bone Joint Surg* 93A:398, 2011.

Nana A, Nelson SB, McLaren A, Chen AF: Specialty update. What's new in musculoskeletal infection: update on biofilms, *J Bone Joint Surg* 98:1226, 2016.

Pae M, Wu D: Nutritional modulaton of age-related changes in the immune system and risk of infection, *Nutr Res* 41:14, 2017.

Parvizi J, Shohat N, Gehrke T: Prevention of periprosthetic joint infection, *Bone Joint J* 99-B(3), 2017.

Perry KI, Hanssen AD: Orthopaedic infection: prevention and diagnosis, *J Am Acad Orthop Surg* 25(Suppl 1):S4–S6, 2017.

Pittet D, Allegranzi B, Boyce J, et al.: The World Health Organization guidelines on hand hygiene in health care and their consensus recommendations, *Infec Control Hosp Epidemiol* 30:611–622, 2009.

Preas MA, O'Hara L, Thom K: 2017 HICPAC-CDC guideline for prevention of surgical site infection: what the infection preventionist needs to know, Available at www.apic.org. Accessed 4 January 2019.

Rezapoor M, Tan TL, Maltenfort MG, Parvizi J: Incise draping reduces the rate of contamination of the surgical site during hip surgery: a prospective, randomized trial, *J Arthroplasty* 33:1891, 2018.

Rondon AJ, Kheir MM, Tan TL, et al.: Cefazolin prophylaxis for total joint arthroplasty: obese patients are frequently underdosed and at increased risk of periprosthetic joint infection, *J Arthroplasty* 33(11):3551, 2018.

Salassa TE, Swiontkowski MF: Surgical attire and the operating room: role in infection prevention, *J Bone Joint Surg* 96A:1485, 2014.

Schwarzkopf R, Takemoto RC, Immerman I, et al.: Prevalence of *Staphylococcus aureus* colonization in orthopaedic surgeons and their patients, *J Bone Joint Surg* 92A:1815, 2010.

Seidl A, Lindeque B: Large joint osteoarticular infection caused by mycobacterium arupense, *Orthopedics* 37:e848, 2014.

Shohat N, Muhsen K, Gilat R, et al.: Inadequate glycemic control is associated with increased surgical site infection in total joint arthroplasty: a systematic review and meta-analysis, *J Arthroplasty* 33:2312, 2018.

Shohat N, Tarabichi M, Tischler E, et al.: Serum fructosamine: a simple and inexpensive test for assessing pre-operative glycemic control, *J Bone Joint Surg Am* 99:1900, 2017.

Singh VK, Hussain S, Javed S, et al.: Sterile surgical helmet system in elective total hip and knee arthroplasty, *J Orthop Surg (Hong Kong)* 19:234, 2011.

Skramm I, Moen AEF, Aroen A, Bukholm G: Surgical site infections in orthopaedic surgery demonstrate clones similar to those in orthopaedic Staphylococcus aureus nasal carriers, *J Bone Joint Surg* 96:882, 2014.

Stefani S, Goglio A: Methicillin-resistant *Staphylococcus aureus:* related infections and antibiotic resistance, *Int J Infect Dis* 14(Suppl 4):S19, 2010.

Taylor AR: Methicillin-resistant Staphylococcus aureus infections, *Prim Care* 40:637, 2013.

Torres EG, Lindmair-Snell JM, Langan JW, Burnikel BG: Is preoperative nasal povidone-iodine as efficient and cost-effective as standard methicillin-resistant Staphylococcus aureus screening protocol in total joint arthroplasty? *J Arthroplasty* 31(1):215, 2016.

Tosti R, Samuelsen BT, Bender S, et al.: Emerging multidrug resistance of methicillin-resistant Staphylococcus aureus in hand infections, *J Bone Joint Surg* 96A:1535, 2014.

Weber DJ, Rutala WA, Sickbert-Bennett EE: Outbreaks associated with contaminated antiseptics and disinfectants, *Antimicrobial Agents and Chemotherapy* 51(12):4217, 2007.

World Health Organization/: Global guidelines on the prevention of surgical site infection. WHO, http://www.who.int/gpsc/ssi-guidelines/en. Accessed 3 January 2019.

World Health Organization: HIV/Aids Fact Sheet N 360, 2014. Available at: http://www.who.int/mediacentre/factsheets/fs360/en/. Accessed 25 September 2015.

World Health Organization: Global Guidelines for the Prevention of Surgical Site Infection. Available at: https://www.who.int/gpsc/ssi-prevention-guidelines/en/. Accessed 4 January 2019.

Wouthuyzen-Bakker M, Benito N, Soriano A: The effect of preoperative antimicrobial prophylaxis on intraoperative culture results in patients with a suspected or confirmed prosthetic joint infection: a systematic review, *J Clin Microbiol* 55(9):2765, 2017.

Yang Y, Reid C, Nambiar M, Penn D: Hydrogen peroxide in orthopaedic surgery – is it worth the risk? *Acta Chir Belg* 116(4):247, 2016.

Yeganeh MH, Kheir MM, Shahi A, Parvizi J: Rheumatoid arthritis, disease modifying agents, and perioprosthetic joint infection: what does a joint surgeon need to know? *J Arthroplasty* 33(4):1258, 2018.

Young SW, Zhu M, Shirley OC, et al.: Do 'surgical helmet systems' or 'body exhaust suits' affect contamination and deep infection rates in arthroplasty? A systematic review, *J Arthroplasty* 31:225, 2016.

Zainul-Abidin S, Amanatullah DF, Anderson MB, et al.: General assembly, prevention, host related general: proceedings of international consensus on orthopedic infections, *J Arthroplasty* 34(2S):S13, 2019.

DIAGNOSIS

Ahmad SS, Hirschmann MT, Becker R, et al.: A meta-analysis of synovial biomarkers in periprosthetic joint infection: Synovasure™ is less effective than the ELISA-based alpha-defensin test, *Knee Surg Sports Traumatol Arthrosc*, 26(10):3039, 2018.

Ascione T, Barrak R, Benito N, et al.: General assembly, diagnosis, pathogen isolation – culture matters: proceedings of international consensus on orthopedic infections, *J Arthroplasty* 34(2S):S197, 2019.

Barrack R, Bhimani S, Blevins JL, et al.: General assembly, diagnosis, laboratory test: proceedings of international consensus on orthopedic infections, *J Arthroplasty* 34(2S):S187, 2019.

Basu S, Kwee TC, Saboury B, et al.: FDG-PET for diagnosing infection in hip and knee prostheses, *Clin Nucl Med* 39:609, 2014.

Belden K, Cao L, Chen J, et al.: Hip and knee section, fungal periprosthetic joint infection, diagnosis and treatment: proceedings of international consensus on orthopedic infections, *J Arthroplasty* 34(2S):S387, 2019.

Browne LP, Guillerman RP, Orth RC, et al.: Community-acquired Staphylococcal musculoskeletal infection in infants and young children: necessity of contrast-enhanced MRI for the diagnosis of growth cartilage improvement, *Am J Radiol* 198:194, 2012.

Corvec S: Clinical and biological features of *Cutibacterium* (formerly *Propionibacterium*) avidum, an underrecognized microorganism, *Clinical Microbiology Reviews* 31(3):1, 2018.

Dailey TA, Berven MD, Vroman PJ: 99mTC-HMPAO-labeled WBC scan for the diagnosis of chronic recurrent multifocal osteomyelitis, *J Nucl Med Technol* 42:299, 2014.

De Fine M, Giavaresi G, Fini M, et al.: The role of synovial fluid analysis in the detection of periprosthetic hip and knee infections: a systematic review and meta-analysis, *Int Orthop* 42(5):983, 2018.

Diaz-Ledezma C, Espinosa-Mendoza R, Gallo J, et al.: General assembly, diagnosis, imaging: proceedings of international consensus on orthopedic infections, *J Arthroplasty* 34(2S):S215, 2019.

Dodson CC, Craig EV, Cordasco FA, et al.: Propionibacterium acnes infection after shoulder arthroplasty: a diagnostic challenge, *J Shoulder Elbow Surg* 19:303, 2010.

Goswami K, Parvii J, Courtney PM: Current recommendations for the diagnosis of acute and chronic PJI for hip and knee – cell counts, alpha-defensin, leukocyte esterase, next-generation sequencing, *Curr Rev Musculoskelet Med* 11:428, 2018.

Govaert GA, Ijpma FF, NcNalley M, et al.: Accuracy of diagnostic imaging modalities for peripheral post-traumatic osteomyelitis – a systematic review of the recent literature, *Eur J Nucl Med Mol Imaging* 44(8):1393, 2017.

Gratz S, Reize P, Kemke B, et al.: Targeting osteomyelitis with complete [99mTc]besilesomab and fragmented [99mTc]sulesomab antibodies: kinetic evaluations, *Q J Nucl Med Mol Imaging* 60(4):413, 2016.

Kheir MM, Tan TL, Ackerman CT, et al.: Culturing periprosthetic joint infection: number of samples, growth duration, and organisms, *J Arthroplasty* 33(11):3531, 2018.

Lee YS, Koo KH, Kim HJ, et al.: Synovial fluid biomarkers for the diagnosis of periprosthetic joint infection: a systematic review and meta-analysis, *J Bone Joint Surg Am* 299(24):2077, 2017.

Liu H, Zhang Y, Li L, Zou HC: The application of sonication in diagnosis of periprosthetic joint infection, *Eur J Clin Microbiol Infect Dis* 36(1):1, 2017.

Palestro CJ: FDG-PET in musculoskeletal infections, *Semin Nucl Med* 43:367, 2013.

Mitchell D, Perez J, Grau L, et al.: Systematic review of novel synovial fluid markers and polymerase chain reaction in the diagnosis of prosthetic joint infection, *Am J Orthop (Bell Mead NJ)* 46(4):190, 2017.

Okroj KT, Calkins TE, Kayupov E, et al.: The alpha-defensin test for diagnosing periprosthetic joint infection in the setting of an adverse local tissue reaction secondary to a failed meta-on-metal bearing or corrosion at the head-neck junction, *J Arthroplasty* 33:1896, 2018.

Parvizi J, Tan TL, Goswami K, et al.: The 2018 definition of periprosthetic hip and knee infection: an evidence-based and validated criteria, *J Arthroplasty* 33:1309, 2018.

Rothenberg AC, Wilson AE, Hayes JP, et al.: Sonication of arthroplasty implants improves accuracy of periprosthetic joint infection cultures, *Clin Orthop Relat Res* 475(7):1827, 2017.

Saleh A, George J, Faour M, Klika AK, Higuera CA: Serum biomarkers in periprosthetic joint infections, *Bone Joint Res* 7(1):85, 2018.

Saleh A, Ramanthan D, Siqueira MBP, et al.: The diagnostic utility of synovial fluid markers in periprosthetic joint infection: a systematic review and metaanalysis, *J Am Acad Orthop Surg* 25(11):763, 2017.

Shohat N, Bauer T, Buttaro M, et al.: Hip and knee section. What is the definition of a periprosthetic joint infection (PJI) of the knee and hip? Can the same criteria be used for both joints?: Proceedings of international consensus on orthopedic infections, *J Arthroplasty* 34(2S):S325, 2019.

Singhal R, Perry DC, Khan FN, et al.: The use of CRP within a clinical prediction algorithm for the differentiation of septic arthritis and transient synovitis in children, *J Bone Joint Surg* 93B(1556), 2011.

Soldatos T, Durand DJ, Subhawong TK, et al.: Magnetic resonance imaging of musculoskeletal infections, *Acad Radiol* 19:1434, 2012.

Sousa R, Massada M, Pereira A, Fontes F, et al.: Diagnostic accuracy of combined 99mTc-sulesomab and 99mTC-nanocolloid bone marrow imaging in detecting prosthetic joint infection, *Nucl med Commun* 32(9):834, 2011.

Suen K, Keeka M, Ailabouni R, Tran P: Synovasure 'quick test' is not as accurate as the laboratory-based a-defensin immunoassay: a systematic review and meta-analysis, *Bone Joint J* 100-B(1):66, 2018.

Turecki MB, Taljanovic MS, Stubbs AY, et al.: Imaging of musculoskeletal soft-tissue infections, *Skeletal Radiol* 39:957, 2010.

Verberne SJ, Raijmakers PG, Temmerman OPP: The accuracy of imaging techniques in the assessment of periprosthetic hip infection, *J Bone Joint Surg Am* 98:1638, 2016.

Wang C, Li R, Wang Q, Wang C: Synovial fluid leukocyte esterase in the diagnosis of periprosthetic joint infection: a systematic review and meta-analysis, *Surg Infect (Larchmt)* 19(3):245, 2018.

TREATMENT

Al-Houraibi RK, Aalirezaie A, Adib F, et al.: General assembly, prevention, wound management: proceedings of international consensus on orthopedic infections, *J Arthroplasty* 34(2S):S157, 2019.

Alt V: Antimicrobial coated implants in trauma and orthopaedics-A clinical review and risk-benefit analysis, *Injury* 48(3):599, 2017.

American Academy of Orthopaedic Surgeons: Appropriate use criteria for the management of patients with orthopaedic implants undergoing dental procedures. 2016, Available at www.OrthoGuidelines.org/auc. Accessed 4 January 2019.

Boisrenout P: *Cutibacterium acnes* prosthetic joint infection: diagnosis and treatment, *Orthop Traumatol Surg Res* 104:S19, 2018.

Boyle K, Kuo FC, Horcajada JP, et al.: General assembly, treatment, antimicrobials: proceedings of international consensus on orthopedic infections, *J Arthroplasty* 34(2S):S225, 2019.

El-Husseiny M, Patel S, MacFarlane RJ, Haddad FS: Biodegradable antibiotic delivery systems, *J Bone Joint Surg* 93B:151, 2011.

Ferguson JY, Dudareva M, Riley ND: The use of a biodegradable antibiotic-loaded calcium sulphate carrier containing tobramycin for the treatment of chronic osteomyelitis, *J Bone Joint Surg* 96B:829, 2014.

Gross L: *AAOS, ADA release CPG for prophylactic antibiotics*, AAOS Now, 2013.

Henry MW, Miller AO, Walsh TJ, Brause BD: Fungal musculoskeletal infections, *Infect Dis Clin North Am* 31(2):353, 2017.

Kaplan SL: Recent lessons for the management of bone and joint infections, *J Infect* 68:S51, 2014.

Kortram K, Bezstarosti H, Metsemakers WJ, et al.: Risk factors for infectious complications after open fractures: a systematic review and meta-analysis, *Int Orthop* 41(10):1964, 2017.

Lee CY, Huang CH, Lu PL, et al.: Role of rifampin for the treatment of bacterial infections other than mycobacteriosis, *J Infect* 75(5):395, 2017.

Lundy D, McLaren A, Sturm PF, et al: American Academy of Orthopaedic Surgeons Board of Directors systematic literature review on the management of surgical site infections June 9, 2018. Available at. www.aaos.org/ssi. Accessed January 4, 2019.

Matsen KLJ, Yoo JY, Maltenfort M, et al.: The effect of implementing a multimodal approach on the rates of periprosthetic joint infection after total joint arthroplasty, *J Arthroplasty* 31(2):451, 2016.

Morata L, Senneville E, Bernard L, et al.: A retrospective review of the clinical experience of Linezolid with or without rifampicin in prosthetic joint infections treated with debridement and implant retention, *Infect Dis Ther* 3(2):235, 2014.

Parker AC, Jennings JA, Bumgardner JD, et al.: Preliminary investigation of crosslinked chitosan sponges for tailorable drug delivery and infection control, *J Biomed Mater Res* 101B:110, 2013.

Pereira LC, Kerr J, Jolles BM: Intra-articular steroid infection for osteoarthritis of the hip prior to total hip arthroplasty: is it safe? A systematic review, *Bone Joint J* 98-B(8):1027.

Pinder EM, Ong JC, Bale RS, Trail IA: Ten questions on prosthetic shoulder infection, *Shoulder Elbow* 8(3):151, 2016.

Rahaman MN, Bal BS, Huang W: Review: emerging developments in the use of bioactive glasses for treating infected prosthetic joints, *Mater Sci Eng C Mater Biol Appl* 41:224, 2014.

Ratta N, Arrigoni C, Rosso F, et al.: Total knee arthroplasty and infection: how surgeons can reduce the risks, 1:339, 2016.

Riesgo AM, Park BK, Herrero CP, et al.: Vancomycin povidone-iodine protocol improves survivorship of periprosthetic joint infection treated with irrigation and debridement, *J Arthroplasty* 33:847, 2018.

Riley LP: Evidence insufficient to recommend routine antibiotics for joint replacement patients who undergo dental procedures. Available at: newsroom.aaos.org/media-resources/Press-releases/evidence-insufficient-to-recommend-routine-antibiotics-for-joint-replacement-patients-who-undergo-dental-procedures.htm.

Romanó CL, DeVecchi E, Bortolin M, et al.: Hyaluronic acid and its composites as a local antimicrobial/antiadhesive barrier, *J Bone Jt Infect* 2(1):63, 2017.

Ruder JA, Springer BD: Treatment of periprosthetic joint infection using antimicrobials: dilute povidone-iodine lavage, *J Bone Joint Infect* 2(1):10, 2017.

Wentao Z, Lei G, Liu Y, et al.: Approach to osteomyelitis treatment with antibiotic loaded PMMA, *Microb Pathog* 102:42, 2017.

HUMAN IMMUNODEFICIENCY VIRUS

American Academy of Orthopaedic Surgeons: Information Statement: Preventing the transmission of bloodborne pathogens. 2001, revised 2008, reviewed 2012. PDF available at www.AAOS.org. Accessed 4 January 2019.

AVERTing AIDS, HIV: Worldwide HIV & AIDS statistics: 2009 AIDS epidemic update. Available at www.avert.org/worldstats.htm. Accessed 5 October 2010.

Bader MS, McKinsey DS: Postexposure prophylaxis for common infectious diseases, *Am Fam Physician* 88:25, 2013.

Centers for Disease Control and Prevention: Surveillance of occupationally acquired HIV/AIDS in healthcare personnel as of December 2006. Available at www.cdc.gov/HAI/organisms/hiv/Surveillance-Occupationally-Acquired-HIV-AIDS.html. Accessed October 5, 2010.

Centers for Disease Control and Prevention: HIV in the United States. Available at www.cdc.gov/hiv. Accessed November 18, 2010.

Centers for Disease Control and Prevention, Hepatitis C: 2010 *STD treatment guidelines*, 2010, Available at http://www.cdc.gov/std/treatment/2010/hepc.htm. .

Centers for Disease Control and Prevention: HIV in the United States: at a glance, Available at http://www.cdc.gov/hiv/statistics/basics/ataglance.html. Accessed January 8, 2015.

Centers for Disease Control and Prevention: Occupational HIV transmission and prevention among health care workers, www.cdc.gov/hiv/risk/other/occupational.html. Accessed January 4, 2019.

Centers for Disease Control: US Public Health Service Preexposure Prophylaxis for the Prevention of HIV Infection in the United States – 2017 Update. A clinical practical guideline. Available at HYPERLINK "https://www.cdc.gov/hiv/pdf/risk/prep/cdc-hiv-prep-guidelines-2017.pdf" https://www.cdc.gov/hiv/pdf/risk/prep/cdc-hiv-prep-guidelines-2017.pdf . Accessed January 4, 2019.

Egro FM, Nwaiwu CA, Smith S, et al.: Seroconversion rates among health care workers exposed to hepatitis C virus-contaminated body fluids: the University of Pittsburgy 13-year experience, *Am J Infect Control* 45:1001, 2017.

Enayatollahi MA, Murphy D, Maltenfort MG, Parvizi J: Human immunodeficiency virus and total joint arthroplasty: the risk for infection is reduced, *J Arthroplasty* 31(10):2146, 2016.

Ford N, Mayer KH: World Health Organization guidelines on postexposure prophylaxis for HIV: recommendations for a public health approach, *CID* 60(Suppl 3):S161, 2015.

Grabowski G, Pilato A, Clark C, Jackson JB: HIV in orthopaedic surgery, *J Am Acad Orthop Surg* 25(8):569, 2017.

Graves N, Wloch C, Wilson J, et al.: A cost-effectiveness modelling study of strategies to reduce risk of infection following primary hip replacement based on a systematic review, *Health Technol Assess* 20:54, 2016.

Henderson DK: Management of needlestick injuries: a house officer who has a needlestick, *JAMA* 307:75, 2012.

Kigera JWM, Straetemans M, Vuhaka SK, et al.: Is there an increased risk of post-operative surgical site infection after orthopaedic surgery in HIV patients? A systematic review and meta-analysis, *PLoS ONE* 8:e42254, 2012.

Kuhar DT, Henderson DK, Struble KA: Updated US public health service guidelines for the management of occupational exposures to human immunodeficiency virus and recommendations for postexposure prophylaxis, Infect Control Hosp Epidemiol 34:875, 2013. Erratum: *Infect Control Hosp Epidemiol* 34:1238, 2013.

Nwaiwu CA, Egro FM, Smith S, et al.: Seroconversion rate among health care workers exposed to HIV-contaminated body fluids: The University of Pittsburgh 13-year experience, *Am J Infect Control* 45:896, 2017.

Pretell-Mazzini J, Subhawong T, Hernandez VH, Campo R: Current concepts review. HIV and orthopaedics, *J Bone Joint Surg Am* 98:775, 2016.

Sacomanno MF, Ammassari A: Bone disease in HIV infection, *Clin Cases Miner Bone Metab* 8:33, 2011.

Weber DJ, Rutala WA: Occupational health update. Focus on preventing the acquisition of infections with pre-exposure prophylaxis and postexposure prophylaxis, *Infect Dis Clin N Am* 30:729, 2016.

Wittmann A, Kralj N, Köver J, et al.: Study of blood contact in simulated surgical needlestick injuries with single or double latex gloving, *Infect Control Hosp Epidemiol* 30:53, 2009.

World Health Organization: HIV/Aids Fact Sheet N 360, 2014. Available at: http://www.who.int/mediacentre/factsheets/fs360/en/. Accessed September 25, 2015.

World Health Organization Regional Office for the Western Pacific: Fact sheets: 3 × 5—responding to a global crisis. Available at www.wpro.who.int/mediacentre/releases/2004/20040916_2/en/.

World Health Organization: HIV/AIDS Guidelines on post-exposure prophylaxis for HIV and the use of co-trimoxazole prophylaxis for HIV-related infections among adults, adolescents, and children. 2014, Available at https://www.who.int/hiv/pub/guidelines/arv2013/arvs2013upplement_dec2014/en/. Accessed 4 January 2019.

Wyzgowski P, Rosiek A, Grzela T, Leksowski K: Occupational HIV risk for health care workers: risk factor and the risk of infection in the course of professional activities, *Ther Clin Risk Manag* 12:989, 2016.

The complete list of references is available online at Expert Consult.com.

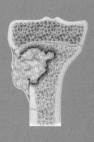

Osteomyelitis has long been one of the most difficult and challenging problems confronted by orthopaedic surgeons. Currently, morbidity and mortality from osteomyelitis are relatively low because of modern treatment methods, including the use of antibiotics and aggressive surgical treatment. The key to successful management is early diagnosis and appropriate surgical and antimicrobial treatment. A multidisciplinary approach is required, involving an orthopaedic surgeon, an infectious disease specialist, and a plastic surgeon in complex cases with significant soft-tissue loss. In addition, these patients may benefit from nutritional and psychological counseling. Osteomyelitis is defined as an inflammation of the bone caused by an infecting organism. The infection may be limited to a single portion of the bone or may involve numerous regions, such as the marrow, cortex, periosteum, and the surrounding soft tissue. The infection generally is due to a single organism, but polymicrobial infections can occur, especially in the diabetic foot.

CLASSIFICATION

Classification of osteomyelitis is based on numerous criteria, such as the duration and mechanism of infection and the type of host response to the infection. Hotchen et al. reviewed 13 different classification systems proposed for osteomyelitis and identified seven different variables in these systems. The authors concluded that the most important of these variables were bone involvement, antimicrobial resistance patterns, need for soft-tissue coverage, and host status. Osteomyelitis is traditionally classified as *acute, subacute,* or *chronic,* depending on the duration of symptoms. The time limits defining these classes are arbitrary, however. The mechanism of infection can be *exogenous* or *hematogenous.* Exogenous osteomyelitis is caused by open fractures, surgery (iatrogenic), or contiguous spread from infected local tissue. The hematogenous form results from bacteremia. Osteomyelitis also can be classified as *pyogenic* or *nonpyogenic,* based on the host response to the disease. Cierny and Mader proposed a classification system for chronic osteomyelitis based on host factors and anatomic criteria. This system is described further in the section on chronic osteomyelitis. Classification in this chapter is based on duration of symptoms (acute, subacute, and chronic) and mechanism of infection (exogenous or hematogenous).

ACUTE HEMATOGENOUS OSTEOMYELITIS

Acute hematogenous osteomyelitis is the most common type of bone infection and usually is seen in children. The incidence of acute hematogenous osteomyelitis has dramatically decreased over the past several decades. A higher standard of living and improved hygiene probably have contributed to this trend. Acute hematogenous osteomyelitis is more common in males in all age groups affected. It is caused by a bacteremia, which is a common occurrence in childhood. The causes of bacteremia are many. Bacteriologic seeding of bone generally is associated with other factors such as localized trauma, chronic illness, malnutrition, or an inadequate immune system. In many cases, the exact cause of the disease cannot be identified.

In children, the infection generally involves the metaphyses of rapidly growing long bones. Bacterial seeding leads to an inflammatory reaction, which can cause local ischemic necrosis of bone and subsequent abscess formation. As the abscess enlarges, intramedullary pressure increases causing cortical ischemia, which may allow purulent material to escape through the cortex into the subperiosteal space. A subperiosteal abscess then develops (Fig. 4.1). If left untreated,

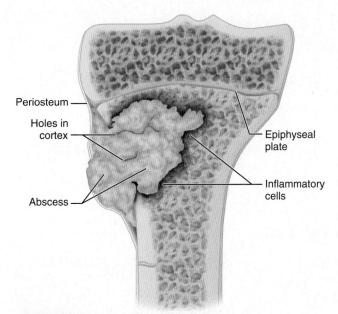

FIGURE 4.1 Pathophysiology of hematogenous seeding. When under pressure, exudate or abscess can extend through Volkmann canals into subperiosteal region and from there into medullary cavity or epiphysis.

this process eventually results in extensive formation of sequestra and in chronic osteomyelitis. The age distribution of acute hematogenous osteomyelitis in children is bimodal, generally affecting children younger than age 2 years and children between the ages of 8 to 12 years. Half of all children with osteomyelitis are younger than 5 years of age. The effects of osteomyelitis in children vary with age based on differences in blood supply and the anatomic structure of the bone.

In children younger than 2 years, some blood vessels cross the physis and may allow the spread of infection into the epiphysis. For this reason, infants are susceptible to limb shortening or angular deformity if the physis or epiphysis is damaged by infection. Otherwise, the physis acts as a barrier that prevents the direct spread of a metaphyseal abscess into the epiphysis. The metaphysis has relatively fewer phagocytic cells than the physis or diaphysis, allowing infection to occur more easily in this area. A resulting abscess breaks through the thin metaphyseal cortex, forming a subperiosteal abscess. The diaphysis rarely is involved, and extensive sequestration occurs infrequently except in the most severe cases.

In children older than 2 years, the physis effectively acts as a barrier to the spread of a metaphyseal abscess. Because the metaphyseal cortex in older children is thicker, the diaphysis is at greater risk in these patients. If the infection spreads into the diaphysis, the endosteal blood supply may be jeopardized. With a concurrent subperiosteal abscess, the periosteal blood supply is damaged and can result in extensive sequestration and chronic osteomyelitis if not properly treated.

After the physes are closed, acute hematogenous osteomyelitis is much less common. Hematogenous seeding of bone in adults is often seen in a compromised host. Although it can occur anywhere and in any part of the bone, generally the vertebral bodies are affected. In these patients, abscesses spread slowly and large sequestra rarely form. If localized destruction of cortical bone occurs, pathologic fracture can result (Fig. 4.2).

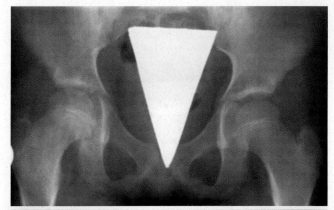

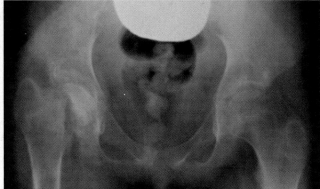

FIGURE 4.2 Pathologic fracture after destruction of cortical bone by infection.

Spread of infection to a contiguous joint also is affected by the patient's age. In children younger than 2 years, the common blood supply of the metaphysis and epiphysis crosses the physis and can allow spread of a metaphyseal abscess into the epiphysis and eventually into the joint. The hip joint is the most commonly affected in young patients; however, the physes of the proximal humerus, radial neck, and distal fibula also are intraarticular, and infection in these areas can lead to septic arthritis as well. In severe infection, epiphyseal separation can occur in children younger than 2 years (Fig. 4.3). In older children, this common circulation is no longer present, and septic arthritis is less common. After the physes are closed, infection can extend directly from the metaphysis into the epiphysis and involve the joint. Septic arthritis resulting from acute hematogenous osteomyelitis is generally seen only in infants and adults.

Staphylococcus aureus is the most common infecting organism found in older children and adults with osteomyelitis. Gram-negative bacteria have been found to cause an increasing number of vertebral body infections in adults. *Pseudomonas* is the most common infecting organism found in intravenous drug abusers with osteomyelitis. Fungal osteomyelitis is seen increasingly in chronically ill patients receiving long-term intravenous therapy or parenteral nutrition. *Salmonella* osteomyelitis has long been associated with sickle cell or sickle cell C hemoglobinopathies. This infection tends to be diaphyseal rather than metaphyseal (Fig. 4.4).

In infants with acute hematogenous osteomyelitis, *S. aureus* is still a frequent isolate, but group B *Streptococcus* and

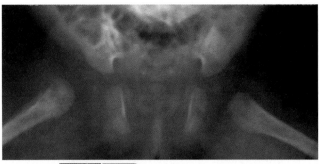
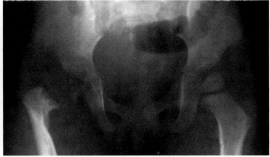

FIGURE 4.3   Epiphyseal separation caused by infection in young child.

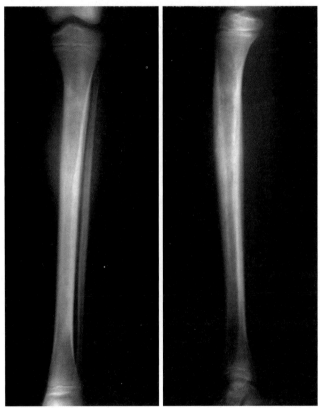

FIGURE 4.4   Osteomyelitis of tibia in sickle cell patient.

BOX 4.1

Evaluation of Acute Hematogenous Osteomyelitis

- History and physical examination
- Laboratory tests: white blood cell count, erythrocyte sedimentation rate, C-reactive protein
- Plain radiographs
- Technetium-99m bone scan ± MRI
- Aspiration for suspected abscess

---

gram-negative coliforms also are commonly found. *S. aureus* or gram-negative organisms are the usual cause of orthopaedic infections found in premature infants undergoing treatment in the neonatal intensive care unit; more than 40% have multifocal involvement. Group B *Streptococcus* is the most likely infecting organism found in otherwise healthy infants 2 to 4 weeks old. *Haemophilus influenzae* infections occur primarily in children 6 months to 4 years old. The incidence of this infection has been reduced dramatically because of routine immunizations against the organism. More recently, there has been a dramatic rise in the number of children with methicillin-resistant *S. aureus* (MRSA), community-acquired MRSA, and *Kingella kingae* infections, which are associated with increased complications. *K. kingae* is a slow growing gram-negative aerobic coccobacillus that is being recognized more frequently as the cause of osteomyelitis, especially in children younger than 4 years. This pathogen is difficult to isolate on routine cultures and often requires molecular

assays such as polymerase chain reaction. For these resistant bacteria, optimizing diagnostic strategies, such as MRI and serum inflammatory markers, is necessary. The white blood cell count, C-reactive protein, erythrocyte sedimentation rate, and absolute neutrophil counts have been found to be significantly higher in resistant bacteria, as well as temperature, respiratory, and heart rate. Dietrich et al., using multivariate regression analysis, determined a set of variables that distinguished MRSA from MSSA with 87% accuracy. They found that elevated temperature, C-reactive protein, and absolute neutrophil counts were copredictors of MRSA osteomyelitis.

DIAGNOSIS

The evaluation of acute hematogenous osteomyelitis should begin with a history and physical examination (Box 4.1). Signs and symptoms can vary significantly. In infants, elderly patients, or immunocompromised patients, clinical findings may be minimal. Fever and malaise may or may not be present in the early stages of the disease, with up to 40% of children reportedly afebrile upon hospital admission, but pain and local tenderness are common findings. Swelling may be significant, and compartment syndrome has been reported in children.

The white blood cell count is often normal, but the erythrocyte sedimentation rate and C-reactive protein level are usually elevated. The C-reactive protein is a measurement of the acute-phase response and is especially useful in monitoring the course of treatment of acute osteomyelitis because it normalizes much sooner than the erythrocyte sedimentation rate.

Standard radiographs are generally negative but may show soft-tissue swelling. Although soft-tissue swelling may be seen 1 to 3 days after the start of the infection, skeletal changes, such as periosteal reaction or bony destruction, are generally not seen on plain films until 10 to 12 days into the infection (Fig. 4.5). Conditions that may be mistaken for osteomyelitis on plain radiographs include septic arthritis, Ewing sarcoma, osteosarcoma, juvenile arthritis, sickle cell crises, Gaucher

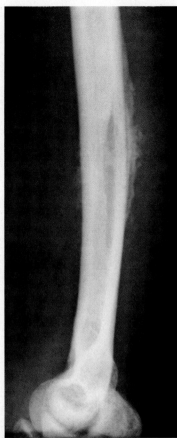

FIGURE 4.5   Radiograph showing bony destruction.

disease, and stress fractures. MRI can show early inflammatory changes in bone marrow and soft tissue and is very useful for detecting intraosseous and subperiosteal abscesses. On T1-weighted MR images, osteomyelitis typically has low signal intensity; on T2-weighted and short-tau inversion recovery (STIR) images, it has a high marrow signal intensity. Although the sensitivity of MRI for the diagnosis of osteomyelitis is high (approximately 98%), the specificity is much lower (around 75%). One study found that nearly 60% of uncomplicated septic joint effusions demonstrated abnormal marrow signal intensity that was mistaken for osteomyelitis. Although MRI is helpful for early diagnosis and is the primary imaging modality for osteomyelitis at our institution, repeat MRI has not been found to be particularly useful in assessing progress of treatment. Repeat MRI may be necessary, however, in patients who have failed to respond to initial treatment or those with persistently high C-reactive protein levels.

Technetium-99m bone scans can confirm the diagnosis 24 to 48 hours after onset in 90% to 95% of patients (Fig. 4.6); a negative technetium-99m bone scan effectively rules out the diagnosis of osteomyelitis. Gallium scans and indium-111-labeled leukocyte scans can also aid in diagnosis when used in conjunction with technetium scanning. The use of bone scans has decreased with the increase in the use of MRI.

Ultrasonography has been used for differentiating acute hematogenous osteomyelitis from cellulitis, soft-tissue abscess, acute septic arthritis, and malignant bone tumors in children; however, this modality is highly operator-dependent, with a diagnostic accuracy of only about 60%. Labbé et al. noted that although ultrasonography only detected osteomyelitis in 64% on the day of admission, by the second day, it positively diagnosed 84%. Other diagnostic modalities currently being investigated include radiolabeled antibiotics scanning, fluorodeoxyglucose-labeled positron emission tomography

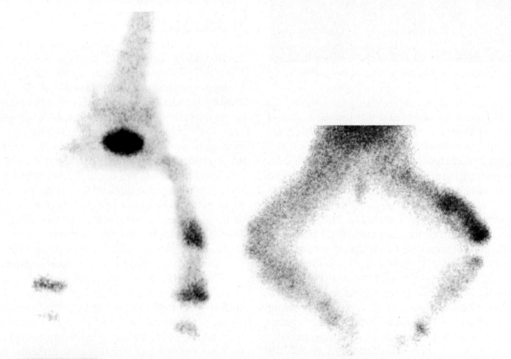

FIGURE 4.6   Bone scan showing increased uptake in area of osteomyelitis.

(FDG-PET), and single photon emission computed tomography (SPECT).

The causative organism can be identified in approximately 50% of patients through blood cultures. Bone aspiration usually gives an accurate bacteriologic diagnosis and should be performed with a 16- or 18-gauge needle in the area of maximal swelling and tenderness, usually the long bone metaphysis. The subperiosteal space should be aspirated first by inserting the needle to the level of the outer cortex. If no purulent material or fluid is encountered, the needle is placed through the cortex to obtain a marrow aspirate. Patients with suspected osteomyelitis of the hip or vertebra should have CT- or ultrasound-assisted aspiration. The sample is sent to the laboratory for Gram stain, culture, and sensitivities.

TREATMENT

Appropriate treatment shortly after onset of acute hematogenous osteomyelitis can significantly lower morbidity. In 2019, Robinette et al. proposed an institutional quality improvement algorithm for children with acute hematogenous osteomyelitis that safely decreased hospital costs but did not alter the overall length of stay. De Ronde et al. described a stewardship approach for pediatric acute osteomyelitis that used clinical pathways, testing algorithms, and monitoring of antibiotic therapy as potential areas of quality care improvement. Surgery and antibiotic treatment are complementary, and in some patients antibiotic treatment alone cures the disease; in others, prolonged antibiotic treatment is doomed to failure without surgical treatment. The choice of antibiotic is based on the highest bactericidal activity, the least toxicity, and the lowest cost.

It has been well established that sequestered abscesses demand surgical drainage. Areas of simple inflammation without abscess formation can be treated with antibiotics alone. In 1983, Nade proposed five principles for the treatment of acute hematogenous osteomyelitis that are still applicable today: (1) an appropriate antibiotic is effective before abscess formation; (2) antibiotics do not sterilize avascular tissues or abscesses, and such areas require surgical removal; (3) if such removal is effective, antibiotics should prevent their reformation, and primary wound closure should be safe; (4) surgery should not damage further already ischemic bone and soft tissue; and (5) antibiotics should be continued after surgery.

A patient suspected to have acute hematogenous osteomyelitis should be evaluated as previously outlined. The patient should receive general supportive care consisting of intravenous fluids, appropriate analgesics, and comfortable positioning of the affected limb. Frequent serial examinations should be done. If an abscess requiring surgical drainage is not found by MRI or ultrasound, empirical intravenous antibiotic therapy should be started, and the patient should be carefully monitored. The C-reactive protein value should be checked every 2 to 3 days after the initiation of antibiotic therapy. If no appreciable clinical response to antibiotic treatment is noted within 24 to 48 hours, occult abscesses must be sought and surgical drainage should be considered. The two main indications for surgery in acute hematogenous osteomyelitis are (1) the presence of an abscess requiring drainage and (2) failure of the patient to improve despite appropriate intravenous antibiotic treatment. One 10-year review of 813 children with *S. aureus* acute hematogenous osteomyelitis found that 44% of patients required surgery and 7% had recurrence; the average length of antibiotic treatment was 44 days.

The objective of surgery is to drain any abscess cavity and remove all nonviable or necrotic tissue. When a subperiosteal abscess is found in an infant, several small holes should be drilled through the cortex into the medullary canal. If intramedullary pus is found, a small window of bone is removed. The skin is closed loosely over drains, and the limb is splinted. The limb is protected for several weeks to prevent pathologic fracture. Intravenous antibiotics should be continued postoperatively. The duration of antibiotic therapy is controversial; however, the current trend is toward a shorter course of intravenous antibiotics, followed by oral antibiotics and monitoring of serum antibiotic levels. This schedule should be determined on an individual basis and in collaboration with an infectious disease consultant.

DRAINAGE OF ACUTE HEMATOGENOUS OSTEOMYELITIS

The technique for draining acute osteomyelitis of the tibia is described. The technique and principles for drainage in other long bones are similar. Approaches for various anatomic areas are described in other chapter.

TECHNIQUE 4.1

- Use a tourniquet whenever possible. Elevate the extremity for a few minutes before inflating the tourniquet. Do not exsanguinate the limb with an elastic bandage if infection is present.
- Make an anteromedial incision 5.0 to 7.5 cm long over the affected part of the tibia.
- Incise the periosteum longitudinally. It may be elevated from bone by a subperiosteal abscess; if so, the compressed pus will escape.
- If no abscess is found, gently elevate the periosteum 1.5 cm on each side. Try to strip as little periosteum as possible; the more periosteum that is stripped, the more an already compromised blood supply to bone is damaged.
- Drill several holes 4 mm in diameter through the cortex into the medullary canal, regardless of whether a subperiosteal abscess is present. If pus escapes through these holes, use a drill to outline a cortical window 1.3 × 2.5 cm and remove the cortex with an osteotome.
- Evacuate the intramedullary pus and gently remove any necrotic tissue.
- Irrigate the cavity with at least 3 L of saline. Antibiotics may be placed in the irrigation solution.
- Close the skin loosely over drains, but do not close the wound if this produces excessive tension on the skin.

POSTOPERATIVE CARE A long leg posterior plaster splint is applied with the foot in a neutral position, the ankle at 90 degrees, and the knee at 20 degrees of flexion. When the wound has healed, the splint is removed and protected weight bearing with crutches is begun. The patient is placed on antibiotics based on culture sensitivities. Generally, a 6-week course of intravenous antibiotics is given. Orthopaedic and infectious disease follow-up is continued for at least 1 year.

SUBACUTE HEMATOGENOUS OSTEOMYELITIS

Compared with acute osteomyelitis, subacute hematogenous osteomyelitis has a more insidious onset and lacks the severity of symptoms, which makes the diagnosis of this disorder difficult. Subacute osteomyelitis is relatively common, reported to occur in over a third of patients with primary bone infections. Currently, no definitive guidelines exist for diagnosis, and recommendations are based on expert opinions and case series.

Because of the indolent course of subacute osteomyelitis, diagnosis typically is delayed for more than 2 weeks. Systemic signs and symptoms are minimal. Temperature is only mildly elevated if at all. Mild-to-moderate pain is one of the only consistent signs suggesting the diagnosis. White blood cell counts generally are normal. The erythrocyte sedimentation rate is elevated in only 50% of patients, and blood cultures usually are negative. Even with an adequate bone aspirate or biopsy specimen, a pathogen is identified only 60% of the time. Plain radiographs and bone scans generally are positive (Fig. 4.7).

The indolent course of subacute osteomyelitis is thought to be the result of increased host resistance, decreased bacterial virulence, or the administration of antibiotics before the onset of symptoms. It is speculated that the combination of an organism of low virulence with a strong host response may allow the inflammation to persist in bone without producing significant signs or symptoms. Nevertheless, correct diagnosis largely depends on clinical suspicion and radiographic findings.

A radiographic classification of subacute hematogenous osteomyelitis was described by Gledhill and modified by Roberts et al. (Table 4.1 and Fig. 4.8). Differentiating these lesions from a primary bone tumor can sometimes be difficult. There are no large series reporting MRI findings in subacute osteomyelitis, but MRI is warranted to help narrow the differential diagnosis and aid surgical planning. The diagnosis often must be established by an open biopsy and culture. Purulent material is not always obtained on biopsy, but granulation tissue is a common finding. *S. aureus* and *Staphylococcus epidermidis* are the predominant organisms identified in subacute osteomyelitis.

Biopsy and curettage followed by treatment with appropriate antibiotics generally are recommended for all lesions

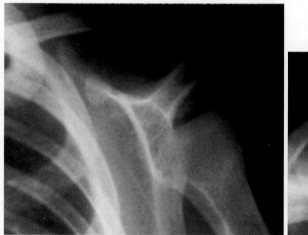
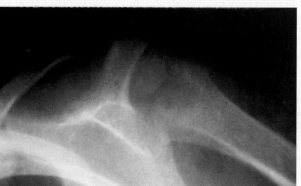

FIGURE 4.7   Subacute osteomyelitis of proximal humerus.

TABLE 4.1

Subacute Osteomyelitis

TYPE	GLEDHILL CLASSIFICATION	ROBERTS ET AL. CLASSIFICATION	DIFFERENTIAL DIAGNOSIS
I	Solitary localized zone of radiolucency surrounded by reactive new bone formation	Ia—Punched-out radiolucency Ib—Punched-out radiolucent lesion with sclerotic margin	Langerhans cell histiocytosis Brodie abscess
II	Metaphyseal radiolucencies with cortical erosion		Eosinophilic granuloma; osteogenic sarcoma
III	Cortical hyperostosis in diaphysis; no onion skin reaction	Localized cortical periosteal reaction	Osteoid osteoma
IV	Subperiosteal new bone and onion skin layering	Onion skin periosteal reaction	Ewing sarcoma
V		Central radiolucency in epiphysis	Chondroblastoma
VI		Destructive process involving vertebral body	Tuberculosis; osteogenic sarcoma

From Willis RB, Rozencwaig R: Pediatric osteomyelitis masquerading as skeletal neoplasia, *Orthop Clin North Am* 27:625, 1996.

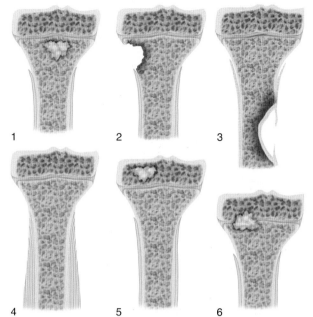

FIGURE 4.8 Classification of subacute osteomyelitis: *type 1*, central metaphyseal lesion; *type 2*, eccentric metaphyseal lesion with cortical erosion; *type 3*, diaphyseal cortical lesion; *type 4*, diaphyseal lesion with periosteal new bone formation, but without definite bony lesion; *type 5*, primary subacute epiphyseal osteomyelitis; and *type 6*, subacute osteomyelitis crossing physis to involve metaphysis and epiphysis.

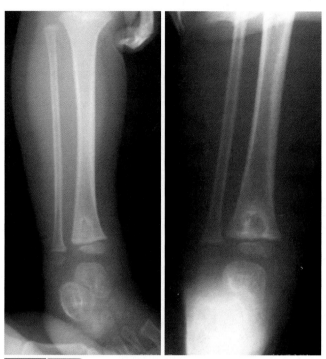

FIGURE 4.9 Brodie abscess in right distal tibial epiphysis of 3-year-old child.

that seem to be aggressive: "biopsy all cultures and culture all biopsies." For lesions that seem to be a simple abscess in the epiphysis or metaphysis, biopsy is not recommended. These lesions, which are characteristic of subacute hematogenous osteomyelitis, should be treated with intravenous antibiotics for 48 hours followed by a 6-week course of oral antibiotics.

Primary epiphyseal or apophyseal subacute osteomyelitis is a rare infection that usually only has mild symptoms and lacks a systemic reaction. In one study of 14 children, C-reactive protein and white blood cell count were normal, and the erythrocyte sedimentation rate was greater than 20 mm in eight of the patients. The pathogen, which included *K. kingae* in eight children and MRSA in one, was not identified on blood tests and required polymerase chain reaction assays for identification. Antibiotic treatment usually is sufficient in treating this infection.

BRODIE ABSCESS

A Brodie abscess is a localized form of subacute osteomyelitis that occurs most often in the long bones of the lower extremities of young adults. Before physeal closure, the metaphysis is most often affected. In adults, the metaphyseal-epiphyseal area is involved. Intermittent pain of long duration is the presenting complaint, along with local tenderness over the affected area. On plain radiographs, a Brodie abscess generally appears as a lytic lesion with a rim of sclerotic bone (Fig. 4.9), but it can have a markedly varied appearance. MRI can be helpful in the diagnosis because a Brodie abscess can be easily mistaken for a variety of neoplasms on plain radiographs.

Organisms of low virulence are believed to cause the lesion. *S. aureus* is cultured in 50% of patients; in 20%, the

culture is negative. This condition often requires an open biopsy with curettage to make the diagnosis. The wound should be closed loosely over a drain.

CHRONIC OSTEOMYELITIS

Chronic osteomyelitis is difficult to eradicate completely. Systemic symptoms may subside, but one or more foci in the bone may contain purulent material, infected granulation tissue, or a sequestrum (Fig. 4.10). Intermittent acute exacerbations may occur for years and often respond to rest and antibiotics. Chronic osteomyelitis is still a major cause of musculoskeletal morbidity in children around the world. The hallmark of chronic osteomyelitis is infected dead bone within a compromised soft-tissue envelope. The infected foci within the bone are surrounded by sclerotic, relatively avascular bone covered by a thickened periosteum and scarred muscle and subcutaneous tissue. This avascular envelope of scar tissue leaves systemic antibiotics essentially ineffective.

In chronic osteomyelitis, secondary infections are common, and sinus track cultures usually do not correlate with cultures obtained at bone biopsy. Multiple organisms may grow from cultures taken from sinus tracks and from open biopsy specimens of surrounding soft tissue and bone. In addition, patients with chronic osteomyelitis have been found to be at higher risk for deep vein thrombosis (DVT). The risk of DVT in patients with chronic osteomyelitis was twice that of controls in one study of over 24,000 patients. The use of daily aspirin therapy should be considered.

Eradication of chronic osteomyelitis generally requires aggressive surgical debridement and dead-space management combined with effective antibiotic treatment. Surgery is not always the best option, however, especially in compromised patients. Consider an ambulatory immunocompromised host

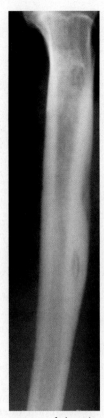

FIGURE 4.10   Sequestrum of chronic osteomyelitis in tibia.

TABLE 4.2

Cierny and Mader Staging System for Chronic Osteomyelitis

ANATOMIC TYPE		
I	Medullary	Endosteal disease
II	Superficial	Cortical surface infected because of coverage defect
III	Localized	Cortical sequestrum that can be excised without compromising stability
IV	Diffuse	Features of I, II, and III plus mechanical instability before or after debridement
PHYSIOLOGIC CLASS		
A host	Normal	Immunocompetent with good local vascularity
B host	Compromised	Local (L) or systemic (S) factors that compromise immunity or healing
C host	Prohibitive	Minimal disability, prohibitive morbidity anticipated, or poor prognosis for cure

Modified from Cierny G III, Mader JT: Adult chronic osteomyelitis: an overview. In: D'Ambrosia RD, Marier RL, editors: *Orthopedic Infections*, Thorofare, NJ, 1989, Slack.

with multiple medical problems, including chronic osteomyelitis of the femur. For this patient, who might not survive the extensive surgical stress required to eradicate the disease, less aggressive alternatives should be considered. Limited surgical debridement combined with suppressive antibiotics and nutritional support may limit the frequency of sinus drainage and pain in these difficult cases. The treatment course and definition of outcome success must be individualized for each patient.

Malignant transformation of chronic osteomyelitis has been reported, albeit rarely now. Although this complication is declining, it still occurs, and new signs of a chronic draining sinus, increased pain, and foul smell should raise the index of suspicion and biopsy should be considered. Squamous cell carcinoma is the most frequent malignancy reported, and definitive treatment is wide local excision or amputation combined with chemotherapy and radiation.

CLASSIFICATION

Cierny and Mader developed a classification system for chronic osteomyelitis, based on physiologic and anatomic criteria, to determine the stage of infection. The physiologic criteria are divided into three classes based on three types of hosts. Class A hosts have a normal response to infection and surgery. Class B hosts are compromised and have deficient wound healing capabilities. When the results of treatment are potentially more damaging than the presenting condition, the patient is considered a class C host.

Anatomic criteria consist of four types. Type I, a medullary lesion, is characterized by endosteal disease. In type II, superficial osteomyelitis is limited to the surface of the bone and infection is secondary to a coverage defect. Type

III is a localized infection involving a stable, well-demarcated lesion characterized by full-thickness cortical sequestration and cavitation (in this type, complete debridement of the area would not lead to instability). Type IV is a diffuse osteomyelitic lesion that creates mechanical instability, either at presentation or after appropriate treatment, and requires complex reconstruction (Table 4.2 and Fig. 4.11).

The anatomic and physiologic classes are combined to designate one of 12 clinical stages of chronic osteomyelitis. A type II lesion in a class A host is designated stage IIA osteomyelitis. This classification system is helpful in determining if treatment should be simple or complex, curative or palliative, and limb sparing or ablative.

Jones et al. later described a classification of chronic hematogenous osteomyelitis in children in which three main types were identified based on radiographic appearance: type A, Brodie abscess; type B, sequestrum involucrum; and type C, sclerotic. Type B, sequestrum involucrum, has four subtypes: B1, localized cortical sequestrum; B2, sequestrum with structural involucrum; B3, sequestrum with sclerotic involucrum; and B4, sequestrum without structural involucrum. Physeal damage is indicated by the addition of "P" (proximal) or "D" (distal) to the classification. Because chronic osteomyelitis is more common in developing countries where CT and MRI might not be available, the classification uses plain radiographs, but CT and MRI can add more information, such as the extent of sclerosis and the presence of sequestra not visible on plain radiographs.

DIAGNOSIS

The diagnosis of chronic osteomyelitis is based on clinical, laboratory, and imaging studies. The "gold standard" is to obtain

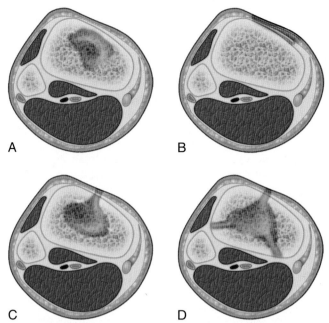

FIGURE 4.11　Anatomic classification of adult osteomyelitis. **A,** Type I, intramedullary osteomyelitis; nidus is endosteal. **B,** Type II, superficial osteomyelitis; limited to bone surface. **C,** Type III, localized osteomyelitis; full thickness of cortex is involved. **D,** Type IV, diffuse osteomyelitis; entire circumference of the bone is involved. (Redrawn from Parsons B, Strauss E: Surgical management of chronic osteomyelitis, *Am J Surg* 188[Suppl]:57S, 2004.)

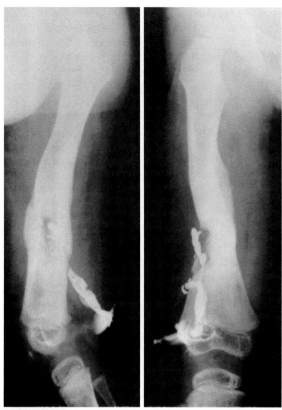

FIGURE 4.12　Radiographs made in two planes after injection of radiopaque liquid into sinus often are helpful in locating focus of infection in chronic osteomyelitis.

a biopsy specimen for histologic and microbiologic evaluation of the infected bone. Chronic osteomyelitis in our practice is most commonly seen after a traumatic injury. These cases are further complicated by the usual presence of implants and a high rate of associated fracture nonunion. Studies evaluating combat-related open femoral and tibial fractures showed that patients with severe muscle damage were at highest risk for osteomyelitis. Jorge et al. studied outcomes and risk factors for patients with polymicrobial posttraumatic osteomyelitis and determined that these infections have worse outcomes than monomicrobial infections. Not surprisingly, risk factors for polymicrobial osteomyelitis included advanced age, farm injuries, Gustilo type III injuries, need for blood transfusions, and need for multiple debridements. Bremmer et al. found a higher rate of osteomyelitis after long-bone fractures in patients with obesity.

Physical examination should focus on the integrity of the skin and soft tissue, determine areas of tenderness, assess bone stability, and evaluate the neurovascular status of the limb. Laboratory studies generally are nonspecific and give no indication of the severity of the infection. Erythrocyte sedimentation rate and C-reactive protein are elevated in most patients, but the white blood cell count is elevated in only 35%.

Multiple imaging studies are available to evaluate chronic osteomyelitis; however, no technique can absolutely confirm or exclude the presence of osteomyelitis. Imaging studies should be done to aid in confirmation of the diagnosis and to prepare for surgical treatment. Plain radiographs can yield valuable information in establishing a diagnosis of chronic osteomyelitis and should be the initial study performed. Signs of cortical destruction and periosteal reaction strongly

suggest the diagnosis of osteomyelitis. Sinography can be performed if a sinus track is present and can be a valuable adjunct to surgical planning (Fig. 4.12).

Isotopic bone scanning is more useful in acute osteomyelitis than in the chronic form because the former typically has negative plain films. Technetium-99m bone scans, which show increased uptake in areas of increased blood flow or osteoblastic activity, tend to lack specificity. This study has a high negative predictive value, although false-negative results have been reported. Gallium scans show increased uptake in areas where leukocytes or bacteria accumulate. A normal gallium scan virtually excludes the presence of osteomyelitis and can be useful as a follow-up examination after surgery. Indium-111–labeled leukocyte scans are more sensitive than technetium or gallium scans and are especially useful in differentiating chronic osteomyelitis from neuropathic arthropathy in the diabetic foot.

CT provides excellent definition of cortical bone and a fair evaluation of the surrounding soft tissues and is especially useful in identifying sequestra. MRI is more useful for soft-tissue evaluation than CT. MRI provides a fairly accurate determination of the extent of the pathologic insult by showing the margins of bone and soft-tissue edema.

In chronic osteomyelitis, MRI may reveal a well-defined rim of high signal intensity surrounding the focus of active disease *(rim sign)*. Sinus tracks and cellulitis appear as areas of increased signal intensity on T2-weighted imaging. Drawbacks include cost, difficulty imaging around metal implants, and poor delineation of cortical bone.

As previously noted, the "gold standard" in the diagnosis of osteomyelitis is a biopsy with culture and sensitivity. A biopsy is not only useful in establishing a diagnosis, but also is helpful in determining the proper antibiotic regimen. Typically, staphylococcal species are identified, especially in posttraumatic infections. Anaerobes and gram-negative bacilli are frequently isolated. Results of bone and soft-tissue biopsies may vary; both soft-tissue and bone specimens should be sent for microbiologic study.

TREATMENT

The treatment of chronic osteomyelitis requires a multifaceted approach. In addition to antibiotic suppression and surgical debridement and reconstruction, host morbidities need to be considered and measures taken to correct these, such as optimization of blood sugar levels in patients with diabetes, smoking cessation, and treatment of liver or renal malfunction. Chronic osteomyelitis generally cannot be eradicated without surgical treatment. Antibiotics alone can rarely eradicate the infection for numerous reasons. Bacteria are able to adhere to orthopaedic implants and bone matrix through various receptors. Some can hide intracellularly. Others can form a slimy coat that protects them from phagocytic cells and antibiotics.

Surgery for chronic osteomyelitis consists of sequestrectomy and resection of scarred and infected bone and soft tissue. For soft-tissue and dead-space management, ring external fixators generally are used after radical debridement. The goal of surgery is eradication of the infection by achieving a viable and vascular environment. Radical debridement often is required to achieve this goal. An oncologic approach of wide excision should be taken because success of treatment depends on adequacy of debridement.

The role of bacterial immunotherapy in the preoperative treatment of chronic osteomyelitis also has been evaluated by Fosco et al. In their study of 154 patients, this treatment was effective (62% healing) in patients with an already normal clinical status but was ineffective in those with a compromised clinical status.

Aytac et al. reported a technique, using irrigation, debridement, temporary hardware maintenance, and a persisting fistula, to control osteomyelitis (acute, subacute, or chronic) until fracture healing in patients who developed bacterial colonization after trauma or surgery. Bone healing was achieved in 89% of patients with no reinfections.

Extensive debridement generally creates a large dead space and bony instability that requires complex reconstruction of bone and soft tissue, often requiring multiple procedures. Antibiotic polymethyl methacrylate (PMMA) or calcium sulfate beads are typically used to fill the dead space created by the initial debridement. Bar-On et al. reported that reaming the intramedullary canal after debridement and lavage and inserting a gentamycin-impregnated rod and beads eradicated infection with minimal tissue loss in a case series of four patients.

Inadequate debridement may be one reason for a high recurrence rate in chronic osteomyelitis. Adequate debridement often leaves a large dead space that must be managed to prevent recurrence and significant bone loss that may result in bony instability. Appropriate reconstruction of the bone and soft-tissue defects is required, combined with culture-specific antibiotic therapy. Reconstruction should be undertaken only after careful planning and identification of sequestra and intraosseous abscesses by plain radiographs, sinography, CT, and MRI. The procedure should be performed in collaboration with an infectious disease consultant and, for the reconstructive phases, a plastic surgeon skilled in coverage techniques, such as skin grafts, muscle and myocutaneous flaps, and occasionally free flaps (Fig. 4.13). Although debridement with reconstruction is complex and costly, it is

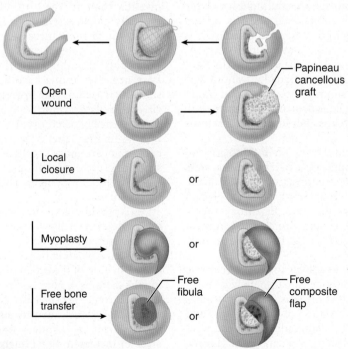

FIGURE 4.13   Four basic methods of immediate biologic management of dead space using living tissue or cancellous bone grafts.

an attractive alternative to amputation or long-term antibiotic treatment and has good clinical outcomes.

Negative-pressure wound therapy (NPWT) devices also may be efficacious in wound closure because not only does it assist in clearing the bacteria, but it promotes granulation tissue and decreases soft-tissue edema. In addition, the use of NPWT may reduce the need for muscle flaps or tissue transfer.

The duration of postoperative antibiotics is controversial. Traditionally, a 6-week course of intravenous antibiotics is prescribed after surgical debridement of chronic osteomyelitis. No solid evidence exists for the long-term use of antibiotics. Fluoroquinolone antibiotics are known to have equivalent serum concentrations whether given orally or intravenously. When deemed appropriate, based on culture sensitivities, oral administration is preferred. The addition of rifampin to other antibiotics also may improve cure rates. Our practice is to place the patient on 6 weeks of antibiotics, typically given intravenously, based on sensitivity and under the direction of an infectious disease specialist, followed by clinical, radiographic, and laboratory examinations.

SEQUESTRECTOMY AND CURETTAGE FOR CHRONIC OSTEOMYELITIS

Sequestrectomy and curettage require more time to perform and result insignificant blood loss. Consequently, appropriate preparation should be made before surgery. Sinus tracks can be injected with methylene blue 24 hours before surgery to make them easier to locate and excise (Fig. 4.12).

TECHNIQUE 4.2

- Expose the infected area of bone and excise all sinus tracks completely.
- Incise the indurated periosteum and elevate it 1.3 to 2.5 cm on each side.
- Use a drill to outline an oval cortical window at the appropriate site and remove it with an osteotome.

- Remove all sequestra, purulent material, and scarred and necrotic tissue (Fig. 4.14A,B). If sclerotic bone seals off a cavity within the medullary canal, open it into the canal in both directions to allow blood vessels to grow into the cavity. Use a high-speed burr to debride necrotic or ischemic bone until the "paprika sign" (active punctate bleeding bone) is achieved, indicating healthy tissue. Tissue obtained at surgical debridement should be sent for culture and pathology studies.
- After removing all suspicious matter, carefully excise the overhanging edges of bone. Subsequent dead space can be filled with antibiotic PMMA or calcium sulfate beads. A soft-tissue, a local muscle flap, or a free-tissue transfer can be performed at the time of bead removal.
- If there is nonunion with any bony instability, the bone must be stabilized, preferably with an Ilizarov-type external frame.
- If possible, close the skin loosely over drains and ensure that no excessive skin tension is present. If closure is impossible, pack the wound open loosely or apply an antibiotic bead pouch and plan for delayed closure or skin grafting at a later time.
- Appropriate antibiotics should be used before, during, and after the operation.

POSTOPERATIVE CARE The limb is splinted until the wound has healed, and then it is protected to prevent pathologic fracture. Antibiotic treatment is continued for a prolonged period and should be monitored by an infectious disease consultant.

■ MANAGEMENT OF DEFECTS

Bony and soft-tissue defects must be filled to reduce the chance of continued infection and loss of function. Several techniques have been described for the management of such defects and have proved successful when properly performed, but they require meticulous surgical technique. The methods described to eliminate this dead space are: (1)

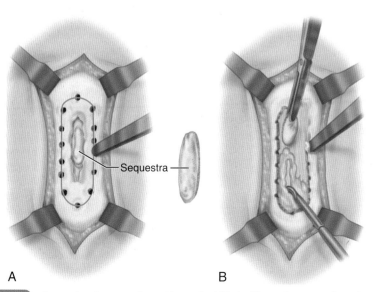

A   B

FIGURE 4.14 Sequestrectomy and curettage. **A,** Affected bone is exposed, and sequestrum is removed. **B,** All infected matter is removed. **SEE TECHNIQUE 4.2.**

bone grafting with primary or secondary closure; (2) use of antibiotic PMMA beads as a temporary filler of the dead space before reconstruction; (3) local muscle flaps and skin grafting with or without bone grafting; (4) microvascular transfer of muscle, myocutaneous, osseous, and osteocutaneous flaps; and (5) the use of bone transport (Ilizarov technique).

- Especially in subcutaneous bones such as the tibia, excise the lips of the wound if the skin tends to cover the granulation tissue before it completely covers the graft.

STAGE III: WOUND COVERAGE
- Apply skin grafts or allow the wound to heal by spontaneous epithelialization.

OPEN BONE GRAFTING

Papineau et al. described an open bone grafting technique for the treatment of chronic osteomyelitis. This procedure relies on the formation of healthy granulation tissue in a bed of bone graft that will become rapidly vascularized. The granulation tissue resists infection and is allowed to adequately drain. This technique is useful when free flaps or soft-tissue transfer options are limited because of anatomic location or in patients who smoke or are medically compromised. Archdeacon and Messerschmitt described a modification of the Papineau technique using NPWT. NPWT has been used extensively in the acute trauma setting and is quite useful for decreasing edema and for closure of soft-tissue dead space. Vacuum-assisted closure (VAC) also stimulates the formation of granulation tissue.

The operation is divided into three stages and usually requires several surgeries: (1) debridement and stabilization, (2) cancellous autografting, and (3) skin closure. Culture-specific intravenous antibiotics should be continued beyond the last surgical procedure.

TECHNIQUE 4.3

(PAPINEAU ET AL.; ARCHDEACON AND MESSERSCHMITT)

STAGE I: DEBRIDEMENT AND STABILIZATION
- Thoroughly debride all sequestra and necrotic bone to healthy and viable soft tissue and bone; thoroughly irrigate the debrided area.
- Stabilize the bone with an external fixator or intramedullary nail if needed.
- Apply VAC.
- Repeat debridement and irrigation with VAC change every 48 to 96 hours until a healthy viable tissue bed is obtained.

STAGE II: GRAFTING
- Harvest cancellous bone graft from the iliac crest or proximal tibia.
- Pack the graft in the bony defect, filling to the subcutaneous level.
- Dress with Adaptic (Smith-Nephew) and VAC sponge.
- Change the VAC every 72 to 96 hours until the wound is covered with healthy-appearing granulation tissue.
- Change the first dressing between the third and fifth days and replace any grafts that adhere to the dressing. Change the dressings until the grafts stabilize.
- If indicated, use local muscle pedicle grafts to enhance the blood supply to the grafts and leave the overlying skin and subcutaneous tissue open.

■ POLYMETHYLMETHACRYLATE ANTIBIOTIC BEAD CHAINS

The use of antibiotic-impregnated PMMA beads in the treatment of chronic osteomyelitis is common practice and is supported by numerous clinical studies. The rationale for this treatment is to deliver levels of antibiotics locally in concentrations that exceed the minimal inhibitory concentrations. Pharmacokinetic studies have shown that the local concentrations of antibiotic achieved are 200 times higher than levels achieved with systemic antibiotic administration. This has the advantage of obtaining very high local antibiotic concentrations while maintaining low serum levels and low systemic toxicity. The antibiotic is leached from the PMMA beads into the postoperative wound hematoma and secretion, which act as a transport medium. High concentrations of the antibiotic can be achieved only with primary wound closure; if such closure cannot be performed, the wound can be covered with a water-impermeable dressing (bead pouch technique). Before the beads are implanted, all infected and necrotic tissue should be adequately debrided surgically and all foreign material removed. Suction drains are not recommended because the concentration level of the antibiotic is diminished when they are used.

Aminoglycosides are the most commonly employed antibiotics for use with PMMA beads. Penicillins, cephalosporins, and clindamycin are eluted well from PMMA beads; vancomycin elutes much less effectively. Antibiotics such as the fluoroquinolones, tetracycline, and polymyxin B are broken down during the exothermic process of cement hardening and should not be used with PMMA beads. Porous, high-viscosity cements, by providing greater surface area, may allow antibiotics to elute more readily than less porous cements. Currently, most commercially available bone cements have a prepackaged form available with gentamicin (500 mg/40-g pack). We generally add 2 to 4 g of vancomycin, with or without 1.2 g of tobramycin, to each 40-g pack of high velocity cement before adding the monomer. Beenken et al. showed that the addition of xylitol, a soluble particulate filler, to PMMA cement enhances the elution of daptomycin in a rabbit model.

Short-term, long-term, or even permanent implantation of PMMA antibiotic beads is possible. In short-term implantation the beads are removed within 10 days, and in long-term implantation they may be left for up to 80 days. The rationale for removal of PMMA beads is based on numerous factors. Local bactericidal antibiotic levels last only 2 to 4 weeks after placement, and when all the antibiotic has leached out of the bead, a foreign body remains that may be colonized by glycocalyx-forming bacteria. PMMA also has been shown to inhibit local immune response by impairing various phagocytic immune cells.

The antibiotic bead pouch technique, described subsequently, has been used with encouraging results for preventing infection in open fractures. It also can be used in the treatment of osteomyelitis if soft-tissue coverage is impossible after initial debridement. The bead pouch must be changed frequently, and repeat debridement should be performed until the wound is ready for a soft-tissue coverage procedure.

ANTIBIOTIC BEAD POUCH

TECHNIQUE 4.4

(HENRY, OSTERMANN, AND SELIGSON)
- Thoroughly debride all necrotic tissue as previously described. Irrigate the wound using a pulsatile lavage system with 9 L of saline solution containing bacitracin.
- Prepare antibiotic PMMA beads by mixing high-viscosity bone cement powder with a powder form of the antibiotic (2 to 4 g of antibiotic per 40-g pack of monomer) in a bowl. Add the activating solution and stir the mixture until the cement is workable.
- Form several beads by rolling them into small spheres. Place the beads on an 18- or 20-gauge wire to form a bead chain. Allow the cement to harden. Record the number of beads on the chain in the operative report to ensure all beads are accounted for on removal.
- Place the PMMA antibiotic bead chains into the bony defect filling the dead space. Close all wound extensions with interrupted nylon sutures.
- Dry the skin edges surrounding the wound and apply a benzoin solution to the skin edges circumferentially.
- Apply an adhesive porous polyethylene wound film to cover the wound. Place a second layer with a larger adhesive porous polyethylene dressing over the first to prevent leakage.

POSTOPERATIVE CARE The limb should be appropriately immobilized. The bead pouch should be changed at 72-hour intervals with repeat debridement and irrigation until the wound is ready for a soft-tissue coverage procedure.

INTRAMEDULLARY ANTIBIOTIC CEMENT NAIL

When debridement of a long bone results in instability, external fixation has been an effective stabilization method; however, more recently, the use of antibiotic-laden PMMA intramedullary rods has been described for use in this situation. Evidence has shown that a reamer-irrigator-aspirator system followed by placement of an antibiotic impregnated PMMA nail along with pathogen-specific systemic antibiotics is safe and efficacious in the treatment of osteomyelitis. In a study of 52 patients with ankle, tibial, femoral, and knee arthrodesis nails, Thonse and Conway reported infection control in 85% of patients, and several small case series have reported no persistent infection with this technique. Reilly et al. reported resolution of infection within 6 months of antibiotic nail insertion in 31 (76%) of 41 patients with postoperative infections

after tibial fractures. Their treatment protocol included removal of the standard intramedullary nail used for fracture fixation, followed by debridement and irrigation of the intramedullary canal, insertion of the antibiotic nail, and intravenous antibiotic administration. After clearance of infection, the antibiotic nail was removed and a standard intramedullary nail implanted.

We have found this to be a useful technique in selected patients. When fabricating an antibiotic cement nail, Kim et al. suggested lubricating the inside of the chest tube with mineral oil before inserting the antibiotic cement and guide rod, then cooling the cemented nail in cold water before peeling off the plastic chest tube. Technical points of nail fabrication suggested by Reilly et al. include use of more than 4 g of antibiotics per 40-g packet of cement and mixing the cement for less time than usual (20 to 30 seconds) and injecting it quickly into the chest tube. For unstable fracture patterns, they recommended use of an Ilizarov threaded rod with nuts at the distal end for a stiffer construct and to avoid residual cement in the canal.

TECHNIQUE 4.5

- After thorough debridement of all necrotic and nonviable soft tissue and bone, prepare the medullary canal with usual reaming technique for intramedullary nail insertion. Send the reamings for culture studies.
- Irrigate the canal and bone with tubing or an irrigating reamer (Fig. 4.15).
- To mold the cement rod, use a T-95 chest tube cut to the desired length. Mix the desired antibiotic with cement and add the monomer. Mix and place in a 60-mL syringe.
- Inject the antibiotic cement mixture into the chest tube. To prevent the cement from extruding from the opposite end of the tube, have an assistant occlude the opening with his or her thumb.
- Before the cement sets up, insert an Ender nail into the chest tube, with the assistant's thumb still occluding the end of the tube. Leave the proximal end of the Ender nail out of the chest tube to be used as a handle.
- Once polymerization is complete, cut and remove the plastic tube and insert the nail with the usual intramedullary nailing technique.
- Apply a long leg, bent-knee bivalved cast.

POSTOPERATIVE CARE The patient is kept non–weight bearing in the cast for 6 to 8 weeks, at which time clinical and laboratory (e.g., erythrocyte sedimentation rate, C-reactive protein) evaluations are done. The cement nail is removed and replaced with a regular intramedullary nail for definitive fixation. Reamings from the nail insertion are sent to the laboratory for culture.

■ BIODEGRADABLE ANTIBIOTIC DELIVERY SYSTEMS

Biodegradable antibiotic delivery systems have significant potential advantages over PMMA in that a second procedure is not required to remove the implant and they have better antibiotic release and compatibility profiles. Several recent studies have reported good results with the use of calcium sulfate as an antibiotic carrier. A biodegradable antibiotic

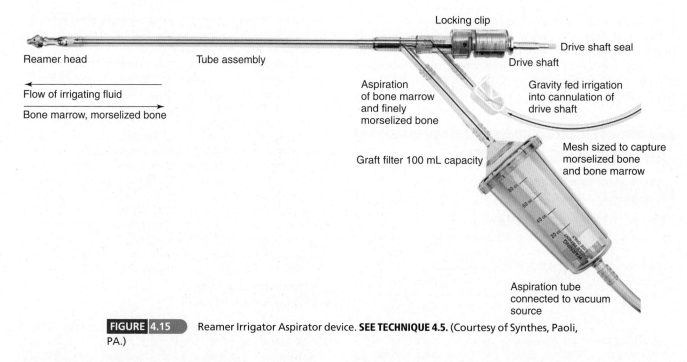

Locking clip

Reamer head   Tube assembly

Flow of irrigating fluid

Bone marrow, morselized bone

Drive shaft seal

Drive shaft

Aspiration
of bone marrow
and finely
morselized bone

Gravity fed irrigation
into cannulation of
drive shaft

Graft filter 100 mL capacity

Mesh sized to capture
morselized bone
and bone marrow

Aspiration tube
connected to vacuum
source

FIGURE 4.15 Reamer Irrigator Aspirator device. **SEE TECHNIQUE 4.5.** (Courtesy of Synthes, Paoli, PA.)

delivery system is especially useful when bony instability is not an issue and soft-tissue coverage is adequate. Some of these biodegradable substrates contain osteoconductive and osteoinductive materials, which can be used to promote new bone formation. A variety of delivery vehicles have been extensively studied in animal models. Currently, no prepackaged biodegradable antibiotic delivery system has been approved for use in the United States; however, such products are available in Europe. Many manufacturers produce a variety of bioabsorbable substrates (calcium sulfate or calcium phosphate) that can be mixed with antibiotics. These kits allow the surgeon to mix powdered antibiotics (generally vancomycin or tobramycin) with the calcium sulfate or calcium phosphate to produce resorbable beads or injectable filler. These beads can be mixed with a variety of available osteoinductive products to fill dead space and act as an osteoconductive and osteoinductive bone graft substitute. These beads typically resorb by about 8 weeks after surgery. Gauland, in a study of 354 patients who had calcium sulfate tablets mixed with a standard antibiotic mixture of vancomycin and gentamicin implanted after surgical debridement, reported healing in 86% without intravenous antibiotic. The use of bioactive glass (BAG) S53P4 has been shown in *in vivo* and *in vitro* studies to be as effective as antibiotic-loaded calcium-based bone substitutes in the treatment of osteomyelitis, with less drainage and without relevant side effects.

The biodegradable substances used as antibiotic delivery systems can be classified into three main categories: proteins, bone graft materials and substitutes, and synthetic polymers. Within the protein category are a variety of substances derived from biologic tissues, including collagen, gelatin, thrombin, and autologous blood clot, all of which provide scaffolding that can be used to contain an antibiotic. Collagen has been the most extensively studied of these, and reports are conflicting as to efficacy of antibiotic-impregnated collagen in the treatment of osteomyelitis. Among the bone graft substitutes, calcium sulfate has long been used because of its low immunoreactivity, ability to be absorbed,

and its structural properties. A comparison study of bioabsorbable bone substitute (BBS; tobramycin-impregnated medical-grade calcium sulfate) and antibiotic-impregnated PMMA cement beads after surgical debridement demonstrated the two to be equivalent in eradicating infection. BBS had the added benefit of eliminating the morbidity associated with additional surgery required for cement bead removal and bone grafting. One problem we have had with calcium-based carriers is that many patients develop a whitish or caseous type of drainage that mimics the drainage of a bacterial infection. These patients generally do not have the pain, cellulitis, fever, or leukocytosis generally associated with a bacterial infection, however. Nevertheless, the situation is bothersome and of concern for the patient and the surgeon. Ferguson et al. reported using a biodegradable calcium sulfate carrier containing tobramycin in 193 patients with osteomyelitis in various locations, but predominantly the tibia and femur, finding it helpful; however, filling of the defect was variable. The prolonged wound exudate was self-limited in their patients and did not lead to recurrent wound infection.

Antibiotic-loaded calcium sulfate pellets with the addition of bone marrow aspirate were used by Badie and Arafa as a one-stage treatment in 30 patients, 77% of whom had eradication of infection. They recommended the use of bone marrow aspirate as an inexpensive, reproducible, and safe addition to calcium sulfate used as a bone substitute. McNally et al. described the use of an injectable, gentamicin-loaded, calcium sulfate/hydroxyapatite biocomposite for one-stage treatment of 105 bone defects in 100 patients, 80 of whom were classified as Cierny-Mader class B hosts. After excision of sinus tracks and implants and debridement until healthy, bleeding bone was exposed, the cavity was washed and dried and filled with the biocomposite. If instability was present, external or internal fixation was used. Infection was eradicated in 96 of the 100 patients by a single-stage operation, with recurrence in four patients; all four remained infection-free at 1 to 2 years after revision surgery. They also reported "white wound drainage" in six of 100 patients; it required no intervention other than dressing changes, and no patients with this drainage developed a recurrence of infection.

More recent biodegradable materials investigated for use in treatment of osteomyelitis are the synthetic polymers. The greatest advantage of these materials is that they can be modified to effectively and accurately release specified drug quantities over a specified amount of time. Polylactide and poly(D,L-lactide-co-glycolic acid) (PLGA) implants have been in use for some time and have been investigated for use as biodegradable antibiotic carriers. These materials, however, have been reported to cause an inflammatory foreign-body reaction that is thought to be caused by their acidic degradation products. Carriers that do not produce acidic breakdown with surface erosion, such as polytrimethylene carbonate (PTMC), are being studied. A monomethyl ether PLGA copolymer biodegradable hydrogel also may hold promise for the future.

As Kluin et al. pointed out, the ideal biodegradable carrier for antibiotics in the treatment of osteomyelitis should have good biocompatibility, controllable degradation, and the ability to release any antibiotic (including vancomycin when resistant bacteria are present) at therapeutic levels for an extended period of time, without releasing acidic byproducts during degradation.

■ CLOSED SUCTION DRAINS

Success rates of approximately 85% have been reported for the modified Lautenbach method of closed suction antibiotic ingress and egress irrigation systems (Fig. 4.16). An advantage of this technique is that it allows a change in local antibiotic delivery based on culture results obtained from surgical biopsies. The technique also aids in the gradual decrease in the size of the soft-tissue dead space. Disadvantages include frequent occlusion of the delivery catheter. This problem has been decreased with the use of frequent doses of streptokinase to the keep the catheter patent. Other disadvantages are the prolonged hospitalization required and the risk of secondary contamination. We have no experience with this method. Hung achieved good results in 77%, fair results in 21%, and poor results in less than 1% using drainage and continuous antibiotic irrigation of 376 tibial medullary canals in children.

A more recent wound closure technique is NPWT, which consists of a pump that generates a vacuum and is capable of creating a negative pressure environment within a sealed wound, dressing material used to pack and seal the wound, tubing for fluid removal from the wound area, and a container to collect waste materials removed from the wound. Most of the published studies on NPWT involve the use of the VAC system (Kinetic Concepts, Inc., San Antonio, TX) (Fig. 4.17A; however, a number of other NPWT systems are available from several manufacturers. Newer designs include canister-less, single-use devices such as the PICO (Smith & Nephew, Memphis TN) and Avelle (ConvaTec, Oklahoma City, OK) (Fig. 4.17B,C).

The efficacy of NPWT for the treatment of complex wounds has been reported by several authors who suggested benefits of edema reduction, increased blood flow, increased granulation tissue, and the possibility of improved bacterial clearance from wounds. Although these studies have emphasized *prevention* of osteomyelitis in complex wounds, there is little information about the *treatment* of osteomyelitis with NPWT. Tan et al., in a study of 68 patients with osteomyelitis, compared NPWT (35 patients) with conventional treatment (33 patients) and found

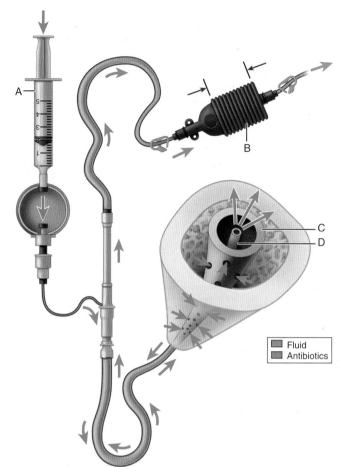

FIGURE 4.16 Lautenbach drainage system. Syringe (**A**) is used to inject every 4 hours. The suction bag (**B**) draws fluid through the outer tube from the bone. Antibiotics enter the bone through the inner tube (**C** and **D**). (Redrawn from Caesar BC, Morgan-Jones RL, Warren RE, et al: Closed double-lumen suction irrigation in the management of chronic diaphyseal osteomyelitis: long-term follow-up, *J Bone Joint Surg* 91B:1243, 2009. Copyright British Editorial Society of Bone and Joint Surgery.)

Fluid
Antibiotics

significantly fewer recurrences of infection, a decreased need for tissue transfers or muscle flaps, and more wounds with bacterial clearance in those treated with NPWT. The most serious complication reported with the use of NPWT is extensive bleeding, which most often occurs with use of the device in the patient's home or in a nursing facility. NPWT should not be used as a replacement for surgical debridement, and it should not be used until all necrotic, nonviable tissue has been removed and appropriate antibiotic therapy initiated. More research is necessary to establish parameters for pressure intensity, duration of treatment, interval between treatments, mode of application, and timing of application that will produce the most efficient and cost-effective therapy.

■ SOFT-TISSUE TRANSFER

Soft-tissue transfers to fill dead space left behind after extensive debridement may range from a localized muscle flap on a vascular pedicle to microvascular free-tissue transfer. The transfer of vascularized muscle tissue improves the local biologic environment by bringing in a blood supply that is important in the host's defense mechanisms and for antibiotic

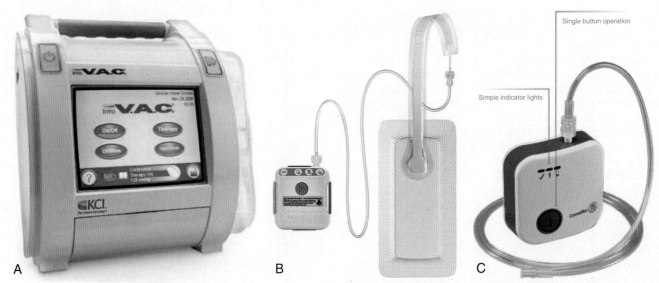

Single button operation

Simple indicator lights

FIGURE 4.17 Negative wound pressure therapy devices. **A,** Kinetic Concepts VAC system. **B,** Smith & Nephew single-use, canister-less PICO. **C,** ConvaTec Group, disposable, canister-less Avelle.

delivery and osseous and soft-tissue healing. The success rates for this technique reported in the literature have ranged from 66% to 100%.

Most commonly, a local muscle flap is used in the treatment of chronic osteomyelitis of the tibia. The gastrocnemius muscle is used for defects around the proximal third of the tibia, and the soleus muscle is used for defects around the middle third. A microvascular free muscle transfer is required for defects around the distal third of the tibia.

Several authors reported a high success rate in the treatment of chronic osteomyelitis with the use of microvascular free tissue transfer. A microvascular transfer of tissue may consist of muscle that is covered with a skin graft or a myocutaneous, osseous, or osteocutaneous flap. Adequate initial debridement of the involved area, so that the flap is placed in a healthy environment, helps to ensure the success of the procedure.

When a microvascular free muscle flap is used, and segmental bone loss has occurred, autogenous cancellous bone grafting can be done about 6 weeks after the initial free-flap transfer. A free fibular graft can be used for segmental bone loss of the tibia. If chronic osteomyelitis involves segmental bone loss of the tibia and the fibula, the results of a free fibular graft are not good, and amputation or reconstruction with external fixation is advised.

■ EXTERNAL FIXATION

The Ilizarov technique of distraction-compression osteogenesis has been helpful in the treatment of chronic osteomyelitis and infected nonunions of long bones or the ankle joint. This technique allows radical resection of the infected bone. A corticotomy is performed through normal bone proximal and distal to the area of disease. The bone is transported until union is achieved. Drózdz et al. reported resolution of infection in 96% of 54 patients with infected nonunions and bone union in 86% with the Ilizarov technique. After the infection is eradicated, many recommend bone grafting if needed and placement of an intramedullary nail after external fixation is removed. Disadvantages of this technique include the time required to achieve a solid union and the high incidence of associated complications. External fixation also has been found to have a negative impact on patients' mental health

that persisted even after removal of the device. Even with these problems, however, the Ilizarov procedure benefits patients who need extensive resection of bone and reconstruction to achieve stability. Use of distraction osteogenesis with ring fixation over an intramedullary rod has been used for the treatment of segmental defects of up to 13 cm.

Qin et al. also described successful treatment of bone defects ranging from 6 to 18.5 cm with radical debridement, antibiotic-impregnated calcium sulfate, and monolateral external fixation. Successful bone union was achieved in 34 of 35 patients with no reinfection; the average length of external fixator wear was 17 months (range, 7 to 32 months), and only six patients required less than a year of external fixator wear. These authors chose monolateral fixators over ring fixators because application is easier to learn and can be done rapidly with minimal equipment; cost is lower, and the device is less cumbersome and better accepted by patients.

■ ADJUNCTIVE THERAPIES

Hyperbaric oxygen therapy has been used for the treatment of chronic osteomyelitis but has not proved to be reliably effective. The use of hyperbaric oxygen can be recommended only as an adjuvant to more traditional methods of treatment. Growth factors, such as bone morphogenic proteins (BMPs) and even platelet-rich plasma (PRP), have been suggested as adjuvant treatments for osteomyelitis because of their ability to accelerate or enhance osteogenesis. We would not consider the use of these products until the infection is eradicated. Some studies of physical energy modalities (pulsed electromagnetic fields [PEMF] and ultrasound) have suggested that they may directly interfere with biofilm formation as well as act synergistically with antibiotics to enhance their activity.

SCLEROSING OSTEOMYELITIS OF GARRÉ

Sclerosing osteomyelitis is a chronic form of disease in which the bone is thickened and distended but abscesses and sequestra are absent (Fig. 4.18). The disease affects children and young adults. Its cause is unknown, but it is thought to be

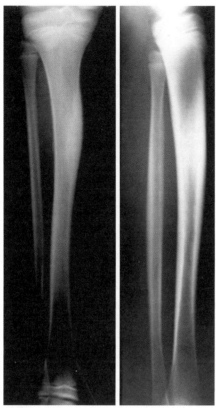

FIGURE 4.18 Sclerosing osteomyelitis of tibia documented by biopsy.

an infection caused by a low-grade, possibly anaerobic bacterium. The condition must be distinguished from osteoid osteoma and Paget disease.

Patients report intermittent pain of moderate intensity and usually of long duration. Swelling and tenderness over the affected bone may be found. Radiographs show an expanded bone with generalized sclerosis. The erythrocyte sedimentation rate usually is slightly elevated. Biopsy specimens show only chronic, low-grade, nonspecific osteomyelitis, and cultures usually are negative. A secondary lesion at a distant site can occur years after onset. No treatment has been predictably helpful, but fenestration of the sclerotic bone and antibiotics are advisable. Schwartz et al. presented a case report of successful surgical treatment of sclerosing osteomyelitis of the humerus using a vascularized fibular osteotomy flap after resection of the diseased bone.

RESIDUAL STAGE OF OSTEOMYELITIS

The residual stage of osteomyelitis is characterized by a complete absence of the signs and symptoms of infection, including drainage. The bone is sclerotic, and its blood supply and strength are normal. During this stage of osteomyelitis, the bone bears the same relation to normal bone that scar tissue bears to normal connective tissue. The adjacent soft tissues are scarred, and if drainage has occurred, the skin often adheres to the bone. Adhesions of skin to bone are more common if the bone is subcutaneous. Injury to such tissues frequently causes skin breakdown and even recurrence of infection. It

is sometimes difficult to know if the disease is in a residual stage or in a remission of the chronic stage. Treatment of the residual stage consists of correcting leg-length inequality or angular and joint deformities. Sometimes contracted scars must be released, and adherent scars must be replaced by myocutaneous flaps.

CHRONIC RECURRENT MULTIFOCAL OSTEOMYELITIS

Chronic recurrent multifocal osteomyelitis (CRMO) is an autoinflammatory bone disease characterized by an insidious onset of mild-to-moderate pain with signs of inflammation over the affected parts, which tend to recur. Symptoms wax and wane for months or years. The cause of CRMO remains unknown, although evidence is accumulating for a genetic cause. Some have suggested that CRMO and Garré syndrome are the same entity. The prevalence of this disease may be underestimated because of the difficulty in its recognition.

The disease is most common in children, with a peak age of 10 years. It most often affects the metaphysis of long bones, especially the tibia, femur, and clavicle. Vertebra plana is frequent in patients with this disease. One study involving 102 children and adolescents with CRMO identified spinal involvement, including vertebral deformities, scoliosis, and kyphosis, in 26%. Another associated condition is palmar-plantar pustulosis, which manifests as a pustular rash on the soles of the feet and palms of the hands. Laboratory testing usually shows a normal or mildly elevated white blood cell count and elevated erythrocyte sedimentation rate and C-reactive protein level; bacterial cultures of the bones and blood are negative. Radiographically, the bony lesions are predominantly lytic and bilaterally symmetric. Varying degrees of sclerosis may be present. Whole-body technetium-99m bone scanning usually shows bilaterally symmetric areas of increased uptake. STIR MRI can facilitate the diagnosis and exclude pyogenic involvement. Whole-body MRI may be useful for showing subclinical edema. The diagnosis is one of exclusion. If the diagnosis is in doubt, a confirmatory biopsy is indicated. The following have been proposed as criteria for the diagnosis of CRMO: two or more bone lesions mimicking osteomyelitis, radiographic and bone scan findings consistent with osteomyelitis, 6 months or more of chronic and relapsing symptoms, failure of response to at least 1 month of appropriate therapy, and a lack of other identifiable cause.

No effective treatment for CRMO has been found, and if the results of cultures are negative, antibiotic treatment is not indicated. Nonsteroidal antiinflammatory medication may help relieve pain. For refractory CRMO, especially with spinal involvement, successful treatment with tumor-necrosis factor-α has been reported. Treatment with bisphosphonates also has been shown to be of benefit. Disease remission after treatment with interferon gamma has been reported, but no absolute proof that the drug caused the remission could be shown. Resolution of symptoms followed by recurrence months later is characteristic of this disease. Generally, the symptoms continue to recur over 2 years, and the disease generally is self-limiting. The long-term prognosis seems to be good; however, one study found that nearly 60% of children diagnosed with CRMO had active disease and pain 6 months to 15 years after diagnosis. Recurrence, however, is common: in a German cohort of 56 patients, 50% relapsed after a median of 2.4 years, and in 70 children from North America, the relapse rate was 83% after a median of 1.8 years.

ANAEROBIC OSTEOMYELITIS

Anaerobic bacteria are recognized increasingly as an important cause of osteomyelitis. In one series, 40 of 182 patients having surgery for osteomyelitis were found to have anaerobic bacteria in their operative cultures. The demonstration of these bacteria requires culturing the clinical material immediately after collection, using fresh media with proper anaerobic conditions, and subculturing the colonies immediately after removing them from the anaerobic environment.

Anaerobic soft-tissue infections usually start in injured or ischemic tissue. Frequently, a putrid discharge and gas production are present, and extensive tissue necrosis tends to burrow through subcutaneous and fascial planes. Anaerobic infections have been frequently associated with diabetic gangrene. Treatment is by surgical drainage and resection of the necrotic tissue, combined with the use of appropriate antibiotics as determined by culture and sensitivity studies.

INCISION AND DRAINAGE FOR OSTEOMYELITIS OF SPECIFIC REGIONS
CALCANEUS

In osteomyelitis of the calcaneus, as of the other tarsal bones, destruction of the cortex usually is not extensive. The periosteum is firmly attached to bone, and it is usually perforated rather than elevated by purulent material; the formation of an involucrum is minimal. One study found *S. aureus* to be the most common bacteria in calcaneal osteomyelitis and *Pseudomonas aeruginosa* in neurologically damaged feet. An American Society of Anesthesiologists score of less than 2, age younger than 65 years, absence of neuropathy and diabetes, and posttraumatic osteomyelitis were associated with better

results. Intravenous and oral antibiotics with surgical debridement (if indicated) can lead to a good clinical outcome.

SPLIT-HEEL INCISION

Medial and lateral approaches to the calcaneus are satisfactory for incision and drainage of localized abscesses, but the Gaenslen approach through the plantar surface of the heel is indicated for resecting the diseased bone of chronic osteomyelitis. The resulting scars usually are painless; they are so deeply situated that the tissues on either side curl inward and form thick cushions (Figs. 4.19 and 4.20).

TECHNIQUE 4.6

(GAENSLEN)
- Place the patient prone with a support beneath the affected ankle.
- Make a longitudinal incision exactly in the midline of the heel, extending 2.5 to 4.0 cm from the level of the base of the fifth metatarsal posteriorly to split the end of the Achilles tendon.
- Incise the plantar aponeurosis in the plane between the abductor digiti quinti and flexor digitorum brevis muscles.
- Retract medially the lateral plantar artery and nerve in the distal angle of the wound.
- Expose the quadratus plantae muscle and split it and the long plantar ligament longitudinally.
- Divide the calcaneus from posterior to anterior with a broad osteotome and retract the two halves to expose the interior of the bone. The subtalar joint can be exposed by increasing the retraction.
- Remove all sequestra and obviously infected matter, but damage the cortex as little as possible.
- Close the wound loosely over drains.

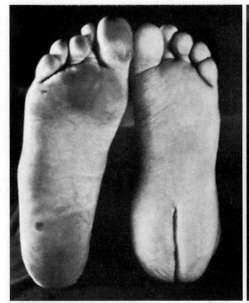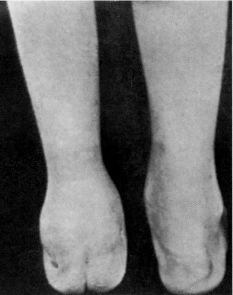

FIGURE 4.19 Retraction of scar prevents pain on weight bearing after complete healing of Gaenslen split-heel incision.

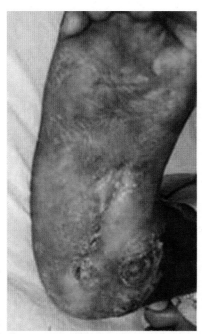

FIGURE 4.20 Healed Gaenslen split-heel incision. The surgical scar is deeply situated, with surrounding tissues forming thick cushions on either side of the incision. (From Jose Jerome JT, Varghese M, Sankaran B, et al: Gaenslen's split-heel incision for calcaneal osteomyelitis: a cast report, *Foot Ankle Online J* 2:3, 2009.)

POSTOPERATIVE CARE A short leg cast is applied with the foot in neutral position and the ankle at 90 degrees. A window is cut over the calcaneus to permit dressing changes.

DISTAL THIRD OF THE FEMUR

Chronic osteomyelitis of the distal third of the femur is difficult to treat. Because the periosteum may become completely separated posteriorly by a subperiosteal abscess, this part of the bone may lose most of its blood supply, and sinuses often persist. A mass of scar tissue forms that interferes with revascularization of the bone; the scar tissue is relatively inaccessible surgically because of the proximity of large vessels and nerves.

TECHNIQUE 4.7

- Make a lateral longitudinal incision on the distal third of the thigh, beginning 5 cm proximal to the joint line of the knee and extend it proximally for 10 cm.
- Incise the iliotibial band, retract the vastus lateralis muscle anteriorly and expose the femur.
- Avoid opening the knee joint in the distal end of the incision. Confine the operation to the lateral and posterolateral surfaces of the bone, or the suprapatellar bursa may be opened and the knee joint could become contaminated.
- Use a drill to outline a cortical window on the posterolateral surface of the bone and remove the window with an osteotome.

- Enter the medullary canal proximal to the metaphysis and place the window so that pus drains posteriorly.
- Remove only necrotic and infected matter.
- Close the wound loosely over rubber drains, which exit through separate incisions and permit direct posterolateral drainage.

POSTOPERATIVE CARE The limb is splinted with the knee straight until the wound has healed, and it is protected during ambulation to prevent pathologic fracture.

PELVIC REGIONS

As in the long bones, osteomyelitis of the pelvis may arise from hematogenous spread, direct inoculation of pathogens from trauma or surgery (e.g., hip implants), or by contiguous spread from the soft tissues (e.g., ulcers). Ramaesh et al. reported a high incidence of pelvic osteomyelitis in neurologically compromised patients. MRI is the most sensitive imaging technique, but culture or bone biopsy is necessary to determine the pathogen as well as to rule out malignancy, such as squamous cell carcinoma. Broad-spectrum antibiotics are necessary because unusual organisms or several pathogens may be present.

▓ ILIUM

In the acute stage of osteomyelitis, the ilium usually is invaded throughout, and large subperiosteal abscesses develop on the medial and lateral cortices. Early symptoms may suggest acute appendicitis or pyogenic arthritis of the hip joint. Before incision and drainage, systemic treatment (especially intravenous antibiotics and blood transfusions, if necessary) should be given. Adequate amounts of blood should be available for use during surgery. Anaerobic bacteria may be involved in osteomyelitis of the pelvis associated with lesions of the intestines.

In chronic osteomyelitis of the ilium, the entire bone often is involved, and infection is so diffuse that it is impossible to remove the individual sequestra and drain all the abscesses. Because most of the iliac wing can be removed without causing significant disability, resecting it usually is preferable to less radical operations (see TECHNIQUE 4.12).

DRAINAGE

TECHNIQUE 4.8

- Begin the incision along the middle third of the iliac crest and extend it as necessary.
- Strip the muscles subperiosteally from the medial and lateral cortices of the iliac wing; usually pus under pressure escapes. Often the muscles will already have been stripped by the subperiosteal abscesses.
- Carefully avoid entering the hip joint.
- Drain each of the abscesses with drains. Bring the drains out through separate incisions to obtain adequate gravity drainage.
- Close the skin loosely.

POSTOPERATIVE CARE Because a flexion contracture of the hip usually develops as a result of irritability of the hip flexor muscles, Buck traction is applied. The patient is turned frequently to the affected side to promote drainage.

ISCHIUM AND PUBIS

In osteomyelitis of the ischium and pubis, an abscess develops either beneath the external or internal obturator muscles or in the ischiorectal fossa. Drainage can be accomplished through an incision located away from the perineum to decrease the possibility of wound contamination and to allow wider retraction of the gracilis and adductor muscles. If necessary, the obturator membrane can be incised and the deep surfaces of the bone explored. Osteomyelitis of the ischial tuberosity is common in bedridden and paraplegic patients who develop pressure sores with secondary infection, necrosis, and osteomyelitis. Effective treatment requires debridement of all necrotic tissue and infected bone, and a soft-tissue transfer usually is required to close the defect. For osteomyelitis in the region of the symphysis, resection of the symphysis may be required when less radical treatment is ineffective.

SPINE

Osteomyelitis of the spine is discussed in other chapter.

RESECTION OR EXCISION FOR OSTEOMYELITIS

It has been shown in many instances that if infection is to be controlled in chronic osteomyelitis, the infected portion of bone must be radically resected, even if this means removing a segment of an essential long bone. Massive resection of a long bone affected by chronic hematogenous osteomyelitis has not been advisable in the past, however, for three reasons: (1) The periosteum may fail to reproduce the entire shaft (Fig. 4.21), (2) the quality of remaining bone usually is unsatisfactory for reconstructive procedures, and (3) a dormant infection may be reactivated if reconstruction is undertaken. With newer techniques of bone and soft-tissue transport, massive resections can be performed and reconstructed without significant disability, although the time needed for reconstruction may be long.

Massive resection of nonessential bones involved by any type of chronic osteomyelitis can be performed safely. Bones such as metatarsals and tarsals and part of the calcaneus, fibula, ilium, ribs, clavicle, and scapula can be resected, and satisfactory function may still be retained.

RESECTION OF THE METATARSALS

TECHNIQUE 4.9

- The first metatarsal should be retained if possible.
- Make a dorsal longitudinal incision over the affected bone from the distal row of tarsals to the middle of the proximal phalanx of the corresponding toe.

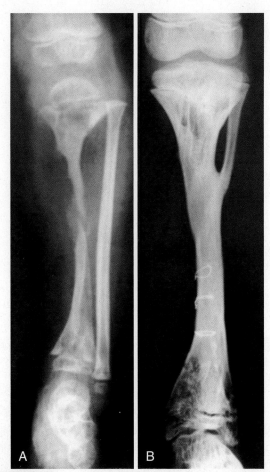

FIGURE 4.21   **A,** Defect in tibia of 4-year-old child after treatment of acute osteomyelitis by removal of large sequestrum before sufficient involucrum had formed to ensure continuity of bone. **B,** After transplantation of fibula to bridge defect.

- Deepen the incision to the periosteum, but do not open the tendon sheaths.
- Incise the periosteum in line with the shaft and strip it completely from the bone.
- Resect the entire shaft, but preserve the physis whenever possible in children.
- Close the wound loosely over a drain.

POSTOPERATIVE CARE A posterior plaster splint is applied and worn until the wound has healed, after which protected weight bearing is started.

RESECTION OF THE TARSALS

Often more than one tarsal bone may be involved in chronic osteomyelitis. If necessary, the affected bone or bones can be excised using dorsolateral and dorsomedial longitudinal incisions. If the calcaneus is to be resected, the approach of Gaenslen is recommended (see TECHNIQUE 4.6).

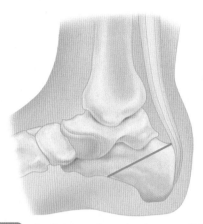

FIGURE 4.22 Partial resection of calcaneus. **SEE TECHNIQUE 4.10.**

PARTIAL CALCANECTOMY

One study of 350 patients with calcaneal osteomyelitis demonstrated higher rates of transtibial amputation when the heel was involved as opposed to just the mid or forefoot. Partial calcanectomy, however, is a useful limb salvage technique in the treatment of large heel ulcerations and calcaneal osteomyelitis.

TECHNIQUE 4.10 *Figure 4.22*

- Tailor the incision to fit the size and shape of the ulcer. If no ulcers are present, use Gaenslen's approach (see TECHNIQUE 4.6). Fisher and Armstrong described a "hurricane incision" that resembles a satellite view of a hurricane to facilitate exposure of the heel (Fig. 4.23).
- Carry the dissection down to the calcaneus to protect the remaining viable heel pad.
- Approach the Achilles tendon in the area of the calcaneus that is to be removed. Release the tendon and allow it to retract proximally.
- Begin an incision 1cm posterior to the edge of the subtalar and calcaneocuboid joints.
- Remove sufficient bone to permit mobilization and approximation of the adjacent healthy soft tissue.
- Close the wounds over suction drains. If primary skin closure is impossible, allow it to heal by secondary wound healing.
- Apply a cast with the ankle in 30 degrees of equinus to reduce tension on the wound.

POSTOPERATIVE CARE When the wounds have healed, the patient is placed in a solid, custom-molded ankle-foot orthosis.

RESECTION OF THE FIBULA

The entire fibula can be resected if necessary, but the distal fourth contributes to ankle stability and should be retained whenever possible. If the proximal end is resected, the lateral collateral ligament of the knee and the biceps femoris tendon should be firmly anchored to the tibia.

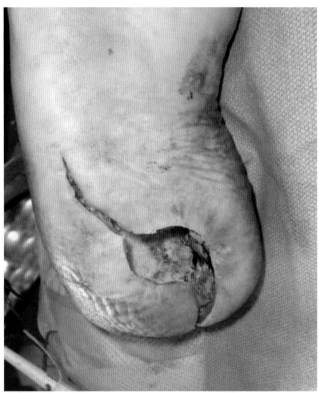

FIGURE 4.23 Hurricane incision. (From Fisher TK, Armstrong DG: Partial calcanectomy in high-risk patients with diabetes: use and utility of a "hurricane" incisional approach, *ePlasty* 10:e17, 2010.)

TECHNIQUE 4.11

- Make a longitudinal incision over the involved portion of the fibula.
- Approach the bone in the interval between the soleus muscle posteriorly and the peroneal muscles anteriorly.
- Expose and protect the peroneal nerve in the proximal end of the wound.
- Incise the periosteum in line with the shaft and strip it from the entire circumference of the part to be resected.
- Resect the diseased portion of the shaft and close the wound loosely over drains.

POSTOPERATIVE CARE A long leg posterior plaster splint is applied with the foot in neutral position, the ankle at 90 degrees, and the knee in 20 degrees of flexion, and it is worn until the wound has healed. Then protected weight bearing is started.

RESECTION OF THE ILIAC WING

Resection of a large part of the iliac wing may be indicated in chronic osteomyelitis of the ilium with prolonged drainage (Fig. 4.24).

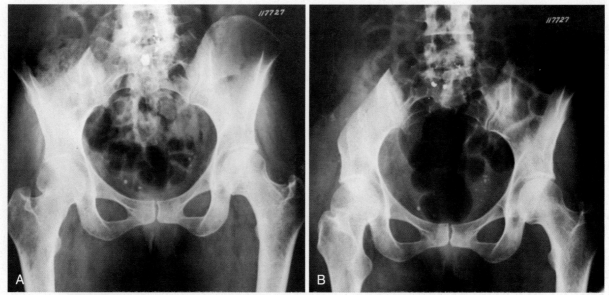

FIGURE 4.24 **A,** Sliding abdominal hernia and osteomyelitis of right iliac crest after removal of bone graft for fusion of lumbar spine. **B,** Appearance of ilium after resection of involved crest and repair of hernia.

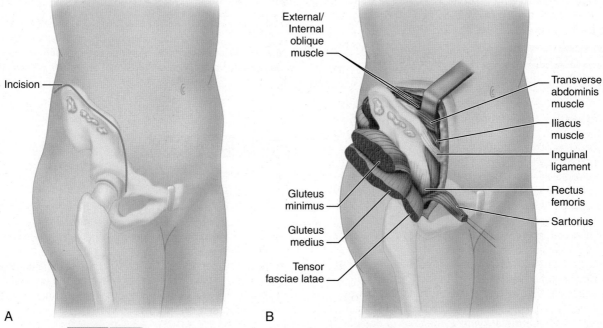

A

B

FIGURE 4.25 **A** and **B,** Subperiosteal exposure for resection of wing of ilium. Poupart ligament can be reflected from ilium, permitting removal of bone from superior ramus of pubis to sacroiliac joint. **SEE TECHNIQUE 4.12.**

TECHNIQUE 4.12

(BADGLEY)

- Make an incision over the iliac crest from the posterior superior iliac spine to the anterior superior iliac spine and distally on the thigh, parallel with the sartorius muscle for 7.5 to 10 cm (Fig. 4.25A).
- Divide the fascia 1.3 cm distal to the crest and incise the periosteum along the crest.

- Detach the gluteal and tensor fasciae latae muscles subperiosteally to the acetabular rim.
- Develop the interval between the tensor fasciae latae and the sartorius muscles and retract the tensor fasciae latae to expose the anterior part of the ilium.
- In children, the cartilaginous iliac crest can be detached easily with the abdominal muscles attached to it.
- Subperiosteally detach the abdominal muscles and the latissimus dorsi, quadratus lumborum, and erector spinae muscles at their insertions.

- Strip the muscles from the medial cortex of the ilium distally to the arcuate line (Fig. 4.25B).
- Resect the ilium as a whole as far distally as the anterior inferior spine and as far posteriorly as the sacroiliac joint if necessary.
- Place drains in the wound and bring them through the skin by a separate incision to establish adequate gravity drainage.
- Close the skin loosely.

POSTOPERATIVE CARE Protected ambulation is begun when the wounds have healed, and the patient's condition permits.

AMPUTATION FOR OSTEOMYELITIS

Amputation is performed infrequently for osteomyelitis. In certain patients, this form of treatment may be preferable, however, to multiple operations and prolonged antibiotic therapy. The prevalence of malignancy arising from chronic osteomyelitis has been reported to be 0.2% to 1.6%. Most of these are squamous cell carcinoma arising from a sinus track, but reticulum cell carcinoma, fibrosarcoma, and other malignancies have been reported. Amputation is the most reliable means of treating osteomyelitis associated with malignant change. Arterial insufficiency, major nerve paralysis, or joint contractures and stiffness that make a limb nonfunctional are indications for amputation.

REFERENCES

GENERAL/MISCELLANEOUS

Birt MC, Anderson DW, Bruce Toby E, et al.: Osteomyelitis: recent advances in pathophysiology and therapeutic strategies, *J Orthop* 14:45, 2016.

Campbell R, Berry G, Deva A, Harris IA: Aggressive management of tibial osteomyelitis shows good functional outcomes, *Eplasty* 11:e3, 2011.

Choi H, McCartney M, Best TM: Treatment of osteitis pubis and osteomyelitis of the pubic symphysis in athletes: a systematic review, *Br J Sports Med* 45:57, 2011.

Faglia E, Clerici G, Caminiti M, et al.: Influence of osteomyelitis location in the foot of diabetic patients with transtibial amputation, *Foot Ankle Int* 34:222, 2013.

Fosco M, Gualdrini G, Ben Ayad R: The role of active immunization therapy as preoperative treatment for chronic osteomyelitis, *Musculoskelet Surg* 98:45, 2014.

Garcia del Pozo E, Collazos J, Carton JA, et al.: Factors predictive of relapse in adult bacterial osteomyelitis of long bones, *BMC Infect Dis* 18:635, 2018.

Lin TY, Chen YG, Huang WY, et al.: Association between chronic osteomyelitis and deep-vein thrombosis. Analysis of a nationwide population-based registry, *Thromb Haemost* 112:573, 2014.

Liu T, Zhang X, Li Z, Peng D: Management of combined bone defect and limb-length discrepancy after tibial chronic osteomyelitis, *Orthopedics* 34:e363, 2011.

Lowenberg DW, DeBaun M, Suh GA: Newer perspectives in the treatment of chronic osteomyelitis: a preliminary outcome report, *Injury* 50(Suppl 1):S56, 2019.

Merlet A, Cazanave C, Dauchy FA, et al.: Prognostic factors of calcaneal osteomyelitis, *Scand J Infect Dis* 46:555, 2014.

Panteli M, Puttaswamaiah R, Lowenberg DW, Giannoudis PV: Malignant transformation in chronic osteomyelitis: recognition and principles of management, *J Am Acad Orthop Surg* 22:586, 2014.

Ramaesh R, Gaston MS, Simpson AH: Chronic osteomyelitis of the pelvis, *Acta Orthop Belg* 79:280, 2013.

DIAGNOSIS/CLASSIFICATION

Chadayammuri V, Herbert B, Hao J, et al.: Diagnostic accuracy of various modalities relative to open bone biopsy for detection of long bone posttraumatic osteomyelitis, *Eur J Orthop Surg Traumatol* 27:871, 2017.

Forsberg JA, Potter BK, Cierny 3rd G, Webb L: Diagnosis and management of chronic infection, *J Am Acad Orthop Surg* 19(Suppl 1):S8, 2011.

Groznik M, Cimerman M, Lusa L, et al.: Increased perioperative C-reactive protein and decreased postoperative albumin is associated with acute posttraumatic osteomyelitis in patients with high-energy tibial fractures, *Injury* 50:827, 2019.

Gursahaney DL, Jesse MK, Stoneback J: Extraosseous marrow fat: an MRI sign of acute aggressive osteomyelitis, *BJR Case Rep* 5:20180050, 2018.

Hoang D, Fisher S, Oz OK, et al.: Percutaneous CT-guided bone biopsy for suspected osteomyelitis: diagnostic yield and impact on patient's treatment change and recovery, *Eur J Radiol* 114:85, 2019.

Hotchen AJ, McNally MA, Sendi P: The classification of long bone osteomyelitis: a systemic review of the literature, *J Bone Jt Infect* 2:167, 2017.

Mijuskovic B, Kuehl R, Widmer AF, et al.: Culture of bone biopsy specimens overestimates rate of residual osteomyelitis after toe or forefoot amputation, *J Bone Joint Surg Am* 100:1448, 2018.

Park BN, Hong SJ, Yoon MA, et al.: MRI diagnosis for post-traumatic osteomyelitis of extremities using conventional metal-artifact reducing protocols: revisited, *Acad Radiol* pii: S1076-6332(19)30020-0, 2019. [Epub ahead of print].

Ryan EC, Ahn J, Wukich DK, et al.: Diagnostic utility of erythrocyte sedimentation rate and C-reactive protein in osteomyelitis of the foot in persons without diabetes, *J Foot Ankle Surgery* 58:484, 2019.

Said N, Chalian M, Fox MG, et al.: Percutaneous image-guided bone biopsy of osteomyelitis in the foot and pelvis has a low impact on guiding antibiotics management: a retrospective analysis of 60 bone biopsies, *Skeletal Radiol*, 2019. https://doi.org/10.1007/s00256-019-3152-4, [Epub ahead of print].

Sethi I, Baum YS, Grady EE: Current status of molecular imaging of infection: a primer, *AJR Am J Roentgenol* 1-9, 2019. https://doi.org/10.2214/AJR.19.21094. [Epub ahead ofprint]

Song Q, Long L, Cui S, et al.: Utility of technetium-99m-methylene diphosphonate single-photon emission computed tomography/computed tomography fusion in detecting post-traumatic chronic-infected nonunion in the lower limb, *Nucl Med Commun*, 2019. https://doi.org/10.1097/MNM.0000000000001027, [Epub ahead ofprint].

Von Kalle T, Heim N, Hospach T, et al.: Typical patterns of bone involvement in whole-body MRI of patients with chronic recurrent multifocal osteomyelitis (CRMO), *Rofo* 185:655, 2013.

ACUTE HEMATOGENOUS OSTEOMYELITIS

Bar-On E, Weigl DM, Bor N, et al.: Chronic osteomyelitis in children: treatment by intramedullary reaming and antibiotic-impregnated cement rods, *J Pediatr Orthop* 30:508, 2010.

Beckles VL, Jones HW, Harrison WJ: Chronic haematogenous osteomyelitis in children: a retrospective review of 167 patients in Malawi, *J Bone Joint Surg* 92B:1138, 2010.

Ceroni D, Belaieff W, Cherkaoui A, et al.: Primary epiphyseal or apophyseal subacute osteomyelitis in the pediatric population: a report of fourteen cases and a systematic review of the literature, *J Bone Joint Surg* 96A:1570, 2014.

Copley LA, Barton T, Garcia C, et al.: A proposed scoring system for assessment of severity of illness in pediatric acute hematogenous osteomyelitis using objective clinical and laboratory findings, *Pediatr Infect Dis J* 33:35, 2014.

Courtney PM, Flynn JM, Jaramillo D, et al.: Clinical indications for repeat MRI in children with acute hematogenous osteomyelitis, *J Pediatr Orthop* 30:883, 2010.

Dartnell J, Ramachandran M, Katchburian M: Haematogenous acute and subacute pediatric osteomyelitis: a systematic review of the literature, *J Bone Joint Surg* 94B:584, 2012.

DeRonde KJ, Girotto JE, Nicolau DP: Management of pediatric acute hematogenous osteomyelitis. Part I: Antimicrobial stewardship approach and review of therapies for methicillin-susceptible Staphylococcus aureus, Streptococcus pyogenes, and Kingella kingae, *Pharmacotherapy* 38:947, 2018.

Dietrich LN, Reid D, Doo D, et al.: Predicting MSSA in acute hematogenous osteomyelitis in a setting with MRSA prevalence, *J Pediatr Orthop* 35:426, 2015.

Eleftheriou D, Gerschman T, Sebire N, et al.: Biologic therapy in refractory chronic non-bacterial osteomyelitis of childhood, *Rheumatology* 49:1505, 2010.

El-Rosasy MA: Ilizarov treatment for pseudarthrosis of the tibia due to haematogenous osteomyelitis, *J Pediatr Orthop B* 22:200, 2013.

Hung NN: Cortical bone fenestrations with continuous antibiotic irrigation to mediate hematogenous tibial osteomyelitis in children, *J Pediatr Orthop B* 19:497, 2010.

Jones HW, Beckles VL, Akinola B, et al.: Chronic haematogenous osteomyelitis in children: an unsolved problem, *J Bone Joint Surg* 93B:1005, 2011.

Kumar J, Ramachandran M, Little D, Zenios M: Pelvic osteomyelitis in children, *J Pediatr Orthop B* 19:38, 2010.

Labbé JL, Peres O, Leclair O, et al.: Acute osteomyelitis in children: the pathogenesis revisited? *Orthop Traumatol Surg Res* 96:268, 2010.

Leigh W, Crawford H, Street M, et al.: Pediatric calcaneal osteomyelitis, *J Pediatr Orthop* 30:888, 2010.

Okubo Y, Nchioka K, Testa M: Nationwide survey of pediatric acute osteomyelitis in the USA, *J Pediatr Orthop B* 26:501, 2017.

Patwardhan S, Shuam AK, Mody RA, et al.: Reconstruction of bone defects after osteomyelitis with nonvascularized fibular graft: a retrospective study in twenty-six children, *J Bone Joint Surg* 95A:e561, 2013.

Peltola H, Pääkkönen M, Kallio P, et al.: Short- versus long-term antimicrobial treatment of acute hematogenous osteomyelitis of childhood: prospective, randomized trial on 131 culture-positive cases, *Pediatr Infect Dis J* 29:1123, 2010.

Pugmire BS, Shailam R, Gee MS: Role of MRI in the diagnosis and treatment of osteomyelitis in pediatric patients, *World J Radiol* 6:530, 2014.

Robinette ED, Brower L, Schaffzin JK, et al.: Use of a clinical care algorithm to improve care for children with hematogenous osteomyelitis, *Pediatrics* 143:pii: e20180387, 2019.

Schlung JE, Bastrom TP, Roocroft JH, et al.: Femoral neck aspiration aids in the diagnosis of osteomyelitis in children with septic hip, *J Pediatr Orthop* 38:532, 2018.

Street M, Puna R, Huang M, Crawford H: Pediatric acute hematogenous osteomyelitis, *J Pediatr Orthop* 35:634, 2015.

Thomsen I, Creech CB: Advances in the diagnosis and management of pediatric osteomyelitis, *Curr Infect Dis Rep* 13:451, 2011.

CHRONIC RECURRENT MULTIFOCAL OSTEOMYELITIS

Chen HC, Wuerdeman MF, Chang JH, et al.: The role of whole-body magnetic resonance imaging in diagnosing chronic recurrent multifocal osteomyelitis, *Radiol Case Rep* 13:485, 2018.

Falip C, Alison M, Boutry N, et al.: Chronic recurrent multifocal osteomyelitis (CRMO): a longitudinal case series review, *Pediatr Radiol* 43:355, 2013.

Hospach T, Langendoerfer M, von Kalle T, et al.: Spinal involvement in chronic recurrent multifocal osteomyelitis (CRMO) in childhood and effect of pamidronate, *Eur J Pediatr* 169:1105, 2010.

Kumar TKJ, Salium J, Shamsudeen TJ: Chronic recurrent multifocal osteomyelitis – a rare clinical presentation and review of the literature, *J Orthop Case Rep* 8(3):3, 2018.

Marangoni RG, Halpern AS: Chronic recurrent multifocal osteomyelitis primarily affecting the spine treated with anti-TNF therapy, *Spine* 35:E253, 2010.

Roderick MR, Ramanan AV: Chronic recurrent multifocal osteomyelitis, *Adv Exp Med Biol* 764:99, 2013.

Wipff J, Adamsbaum C, Kahan A, Job-Deslandre C: Chronic recurrent multifocal osteomyelitis, *Joint Bone Spine* 78:555, 2011.

Zhao Y: Ferguson: Chronic nonbacterial osteomyelitis and chronic recurrent multifocal osteomyelitis in children, *Pediatr Clin North Am* 65:783, 2018.

CHRONIC NONBACTERIAL OSTEOMYELITIS

Buch K, Thuesen ACB, Brøns C, et al.: Chronic non-bacterial osteomyelitis: a review, *Calcif Tissue Int* 104:544, 2019.

Gupta V, Jain A, Aggarwal A: Chronic nonbacterial osteomyelitis from a tertiary care referral center, *J Postgrad Med* 64:170, 2018.

Hofmann SR, Schnabel A, Rösen-Wolff A, et al.: Chronic nonbacterial osteomyelitis: pathophysiological concepts and current treatment strategies, *J Rheumatol* 43:1956, 2016.

POSTTRAUMATIC OSTEOMYELITIS

Aytac S, Schnetzke M, Swartman B, et al.: Posttraumatic and postoperative osteomyelitis: surgical revision strategy with persisting fistula, *Arch Orthop Trauma Surg* 134:159, 2014.

Bremmer D, Bookstaver B, Cairns M, et al.: Impact of body mass index and bacterial resistance in osteomyelitis after antibiotic prophylaxis of open lower-extremity fractures, *Surg Infect (Larchmt)* 18:368, 2017.

Jorge LS, Fucuta PS, Oliveira MGL, et al.: Outcomes and risk factors for polymicrobial posttraumatic osteomyelitis, *J Bone Jt Infect* 3:20, 2018.

Kim JH, Lee DH: Negative pressure wound therapy vs. conventional management in open tibia fractures: systematic review and meta-analysis, *Injury* pii: S0020, 2019. [Epub ahead of print].

Lewandowski LR, Potter BK, Murray CK, et al.: Osteomyelitis risk factors related to combat trauma in open femur fractures: a case-control analysis, *J Orthop Trauma* 33:e110, 2019.

Tribble DR, Lewandowski LR, Potter BK, et al.: Osteomyelitis risk factors related to combat trauma open tibia fractures: a case-control analysis, *J Orthop Trauma* 32:e344, 2018.

TREATMENT
EXTERNAL FIXATION

Abulaiti A, Yilihamu Y, Yasheng T, et al.: The psychological impact of external fixation using the Ilizarov or Orthofix LRS method to treat tibial osteomyelitis with a bone defect, *Injury* 48:2842, 2017.

Chen CM, Su AW, Chiu FY, Chen TH: A surgical protocol of ankle arthrodesis with combined Ilizarov's distraction-compression osteogenesis and locked nailing for osteomyelitis around the ankle joint, *J Trauma* 69:660, 2010.

Dróżdz M, Rak S, Bartosz P, et al.: Results of the treatment of infected nonunions of the lower limbs using the Ilizarov method, *Ortop Traumatol Rehabil* 19:111, 2017.

Lin CC, Chen CM, Chiu FY, et al.: Staged protocol for the treatment of chronic tibial shaft osteomyelitis with Ilizarov's technique followed by the application of intramedullary locked nail, *Orthopedics* 35:31769, 2012.

Yilihamu Y, Keremu A, Abulaiti A, et al.: Outcome of post-traumatic tibial osteomyelitis treated with an Orthofix LRS versus an Ilizarov external fixator, *Injury* 48:1636, 2017.

ANTIBIOTIC-LOADED IMPLANTS

Badie AA, Arafa MS: One-stage surgery for adult chronic osteomyelitis: concomitant use of antibiotic-loaded calcium sulphate and bone marrow aspirate, *Int Orthop* 43:1061, 2018.

Beenken KE, Bradney L, Bellamy W, et al.: Use of xylitol to enhance the therapeutic efficacy of polymethylmethacrylate-based antibiotic therapy in treatment of chronic osteomyelitis, *Antimicrob Agents Chemother* 56:5839, 2012.

El-Husseiny M, Patel S, MacFarlane RJ, Haddad FS: Biodegradable antibiotic delivery systems, *J Bone Joint Surg* 93B:151, 2011.

Ferguson JY, Dudareva M, Riley ND, et al.: The use of a biodegradable antibiotic-loaded calcium sulphate carrier containing tobramycin for the treatment of chronic osteomyeliitis: a series of 195 cases, *Bone Joint J* 96B:829, 2014.

Gauland C: Managing lower-extremity osteomyelitis locally with surgical debridement and synthetic calcium sulfate antibiotic tablets, *Adv Skin Wound Care* 24:515, 2011.

Kim JW, Cuellar DO, Hao J, et al.: Custom-made antibiotic cement nails: a comparative study of different fabrication techniques, *Injury* 45:1179, 2014.

Kluin OS, Busscher HJ, Neut D, van der Mei HC: Poly(trimethylene carbonate) as a carrier for rifampicin and vancomycin to target therapy recalcitrant staphylococcal biofilms, *J Orthop Res* 34(10):1828, 2016.

Kluin OS, van der Mei HC, Busscher HJ, Neut D: Biodegradable vs non-biodegradable antibiotic delivery devices in the treatment of osteomyelitis, *Expert Opin Drug Deliv* 10(3):341, 2013.

Koury KL, Hwang JS, Sirkin M: The antibiotic nail in the treatment of long bone infection: technique and results, *Orthop Clin North A* 48:155, 2017.

Lluin OS, van deer Mei HC, Busscher HJ, Neut D: Biodegradable vs nonbiodegradable antibiotic delivery devices in the treatment of osteomyelitis, *Expert Opin Drug Deliv* 10:341, 2013.

Mauffrey C, Butler N, Hake ME: Fabrication of an interlocked antibiotic/cement-coated carbon fiber nail for the treatment of long bone osteomyelitis, *J Orthop Trauma* 30(Suppl 2):S23, 2016.

McKee MD, Li-Bland EA, Wild LM, Schemitsch EH: A prospective, randomized clinical trial comparing an antibiotic-impregnated bioabsorbable bone substitute with standard antibiotic-impregnated cement beads in the treatment of chronic osteomyelitis and infected non-union, *J Orthop Trauma* 24:483, 2010.

McNally MA, Ferguson JY, Lau ACK, et al.: Single-stage treatment of chronic osteomyelitis with a new absorbable, gentamicin-loaded, calcium sulphate/ hydroxyapatite biocomposite, *Bone Joint J* 98-B:1289, 2016.

Niazi NS, Drampalos E, Morrissey N, et al.: Adjuvant antibiotic loaded biocomposite in the management of diabetic foot osteomyelitis – a multicenter study, *Foot (Edinb)* 39(22), 2019.

Peng KT, Chen CF, Chu IM: Treatment of osteomyelitis with teicoplanin-encapsulated biodegradable thermosensitive hydrogel nanoparticles, *Biomaterials* 19:5227, 2010.

Qin C, Xu L, Liao J, et al.: Management of osteomyelitis-induced massive tibial bone defect by monolateral external fixator combined with antibiotics-impregnated calcium sulphate: a retrospective study, *Biomed Res Int* 9070216, 2018.

Qin CH, Zhang HA, Chee YH, et al.: Comparison of the use of antibiotic-loaded calcium sulphate and wound irrigation-suction in the treatment of lower limb chronic osteomyelitis, *Injury* 50:508, 2019.

Qin CH, Zhou CH, Song HJ, et al.: Infected bone resection plus adjuvant antibiotic-impregnated calcium sulfate versus infected bone resection alone in the treatment of diabetic forefoot osteomyelitis, *BMC Musculoskelet Disord* 20:246, 2019.

Reilly RM, Robertson T, O'Toole RV, et al.: Are antibiotic nails effective in the treatment of infected tibial fractures? *Injury* 47:2809, 2016.

Romanó CL, Logoluso N, Meani E, et al.: A comparative study of the use of bioactive glass S53P4 and antibiotic-loaded calcium-based bone substitutes in the treatment of chronic osteomyelitis: a retrospective comparative study, *Bone Joint* 96B:845, 2014.

OTHER PROCEDURES/MODALITIES

Cierny 3rd G: Surgical treatment of osteomyelitis, *Plast Reconstr Surg* 127(Suppl 1):1905, 2011.

Clutton JM, Donaldson O, Perera A, et al.: Treating osteomyelitis of major limb amputations with a modified Lautenbach technique, *Injury* 48:2496, 2017.

Cox G, Jones E, McGonagle D, Giannoudis PV: Reamer-irrigator-aspirator indications and clinical results: a systematic review, *Int Orthop* 35:951, 2011.

Drago L, Romanó D, De Vecchi E, et al.: Bioactive glass BAG-S53P4 for the adjunctive treatment of chronic osteomyelitis of the long bones: an in vitro and prospective clinical study, *BMC Infect Dis* 13:584, 2013.

Fisher TK, Armstrong DG: Partial calcanectomy in high-risk patients with diabetes: use and utility of a "hurricane" incision approach, *Eplasty* 10:e17, 2010.

Kanakaris N, Gudipati S, Tosounidis T, et al.: The treatment of intramedullary osteomyelitis of the femur and tibia using the Reamer-Irrigator-Aspirator system and antibiotic cement rods, *Bone Joint J* 96B:783, 2014.

Savvidou OD, Kaspiris A, Bolia IK, et al.: Effectiveness of hyperbaric oxygen therapy for the management of chronic osteomyelitis: a systematic review of the literature, *Orthopedics* 41:193, 2018.

Schwartz AJ, Jones NF, Seeger LL, et al.: Chronic sclerosing osteomyelitis treated with wide resection and vascularized fibular autograft: a case report, *Am J Orthop* 39:E28, 2010.

Segreto FA, Beyer GA, Brieco P, et al.: Vertebral osteomyelitis: a comparison of associated outcomes in early versus delayed surgical treatment, *Int J Spine Surg* 12:703, 2018.

Sun Y, Zhang C, Jin D, et al.: Free vascularised fibular grafting in the treatment of large skeletal defects due to osteomyelitis, *Int Orthop* 34:425, 2010.

Tan Y, Wang X, Li H, et al.: The clinical efficacy of the vacuum-assisted closure therapy in the management of adult osteomyelitis, *Arch Orthop Trauma Surg* 131:255, 2011.

Waibel FWA, Klammer A, Götschi T, et al.: Outcome after surgical treatment of calcaneal osteomyelitis, *Foot Ankle Int* 40:562, 2019.

Walsh TP, Yates BJ: Calcanectomy: avoiding major amputation in the presence of calcaneal osteomyelitis – a case series, *Foot* 23:130, 2013.

ANTIBIOTIC TREATMENT

Haidar R, Boghossian AD, Atiyeh B: Duration of post-surgical antibiotics in chronic osteomyelitis: empiric or evidence-based? *Int J Infect Dis* 14:e752, 2010.

Rao N, Ziran BH, Lipsky BA: Treatment osteomyelitis: antibiotics and surgery, *Plast Reconstr Surg* 127(Suppl 1):1775, 2011.

Rod-Fleury T, Dunkel N, Assal M, et al.: Duration of post-surgical antibiotic therapy for adult chronic osteomyelitis: a single-centre experience, *Int Orthop* 35:1725, 2011.

Spellberg B, Lipsky BA: Systemic antibiotic therapy for chronic osteomyelitis in adults, *Clin Infect Dis* 54:393, 2012.

The complete list of references is available online at Expert Consult.com.

CHAPTER 5

INFECTIOUS ARTHRITIS

Anthony A. Mascioli, Ashley L. Park

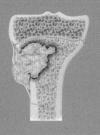

Acute septic arthritis results from bacterial invasion of a joint space, which can occur through hematogenous spread, direct inoculation from trauma or surgery, or contiguous spread from an adjacent site of osteomyelitis or cellulitis. Despite in-depth research into the pathophysiology and treatment of acute septic arthritis, the morbidity and mortality are still significant, especially in patients at the extremes of age. The bacterial strain and the individual's immune system determine whether a septic joint or a less severe infection develops. Even with currently available antibiotics and treatment regimens, serious complications may result. Delay in diagnosis and failure to begin treatment promptly are the most common reasons for late complications of infection.

A systematic review of the literature by Mathews et al. found that the risk factors for developing joint sepsis included rheumatoid arthritis, osteoarthritis, a prosthetic joint, low socioeconomic status, intravenous drug abuse, alcoholism, diabetes, previous intraarticular corticosteroid injection, and cutaneous ulcers.

CLINICAL PRESENTATION

Acute septic arthritis can occur at any age, but young children and elderly adults are most susceptible, especially if they have an already abnormal joint from previous trauma or from conditions such as hemophilia, osteoarthritis, or rheumatoid arthritis. Immune compromise for any reason and diseases such as cancer, diabetes, alcoholism, cirrhosis, and uremia increase the risk for infection. Usually, predisposing conditions are associated with particular types of causative

organisms (Table 5.1); a thorough history and physical examination should be done.

Septic arthritis occurs most frequently in adults; however, the most serious sequelae from infection occur in children, especially if a hip joint is involved and treatment has been delayed. Age-dependent anatomic variables may be responsible for the serious complications in children, such as destruction of the epiphysis and associated osteonecrosis from increased intracapsular pressure and septic effusion. Using immature avian models, Alderson et al. provided evidence that transepiphyseal vessels do exist and provide a direct connection between the physis and epiphyseal cartilage, supplying a route for bacteria to spread from an osteomyelitic focus in the metaphysis to the epiphysis and subsequently to the joint space.

The lower extremity weight-bearing joints are predominantly affected (61% to 79%); however, any joint can be involved, and multiple joint infections do occur. A thorough examination to determine if there is monoarticular or polyarticular infection is necessary before treatment is initiated. Inflammation of a single joint can be caused by numerous diseases (Box 5.1). Joint sepsis should be an early consideration, however, because failure to diagnose this condition promptly may result in irreversible joint damage or death.

Acute septic arthritis can be difficult to diagnose in neonates because the inflammatory response is blunted and signs such as fever, swelling, erythema, and pain may be minimal or lacking. The only finding in a neonate may be infection at another site (e.g., the umbilical catheter), irritability, failure to thrive, asymmetry of limb position, or displeasure at being handled.

TABLE 5.1

Organisms Found in Common Clinical Settings of Infectious Arthritis

CLINICAL FACTOR	ORGANISM
PATIENT AGE	
Neonate	*Staphylococcus aureus*
<2 yr	*Haemophilus influenzae, S. aureus*
>2 yr	*S. aureus*
Young adults (healthy, sexually active)	*Neisseria gonorrhoeae*
Elderly adults	*S. aureus* (50%), streptococci, gram-negative bacilli
STRUCTURAL ABNORMALITIES	
Aspiration or injection	*S. aureus*
Trauma	Gram-negative bacilli, anaerobes, *S. aureus*
PROSTHESIS	
Early infection	*S. epidermidis*
Late infection	Gram-positive cocci, anaerobes
MEDICAL CONDITIONS	
Injecting drug use	Atypical gram-negative bacilli (e.g., *Pseudomonas* species)
Rheumatoid arthritis	*S. aureus*
Systemic lupus erythematosus, sickle cell anemia	*Salmonella* species
Hemophilia	*S. aureus* (50%), streptococci, gram-negative bacilli
Immunosuppression	*S. aureus, Mycobacterium* species, fungi

Modified from Stimmler MM: Infectious arthritis: tailoring initial treatment to clinical findings, *Postgrad Med* 99:127–131, 1996.

BOX 5.1

Differential Diagnostic Considerations in Monoarticular Arthritis

- Infection
- Crystal-induced arthritis (gout, calcium pyrophosphate dihydrate deposition disease)
- Trauma
- Hemarthrosis (hemophilia, sickle cell anemia)
- Osteomyelitis
- Periarticular syndrome (bursitis, tendinitis)
- Ruptured Baker cyst
- Deep vein thrombosis
- Pigmented villonodular synovitis
- Mechanical derangement
- Foreign body

Adapted from Stimmler MM: Infectious arthritis: tailoring initial treatment to clinical findings, *Postgrad Med* 99:127–131, 1996.

TABLE 5.2

Probability Algorithm for Two-Variable Model

C-REACTIVE PROTEIN	UNABLE TO BEAR WEIGHT	PROBABILITY
Yes	Yes	0.74
Yes	No	0.15
No	Yes	0.06
No	No	0.01

From Singhal R, Perry DC, Khan FN, et al: The use of CRP within a clinical prediction algorithm for the differentiation of septic arthritis and transient synovitis in children, *J Bone Joint Surg Br* 93:1156–1161, 2011.

Clinical predictor algorithms have been used to differentiate transient synovitis from septic arthritis in children. A C-reactive protein greater than 20 mg/L and inability to bear weight yielded a 74% probability of septic arthritis, and patients with neither predictor had a less than 1% probability of septic arthritis (Table 5.2).

SYNOVIAL FLUID STUDIES

The importance of early diagnosis and treatment of septic arthritis prior to destruction of an affected joint is well established. The organisms and/or the cytotoxins they may produce can irreversibly damage cartilage and subchondral bone within only a few days. An estimated 25% to 50% of patients with septic arthritis end up with irreversible loss of joint function. Therefore, early diagnosis is the most important factor for functional prognosis in patients with septic arthritis.

The current benchmark for identification of the causative microorganism and ascertaining its antimicrobial susceptibility is the conventional culture of aspirated joint fluid. The synovial fluid obtained should be sent for immediate Gram staining, culture, cell counts, and crystal analysis. Measuring erythrocyte sedimentation rates or C-reactive protein levels may be helpful in following the treatment course. A C-reactive protein of more than 10.5 mg/dL is predictive of infection. A leukocyte count greater than 2000/mm³ points toward inflammation, whereas lower counts suggest a mechanical disorder. However, features classically taken to indicate septic arthritis include cloudy or turbid joint fluid, a nucleate cell count greater than 50,000/mm, or a high percentage of neutrophils; leukocyte counts of 28,000/mm or less also have been implicated, especially in immunocompromised patients. In addition to the total leukocyte count, the proportion of polymorphonuclear neutrophils (PMNs), if greater than 90%, indicates infection.

Crystal-induced arthritis is the main differential diagnosis in septic arthritis, as the clinical manifestations may be similar and the joint fluid findings comparable. Furthermore, infection developing concomitantly with crystal-induced arthritis may be overlooked when the joint fluid examination shows microcrystals. Combining standard joint fluid markers with the absence of microcrystals improves diagnosis of septic arthritis compared to standard cytologic features used alone.

Although synovial fluid culture is useful in the diagnosis of septic arthritis, both false negatives and false positives can occur. Cultures can be negative in up to 75% of patients with septic arthritis. The use of empirical antibiotics may obscure results. Studies are being conducted to develop tests for rapid and accurate diagnosis of septic arthritis. Molecular methods such as polymerase chain reaction (PCR) technique are used to identify bacteria by their genotypes. The advantage of automated multiplex PCR (MPCR) lies in the rapid identification of causative pathogens and their antibiotic sensitivities (5 hours compared with several days in standard tissue culture techniques). Results appear promising for the diagnosis of periprosthetic joint infection in sonication and synovial fluid as well as septic arthritis in synovial fluid of native joints.

IMAGING STUDIES

Numerous imaging techniques are available to help detect joint infections, and although they can help confirm the suspicion of septic arthritis, they are not diagnostic. In the first few days of infection, radiographs usually are normal; however, they may be helpful in that they may show soft-tissue swelling, displacement of the fat pad, or joint space widening from localized edema. As the infection progresses, joint space narrowing from the destruction of cartilage may become evident. Radiographs may be used to monitor the response to treatment and to detect inadequately treated stages of the disease, such as generalized joint destruction, osteomyelitis, osteoarthritis, joint fusion, or bone loss.

Ultrasonography, in contrast to radiographs, can be used to detect even small collections of fluid deep in the joints. Non-echo-free effusions from clotted hemorrhagic collections are characteristic of a septic joint. Ultrasonography can be used to guide initial joint aspiration and drainage and to monitor the status of intraarticular compartments, joint capsules, bone surface, or adjacent soft tissues. It is noninvasive, inexpensive, and easy to use but is heavily operator-dependent. Ultrasound-guided percutaneous needle aspiration has also proved useful in obtaining biopsy and to decompress the infection; in cases of acute arthritis when joint aspiration is not possible or in the absence of synovial fluid, the biopsy can confirm the diagnosis by determining the causal pathogen or can improve it when there is perivascular PMN infiltration.

Computed tomography (CT), magnetic resonance imaging (MRI), and bone scans also may be obtained to diagnose septic arthritis; however, these tests are not always necessary. CT, which is more sensitive than radiography, has limited use in the early stages of infection. It can show soft-tissue swelling, joint effusion, and abscess formation and can be used to guide joint aspiration, monitor therapy, and help select operative approaches. MRI can detect infection, and the extent of infection, and is particularly useful in diagnosing infections that are difficult to access. MRI has a greater resolution than CT and shows better anatomic detail than bone scans, making it useful in differentiating between bone and soft-tissue infections and showing joint effusion. In addition, patients are not exposed to radiation. MRI is costly, has limited value in the presence of metal implants, and has a lower resolution than CT in calcified bone structures and cortices. Similar to other imaging techniques, MRI is nonspecific and cannot differentiate between infectious and noninfectious inflammatory arthropathies.

Radionuclide bone scans often can detect localized areas of inflammation. Although the technetium-99m (^{99m}Tc)-methylene diphosphonate scan shows increases in isotope accumulation in areas of osteoblasts and increased vascularity, it may be normal in the early stages of septic arthritis. Other radiopharmaceuticals, including gallium citrate and indium-111 (^{111}In) chloride, are more specific and sensitive in the detection of active infection than ^{99m}Tc-methylene diphosphonate, but they do not show bone or joint detail well, and it is often difficult to distinguish between bone, joint, or soft-tissue inflammation.[111] In-labeled leukocytes localize in the areas of acute infection, but although this scan is positive in approximately 60% of patients with septic arthritis, false-positive results may occur in patients with osteoarthritis.

PATHOGENESIS

Hematogenous infection of a joint begins with a systemic bacteremia that ultimately invades the synovial cartilaginous junction from the intravascular space and spreads throughout the synovium and synovial fluid. Why joints are affected and other vulnerable organs are not is unclear; however, collagen receptors found on *Staphylococcus aureus* (the most common nongonococcal infecting cause of hematogenous septic arthritis) may play a role. Also, the lack of a limiting basement membrane in the capillaries of synovia may allow intravascular bacteria to reach the extravascular space of synovial tissue through gaps between capillary endothelial cells. In addition, synovial fibroblasts inhibit phagocytosis of bacteria.

Soon after the synovium has been infected it becomes hyperemic and infiltrated with polymorphonuclear leukocytes that rapidly increase over the next several days. Histologically, the appearance changes from acute to chronic inflammation with an increase in mononuclear leukocytes and lymphocytes, which become the predominant inflammatory cells by 3 weeks.

Destruction of the articular cartilage, which results from degradation of ground substance, is apparent 4 to 6 days after infection. Depletion of ground substance, according to Perry, begins approximately 2 days after inoculation and is caused by activation of enzymes from the acute inflammatory response, production of toxins and enzymes by bacteria, and stimulation of T lymphocytes during the delayed immune response. Bacterial antigens deposited in the synovium and specific toxins, such as staphylococcal enterotoxin, produced by bacteria stimulate proliferation of T lymphocytes. As the T lymphocytes increase and degrade the ground substance, collagen is exposed to collagenases, altering the mechanical properties of the articular cartilage and increasing its susceptibility to wear. Complete destruction of articular cartilage occurs at approximately 4 weeks. Joint dislocation or subluxation and osteomyelitis also may occur.

MICROBIOLOGY

Age is an important factor in determining the causative agent in bacterial infection. *S. aureus* is the leading cause in all ages followed by group *A. streptococcus* and *Enterobacter*. Until the development of a vaccine, *Haemophilus influenzae* was the main pathogen in infants and toddlers and is still recognized in the literature as such. *S. aureus* (including methicillin-resistant strains) is the most common pathogen of septic arthritis in hospitalized neonates. Intravenous catheters and hyperalimentation have been implicated in the transmission of this organism.

Kingella kingae, an organism difficult to recover by joint cultures on solid media, may be a more common cause of septic arthritis than previously recognized, especially in children between the ages of 6 and 36 months. Infections caused by

K. kingae are milder, and fever may even be absent. This organism is susceptible to most penicillins and cephalosporins.

Neisseria gonorrhoeae causes approximately 75% of septic arthritis cases in healthy, sexually active young adults, although a septic joint develops in less than 3% of patients infected with *N. gonorrhoeae*. This infection has a slightly different presentation than other types of infectious arthritis. Often the infection is polyarticular and may be associated with a papular rash. Joint cultures often are negative, but cultures from the pharynx or urethra may be positive. PCR may help identify *N. gonorrhoeae* in culture-negative synovial fluid. Gonococcal arthritis generally has a favorable outcome if treated with appropriate antibiotics, and drainage usually is unnecessary.

There has been a noted increase in the number of community-acquired methicillin-resistant *S. aureus* infections in the pediatric population in several large communities. This includes osteomyelitis and septic arthritis. At our pediatric institution, community-acquired methicillin-resistant *S. aureus* infection accounted for 26% of all septic arthritis and acute hematogenous osteomyelitis admissions. The community-acquired methicillin-resistant *S. aureus* infections are more likely to have positive blood cultures after appropriate treatment has been initiated and to require multiple surgical procedures.

In older adults with nongonococcal disease, *S. aureus* infections cause about half of the cases of septic arthritis, and streptococci and gram-negative bacilli are responsible for the other half. Polyarticular sepsis caused by *S. aureus* is extremely serious in patients with rheumatoid arthritis, hemophilia, or immunosuppression, and mortality rates have been reported to be 56%. Hallmark findings in acute septic arthritis, such as pain with passive motion, swelling, and erythema, also may be difficult to interpret in patients with rheumatoid arthritis. Adults with systemic lupus erythematosus have an increased likelihood of *Salmonella* infection, and individuals with a history of intravenous drug use are predisposed to gram-negative infections, including those caused by *Pseudomonas* organisms.

TREATMENT

The principles in the management of acute septic arthritis include (1) adequate drainage of the joint and resection of infected tissue, (2) antibiotics to diminish the systemic effects of sepsis, and (3) resting the joint in a stable position. Prompt drainage and evaluation of purulent joint fluid is crucial for preservation of articular cartilage and for resolution of the infection.

If a joint is suspected of being infected, aspiration with a large-bore needle should be done before antibiotic therapy is initiated. Treatment in children should be aggressive whether or not a causative organism is identified.

Empirical antibiotic treatment is based on the patient's age and risk factors (Table 5.3). Empirical antibiotic therapy should be given until culture and sensitivity results are available, at which time definitive treatment is initiated (Table 5.4). If no organism is isolated, empirical therapy should be continued. In general, the decision regarding duration of therapy is left up to the physician and depends on the type of infecting organism, the condition of the patient, and the response to therapy. Infections caused by *H. influenzae* type b, *Neisseria,* or *Streptococcus* generally respond rapidly to

TABLE 5.3

Empirical Antimicrobial Therapy

PATHOGEN	EMPIRICAL ANTIMICROBIAL
Gram-positive cocci in clusters with MRSA risk factor* or β-lactam allergy	Vancomycin 15 mg/kg IV q12h
Gram-positive cocci in clusters, no MRSA risk factors	Nafcillin or oxacillin 2 g IV q4h
Gram-positive cocci, no MRSA risk factors	Cefazolin 2 g IV q8h
Gram-positive cocci in chains (*Streptococci* presumed)	Penicillin G 12-18 MU/day or ampicillin 2 g IV q4h
Gram-negative cocci (presumptive *Neisseria*)	Ceftriaxone 1-2 g IV/IM q12-24h or cefotaxime 2 g IV q8h
Gram-negative rods	Ceftazidime 2 g IV q 8 h or cefepime 2 g IV q8h
Negative Gram stain, previously healthy, no MRSA risk factors	Cefazolin 2 g IV q8h
Negative Gram stain, healthcare associated or other MRSA risk factors	Vancomycin 15 mg/kg IV q12h plus ceftazidime 2 g IV q8h, cefepime 2 g IV q8h or piperacillin/tazobactam 4.5 g IV q6h
Human, dog, or cat bite	Ampicillin sulbactam 1.5-3 g IV q4h

*Risk factors for methicillin-resistant *Staphylococcus aureus*: recent hospitalization or nursing home admission, hemodialysis, diabetes, intravenous drug use, recent antibiotic exposure, recent incarceration, recent skin or soft-tissue infection in patient, or close contact. Community-acquired MRSA often occurs without preexisting risk factors. *MRSA*, Methicillin-resistant *Staphylococcus aureus*.

Data from Nuermberger E: Septic arthritis community acquired. In Bartlett JG, Auwaerter PG, Pham PA, editors: *John Hopkins ABX guide to diagnosis and treatment of infectious diseases*, ed 3, Burlington, 2012, Jones and Bartlett.

appropriate antibacterial management, and duration of therapy can be brief (<2 weeks). Infections caused by staphylococci and gram-negative bacilli respond more slowly, however, often requiring 4 to 6 weeks of treatment. A longer period of therapy is required if the hip or shoulder is involved, if the patient is immunocompromised, or if the response to treatment has been poor. In general, if laboratory findings do not improve after treatment, an infectious disease consultation is warranted.

There is strong evidence to support the beneficial effect of corticosteroids as adjunctive therapy with antibiotics in the treatment of septic arthritis. This is consistent with data that show improved outcomes associated with steroid use in severe sepsis, severe pneumonia, bacterial meningitis, and acute pyelonephritis.

We believe that if the diagnosis is made early and the involved joint is superficial, such as the elbow or ankle, aspiration should be performed and repeated if necessary. Appropriate antibiotics should be administered, and the joint should be splinted in a position of function. The patient should be observed for a decrease in pain, swelling, and temperature and for improved joint mobility. Infections caused by less virulent organisms usually respond promptly to treatment. If the response is not favorable and repeat aspiration does not

TABLE 5.4

Pathogen-Directed Antimicrobial Therapy

PATHOGEN	ANTIMICROBIAL THERAPY
Staphylococcus aureus (methicillin sensitive)	Nafcillin or oxacillin 2 g IV q4h × 3 wk Cefazolin 2 g IV q8h × 3 wk
S. aureus (methicillin resistant or type I penicillin allergy)	Vancomycin 15 mg/kg IV q12h × 3 wk
Streptococci including penicillin-sensitive *Streptococcus pneumoniae* ([MIC <4 mg/L])	Penicillin G 12-18 MU IV qd divided dose or ampicillin 2 g IV q4h × 2 wk
S. pneumoniae (penicillin-resistant)	Ceftriaxone 1-2 g IV q12h or cefotaxime 2 g IV q8h if susceptible, or vancomycin 15 mg/kg IV q12h × 2 wk
Enteric gram-negative bacilli	Ceftriaxone 1-2 g IV q12h or cefotaxime 2 g IV q8h × 3 wk
Gram-negative bacilli (*Pseudomonas aeruginosa*)	Ceftazidime 2 g IV q8h or cefepime 2 g IV q8h, plus gentamicin or tobramycin 5 mg/kg IV q24h × 3 wk
Gram-negative bacilli	Ciprofloxacin 400 mg IV q8-12h or 750 mg PO q12h or levofloxacin 750 mg IV or 750 mg PO qd × 3 wk
Polymicrobial	Ampicillin/sulbactam 1.5-3 g IV q4h × 3 wk Clindamycin 600 mg IV q6-8h × 3 wk plus ciprofloxacin 400 mg IV or 750 mg PO q12h or levofloxacin 750 mg IV or 750 mg PO qd × 3 wk
Gram-positive etiology and type I penicillin allergy	Vancomycin 15 mg/kg IV q12h × 3 wk
Vancomycin resistance	Linezolid 600 mg IV or PO q12h. For ages younger than 12 years 10 mg/kg q8h.

MIC, Minimal inhibitory concentration.
Data from Nuermberger E: Septic arthritis community acquired. In Bartlett JG, Auwaerter PG, Pham PA, editors: *John Hopkins ABX guide to diagnosis and treatment of infectious diseases*, ed 3, Burlington, 2012, Jones and Bartlett.

show a decrease in the synovial leukocyte count within 24 to 48 hours, drainage is necessary. If purulent material is deeply situated in a joint, such as the shoulder or hip, open surgical drainage may be necessary. Arthroscopic drainage is a good alternative to open drainage in many instances. Clinical comparisons of aspiration with arthroscopy or through open procedures have shown comparable results. Stutz et al. reported a 91% cure rate in 78 joints with arthroscopic irrigation and debridement, with only 4% requiring open procedures. The efficacy of treatment, however, was dependent on the stage of the joint infection. Numerous other studies have reported lower infection rates, fewer repeat debridements, shorter hospital stays, and better functional results in patients who have had arthroscopic irrigation and debridement compared to

open drainage of the knee, hip, shoulder, wrist, elbow, and ankle. In one study of 161 patients with septic arthritis of the knee, 71% in the open drainage group required repeat drainage compared with 50% in the arthroscopic group. Jiang et al. analyzed 7145 cases from a nationwide database of septic arthritis of the shoulder and found higher incidences of septicemia and urinary tract infections perioperatively in arthroscopically treated patients than in those treated with an open procedure, but they had significantly fewer incidences of osteomyelitis. These authors noted that the patients in the arthroscopic group had substantially more preexisting conditions than those in the open group, which was likely a contributing factor. As Abdel et al. pointed out in their study of 50 patients with native shoulder sepsis, most patients were elderly, with 57% being immunocompromised. One in three required additional intervention. Kang and Lee agreed that host factors, age, comorbidities, and causative organisms are all related to outcome of arthroscopic debridement in septic arthritis. A systematic review of septic arthritis of the hip showed that arthroscopic native hip irrigation was safe and effective in select patients (those without deformity, with no bacterial infection, or those who were immunocompromised). The most important factor for a good outcome remains early diagnosis and treatment and patient selection. Patients with advanced arthroscopic findings have been shown to have worse outcomes.

As the infection resolves, therapy to restore normal joint function is begun, including functional splinting initially to prevent deformity, isometric muscle strengthening, and active range-of-motion exercises. Patients being treated for infectious arthritis often have varying degrees of deformity, and treatment with traction, dynamic splints, serial casting, and passive exercises may be useful. In the residual stage, the infection has completely subsided but the joint or joints involved are left with deformity or limitation of motion, so treatment is directed at correction and functional restoration of the joint. The possibility of reactivating the infection should be considered, however, when any necessary procedure is undertaken at this stage.

TARSAL JOINTS

Primary septic arthritis of the tarsal joints is rare. An uncontrolled infection in the tarsal joints requires wide surgical drainage.

SURGICAL DRAINAGE OF THE TARSAL JOINT

TECHNIQUE 5.1

- Make a medial or lateral longitudinal incision 5 to 7.5 cm long.
- Deepen the incision to the joint capsules and open them widely.
- Take appropriate material for Gram stain and cultures and evacuate the pus by copious saline irrigation.
- Close the wound loosely over drains.

- Carry the dissection through the fascia just lateral to the sheath of the extensor tendons and the peroneus tertius tendon.
- Incise the joint capsule longitudinally.

POSTEROLATERAL DRAINAGE OF THE ANKLE

TECHNIQUE 5.3

- Hold the foot in dorsiflexion. This tends to obliterate the anterior compartment and enlarge the posterior compartment; consequently, the purulent material may be evacuated more thoroughly.
- Begin the incision 5 cm proximal to the tip of the lateral malleolus and just lateral to the Achilles tendon. Extend the incision distally to the calcaneus and curve it along the superior border of that bone for 2.5 cm.
- Retract the sural nerve and small saphenous vein laterally. Press the thick pad of fatty tissue over the posterior part of the capsule distalward against the subtalar joint to protect that joint.
- Retract the peroneal tendons laterally and incise the joint proximal to the shining, cord-like, posterior talofibular ligament.
- Be sure to incise the posterior capsule under direct vision. This approach also is excellent for draining the subtalar joint.

ANTEROMEDIAL DRAINAGE OF THE ANKLE

TECHNIQUE 5.4

- Make an incision 7.5 cm long on the anterior aspect of the ankle parallel with the medial border of the anterior tibial tendon.
- Carry the dissection directly into the capsule of the joint.
- Do not disturb the tendon sheaths.

POSTEROMEDIAL DRAINAGE OF THE ANKLE

TECHNIQUE 5.5

- Make an incision 7.5 to 10 cm long medial to and parallel with the Achilles tendon.
- Retract the flexor hallucis longus tendon and the neurovascular bundle medially.

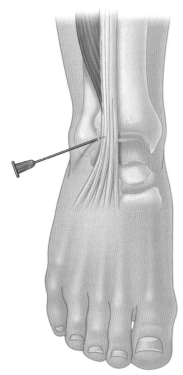

FIGURE 5.1 Aspiration of ankle, anterolateral view.

POSTOPERATIVE CARE A posterior plaster splint is applied with the foot in neutral position and the ankle at 90 degrees. The splint is worn until the wound has healed; then graduated weight bearing is started.

ANKLE

ASPIRATION

Swelling around the ankle often makes fluctuation difficult to locate. To avoid injuring important structures, the needle is inserted 2.5 cm proximal and 1.3 cm anterior to the tip of the lateral malleolus. This is just lateral to the peroneus tertius tendon (Fig. 5.1).

DRAINAGE

The ankle may be drained through any of the following approaches: anterolateral, anteromedial, posterolateral, and posteromedial (see Figs. 1.34, 1.36, and 1.38). The posterolateral approach has proved safer and more effective than any other approach.

ANTEROLATERAL DRAINAGE OF THE ANKLE

TECHNIQUE 5.2

- Make an incision 5 to 7.5 cm long over the joint and 1.3 to 2.5 cm anterior to the lateral malleolus.

■ Continue the dissection down to the ankle joint capsule. Incise the capsule. If the dissection is kept lateral to the flexor hallucis longus tendon, the nerve, vessels, and tendons that lie posterior to the medial malleolus are avoided.

POSTOPERATIVE CARE After the capsule has been incised by any of the previous approaches, the wound is closed loosely over drains. A posterior splint is applied with the foot in neutral position and the ankle at 90 degrees. The splint is worn until the wound has healed; then graduated weight bearing and active range-of-motion exercises are begun.

ANKLE ARTHROSCOPY

Ankle arthroscopy has been shown to be successful in treating early septic arthritis. Arthroscopic synovectomy was added to the protocol in addition to irrigation, yielding similar outcomes to a traditional open approach. Ankle arthroscopy is described in other chapter.

KNEE

The incidence of bacterial infections in the large joints is 2 in 100,000 per year. The knee joint is the most frequently affected.

ASPIRATION

Because the knee is a superficial joint, it can be aspirated easily. The needle is inserted on the lateral side at the level of the superior pole of the patella. It is advanced through the lateral retinaculum and into the joint (Fig. 5.2).

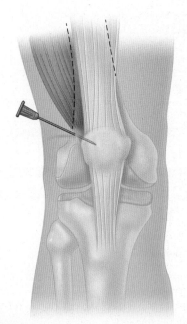

FIGURE 5.2 Aspiration of knee, anteroposterior view.

DRAINAGE

In acute septic arthritis, usually anteromedial arthrotomy or arthroscopic drainage and antibiotic treatment are adequate. In more difficult cases, the following approaches may be used. If the posterior compartment of the knee is distended and a popliteal abscess is well established, parallel anterior incisions combined with posterolateral and posteromedial (Henderson) incisions usually are best. If possible, posterior drainage should be avoided because the infection may spread through the fascial planes of the thigh and leg. When fluctuation indicates a pocket of pus in the posterior compartment of the joint that has not been or that cannot be drained effectively through Henderson incisions, posterior drainage is necessary. The posterior compartment may be divided by a median septum into medial and lateral compartments. These may be drained effectively by the Klein or Kelikian approach (both described subsequently). A posterior midline approach should not be used to drain an infected knee because it exposes the popliteal vessels to pus and to pressure from the drain and creates a potentially contracting scar across the joint.

■ ARTHROSCOPIC DRAINAGE OF THE KNEE

Arthroscopic drainage is the preferred treatment for acute septic arthritis of the knee in adults. Several studies have reported good results with this technique, which combines the advantages and avoids the disadvantages of needle aspiration and arthrotomy. With arthroscopy, purulent material can be removed and the joint can be irrigated. The joint cartilage can be inspected, and loculations or adhesions can be removed with the arthroscope. A partial synovectomy can be performed if necessary. Drains can be placed into the joint through the portal sites for drainage or for a continuous suction drainage system. Arthroscopy also has the advantage of allowing much earlier range of motion and rehabilitation of the knee joint compared with arthrotomy. Arthroscopic drainage has been reported to be a more successful index procedure and requires fewer repeat irrigation and debridements than open drainage.

ARTHROSCOPIC DRAINAGE OF THE KNEE

TECHNIQUE 5.6

■ After sterile preparation of the knee, with the patient under general or regional anesthesia, insert a large-bore inflow cannula into the suprapatellar pouch (Fig. 5.3A).

■ Place the arthroscope through a standard anterolateral portal and irrigate the joint with saline or lactated Ringer solution (preferably Neosporin G.U. solution) until the fluid coming out of the joint cavity is clear.

■ Inspect the joint for any evidence of fibrinous debris or loculations and note the condition of the joint cartilage.

■ Use other portals for debridement and irrigation as necessary.

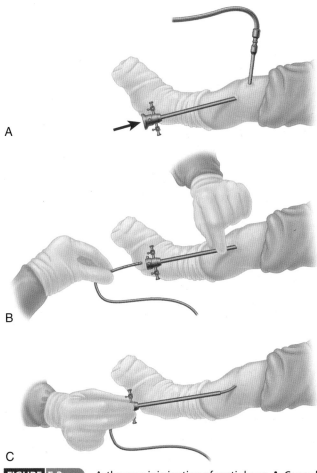

A

B

C

FIGURE 5.3 Arthroscopic irrigation of septic knee. **A,** Cannula is inserted in suprapatellar pouch for outflow, and knee is irrigated through arthroscopic sheath. **B,** Small suction drain is inserted through arthroscopic sheath. **C,** Sheath is removed as drain is held in place. **SEE TECHNIQUE 5.6.**

- After the joint has been visually inspected and debrided, continue joint irrigation.
- After the arthroscope has been removed, insert a small drain through the arthroscopic sheath (Fig. 5.3B), and remove the sheath as the drain is held in place (Fig. 5.3C).
- Splint the knee in a functional position.

POSTOPERATIVE CARE An active exercise regimen beginning with straight-leg raising and quadriceps setting is begun immediately postoperatively. Active range of motion is started as soon as the patient is comfortable, generally 24 hours after anteromedial arthrotomy or arthroscopic drainage. The drains, if present, are removed at 24 to 48 hours after surgery. Functional splinting is maintained for 1 week except for periods of exercise.

ANTERIOR DRAINAGE OF THE KNEE

TECHNIQUE 5.7

- Make parallel anterior incisions 7.5 to 10 cm long on each side of the patella and sufficiently medial or lateral to the sides of the patellar tendon.
- Incise the capsule and synovium, carefully evacuate the purulent material, and disrupt any loculations or adhesions. Use copious saline irrigation.
- Leave the synovium open, but loosely close the capsule and skin over drains. Use absorbable monofilament sutures for closing the capsule.
- When this approach is used for drainage, patients must spend most of their time in the prone position for adequate drainage, or they must be allowed to carry out either early active range of motion of the knee or continuous passive motion.

POSTEROLATERAL AND POSTEROMEDIAL DRAINAGE OF THE KNEE

TECHNIQUE 5.8

(HENDERSON)
- With the knee flexed, make an incision 7.5 cm long on the posterolateral aspect of the knee just anterior to the fibular head and biceps tendon. This approach avoids the peroneal nerve, which parallels the posteromedial border of the biceps tendon and passes around the neck of the fibula. Continue the incision through the iliotibial band to the joint capsule.
- Incise the capsule and enter the lateral part of the posterior compartment of the knee (see Fig. 1.62).
- Make a similar posteromedial incision anterior to the relaxed tendon of the semimembranosus, semitendinosus, sartorius, and gracilis muscles (see Fig. 1.63).
- Carry the dissection down through the capsule into the medial part of the posterior compartment. This longitudinal capsular incision is made just posterior to the tibial collateral ligament.

POSTEROMEDIAL DRAINAGE OF THE KNEE

Klein's approach to the posteromedial aspect of the joint takes advantage of the fact that the bursae between the semimembranosus tendon and the medial head of the gastrocnemius muscle often communicate with the knee joint. Consequently, an incision into these bursae often leads directly into that joint.

TECHNIQUE 5.9

(KLEIN)
- With the knee slightly flexed, make a longitudinal incision 10 cm long centered over the knee joint and located just lateral to the semimembranosus tendon.
- Incise the superficial fascia and expose the tendons of the medial hamstrings.
- Identify the interval between the gastrocnemius and semimembranosus and follow the gastrocnemius proximally to its insertion on the medial femoral condyle.
- Expose and incise the capsule in this interval.

POSTEROMEDIAL AND POSTEROLATERAL DRAINAGE OF THE KNEE

TECHNIQUE 5.10

(KELIKIAN)
- Make a posterior longitudinal incision 7.5 to 10 cm long centered over the joint and the semimembranosus tendon.
- Develop the interval between this tendon and the medial head of the gastrocnemius muscle.
- Divide the semimembranosus and suture its proximal end to the deep fascia (Fig. 5.4A).
- Make a generous window in the joint capsule and excise the posterior horn of the medial meniscus.

- If the posterior compartment is divided by a median septum and complete drainage is impossible through the posteromedial incision, or if drainage of only the lateral compartment is desired, make a longitudinal incision 7.5 to 10 cm long over the biceps femoris tendon.
- Incise the deep fascia lateral and anterior to this tendon and free the tendon from the head of the fibula. Also free the popliteus tendon from its insertion on the lateral femoral condyle.
- Suture the free ends of both tendons to the deep fascia (Fig. 5.4B).
- Window the joint capsule and remove a wedge of the lateral meniscus.
- Kelikian advises that drains not be used but rather that skeletal traction be applied to separate the joint surfaces.

HIP

Acute septic arthritis of the hip is a more serious disease in children than in adults, and severe complications are much more common in children. In many cases, infection begins first in the metaphysis or epiphysis and is carried into the joint. As a result of the peculiar circulation of the femoral head, a septic hip places the femoral head at high risk for osteonecrosis. Epiphyseal separation also has been reported as a complication of septic arthritis of the hip in children. If a septic hip goes undiagnosed in an infant, a pathologic dislocation may occur. After an infected hip in an infant or child has been surgically drained, the hip should be

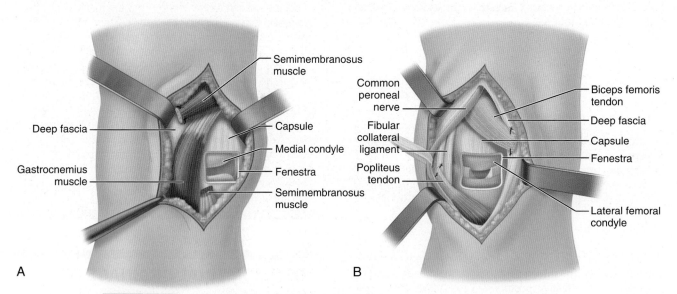

A

B

FIGURE 5.4 **A,** Kelikian approach to drain medial half of posterior compartment of knee. Semimembranosus tendon has been divided, and its proximal end has been sutured to deep fascia. Capsule has been windowed, and posterior horn of medial meniscus has been excised. **B,** Kelikian approach to drain lateral half of posterior compartment of knee. Incision has been made medial to biceps femoris tendon to protect common peroneal nerve. Biceps tendon has been divided at its insertion, popliteus tendon has been freed from its origin, and free ends of tendons have been sutured to deep fascia. Capsule has been windowed, and wedge of lateral meniscus has been excised. **SEE TECHNIQUE 5.10.**

supported in abduction to reduce the risk of pathologic dislocation. Bilateral septic arthritis is seen more often in the hip than in other joints and occasionally is associated with spinal infection. Independent risk factors for repeat surgical procedures in children include a C-reactive protein greater than 10 mg/L, an erythrocyte sedimentation rate of greater than 40 mm/hr, osteomyelitis, and methicillin-resistant *S. aureus* infection.

ASPIRATION

A lateral, anterior, or medial approach can be used to aspirate the hip joint. The use of image intensification makes needle placement more certain. If fluid cannot be aspirated, an arthrogram should be made to verify the needle's position. At times, pus cannot be aspirated, although later it is proved to be present by open drainage. In these circumstances, the hip should be explored if local and systemic symptoms cannot be otherwise controlled.

LATERAL ASPIRATION OF THE HIP

TECHNIQUE 5.11

- Insert the needle at a 45-degree angle with the surface of the thigh just inferior and anterior to the greater trochanter (Fig. 5.5).
- Advance the needle medially and proximally close to the bone for 5 to 10 cm, depending on the size of the patient, and into the joint.

ANTERIOR ASPIRATION OF THE HIP

TECHNIQUE 5.12

- Palpate the femoral artery in line with the inguinal ligament (Fig. 5.5).
- Insert the needle 2.5 cm lateral and 2.5 cm distal to this point at a 45-degree angle to the skin surface.
- Advance the needle 5 to 7.5 cm medially and proximally into the joint.

MEDIAL ASPIRATION OF THE HIP

TECHNIQUE 5.13

- Flex and abduct the leg; this is usually a more comfortable position for patients with septic arthritis.
- Place the needle inferior to the adductor longus tendon and using image intensification advance it in a plane below the palpated femoral artery until the femoral head or neck is reached (Fig. 5.6).
- Aspirate the joint.

DRAINAGE

Drainage of the hip may be accomplished through a posterior, medial, lateral, or anterior approach. The anterior approach is preferred in small children for several reasons: (1) damage to the major blood supply to the femoral head is avoided, (2) the chance of postoperative dislocation is reduced, and (3) the landmarks for the surgical approach are much clearer in a small child. In an adult, the posterior approach allows dependent drainage and is a more familiar approach for most orthopaedic surgeons.

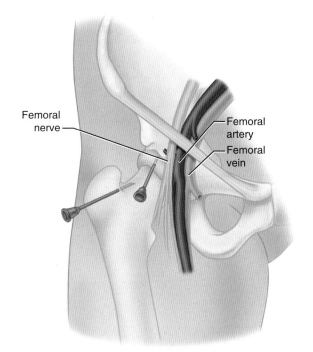

Femoral nerve
Femoral artery
Femoral vein

FIGURE 5.5 Aspiration of hip, two approaches. **SEE TECHNIQUES 5.11 AND 5.12.**

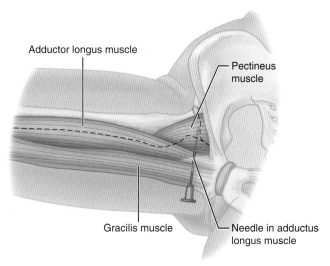

Adductor longus muscle
Pectineus muscle
Gracilis muscle
Needle in adductus longus muscle

FIGURE 5.6 Aspiration of hip, medial approach. **SEE TECHNIQUES 5.13 AND 5.17.**

POSTERIOR DRAINAGE OF THE HIP

TECHNIQUE 5.14

(OBER)

- Make an oblique incision in the line of the femoral neck extending from the greater trochanter toward the posterior superior iliac spine (see Fig. 1.92).
- Split the gluteus maximus muscle in line with its fibers, ligating branches of the inferior gluteal vessels as they are encountered.
- Identify and protect the sciatic nerve in the medial angle of the incision.
- Divide the external rotators of the hip at their insertions on the greater trochanter. Protection of the quadratus femoris is crucial because it contains the vasculature for the femoral head.
- Incise the capsule, preferably at its pelvic attachment, to protect the blood supply of the femoral head.
- Irrigate the joint profusely with saline to remove the pus completely.
- Leave the capsule open, but close the skin loosely over drains.

ANTERIOR DRAINAGE OF THE HIP

TECHNIQUE 5.15

- Make a vertical incision beginning about 1 cm below the anterior superior iliac spine inferiorly.
- Expose the sartorius muscle on the medial side and the tensor fasciae latae and vastus lateralis muscles on

the lateral side. Use blunt dissection to separate these muscles.
- Identify the lateral border of the rectus femoris and retract this muscle medially (Fig. 5.7); this exposes the hip joint capsule.
- Incise the capsule, evacuate the pus, and irrigate the joint with saline.
- Leave the capsule open, but close the skin loosely over drains.
- If wider exposure is required, extend the skin incision proximally onto the iliac crest and subperiosteally detach the origins of the tensor fasciae latae and gluteal muscles from the ilium.
- Protect the lateral femoral cutaneous nerve proximally and the branches of the lateral femoral circumflex artery distally, if possible.

LATERAL DRAINAGE OF THE HIP

TECHNIQUE 5.16

- Make a longitudinal incision 7.5 to 12.5 cm long parallel with the anterior border of the greater trochanter.
- Incise the tensor fasciae latae, exposing the vastus lateralis.
- Detach the anterior portion of the vastus lateralis and retract the abductor muscles proximally to gain access to the anterior capsule of the hip.
- Incise the capsule, evacuate the pus, and irrigate the joint with saline.
- Close the skin loosely over drains.

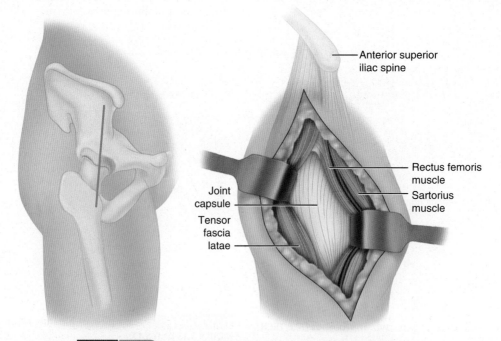

FIGURE 5.7   Anterior approach to septic hip. **SEE TECHNIQUE 5.15**.

MEDIAL DRAINAGE OF THE HIP

TECHNIQUE 5.17

(LUDLOFF)

- Make a longitudinal incision 7.5 to 10 cm long on the medial aspect of the proximal thigh and expose the proximal one fourth of the gracilis and adductor longus muscles (see Fig. 5.6).
- Bluntly dissect posterior to the adductor longus and pectineus muscles and into the abscess cavity, which communicates with the hip joint behind the iliopsoas muscle.
- Evacuate the pus and irrigate the wound with saline.
- Close the skin loosely over drains.

POSTOPERATIVE CARE An infant usually is best treated after surgery in a double spica cast with the affected extremity in moderate abduction. Adequate windows are made in the cast for wound inspection and care. Older children and adults are confined to bed rest in Buck traction until the wound has healed and the patient can control the leg (i.e., can raise the limb from the bed against gravity). Protective weight bearing using crutches is permitted, and active range-of-motion exercises are started.

■ ARTHROSCOPIC DRAINAGE

Arthroscopic drainage for acute septic arthritis of the hip has been reported, with a few small studies showing good results.

ARTHROSCOPIC DEBRIDEMENT AND PARTIAL SYNOVECTOMY OF THE HIP IN AN ADULT

TECHNIQUE 5.18

(SCHRÖDER ET AL.)

- Place the patient supine.
- Using four portals as described by Byrd, carry out debridement and lavage without traction in the peripheral compartment and then in the central compartment. High-volume lavage (minimum of 30 L physiologic saline) should be used. Antibacterial agents should not be used due to possible chondrotoxicity.
- To avoid fluid leakage and potential spread of infection, capsulotomy is NOT performed.
- After synovectomy and irrigation, insert two suction drains into the peripheral compartment, placing the first drain into the anterior portal encircling the femoral neck medially and the second drain into the anterolateral portal to ensure sufficient drainage for the lateral and posterior side.

POSTOPERATIVE CARE The suction drains are removed depending on the amount of fluid draining. Patients are allowed to mobilize the first day after surgery. Partial weight bearing is indicated for 3 weeks with crutches. Continuous passive motion is applied after drain removal. Intravenous antibiotics followed by oral antibiotics are administered for 4 weeks postoperatively.

COMPLICATIONS OF ACUTE SEPTIC ARTHRITIS OF THE HIP
■ PATHOLOGIC DISLOCATION

Pathologic dislocation occurs predominantly in children; it is rare in adults. When dislocation is recognized before severe contracture of the soft tissue has occurred, reduction is accomplished easily at the time of drainage and satisfactory function may result (Fig. 5.8). If the femoral head has been damaged by the infection, however, skeletal traction should be applied through the distal femur and continued until the femoral head is at the level of the acetabulum. The dislocation is reduced by abduction and gentle rotation; manipulation before the femur is displaced distally should not be attempted because the femoral head or neck may be fractured. After the dislocation has been reduced, the hip is immobilized in a spica cast until it is stable or until fibrous or bony ankylosis develops.

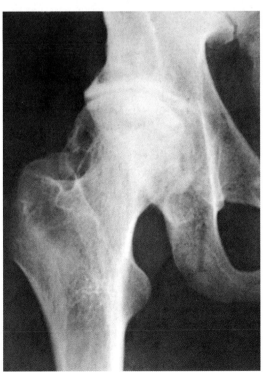

FIGURE 5.8 Appearance of hip 21 years after pathologic dislocation and treatment of septic arthritis. Joint space is slightly narrowed, and acetabulum and femoral head are slightly incongruous, but seldom is result so satisfactory. Usually, it is more satisfactory than that shown in Figure 5.9.

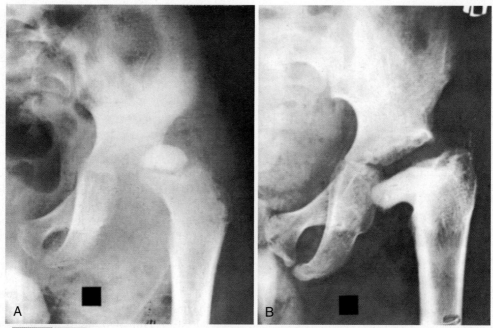

FIGURE 5.9 Pathologic dislocation of hip. **A,** Early sequestration of epiphysis, as shown by apparent increase in density. **B,** After 16 months, note absorption of epiphysis and part of neck.

■ OSTEOMYELITIS

When the infection is confined to the joint, prompt drainage and appropriate antibiotic therapy should prevent osteomyelitis of the proximal femur. If osteomyelitis results in sequestration of the femoral head in children younger than 12 years old, however, the head may be totally reabsorbed (Fig. 5.9), or it may be replaced by new bone after its circulation is restored. In older children and adults, it usually remains as an infected sequestrum and requires excision. Any of the approaches described for draining the hip may be used, but the anterior approach gives better exposure of the joint. In a child, osteomyelitis of the ilium may complicate acute septic arthritis of the hip or the joint infection may be secondary to infection in the bone; in each case, the hip joint and ilium require drainage. In adults, osteomyelitis of the ilium is a less common complication, but impairment of the circulation of the femoral head may lead to pathologic fracture of the neck and sequestration of the femoral head.

■ PELVIC ABSCESS

Pelvic abscess complicating acute septic arthritis of the hip is caused by suppurative infection of the iliac lymph nodes or by spread from the joint into the sheath of the iliopsoas, which may communicate with the joint. The abscess is retroperitoneal and tends to gravitate along the iliopsoas muscle beneath the inguinal ligament, eventually pointing in the medial thigh. In large abscesses, the pus may track proximally along the iliopsoas and point proximal to the posterior iliac crest. MRI may help locate and determine the true extent of psoas involvement. Often this can be drained by CT-directed aspiration.

Freiberg and Perlman advised draining pelvic abscesses as follows. When the abscess points to the medial thigh, a Ludloff incision is made (see Fig. 1.95). By blunt dissection between the adductor longus and brevis muscles, the abscess is found anterior or posterior to the pectineus muscle. When the abscess points subcutaneously anterior to the pectineus, the incision

may be made directly over it, but care must be taken to avoid injuring the femoral vessels and nerve. Drainage above the inguinal ligament is not advised because a fecal fistula may result, and the abscess cannot be thoroughly evacuated. If the abscess points proximal to the iliac crest posteriorly, the incision is made parallel with the crest and just proximal to it. The abdominal muscles are detached from the crest, and the abscess is opened by blunt dissection. Any associated septic arthritis of the hip is drained through a posterior approach (see Fig. 1.94).

■ PERSISTENT INFECTION

Persistent infection around the hip, although rare, is difficult to treat. Usually, scarring is extensive, and draining sinuses have become established. Often the sinuses become blocked, causing recurring abscesses. Unless aggressive surgery is performed, chronic sepsis and its sequelae result. Girdlestone described a radical operation for chronic pyogenic infection around the hip. In this operation, the infected area around the hip is almost completely saucerized. In addition to resecting all of the infected bone, a mass of muscle is resected to ensure drainage. This operation may result in a nearly useless pseudarthrosis or ankylosis. Marked shortening of the affected extremity results. For these reasons, this operation is a last resort.

RESECTION OF THE HIP

TECHNIQUE 5.19

(GIRDLESTONE)

- Begin a transverse incision 2.5 cm posterior and distal to the anterior superior iliac spine and extend it laterally until the center of the incision is about 2.5 cm proximal to the greater trochanter (Fig. 5.10).

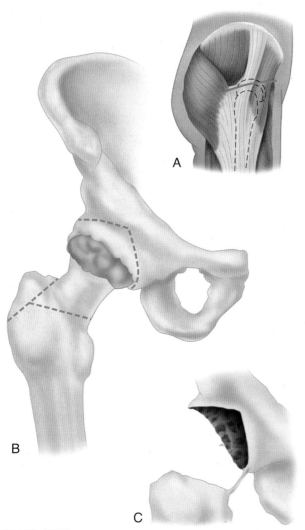

adequately and leave only raw surfaces of vascular cancellous bone (Fig. 5.10C).
- Partially advance skin flaps over healthy muscle at closure.
- If an abscess is found that extends from the lesser trochanter into the adductor region, make another incision on the medial side of the proximal thigh and resect enough of the pectineus, adductor longus, and adductor brevis muscles to provide free drainage.
- Insert two or three drains and fill the cavity loosely with petrolatum gauze.

POSTOPERATIVE CARE The hip is immobilized in a cast or with traction in 20 to 30 degrees of flexion. According to Girdlestone, it is especially important that proximal displacement of the femur be prevented; otherwise, the purpose of the operation (saucerization of the area) would be defeated and drainage from the acetabulum would be blocked.

FIGURE 5.10 Girdlestone resection of hip for chronic or persistent deep-seated sepsis. **A,** Line of incision. **B,** *Broken lines* depict amount of bone to be resected. **C,** Procedure completed. **SEE TECHNIQUE 5.19**.

Klein et al. described a technique for the treatment of chronic sepsis of the hip in paraplegic patients; it consists of three separate measures to control the infection: (1) a Girdlestone procedure, (2) transposition of the vastus lateralis muscle into the void left by the removal of the femoral head and neck and acetabular wall, and (3) external fixation to prevent unrestrained motion of the femoral shaft that might damage the transposed muscle. The external fixator spans the hip joint with a posterior pelvic-femoral frame.

SACROILIAC JOINT

Acute septic arthritis of the sacroiliac joint is uncommon but not rare. Patients have buttock pain and commonly also have low back, thigh, and abdominal pain. The iliac compression, Patrick, and Gaenslen tests all elicit pain in the involved sacroiliac joint. Routine radiographs usually are normal. ^{99m}Tc and ^{67}Ga scans usually show increased activity, but the most sensitive diagnostic study is CT. MRI also may be helpful. Miskew, Block, and Witt published a technique for joint aspiration that successfully obtained diagnostic material in seven of eight patients. Ultrasound usually is employed to isolate the sacroiliac joint. An 18-gauge spinal needle is introduced in the midline at the level of the sacroiliac joint at a 45-degree angle with the transverse plane and at a 30-degree angle with the sagittal plane. The needle is passed laterally and distally at these angles, and image intensification is used to guide it into the sacroiliac joint 0.5 cm from its most inferior margin. Most of the reported patients responded well to appropriate antibiotic treatment. Patients who develop an abscess require open drainage. Osteomyelitis of the adjacent sacrum or ilium is a common complication.

- Retract the skin edges and expose the fascia overlying the gluteus medius and a part of the gluteus maximus.
- Make two deep incisions in line with the edges of the retracted skin incision. In the proximal incision, divide the glutei down to the ilium just proximal to the acetabulum; in the distal incision, expose the lateral aspect of the greater trochanter.
- With an osteotome directed proximally and obliquely toward the superior aspect of the base of the femoral neck, resect the greater trochanter and remove it and the incised mass of gluteal muscles.
- Incise the capsule and expose the femoral head and neck and the acetabular rim (Fig. 5.10B).
- Do not resect the femoral head if it is not necrotic or if the hip is ankylosed. Otherwise, divide the femoral neck and acetabular rim and remove the femoral head and neck.
- Curet all necrotic and infected bone from the acetabulum and ilium. Ensure that any intrapelvic abscess is drained

SPINE

Infections of the spine are discussed in other chapter.

STERNOCLAVICULAR AND ACROMIOCLAVICULAR JOINTS

Usually the sternoclavicular and acromioclavicular joints are affected only when acute septic arthritis involves other joints or in heroin addicts, in whom the causative organism now is predominantly *S. aureus*. *Pseudomonas aeruginosa* infections in injection drug users declined dramatically in the 1980s. Isolated cases have been described in healthy adults, however. Because these joints are subcutaneous, aspiration and surgical drainage can be accomplished. Occasionally, a portion of the clavicle needs to be excised for associated osteomyelitis.

SHOULDER

Septic arthritis of the shoulder rarely occurs in young, healthy individuals of any age. Usually, acute septic arthritis of the shoulder in children is a complication of osteomyelitis of the proximal humeral metaphysis; in adults, it usually is associated with a debilitating disease and rarely responds well to treatment. The joint should be aspirated whenever an infection is suspected, and early surgical drainage is indicated if frank pus is obtained. CT or MRI can be helpful in determining if an abscess is present.

ASPIRATION

The shoulder may be aspirated anteriorly, posteriorly, or laterally. Because the fluctuant area usually is palpable anteriorly, and the bony landmarks can be identified more easily (Fig. 5.11), the needle is inserted here most often. The aspiration site is located half the distance between the coracoid process and the anterolateral edge of the acromion. The needle is directed posteriorly through the joint capsule, and the joint is aspirated.

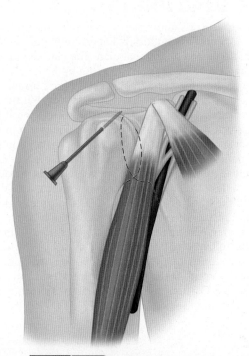

FIGURE 5.11 Aspiration of shoulder.

DRAINAGE

The shoulder may be drained through an anterior incision or a posterior incision, but the anterior incision is preferable. In a review of adult patients treated for septic arthritis of the shoulder, Leslie et al. found that arthrotomy yielded better results than repeat aspirations.

ANTERIOR DRAINAGE OF THE SHOULDER

TECHNIQUE 5.20

- Begin an anterior longitudinal incision at the anterior border of the acromion and extend it 5 to 7.5 cm over the center of the humeral head.
- Split the fibers of the deltoid muscle 5 cm from the acromion, divide the subscapularis tendon, and open the capsule under direct vision.
- Open the synovial sheath of the long head of the biceps tendon. Evacuate the pus and irrigate the joint copiously with saline.
- In children, drill the proximal humeral metaphysis to decompress any abscess but take care not to injure the physis.
- Close the wound loosely over drains.

POSTERIOR DRAINAGE OF THE SHOULDER

TECHNIQUE 5.21

- Begin the incision at the base of the spine of the scapula and extend it distally and laterally for 7.5 cm in line with the fibers of the deltoid muscle.
- Split the fibers of the deltoid, expose the external rotators of the shoulder and dissect between the infraspinatus and teres minor muscles just medial to the greater tuberosity of the humerus.
- Incise the capsule and evacuate the pus.
- Irrigate the joint with copious amounts of saline and close the skin loosely over drains.

POSTOPERATIVE CARE The shoulder is supported on a splint at 45 degrees of abduction until the wound has healed. Then active and active-assisted range-of-motion exercises are started.

■ ARTHROSCOPIC DRAINAGE OF THE SHOULDER

Arthroscopic drainage has been reported and is seen in increasing frequency for the treatment of acute septic arthritis of the shoulder. Arthroscopic drainage should be reserved for treatment of septic arthritis early in the disease process, particularly before 2 weeks of onset of Gächter stage I or II infections (Table 5.5). With arthroscopy, washout is done

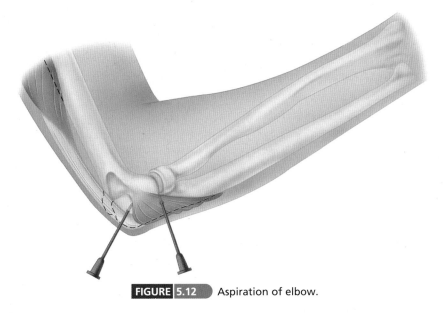

FIGURE 5.12 Aspiration of elbow.

TABLE 5.5	
Gächter Stages of Infection	
Stage I	Opacity of fluid, redness of the synovial membrane, possible petechial bleeding, no radiographic alterations
Stage II	Severe inflammation, fibrinous deposition, pus, no radiologic alterations
Stage III	Thickening of the synovial membrane, compartment formation, no radiologic alterations
Stage IV	Aggressive pannus with infiltration of the cartilage, undermining the cartilage, radiologic signs of subchondral osteolysis, possible osseous erosions and cysts

From Gächter A: Der Gelenkinfektion, *Inform Arzt* 6:35–43, 1985.

under direct vision with the patient in the lateral decubitus position and the arm suspended in skin traction. A three-portal technique (anterior, posterior, and superior) affords almost complete access. Accessory posterior and inferior operating portals may be necessary for involvement of the inferior recess. Lavage of the joint with saline or a mixture of saline and antibiotic can be performed, with loculations and adhesions debrided. A near-total synovectomy can be accomplished with a motorized synovial resector without disrupting the deltoid or rotator cuff. If necessary drains are placed through portal sites and intravenous antibiotics administered. (see other chapter for an arthroscopic technique using standard anterior and posterior portals.) Early active mobilization may be initiated sooner than with an open technique.

ELBOW
ASPIRATION

For elbow aspiration, the physician flexes the elbow and inserts the needle on its posterior aspect just lateral to the olecranon (Fig. 5.12). The needle is advanced through the skin and joint capsule, and the joint is aspirated.

DRAINAGE

The elbow is best drained through a medial or lateral approach or both.

MEDIAL DRAINAGE OF THE ELBOW
TECHNIQUE 5.22

- Make an incision over the medial humeral epicondyle and extend it 5 cm proximally and 2.5 cm distally.
- Develop the interval between the triceps posteriorly and the brachialis anteriorly, taking care not to injure the ulnar nerve.
- Elevate the periosteum laterally and distally until the capsule is exposed.
- Incise the capsule and evacuate the pus.
- Irrigate the joint with saline and close the skin loosely over drains.

LATERAL DRAINAGE OF THE ELBOW
TECHNIQUE 5.23

- Make an incision over the lateral humeral epicondyle and extend it 5 cm proximally and 2.5 cm distally.
- Separate the triceps muscle posteriorly from the extensor carpi radialis longus anteriorly and expose the joint capsule. Dissect close to the bone to avoid injuring the radial nerve.
- Incise the capsule, evacuate the pus, and irrigate the joint with saline.
- Close the skin loosely over drains.

- The posterior compartment of the joint also may be drained through this incision by dissecting posteriorly on the humerus and elevating the attachment of the triceps from the lateral surface of the bone.

POSTERIOR DRAINAGE OF THE ELBOW

TECHNIQUE 5.24

- Begin parallel longitudinal incisions on each side of the olecranon and continue them proximally for 7.5 cm (Fig. 5.13).
- Deepen the incisions through the medial and lateral borders of the triceps aponeurosis into the posterior compartment of the joint. Avoid injuring the ulnar nerve as it crosses the posterior aspect of the medial humeral epicondyle.

POSTOPERATIVE CARE The elbow is splinted at 90 degrees with the forearm in neutral rotation until the wound has healed. Then active range-of-motion exercises are started.

ARTHROSCOPY OF THE ELBOW

Arthroscopic irrigation and synovectomy are safe and effective in the elbow, producing good functional results in patients who are immunocompetent with septic arthritis (see other chapter for arthroscopic elbow examination and treatment of pyarthrosis).

WRIST

Septic arthritis of the wrist is seen less frequently than in other joints and usually occurs after penetrating trauma. Signs may be subtle, and the diagnosis is easily missed. Early incision and drainage should be performed to avoid the complications of joint ankylosis, periarticular osteomyelitis, or suppurative flexor tenosynovitis.

ASPIRATION

Aspiration is performed on the dorsal side of the wrist. Several aspiration sites on the dorsum of the wrist can be used. The most common site of aspiration is between the first and second extensor compartments at the radiocarpal level, immediately adjacent to the point where the extensor pollicis longus crosses the extensor carpi radialis longus. Other aspiration sites are between the third and fourth extensor compartments or between the fourth and fifth extensor compartments (Fig. 5.14).

DRAINAGE

The wrist can be drained by a medial, lateral, or dorsal approach. Avoid opening the tendon sheaths.

LATERAL DRAINAGE OF THE WRIST

TECHNIQUE 5.25

- Make a longitudinal incision 5 cm long between the abductor pollicis longus and extensor pollicis brevis tendons volarly and the extensor pollicis longus tendon dorsally.
- Deepen the incision into the anatomic snuffbox, taking care to avoid injuring the radial artery.
- Incise the radial collateral ligament and synovium and evacuate the pus.
- Irrigate the joint and close the skin loosely over drains.

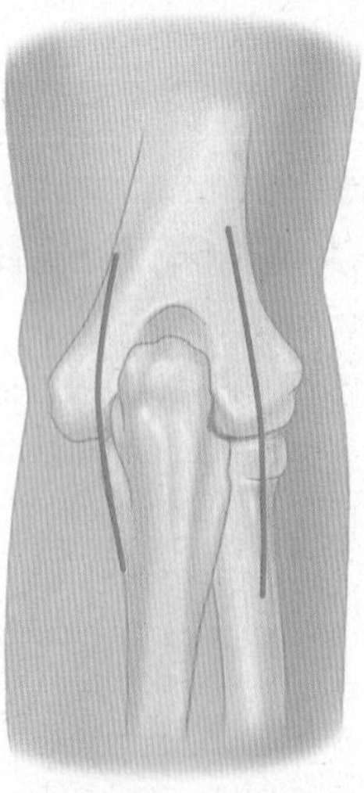

FIGURE 5.13 Incision on each side of triceps aponeurosis for posterior drainage of elbow. **SEE TECHNIQUE 5.24.**

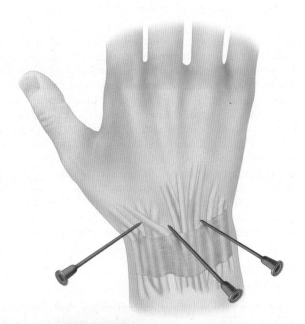

FIGURE 5.14 Aspiration of wrist.

MEDIAL DRAINAGE OF THE WRIST

TECHNIQUE 5.26

- Make an incision 5 cm long over the ulnar head between the tendons of the flexor and extensor carpi ulnaris. Avoid injuring the dorsal branch of the ulnar nerve.
- Expose the ulnar collateral ligament and synovium and incise them distal to the ulnar styloid. Do not detach the triangular fibrocartilage.

DORSAL DRAINAGE OF THE WRIST

TECHNIQUE 5.27

- Make a dorsal longitudinal incision 5 cm long between the extensor pollicis longus and extensor indicis proprius tendons or between the extensor carpi ulnaris and extensor digiti quinti proprius tendons.
- Incise the dorsal carpal ligament and enter the joint (see chapter 1).

POSTOPERATIVE CARE The wrist is splinted in the position of function until the wound has healed, and then active range-of-motion exercises are started.

ARTHROSCOPY OF THE WRIST

Arthroscopic irrigation has been reported to be an effective treatment in patients with isolated septic arthritis of the wrist, with fewer procedures required than with open treatment. However, there are several contraindications, including multiple sites of infection, prior surgery, osteomyelitis, small wrist size, severe joint destruction, and infection that has spread outside of the radiocarpal and midcarpal joints. (see other chapter for patient positioning and arthroscopic portal placement for wrist examination.) Antibiotics are not started unless cultures have already been obtained. Once the arthroscope has been introduced, gravity inflow is started and outflow provided with low suction through a joint shaver. Gravity inflow rather than a mechanical pump should be used in the presence of septic arthritis to avoid extravasation of the joint fluid. Synovitis, loculations, and purulence are debrided using the joint shaver. After debridement, the joint is irrigated thoroughly. Each joint in turn undergoes the same inspection and debridement process. The wrist is immobilized in 20 degrees of extension.

OPERATIONS TO CORRECT DEFORMITIES AFTER SEPTIC ARTHRITIS

ANKLE

When the ankle is fixed in equinus by soft-tissue contracture, treatment by Quengel casting or serial wedged casts or by operations such as lengthening of the Achilles tendon with or without posterior capsulotomy generally is effective in restoring plantigrade position of the foot. When fixed equinus is caused by bony ankylosis, cuneiform osteotomy through the joint is indicated.

OSTEOTOMY OF THE ANKLE

TECHNIQUE 5.28

- Expose the ankle through an anterolateral approach (see Fig. 1.34). With an osteotome, remove from the joint a cuneiform wedge of bone with its base anterior.
- If necessary, lengthen the Achilles tendon and perform a posterior capsulotomy to avoid resecting excessive bone, which would cause too much shortening.
- Dorsiflex the foot to the neutral position and see that the bony surfaces of the osteotomy are accurately apposed in this position.
- Apply an external fixation device, such as is used for ankle arthrodesis.

POSTOPERATIVE CARE The postoperative care is the same as that for compression arthrodesis of the ankle.

KNEE

Soft-tissue flexion contractures of the knee can be managed by Quengel or serial wedged casts or may require soft-tissue operations such as those described in other chapter. For bony or rigid fibrous ankylosis or severe soft-tissue contractures, the following procedures may be considered in addition to techniques for complex deformity correction, using circular fixators or other external fixation compression devices. A flexion deformity can be corrected indirectly by a supracondylar osteotomy that causes a compensatory deformity in the opposite direction. This operation should be considered when the flexion deformity is not severe but the joint is unsuitable for manipulation or soft-tissue release. In children, the osteotomy should be made well proximal to the physis.

TRANSVERSE SUPRACONDYLAR OSTEOTOMY OF THE FEMUR

TECHNIQUE 5.29

- Make a lateral longitudinal incision 2.5 cm long just proximal to the lateral femoral condyle. Incise the fascia lata and vastus lateralis, exposing the femur.
- Insert an osteotome and turn it to cut transversely.
- Divide the femur laterally and posteriorly through two thirds of its thickness.

- By manipulation, create a greenstick fracture in the remaining bone and correct the deformity (Fig. 5.15).
- If the flexion contracture is greater than 45 degrees, the hamstring tendons should be lengthened before the osteotomy.

POSTOPERATIVE CARE After the extremity is aligned, a long-leg cast with a pelvic band is applied. At 2 weeks, the cast is changed to permit any necessary further correction of the deformity. At 8 to 12 weeks, the second cast is removed and a long-leg orthosis with the knee fixed in neutral position is applied to maintain the corrected position. If the knee had functional range of motion before surgery, the orthosis is omitted. Active motion and quadriceps exercises are begun as soon as possible and are continued until the range of motion present before surgery is regained.

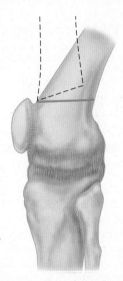

FIGURE 5.15 Supracondylar osteotomy for ankylosis of knee in flexion. Transverse osteotomy. *Dotted line* indicates the femur after correction, with subsequent wedge-shaped space based posteriorly. Telescoping actually occurs to sufficient degree to close defect. **SEE TECHNIQUE 5.28**.

Ankylosis of the knee in flexion may be corrected by the V-osteotomy described by Thompson.

V-OSTEOTOMY OF THE FEMUR

TECHNIQUE 5.30

(THOMPSON)
- Divide the anterior cortex of the femur by V-osteotomy, divide the medial and lateral cortices obliquely, and divide the posterior cortex transversely (Fig. 5.16).
- Make an excavation in the distal fragment and insert the pointed end of the proximal fragment into it.
- Resect a portion of the proximal fragment, if necessary, to reduce tension on the neurovascular structures.

POSTOPERATIVE CARE The postoperative care is the same as that described for transverse osteotomy. When the flexion contracture is greater than 60 degrees, transverse osteotomy allows only limited bony apposition after the deformity has been corrected. Cuneiform osteotomy is preferable, especially in adults.

SUPRACONDYLAR CUNEIFORM OSTEOTOMY OF THE FEMUR

TECHNIQUE 5.31

- Make a lateral longitudinal incision 7.5 cm long starting just proximal to the lateral femoral condyle.
- Divide the fascia lata and the vastus lateralis muscle and retract the latter anteriorly.
- Remove a wedge-shaped section of bone from the anterior surface of the femoral metaphysis. The angle of the wedge should be approximately half the angle of the flexion contracture (Fig. 5.17).
- After the deformity has been corrected, the gap that was created is closed and a small gap is created posteriorly.

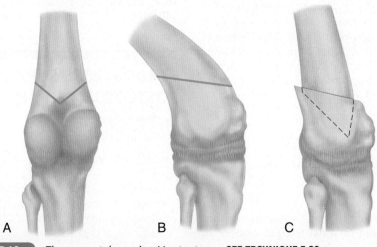

A   B   C

FIGURE 5.16 Thompson telescoping-V osteotomy. **SEE TECHNIQUE 5.29**.

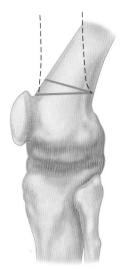

FIGURE 5.17 Cuneiform osteotomy based anteriorly. Section of bone removed is indicated by *green area*. *Dotted lines* show position of femur after osteotomy, with complete apposition of raw surfaces of fragments. **SEE TECHNIQUE 5.31.**

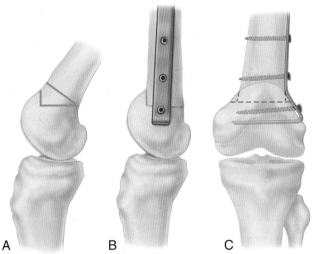

FIGURE 5.18 Modification of Osgood supracondylar controlled rotation osteotomy of femur. **A,** *Green area* illustrates section of bone to be removed. **B** and **C,** After osteotomy, corrected position is maintained by blade plate. **SEE TECHNIQUE 5.32.**

- When satisfactory correction has been obtained at the time of surgery, the fragments are immobilized better and union is hastened by applying a compression clamp or some other external fixation compression device. This is especially applicable when the knee is solidly ankylosed.

POSTOPERATIVE CARE The postoperative care is the same as that for compression arthrodesis of the knee.

Femoral osteotomy is indicated when a functional range of flexion remains beyond the flexion contracture. The osteotomy should be made as near the joint as possible. Full extension can be regained by this operation, but the preoperative range of flexion may be reduced.

SUPRACONDYLAR CONTROLLED ROTATIONAL OSTEOTOMY OF THE FEMUR

TECHNIQUE 5.32

- Through a lateral incision 10 cm long, subperiosteally expose the supracondylar area of the femur laterally and anteriorly.
- With a reciprocating motor saw, remove a small quadrilateral segment of bone. Cut the distal end of the proximal fragment transversely and the proximal end of the distal fragment at an angle (Fig. 5.18A), then rotate the femoral condyles anteriorly.
- Bend a Blount blade plate to slightly more than a right angle, insert the blade transversely through the distal fragment,

and fix the plate to the femur with screws. Other blade plate devices that are contoured to fit and provide rigid fixation can be used as alternatives (Fig. 5.18B,C).

POSTOPERATIVE CARE If the internal fixation is secure, the extremity is supported in a knee extension splint until the wound has healed; otherwise, a long-leg cast is applied with the knee extended and is worn for 4 weeks.

■ INTRAARTICULAR OSTEOTOMY

Sometimes intraarticular osseous ankylosis occurs in so much flexion that weight bearing is impossible. If arthroplasty is contraindicated because of the patient's age or occupation, intraarticular osteotomy to correct the flexion contracture is indicated. In children, the physes must be protected (Fig. 5.19). When the joint is ankylosed in extreme flexion, correcting the deformity completely by surgery is not advisable. If enough bone were removed to allow full correction, it would cause too much shortening; if not enough bone were removed and the joint were forced into extension, vascular or neurologic complications would be likely. A severe deformity should be only partly corrected at the time of surgery, and the contracted structures on the posterior surface of the joint should be stretched gradually by conservative measures.

INTRAARTICULAR OSTEOTOMY

TECHNIQUE 5.33

- Make a medial parapatellar incision.
- Free the patella from the femur and strip the soft tissues subperiosteally from the anterior surface of the femur and tibia.

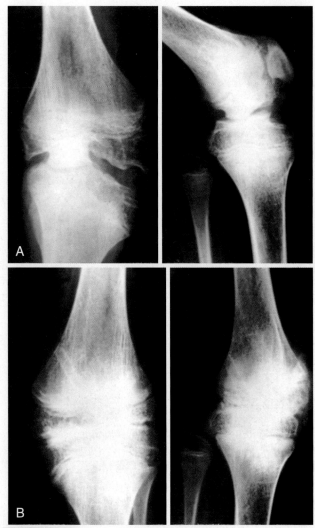

FIGURE **5.19** **A,** Ankylosis and deformity of knee after pyogenic arthritis. **B,** After intraarticular osteotomy and arthrodesis. Physes were not injured by surgery.

- For moderate deformity, make the osteotomy parallel to the contour of the femoral condyles (Fig. 5.20).
- If the deformity is extreme, remove an anterior wedge of bone (Fig. 5.21).
- In children with extreme flexion contracture, full correction may be impossible without damaging the physes; the deformity should be partly corrected by excising bone, and 2 weeks later a posterior capsulotomy and hamstring lengthening procedure should be performed.
- When the deformity can be corrected completely during surgery, immobilize the joint with a compression clamp or some other form of external fixation compression device.

POSTOPERATIVE CARE If the deformity has been corrected by surgery, apply a long-leg cast incorporating the fixation device. If the deformity can be corrected only partly, apply a splint maintaining the knee in maximal extension, and apply a series of wedging casts until full correction is achieved.

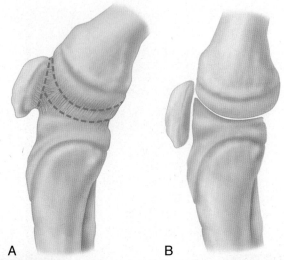

FIGURE **5.20** Intraarticular osteotomy for ankylosis of knee in flexion. **A,** *Broken lines* show where bone is divided, conforming to general contour of joint surfaces. **B,** After correction. **SEE TECHNIQUE 5.33**.

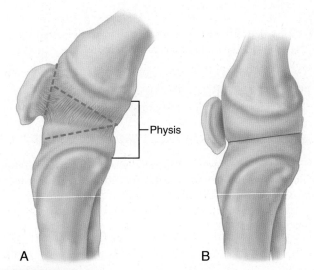

FIGURE **5.21** Cuneiform intraarticular osteotomy for ankylosis of knee in flexion. **A,** *Dotted lines* show where bone is divided, wedge-shaped section being removed. **B,** After correction of deformity. **SEE TECHNIQUE 5.33**.

HIP

The goal in treating acute septic arthritis of the hip is to achieve normal function with no residual deformity or disability. This goal may not be achieved, however, even with the best of treatment. Choi et al. found several poor prognostic factors related to septic arthritis of the hip in infants, including: (1) an infection that occurred before 22 weeks of age, (2) prematurity, and (3) symptoms that lasted longer than 4 days. The most important factor was delay in diagnosis.

Disability after acute septic arthritis of the hip may be the result of any of the following:
1. Pain may be caused by incongruous articular surfaces or by pathologic dislocation.

2. Stiffness from partial or complete ankylosis may cause moderate or severe disability, depending on whether a significant contracture also is present.

3. Deformity may consist of abnormal angulation, as in coxa vara, or of shortening. Flexion and adduction deformities in children are common even if spontaneous bony ankylosis in optimal position is initially achieved.

4. Instability may result from bone destruction in the proximal femur or from pathologic dislocation.

Reconstructive operations usually should be delayed for months and sometimes years after the infection has subsided. The reasons for this delay are as follows: (1) the danger of reactivating the old infection is reduced; (2) the status of the proximal femur and femoral head should be definitely determined in children because early radiographs may show what appears to be destruction of the proximal femur with separation and osteonecrosis of the femoral head epiphysis, only to show satisfactory reconstitution on later films; and (3) the strength and general character of the bone improve with time, especially in children, as necrotic bone is revascularized, and abscess cavities are filled in, increasing the likelihood of success after reconstructive surgery. It generally is accepted that an unstable hip should not go untreated during the period of growth, and a fixed deformity should not be allowed to persist for many years. However, some authors have noted that reconstructive surgery after hip sepsis may not yield results comparable to nonoperative treatment.

■ ARTHROPLASTY

Interposition or cup arthroplasty still may be useful in younger patients with an ankylosed hip. Total hip arthroplasty should be considered only for older patients. These operations probably should be performed in collaboration with an infectious disease consultant and with the administration of appropriate perioperative antibiotics.

■ OPERATIONS TO STABILIZE THE HIP

The hip may be stabilized after acute septic arthritis by (1) arthrodesis, (2) pelvic osteotomy, (3) proximal femoral osteotomy, (4) trochanteric arthroplasty (Colonna) combined with proximal femoral osteotomy, and (5) Harmon or L'Episcopo reconstruction. Although many of these osteotomy and arthroplasty procedures seem to be antiquated, they are mentioned here for completeness and because they may be useful in the rare catastrophic situation.

Arthrodesis provides a stable and painless hip with moderate inconvenience. It is probably more useful in adults or older children.

Pelvic osteotomy, such as acetabuloplasty or the Salter or Chiari procedures, may be useful in children to provide a support for the proximal femur when the head and neck have been absorbed. The limp is decreased, and mobility is preserved, but pain may persist. These operations are less helpful in adults.

A Schanz or proximal femoral osteotomy may be useful when the remnant of the neck remaining in the acetabulum is large enough. It usually is not indicated unless some part of the femur articulates with the acetabulum. The operation often decreases lurch and increases the functional length of the limb by abducting the distal fragment.

Trochanteric arthroplasty for instability after septic arthritis is performed in stages, with the greater trochanter placed into the acetabulum and the hip abductors moved distally on the femur. A proximal femoral osteotomy is performed about 1 month later, accompanied in some cases by acetabuloplasty. The operation is performed in children younger than 10 years.

In the L'Episcopo or Harmon reconstruction, a new femoral neck is fashioned to articulate with the acetabulum (Fig. 5.22). These operations are useful for young children in whom the femoral head and neck have been absorbed.

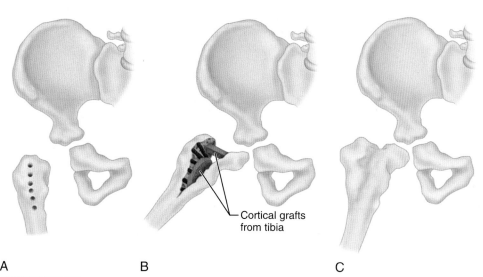

Cortical grafts from tibia

A   B   C

FIGURE 5.22 Harmon reconstruction for loss of femoral head and neck in child as result of acute infectious arthritis. Period of growth and of weight bearing produces substantial neck and trochanter (see text). **SEE TECHNIQUE 5.34.**

RECONSTRUCTION AFTER HIP SEPSIS

TECHNIQUE 5.34

(HARMON)

- Expose the acetabulum and proximal femur through an anterior iliofemoral incision (see Fig. 1.99).
- Strip the periosteum from the anterior aspect of the proximal femur, but do not disturb the muscles attached to the greater trochanter.
- With the extremity in neutral rotation, drill four to six holes through the bone in an anteroposterior direction (Fig. 5.22A). Using the holes as a guide, osteotomize the proximal femur longitudinally, then pry the medial fragment medially, creating a greenstick fracture.
- Obtain cortical tibial grafts from the opposite limb and place them in the osteotomy to keep the fragment angulated medially (Fig. 5.22B).
- Remove the scar tissue from the acetabulum, taking care not to injure its cartilaginous surface.
- Place the medial fragment of the femur into the acetabulum by manipulating the limb (Fig. 5.22C).

POSTOPERATIVE CARE A cast is applied from the nipple line to the toes on the affected side and to above the knee on the opposite side, holding the affected hip in neutral rotation and slight abduction. Immobilization is continued for 3 months, and then graduated weight bearing with crutches is begun.

■ OPERATIONS TO CORRECT DEFORMITY

Deformities should be corrected as soon as possible after the infection has subsided. A flexion and adduction contracture is treated by transferring the crest of the ilium and, when necessary, by an adductor tenotomy. A hip ankylosed in flexion and adduction is treated by intertrochanteric osteotomy, as described here, fixing the hip in neutral rotation, 0 degrees of flexion, and 20 to 30 degrees of abduction (in children). Because the deformity may recur before the child reaches maturity, all concerned should be informed that a second osteotomy may be required later. In adults, 25 degrees of flexion and neutral abduction is the best position.

One of three types of intertrochanteric osteotomies can be used alone or combined with such operations as adductor tenotomy: a transverse opening wedge osteotomy, a transverse closing wedge osteotomy, or the Brackett ball-and-socket osteotomy (Fig. 5.23). These are basic operations used for many years and have been modified as improvements in technique have occurred (Fig. 5.24). The transverse opening wedge osteotomy is simple, and it lengthens the extremity; however, bony apposition is limited, union is delayed in adults, and it is initially unstable.

TRANSVERSE OPENING WEDGE OSTEOTOMY OF THE HIP

TECHNIQUE 5.35

- Expose the lateral aspect of the proximal femur by a lateral longitudinal incision.

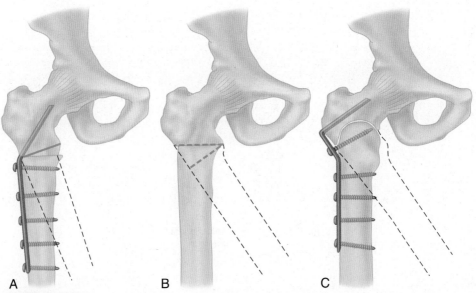

FIGURE 5.23   Trochanteric osteotomy. **A,** Gant opening wedge osteotomy fixed by blade plate. **B,** Whitman closing wedge osteotomy. **C,** Brackett ball-and-socket osteotomy fixed by Blount blade plate. **SEE TECHNIQUES 5.35 TO 5.37.**

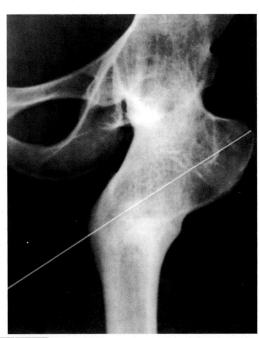

FIGURE 5.24 Satisfactory weight-bearing hip after osteotomy for adduction deformity with ankylosis of hip. *Line* shows adduction deformity of femur before operation.

- Insert a drill point perpendicular to the femoral shaft at a level slightly proximal to the lesser trochanter. Verify its position by radiographs.
- Divide the femur at the level of the drill point with an osteotome.
- Place the extremity in the corrected position and insert a rigid internal fixation device, such as those used for intertrochanteric fractures (Fig. 5.23A see other chapter).

POSTOPERATIVE CARE A one and one-half spica cast is applied and is worn for 8 to 12 weeks. Range-of-motion and strengthening exercises are then started, and protected weight bearing using crutches is begun.

The transverse closing wedge osteotomy provides good bony apposition and is stable; however, it shortens the extremity.

TRANSVERSE CLOSING WEDGE OSTEOTOMY OF THE HIP

TECHNIQUE 5.36

- Expose the lateral aspect of the proximal femur through a longitudinal incision.
- Use an osteotome to outline a laterally based wedge with the apex at the upper border of the lesser trochanter.
- The size of the wedge is determined by the deformity. Paper cutouts of tracings made from radiographs taken before surgery are helpful in determining the proper angles and position of the wedge (Fig. 5.23B).

- Remove the wedge of bone and abduct the distal fragment.
- With the defect closed, the alignment of the extremity should be correct.
- Insert a rigid internal fixation device, such as the one used for intertrochanteric fractures.

POSTOPERATIVE CARE Protected weight bearing with crutches is begun after the reaction has subsided and is continued until union is mature.

The Brackett osteotomy achieves stability without shortening the extremity; however, extensive dissection is required. In severe biplane deformities, an accurate and stable osteotomy is difficult to perform.

BRACKETT OSTEOTOMY OF THE HIP

TECHNIQUE 5.37

(BRACKETT)
- Expose the anterior surface of the intertrochanteric region, the base of the neck, and the proximal shaft of the femur through a straight incision 12.5 cm long, beginning at the anterior superior iliac spine and extending distally, or through a lateral Watson-Jones (see chapter 1) approach.
- Retract the tensor fasciae latae muscles laterally and the sartorius and rectus femoris muscles medially.
- With a narrow osteotome or a reciprocating motor saw, make an osteotomy through the bone convex superiorly and medially (Fig. 5.23C). Begin it on the lateral side of the greater trochanter and continue it to the junction of the lesser trochanter with the neck.
- Complete the osteotomy and abduct the distal fragment. As the distal fragment rotates within the hollow of the proximal fragment, the deformity is corrected.
- When the adduction deformity is mild, the lateral margin of the osteotomy should be level with the medial margin; however, when it is severe, the lateral margin should be slightly more proximal than the medial margin.
- When there is a severe flexion deformity, the anteroposterior plane of the osteotomy should be directed so that it provides a slight roof over the anterior edge of the proximal fragment.
- After the fragments have been aligned properly, insert a rigid internal fixation device, such as one used for intertrochanteric fractures.

POSTOPERATIVE CARE Protected weight bearing with crutches is begun after the reaction has subsided and is continued until the union is mature.

■ OPERATIONS TO EQUALIZE LEG LENGTHS
Operations to correct leg-length inequality are performed only after all reconstructive operations on the affected limb have been completed.

REFERENCES

Abdel MP, Perry KI, Morrey ME, et al.: Arthroscopic management of native shoulder septic arthritis, *J Shoulder Elbow Surg* 22(3):418, 2013.

Acher Y, Vogt M, Leunig Wüst J, Trampuz A: Improved diagnosis of periprosthetic joint infection by multiplex PCR of sonication fluid from removed implants, *J Clin Microbiol* 48:1208, 2010.

Achermann Y, Vogt M, Leunig M, Wust J, Trampuz A: Improved diagnosis of periprosthetic joint infection by multiplex PCR of sonication fluid from removed implants, *J Clin Microbiol* 48:1208, 2010.

Aim F, Delambre J, Bauer T, Hardy P: Efficacy of arthroscopic treatment for resolving infection in septic arthritis of native joints, *Orthop Traumatol Surg Res* 101(1):61, 2015.

Annane D, Bellissant E, Bollaert PE, et al.: Corticosteroids in the treatment of severe sepsis and septic shock in adults: a systematic review, *JAMA* 301:2362, 2009.

Baran S, Price C, Hak DJ: Diagnosing joint infections: synovial fluid differential is more sensitive than white blood cell count, *Eur J Orthop Surg Traumatol* 24:1469, 2014.

Bauer TW, Resnick L: Causes and conditions associated with septic arthritis, *JBJS Case Connect* 8(4):e103, 2018.

Böhler C, Dragana M, Puchner S, Windhager R, Holinka J: Treatment of septic arthritis of the knee: a comparison between arthroscopy and arthrotomy, *Knee Surg Sports Traumatol Arthrosc* 24910:3147, 2016.

Borde JP, Häcker GA, Guschl S, et al.: Diagnosis of prosthetic joint infections using UMD-Universal Kit and the automated multiplex-PCR Unyvero i60 ITI cartridge system: a pilot study, *Infection* 43:551, 2015.

Brouwer MC, McIntyre P, Prasad K, van de Beek D: Corticosteroids for acute bacterial meningitis, *Cochrane Database Syst Rev* 6:CD004405, 2013.

Claiborne JR, Branch LG, Reynolds M, Defranzo AJ: An algorithmic approach to suspected septic wrist, *Ann Plast Surg* 78(6):659, 2017.

Coiffier G, Ferreyra M, Albert JD, et al.: Ultrasound-guided synovial biopsy improves diagnosis of septic arthritis in acute arthritis without enough analyzable synovial fluid: a retrospective analysis of 176 arthritis from a French rheumatology department, *Clin Rheumatol* 37(8):2241, 2018.

Courtney P, Doherty M: Joint aspiration and infection and synovial fluid analysis, *Best Pract Res Clin Rheumatol* 27:137, 2013.

de SA D, Cargnelli S, Catapano M, et al.: Efficacy of hip arthroscopy for the management of septic arthritis: a systematic review, *Arthroscopy* 31(7):1358, 2015.

De Souza Miyahara H, Helito CP, Oliva GB, et al.: Clinical and epidemiological characteristics of septic arthritis of the hip, 2006 to 2012, a seven-year review, *Clinics (Sao Paolo)* 69:464, 2014.

Faour M, Sultan AA, George J, et al.: Arthroscopic irrigation and debridement is associated with favourable short-term outcomes vs. open management: an ACS-NSQIP database analysis, *Knee Surg Sports Traumatol Arthrosc* 2019 Jan 2, [Epub ahead of print].

Farrow L: A systematic review and meta-analysis regarding the use of corticosteroids in septic arthritis, *BMC Musculoskelet Disord* 16:241, 2015.

Ferreyra M, Coiffier G, Albert JD, et al.: Combining cytology and microcrystal detection in nonpurulent joint fluid benefits the diagnosis of septic arthritis, *Joint Bone Spine* 84(1):65, 2017.

Flores-Robles BJ, Jiménez Palop M, Sanabria Sanchinel AA, et al.: Medical versus surgical approach to initial treatment in septic arthritis: a single Spanish center's 8-year experience, *J Clin Rheumatol* 25(1):4, 2019.

Hischebeth GT, Randau TM, Buhr JK, et al.: Unyvero i60 implant and tissue infection (ITI) multiplex PCR system in diagnosing periprosthetic joint infection, *J Microbio Methods* 121:27, 2016.

Huang TW, Huang KC, Lee PC, et al.: Encouraging outcomes of staged, uncemented arthroplasty with short-term antibiotic therapy for treatment of recalcitrant septic arthritis of the native hip, *J Trauma* 68:965, 2010.

Imagama T, Tokushige A, Seki K, et al.: Early diagnosis of septic arthritis using synovial fluid presepsin: a preliminary study, *J Infect Chemother* 25(3):170, 2019.

Jiang JJ, Piponov HI, Mass DP, Angeles JG, Shi LL: Septic arthritis of the shoulder: a comparison of treatment methods, *J Am Acad Orthop Surg* 25(8):e175, 2017.

Johns BP, Loewenthal MR, Dewar DC: Open compared with arthroscopic treatment of acute septic arthritis of the native knee, *J Bone Joint Surg Am* 99(6):499, 2017.

Kang T, Lee JK: Host factors affect the outcome of arthroscopic lavage treatment of septic arthritis of the knee, *Orthopedics* 41(2):e184, 2018.

Kil HR, Lee JH, Lee KY, et al.: Early corticosteroid treatment for severe pneumonia caused by 2009 H1N1 influenza virus, *Crit Care* 15:413, 2011.

Kuo CL, Chang JH, Wu CC, et al.: Treatment of septic knee arthritis: comparison of arthroscopic debridement alone or combined with continuous closed irrigation-suction system, *J Trauma* 71(2):454, 2011.

Lauper N, Davat M, Gjika E, et al.: Native septic arthritis is not an immediate surgical emergency, *J Infect* 77(1):47, 2018.

Lee KH, Choi ST, Lee SK, et al.: Application of a novel diagnostic rule in the differential diagnosis between acute gouty arthritis and septic arthritis, *J Korean Med Sci* 30:700, 2015.

Lee YK, Park KS, Ha YC, Koo KH: Athroscopic treatment for acute septic arthritis of the hip joint in adults, *Knee Surg Sports Traumatol Arthrosc* 22(4):942, 2014.

Mankovecky MR, Roukis TS: Arthroscopic synovectomy, irrigation, and debridement for treatment of septic ankle arthrosis: a systematic review and case series, *J Foot Ankle Surg* 53:615, 2014.

Moon JG, Biraris S, Jeong WK, Kim JH: Clinical results after arthroscopic treatment for septic arthritis of the elbow joint, *Arthroscopy* 30:673, 2014.

Morgenstern C, Cabric S, Perka C, Trampuz A, Renz N: Synovial fluid multiplex PCR is superior to culture for detection of low-virulent pathogens causing periprosthetic joint infection, *Diagn Microbiol Infect Dis* 90:115, 2018.

Morgenstern C, Renz N, Cabric S, Perka C, Trampuz A: Multiplex polymerase chain reaction and microcalorimetry in synovial fluid: can pathogen-based detection assays improve the diagnosis of septic arthritis? *J Rheumatol* 45(11):1588, 2018.

Murgai RR, Compton E, Illingworth KD, Kay RM: The incidence of pin tract infections and septic arthritis in percutaneous distal femur pinning, *J Pediatr Orthop* 39(6):e462, 2019.

Murphy RF, Plumblee L, Barfield WB, et al.: Septic arthritis of the hip-risk factors associated with secondary surgery, *J Am Acad Orthop Surg* 27(9):321, 2019.

Nuermberger E: Septic arthritis community acquired. In Bartlett JG, Auwaerter PG, Pham PA, editors: John Hopkins ABX guide to diagnosis and treatment of infectious diseases, ed 3, Burlington, 2012, Jones and Bartlett.

Pääkkönen M: Septic arthritis in children: diagnosis and treatment, *Pediatr Health Med Ther* 8:65, 2017.

Peres LR, Marchitto RO, Pereira GS, et al.: Arthrotomy versus arthroscopy in the treatment of septic arthritis of the knee in adults: a randomized clinical trial, *Knee Surg Sports Traumatol Arthrosc* 24(10):3155, 2016.

Pupaibool J, Vasoo S, Erwin PJ, Murad MH, Berbari EF: The utility of image-guided percutaneous needle aspiration biopsy for the diagnosis of spontaneous vertebral osteomyelitis: a systematic review and meta-analysis, *Spine J* 15(1):122, 2015.

Quin YF, Li ZJ, Li H: Corticosteroids as adjunctive therapy with antibiotics in the treatment of children with septic arthritis: a meta-analysis, *Drug Des Devel Ther* 12:2277, 2018.

Renz N, Feihl S, Cabric S, Trampuz A: Performance of automated multiplex PCR using sonication fluid for diagnosis of periprosthetic joint infection: a prospective cohort, *Infection* 45:877, 2017.

Roberts J, Schaefer E, Gallo RA: Indicators for detection of septic arthritis in the acutely swollen joint cohort of those without joint prostheses, *Orthopedics* 37:e98, 2014.

Sammer DM, Shin AY: Arthroscopic management of septic arthritis of the wrist, *Hand Clin* 27(3):331, 2011.

Sanpera I, Raluy-Collado D, Sanpera-Iglesias J: Arthroscopy for hip septic arthritis in children, *Orthop Traumatol Surg Res* 102(1):87, 2016.

Saper M, Stephenson K, Heisey M: Arthroscopic irrigation and debridement in the treatment of septic arthritis after anterior cruciate ligament reconstruction, *Arthroscopy* 30(6):747, 2014.

Schröder JH, Krüger D, Perka C, Hufeland M: Arthroscopic treatment for primary septic arthritis of the hip in adults, *Adv Orthop* 8713037, 2016, [Epub ahead of print].

Sigmund IK, Holinka J, Sevelda F, et al.: Performance of automated multiplex polymerase chain reaction (mPCR) using synovial fluid in the diagnosis of native joint septic arthritis in adults, *Bone Joint J* 101-B(3):288, 2019.

Singhal R, Perry DC, Khan FN, et al.: The use of CRP within a clinical prediction algorithm for the differentiation of septic arthritis and transient synovitis in children, *J Bone Joint Surg* 93B:1556, 2011.

Thompson RM, Gourineni P: Arthroscopic treatment of septic arthritis in very young children, *J Pediatr Orthop* 37(1):353, 2017.

Yagupsky P: Kingella kingae: carriage, transmission and disease, *Clin Microbiol Rev* 28(1):54, 2015.

Yagupsky P, Dubnov-Raz G, Gené A, Ephros M, Israeli-Spanish Kingella kingae Research Group: Differentiating Kingella kingae septic arthritis of the hip from transient synovitis in young children, *J Pediatr* 165(5):985, 2014.

Yanmis I, Ozkan H, Koca K, et al.: The relation between the arthroscopic findings and functional outcomes in patients with septic arthritis of the knee joint treated with arthroscopic debridement and irrigation, *Acta Orthop Traumatol Turc* 45(2):94, 2011.

The complete list of references is available online at ExpertConsult.com.

CHAPTER 6

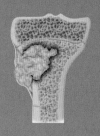

TUBERCULOSIS AND OTHER UNUSUAL INFECTIONS

Andrew H. Crenshaw Jr.

TUBERCULOSIS

Tuberculosis is transmitted primarily through inhalation or ingestion of *Mycobacterium tuberculosis* or *Mycobacterium bovis*. After exposure, the infection may be cleared by the host, lead to a primary infection, or can later be reactivated from a latent infection. Thereafter, lymphogenous, hematogenous, or contiguous extension to other tissues and organ systems may occur. The clinical presentation depends on the presence of isolated musculoskeletal involvement or miliary disease. Miliary disease has a rapid course, and constitutional symptoms include fever, chills, and cough, with accompanying pleuritic pain, weight loss, and fatigue. The patient may have acute or chronic symptoms. The mortality rate for miliary disease is 20% to 30%. The term "miliary" refers to the chest radiograph appearance of tiny lesions (1 to 5 mm) scattered throughout the lung fields that resemble millet seeds.

Current estimates of the worldwide rate of tuberculosis infection are as high as one third of the world's population. Even though the incidence of tuberculosis has been falling globally for several years, it remains one of the most frequent causes of death worldwide; the World Health Organization reported 1.1 million deaths in 2013. The highest rate of new cases is in Southeast Asia, but the highest rates of infection and mortality are in sub-Saharan Africa.

NORTH AMERICAN DEMOGRAPHICS

According the Centers for Disease Control and Prevention (CDC), there were 9093 new cases of tuberculosis reported in the United States in 2017. Since 1992, there has been a 67% decrease in the rate of cases in the United States. There were 544 deaths in the United States attributed to tuberculosis in 2013, an 8% decrease from 2012. The provisional tuberculosis case count and incidence in 2017 were the lowest in the United States since surveillance began in 1953 at 2.8 cases per 100,000 population. Since 2014, the annual percentage rate has decreased 2.0% per year. However, to eliminate tuberculosis by 2100, the annual rate of decline should be 3.9%.

More than 80% of percent tuberculosis cases in the United States represent reactivation of latent tuberculosis infections rather than recent transmissions. There are older chemotherapeutic drugs, such as methotrexate, now used for various autoimmune diseases that can lower the immune system, leading to reactivation of latent tuberculous infection in an otherwise healthy patient.

Minozzi et al. reviewed 78 controlled trials involving 24,996 patients with rheumatoid arthritis, psoriatic arthritis, and ankylosing spondylitis involving treatment with antitumor necrosis factor agents (adalimumab, golimumab, infliximab, certolizumab, and etanercept). Their meta-analysis showed increases in general infections (20%), serious infections (40%), and tuberculosis (250%).

In a systematic literature review by Cantini et al., it was found that non-antitumor necrosis factor agents used for the treatment of rheumatoid arthritis, psoriatic arthritis, and ankylosing spondylitis had a negligible latent tuberculosis reactivation rate, raising the question as to the need for pretreatment screening.

Populations most at risk include individuals with acquired immunodeficiency syndrome (AIDS) or other immunodeficiencies, patients with chronic renal failure, substance abusers, homeless or incarcerated individuals, and immigrants from developing countries. Foreign-born individuals account for approximately two thirds of recent tuberculosis cases in the United States. The high-risk period for developing the disease is within the first 5 years of immigration. Population density continues to be a risk factor; 75% of newly reported cases occur in metropolitan areas with a population of more than 500,000. In 2016, 1.0% of culture-confirmed cases were multidrug-resistant; 80.4% of those were primary tuberculosis cases, and 92% were in non-US-born persons.

MUSCULOSKELETAL INVOLVEMENT

Tuberculosis commonly affects the pulmonary system but can affect virtually any organ system of the body. Skeletal tuberculosis accounts for 10% to 20% of cases of tuberculosis. Approximately 50% of patients with osseous tuberculosis have pulmonary involvement, and 30% to 50% of patients with osseous disease have vertebral involvement, most often in the lower thoracic spine. Frequently, a primary extraosseous lesion is not well delineated. Less frequently observed appendicular involvement usually affects major weight-bearing joints of the lower extremity, most commonly the hip and knee, followed in frequency by the foot, elbow, and hand. Virtually any other bone or joint can be involved. Soft-tissue abscesses with sinus tracks have been described, as has tenosynovitis.

The spine is the most common (30% to 50%) site of osseous involvement, especially in elderly individuals; however, spinal involvement is also common in children and in young adults from developing countries. A primary accompanying lesion may be discovered from the pulmonary or urogenital system or from an unknown source. Lymphogenous and hematogenous spread have been implicated in thoracolumbar lesions but less often in cervical or sacral lesions. Usually, active spinal lesions involve a particular segment: two vertebral bodies and the corresponding disc. Some authors have speculated that these areas are affected most often because of the generous arterial and venous supply and the high oxygen pressure requirement of the tuberculosis bacilli. A peridiscal presentation occurs in approximately 80% of patients, with the anterior vertebral body affected and contiguous progression through subligamentous burrowing (anterior longitudinal ligament) and eventual extension to the adjacent vertebrae. Less frequently, lesions occur centrally in the vertebral body. These lesions are more difficult to diagnose and may mimic a tumor or contribute to significant spinal deformities. Patients may have intramedullary granulomas, arachnoiditis, segmental collapse with anterior wedging, and gibbus formation (Pott disease). The posterior elements of the spine are rarely the only sites affected. Perispinal abscesses with sinus extension to the skin may also arise and extend through tissue planes to reach intraperitoneal structures. They have been reported to occur as far distally as the popliteal fossa. Patients present with pain, weakness, and, in the late stages, paralysis. Operative treatment of Pott disease is found in other chapter.

Appendicular joint involvement typically affects the major weight-bearing joints of the lower extremities. Lesions involve the articular cartilage, which eventually is separated by granulomatous tissue. The trabecular zones of the bone are affected, with subchondral involvement affecting the weight-bearing capability of the joint, which may progress to significant accelerated joint surface degeneration. Pathologic assessment reveals a central caseating lesion within necrotic tissue and multinucleated giant cells.

Other, less frequently involved joints include the ankle, foot, and upper extremity joints. Patients may present with a limp and a joint that is warm and swollen and has a decreased range of motion. Tuberculosis in a joint markedly decreases its functional use; even when adequately treated, the disease may reactivate in isolated regions. Peripheral joint involvement from tuberculosis can be confused with other rheumatologic conditions (e.g., gout and rheumatoid arthritis). Periprosthetic joint infections have also been reported after hip, knee, and wrist arthroplasty in patients without a history of tuberculosis, with a delay in diagnosis of approximately 4 months.

LABORATORY FINDINGS

Patients may have a normochromic or normocytic anemia, pancytopenia, or thrombocytopenia. Frequently, the white blood cell count is normal, and the sedimentation rate may be elevated or normal. The patient may have the syndrome of inappropriate antidiuretic hormone. Tuberculosis skin testing is usually effective in diagnosing this condition; however, false-negative rates can be 20% to 30%. Immunocompromised individuals frequently have an unreliable skin test result. The hallmark of the diagnosis is demonstration of the tuberculosis acid-fast bacilli from a tissue or fluid source. Bone cultures taken from disc involvement are positive in 60% to 80% of cases. Sputum and gastric cultures of patients with pulmonary involvement usually are positive in more than 50%. The clinical utility of newer T-cell-based assays to detect skeletal and other forms of extrapulmonary tuberculosis has been studied in large cohorts of patients, which, in general, have shown the same results as testing in patients with pulmonary tuberculosis: such assays lack sufficient sensitivity and specificity to rely on them singly in the absence of traditional diagnostic testing such as biopsy and culture and imaging studies.

Tang et al. reported that the T-cell-based interferon gamma release assay (IGRA[T-SPOT.TB]), when used along with the rifampin resistance fluorescence test, Xpert MTB/RIF assay, produced a combined sensitivity of 91.9%.

Transbronchial biopsy specimens in patients with pulmonary involvement are positive in 70% to 86% of patients. Pulmonary exudates may reveal predominantly lymphocytic exudate or polymorphonuclear leukocytes and have a low pH that is slightly-to-moderately acidic. Molecular subtyping has also been used to assess infection patterns and sensitivities to medications.

IMAGING

Plain radiographs of involved joints assist in guiding treatment. When a joint is involved, synovial infiltration that affects the subarticular bone is usually present. Periarticular erosions observed radiographically have an almost lytic appearance and can mimic infection, noninfectious arthropathy, or malignancy. Periarticular bone mass is decreased and may mimic juvenile arthritis. Progression to fusion is rare but can occur. Characteristics of typical spinal involvement have been described previously. Anterior vertebral involvement occurs more commonly than central vertebral involvement. There is a relative sparing of the intervertebral disc space. Later stages include a focal segmental collapse with anterior wedging and gibbus formation, characteristic of Pott disease.

Other imaging studies include a bone scan or a gallium scan, which can detect 88% to 96% of osseous tuberculosis lesions. Such scans are quite sensitive but not particularly specific for tuberculosis. MRI and CT can provide more detail and delineate the disease in earlier phases and are helpful in defining soft-tissue abscesses. MRI findings are nonspecific for tuberculosis and may be consistent with osteomyelitis, tumor, osteonecrosis, or neuropathic joint. If tuberculosis is a consideration, tissue or bone biopsy is indicated. Calcifications (best seen on CT) within paraspinous abscesses indicate bone destruction and are characteristic of spinal tuberculosis. CT or ultrasound-guided fluoroscopy can assist in obtaining appropriate tissue or fluid samples for additional studies. Arthrography and other imaging studies for tendon sheaths have been described but are used less frequently.

NONOPERATIVE TREATMENT OF APPENDICULAR TUBERCULOUS INFECTIONS

The primary treatment objectives for tuberculosis of bone include halting the infection, limiting deformity, maintaining mobility, and reducing discomfort. A multidisciplinary approach with the assistance of infectious disease and pain management specialists is ideal. Other affiliated team members should include nurses, physical therapists, occupational therapists, and orthotists. Approximately 90% of patients can be treated conservatively with chemotherapy, relative rest, and guided remobilization. Adjunctive splinting (passive, dynamic, functional) and casting techniques are useful

for marked or painful and progressive joint involvement. At times, destructive changes are markedly progressive and eventually may lead to fusion of the joint (e.g., elbow), so it is crucial to place the extremity in a position of function (elbow flexion 70 to 90 degrees) to obtain an optimal range for future functional use.

A judicious, well-guided chemotherapeutic approach to tuberculosis along with the assistance of an infectious disease specialist yields optimal results. The pharmacologic agents and duration of treatment depend on the patient's age, dissemination of disease, and accompanying medical conditions (e.g., AIDS, chronic renal failure). Several agents interact with medications typically used for immunosuppressed individuals, especially patients infected with human immunodeficiency virus (HIV). In these patients, it may be necessary to adjust dosages and modify treatment regimens. Various combinations of medications are used to treat tuberculosis: first-line drugs include isoniazid, rifampin, ethambutol, and pyrazinamide (Table 6.1). Drug-resistant tuberculosis may

TABLE 6.1

Doses* of Antituberculosis Drugs for Adults and Children†

DRUG	PREPARATION	POPULATION	DAILY	ONCE-WEEKLY	TWICE-WEEKLY	THRICE-WEEKLY
FIRST-LINE DRUGS						
Isoniazid	Tablets (50 mg, 100 mg, 300 mg); elixir (50 mg/5 mL); aqueous solution (100 mg/mL) for intravenous or intramuscular injection. Note: Pyridoxine (vitamin B6), 25–50 mg/day, is given with INH to all persons at risk of neuropathy (e.g., pregnant women, breastfeeding infants; persons with HIV; patients with diabetes, alcoholism, malnutrition, or chronic renal failure; or patients with advanced age). For patients with peripheral neuropathy, experts recommend increasing pyridoxine dose to 100 mg/day.	Adults	5 mg/kg (typically 300 mg)	15 mg/kg (typically 900 mg)	15 mg/kg (typically 900 mg)	15 mg/kg (typically 900 mg)
		Children	10–15 mg/kg	—	20–30 mg/kg	—†
Rifampin	Capsule (150 mg, 300 mg). Powder may be suspended for oral administration.	Adults‡	10 mg/kg (typically 600 mg)	—	10 mg/kg (typically 600 mg)	10 mg/kg (typically 600 mg)
	Aqueous solution for intravenous injection	Children	10–20 mg/kg		10–20 mg/kg	—†
Rifabutin	Capsule (150 mg)	Adults§	5 mg/kg (typically 300 mg)	—	Not recommended	Not recommended
		Children	Appropriate dosing for children is unknown. Estimated at 5/mg/kg.			

TABLE 6.1

Doses* of Antituberculosis Drugs for Adults and Children†—cont'd†

DRUG	PREPARATION	POPULATION	DAILY	ONCE-WEEKLY	TWICE-WEEKLY	THRICE-WEEKLY
Rifapentine	Tablet (150 mg film coated)	Adults	10 mg/kg$^{\|}$			
		Children	Active tuberculosis: for children ≥12 years of age, same dosing as for adults, administered once weekly, Rifapentine is not FDA-approved for the treatment of active tuberculosis in children <12 years of age			
Pyrazinamide	Tablet (500 mg scored)	Adults	18.2–26.3 mg/kg based on weight	—	36.4–52.6 mg/kg based on weight	27.3–39.5 mg/kg based on weight
		Children	35 (30–40) mg/kg	—	50 mg/kg	—†
Ethambutol	Tablet (100 mg; 400 mg)	Adults	14.5–21.1 mg/kg based on weight	—	36.4–52.6 mg/kg based on weight	21.8–31.6 mg/kg based on weight
		Children¶	20 (15–25) mg/kg	—	50 mg/kg	—†

SECOND-LINE DRUGS

DRUG	PREPARATION	POPULATION	DAILY	ONCE-WEEKLY	TWICE-WEEKLY	THRICE-WEEKLY
Cycloserine	Capsule (250 mg)	Adults**	10–15 mg/kg total (usually 250–500 mg) once or twice daily	There are inadequate data to support intermittent administration.		
		Children	15–20 mg/kg total (divided 1–2 times daily)			
Ethionamide	Tablet (250 mg)	Adults††	15–20 mg/kg total (usually 250–500 mg once or twice daily)	There are inadequate data to support intermittent administration.		
		Children	15–20 mg/kg total (divided 1–2 times daily)			
Streptomycin	Aqueous solution (1 g vials) for IM or IV administration	Adults	15 mg/kg daily. Some clinicians prefer 25 mg/kg 3 times weekly. Patients with decreased renal function may require the 15 mg/kg dose to be given only 3 times weekly to allow for drug clearance.			
		Children	15–20 mg/kg	—	25–30 mg/kg‡‡	—
Amikacin/ kanamycin	Aqueous solution (500 mg and 1 g vials) for IM or IV administration	Adults	15 mg daily. Some clinicians prefer 25 mg/kg 3 times weekly. Patients with decreased renal function, including older patients, may require the 15 mg/kg dose to be given only 3 times weekly to allow for drug clearance.			
		Children	15–20 mg/kg	—	25–30 mg/kg‡‡	—
Capreomycin	Aqueous solution (1 g vials) for IM or IV administration	Adults	15 mg/kg daily. Some clinicians prefer 25 mg/kg 3 times weekly. Patients with decreased renal function, including older patients, may require the 15 mg/kg dose to be given 3 times weekly to allow for drug clearance.			
		Children	15–20 m/kg	—	25–30 mg/kg‡‡	—

Continued

TABLE 6.1

Doses* of Antituberculosis Drugs for Adults and Children†—cont'd†

DRUG	PREPARATION	POPULATION	DAILY	ONCE-WEEKLY	TWICE-WEEKLY	THRICE-WEEKLY
Para-amino-salicylic acid	Granules (4 g packets) can be mixed in and ingested with soft food (granules should not be chewed). Tablets (500 mg) are still available in some countries, but not in the United States. A solution for IV administration is available in Europe.	Adults	8–12 g total (usually 4000 mg) 2–3 times daily	There are inadequate data to support intermittent administration.		
		Children	200–300 mg/kg total (usually divided 100 mg/kg given 2–3 times daily)			
Levofloxacin	Tablets (250 mg, 500 mg, 750 mg); aqueous solution (500 mg vials) for IV injection	Adults	500–1000 mg daily	There are inadequate data to support intermittent administration.		
		Children	The optimal dose is not known, but clinical data suggest 15–20 mg/kg.			
Moxifloxacin	Tablets (400 mg); aqueous solution (400 mg/250 mL) for IV injection	Adults	400 mg daily	There are inadequate data to support intermittent administration.§§		
		Children	The optimal dose is not known. Some experts use 10 mg/kg daily dosing, though lack of formulations makes such titration challenging. Aiming for serum concentrations of 3–5 uL/mL 2 h post dose is proposed by experts as a reasonable target.			

*Dosing based on actual weight is acceptable in patients who are not obese. For obese patients (>20% above ideal body weight [IBW]), dosing based on IBW may be preferred for initial doses. Some clinicians prefer a modified IBW (IBW + [0.40 × (actual weight – IBW)]) as is done for initial aminoglycoside doses. Because tuberculosis drug dosing for obese patients has not been established, therapeutic drug monitoring may be considered for such patients.
†For purposes of this document, adult dosing begins at the age of 15 years or at a weight of greater than 40 kg in younger children. The optimal doses for thrice-weekly therapy in children and adolescents have not been established. Some experts use in adolescents the same doses as recommended for adults, and for younger children the same doses as recommended for twice weekly therapy.
‡Higher doses of rifampin, currently as high as 35 mg/kg, are being studied in clinical trials.
§Rifabutin dose may need to be adjusted when there is concomitant use of protease inhibitors or nonnucleoside reverse transcriptase inhibitors.
‖TBTC Study 22 used rifapentine (RPT) dosage of 10 mg/kg in the continuation phase of treatment for active disease. However, RIFAQUIN and PREVENT TB safely used higher dosages of RPT, administered once weekly. Daily doses of 1200 mg RPT are being studied in clinical trials for active tuberculosis disease.
¶As an approach to avoiding ethambutol (EMB) ocular toxicity, some clinicians use a 3-drug regimen (INH, rifampin, and pyrazinamide) in the initial 2 months of treatment for children who are HIV-uninfected, have no prior tuberculosis treatment history, are living in an area of low prevalence of drug-resistant tuberculosis, and have no exposure to an individual from an area of high prevalence of drug-resistant tuberculosis. However, because the prevalence of and risk for drug-resistant tuberculosis can be difficult to ascertain, the American Academy of Pediatrics and most experts include EMB as part of the intensive-phase regimen for children with tuberculosis.
**Clinicians experienced with using cycloserine suggest starting with 250 mg once daily and gradually increasing as tolerated. Serum concentrations often are useful in determining the appropriate dose for a given patient. Few patients tolerate 500 mg twice daily.
††Ethionamide can be given at bedtime or with a main meal in an attempt to reduce nausea. Clinicians experienced with using ethionamide suggest starting with 250 mg once daily and gradually increasing as tolerated. Serum concentrations may be useful in determining the appropriate dose for a given patient. Few patients tolerate 500 mg twice daily.
‡‡Modified from adult intermittent dose of 25 mg/kg, and accounting for larger total body water content and faster clearance of injectable drugs in most children. Dosing can be guided by serum concentrations.
§§Rifaquin trial studied at 6-month regimen. Daily isoniazid was replaced by daily moxifloxacin 400 mg for the first 2 months followed by once-weekly doses of moxifloxacin 400 mg and RPT 1200 mg for the remaining 4 months. Two hundred twelve patients were studied (each dose of RPT was preceded by a meal of 2 hard-boiled eggs and bread). This regimen was shown to be noninferior to a standard daily administered 6-month regimen.
FDA, US Food and Drug Administration; *HIV*, human immunodeficiency virus; *IM*, intramuscular; *INH*, isoniazid; *IV*, intravenous.
From Nahid P, Dorman SE, Alipanah N, et al: Official American Thoracic Society/Centers for Disease Control and Prevention/Infectious Diseases Society of America clinical practice guidelines: treatment of drug-susceptible tuberculosis, *Clin Infect Dis* 63(7):147, 2016.

require fluoroquinolones and injectable medications such as amikacin, kanamycin, or capreomycin, which typically are used for 20 to 30 months. Some types of tuberculosis are developing resistance to these drugs. Several new drugs are in development to be used as an add-on therapy. Bedaquiline, delamanid, and PA-824 target pulmonary tuberculosis, whereas linezolid and sutezolid are antibiotics for extensively drug-resistant tuberculosis infection. The efficacy and safety of these drugs are still being established. Traditionally, 12- to 18-month courses of therapy have been advocated for musculoskeletal tuberculosis because of concerns about poor drug penetration into osseous and fibrous tissues; however, more recent studies have suggested that shorter courses of treatment (6 to 9 months) with regimens containing rifampin are as effective as longer courses of treatment without rifampin.

Because treatment for tuberculosis is frequently modified, readily available guidelines from the CDC should be consulted. Although primary and secondary resistance to multiple medications has been reported, especially in countries outside the United States, most are isolated cases. Generally, only a small percentage of new patients (<1%) are resistant to multiple chemotherapeutic agents.

Treatment should not be limited to the patient, but chemoprophylaxis should be considered in family members and other close contacts who have a positive tuberculosis skin test. Chemoprophylaxis is particularly important in individuals who are younger than 50 to 55 years of age. Older individuals may not tolerate some of the medications typically used for prophylaxis. Treatment for chemoprophylaxis may last 3 to 12 months, depending on the conversion of the tuberculosis skin test.

Patients may require analgesics for pain. In severe cases, a pain management specialist should be consulted. Although the use of systemic corticosteroids to reduce symptoms in severe cases has been described, their use may mask a septic joint, and intraarticular corticosteroid injections can accelerate the destructive articular changes.

OPERATIVE TREATMENT

Operations applicable to bone and joint tuberculosis include (1) arthrotomy, including biopsy, synovectomy, and curettage with bone grafting of articular erosions; (2) curettage and bone grafting of extraarticular skeletal lesions; (3) resection of joints; (4) resection of bones; (5) evacuation or excision of soft-tissue abscesses; (6) arthrodesis; and (7) amputation. Arthroscopic debridement of joint tuberculosis has been shown to be effective.

Most authorities agree that effective antibiotic therapy should be started before surgery for tuberculosis. Miliary dissemination of the disease has been reported when surgery was done without adequate chemotherapeutic coverage. Long duration multi-antibiotic release scaffolds are under development using methylmethacrylate and hydroxyapatite.

■ FOOT

In tuberculosis of the foot (Fig. 6.1), many bones may become involved, and a delay in diagnosis increases the risk of joint involvement. Operative indications include juxtaarticular focus or joint destruction. Bones with cystic changes typically respond better than rheumatologic-appearing joints. When present, isolated lesions usually involve the calcaneus or talus. When several bones are involved, especially in adults, amputation is the procedure of choice. Curettage is indicated for isolated lesions even when sinuses are present.

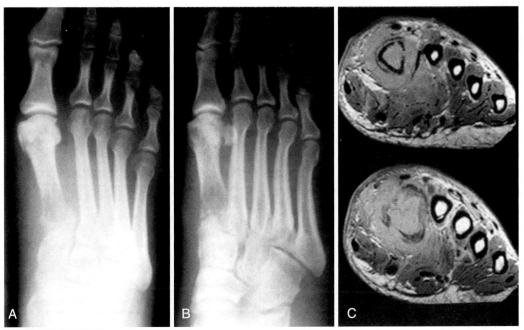

FIGURE 6.1   **A** and **B,** Anteroposterior and oblique radiographs of tuberculous lesion involving base of first metatarsal. Medial and lateral cortices are eroded. **C,** MR image shows circumferential destruction of base of first metatarsal with extension into soft tissues. (From Lonner JH, Sheskier SC: Tuberculosis of the foot as the initial manifestation of acquired immune deficiency syndrome: a report of two cases, *Foot Ankle Int* 16:167, 1995.)

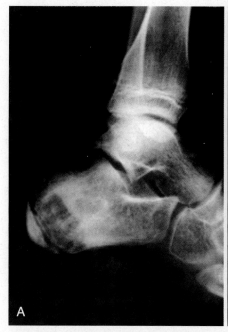
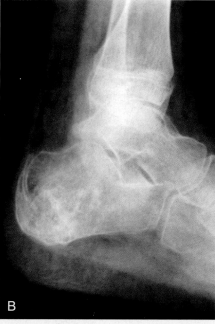

FIGURE 6.2 Tuberculosis of calcaneus before **(A)** and 6 months after **(B)** curettage, grafting with cancellous bone chips, and primary closure of wound. The calcaneus healed without drainage, an excellent result. **SEE TECHNIQUE 6.1.**

CURETTAGE FOR TUBERCULOUS LESIONS IN THE FOOT

TECHNIQUE 6.1

- Make an incision directly over the lesion or directly through a sinus or abscess, if present.
- Remove all necrotic and scarred tissue but not uninvolved osteopenic bone.
- Pack the cavity with autogenous cancellous bone and close the incision (Fig. 6.2).
- In the presence of secondary infection, omit the bone grafts and close the incision loosely over drains.

POSTOPERATIVE CARE A short leg cast is applied with appropriate windows cut out for dressing the wound. Immobilization is continued for 3 to 4 months, and weight bearing is permitted during the latter part of this period.

When lesions involve the subtalar or midtarsal joints, a triple arthrodesis is indicated. When the subtalar and the ankle joints are affected, posterior arthrodesis of these joints can be done.

EXCISION OF BONES

When the disease is extensive, especially when complicated by sinuses or secondary infection, excision of bones or amputation is indicated. Involvement of a phalanx or metatarsal often is best treated by excision. When a tarsal bone is excised, a proportionate amount of bone is taken from the opposite side of the foot so that proper alignment can be maintained.

When a metatarsal is excised, amputation of the corresponding toe permits better approximation of adjacent metatarsals and provides a foot with a better appearance and function. Excision of the first metatarsal should be avoided, if possible.

EXCISION OF METATARSAL

TECHNIQUE 6.2

- In the presence of secondary infection, make a longitudinal incision over the affected bone extending from the distal row of the tarsus to the middle of the proximal phalanx.
- Expose the bone without injuring the extensor tendons.
- Excise the bone with the periosteum intact and close the wound loosely over drains.

POSTOPERATIVE CARE A short leg cast is applied. When the wound has healed, protective weight bearing is begun.

Usually, more than one bone is involved, so an anterior tarsectomy is required. To obtain satisfactory alignment of the foot, part of the cuboid must also be removed.

EXCISION OF CUNEIFORM BONES

TECHNIQUE 6.3

- Make a 5-cm longitudinal incision laterally and expose the joint between the cuboid and fifth metatarsal.
- Approach the first cuneiform and the base of the first metatarsal through a similar medial incision.
- Expose the second and third cuneiforms by subperiosteal dissection.
- Excise the anterior half of the cuboid and the three cuneiforms with an osteotome.
- Resect the articular cartilage from the anterior surface of the navicular and the bases of all five metatarsals.

- Approximate the denuded surfaces of the metatarsals to those of the navicular and cuboid.
- Close the incisions.

POSTOPERATIVE CARE A short leg cast is applied, and protected weight bearing is begun when the wound has healed.

EXCISION OF NAVICULAR

TECHNIQUE 6.4

- Expose the midtarsus through an anterolateral approach.
- Make an additional medial incision to expose the navicular.
- Excise the navicular by sharp subperiosteal dissection. Avoid injuring the dorsalis pedis artery and the branches of the deep peroneal nerve on the dorsum of the foot.
- Expose the calcaneocuboid joint and excise the articular cartilage and subchondral bone from the distal end of the calcaneus and the proximal one third of the cuboid.
- Remove the articular cartilage from the head of the talus and from the proximal surfaces of the cuneiforms.
- Approximate the raw surfaces of the denuded bones, obliterating the space. The position can be maintained by crossed, threaded wires.
- After excision of the navicular, a midtarsal arthrodesis should be performed to stabilize the foot in satisfactory alignment.

POSTOPERATIVE CARE A short leg cast is applied, and protected weight bearing is begun when the wound has healed.

EXCISION OF CUBOID

TECHNIQUE 6.5

- Approach the cuboid through an anterolateral approach and excise it by sharp subperiosteal dissection.
- Resect the articular surfaces and adjacent bone from the proximal aspect of the cuneiforms and the fifth metatarsal and from the distal surface of the calcaneus.
- Excise the navicular and remove the articular surface and superficial bone from the head of the talus.
- Approximate the denuded surfaces of the bones and maintain the position by crossed, threaded wires.

POSTOPERATIVE CARE Postoperative care is the same as for excision of the navicular just described.

Calcanectomy produces considerable disability, but the result may be preferable to amputation. Partial calcanectomy has long been used for the treatment of osteomyelitis of the calcaneus, with less disability and better cosmetic and functional

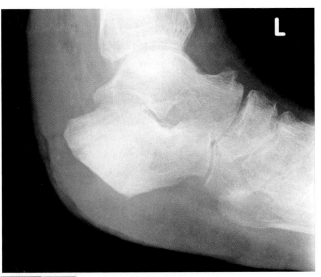

FIGURE 6.3   Partial calcanectomy. (From Walsh TP, Yates BJ: Calcanectomy: avoiding major amputation in the presence of calcaneal osteomyelitis—a case series, *Foot* 23:130, 2013.)

results than total calcanectomy (Fig. 6.3), although there are few reports of its use in patients with tuberculous infection.

EXCISION OF CALCANEUS

TECHNIQUE 6.6

- Begin a Kocher incision (see Technique 1.18) 10 cm proximal to the lateral malleolus and follow the lateral border of the Achilles tendon to the superior surface of the calcaneus; continue it inferiorly to the lateral malleolus and end it 2.5 cm distal to the calcaneocuboid joint.
- Divide the calcaneofibular ligament and displace the peroneal tendons superiorly and anteriorly.
- Incise the capsule of the calcaneocuboid joint and divide the ligamentous attachments of the calcaneus in this area.
- Insert a periosteal elevator or lamina spreader into the subtalar joint and divide the interosseous talocalcaneal ligaments.
- Dislocate the subtalar joint; use sharp subperiosteal dissection to free the soft tissues from the medial, anterior, and posterior surfaces; and divide the attachment of the Achilles tendon.
- Deliver the calcaneus from the wound. Avoid injuring the tibial nerve and vessels on the medial side of the bone.
- Suture the Achilles tendon to the inferior surface of the talus and to the short muscles of the foot.

POSTOPERATIVE CARE

A long leg cast is applied with the knee in 30 degrees of flexion and the ankle in moderate equinus. At 3 weeks, the cast is changed to a short leg cast, and the foot is maintained in mild equinus. Protective weight bearing is begun at 8 weeks, and cast immobilization is continued for 4 months. A shoe insert with heel elevation is required later.

Hutson et al. described excision of the talus through an anteromedial approach, followed by insertion of antibiotic beads, for the treatment of infection before tibiocalcaneal arthrodesis.

EXCISION OF TALUS

TECHNIQUE 6.7

- Approach the talus through a Kocher (see Technique 1.18) or anterolateral (see Technique 1.19) approach.
- Divide the capsule of the talonavicular joint on its dorsolateral and inferior aspects.
- Divide the components of the fibular collateral ligament of the ankle at their fibular attachments.
- Dislocate the ankle and displace the foot medially.
- Grasp the neck of the talus and apply slight traction; use sharp subperiosteal dissection to sever all soft tissues and ligamentous attachments on the posterior and inferior aspects from anteriorly to posteriorly and remove the talus. If the bone is necrotic, it must be removed in pieces.
- Use subperiosteal dissection to free the soft tissues on both malleoli and both sides of the anterior aspect of the calcaneus.
- Displace the foot posteriorly, placing the anterior aspect of the calcaneus between the malleoli. The articular surfaces of the calcaneus should approximate the articular surface of the tibia.
- Close the wound while the foot is held in equinus (Fig. 6.4).

POSTOPERATIVE CARE A long leg cast is applied with the knee in 30 degrees of flexion and the ankle in moderate equinus. A window is removed from the cast on the dorsum of the foot and ankle and is loosely replaced. At 2 or 3 weeks, the cast is changed to a short-leg cast and the foot is maintained in equinus. Protective weight bearing is begun at 8 weeks, and cast immobilization is continued for 4 months. A comfortable shoe with heel elevation is fitted.

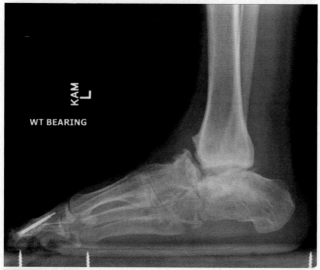

FIGURE 6.4 After talectomy for infection. **SEE TECHNIQUE 6.7.**

ANKLE

If the disease is confined to the synovial membrane, immobilization and chemotherapy may suffice. An abscess can be drained, or a localized bone lesion can be curetted. However, tuberculosis of the ankle is often best treated by arthrodesis (Fig. 6.5).

KNEE

Determination of the extent of joint involvement is paramount in the treatment of tuberculosis of the knee. At times, a patient may have a relatively benign-appearing periarticular soft-tissue inflammation (which represents tuberculous bursitis), purulent popliteal cystic changes, or abscess formation. The radiographic appearance of the knee may help to guide the treatment regimen. A knee with a normal-appearing radiograph or with mildly confined osteomyelitic changes frequently responds to multidrug chemotherapy. These patients usually tolerate early range-of-motion and mobilization procedures. If a patient does not respond adequately to chemotherapy alone, a synovectomy (at times performed arthroscopically), sequestrectomy, or both, or curettage of the bony lesion may be required. When the joint shows significant degenerative involvement and apparent radiographic changes, the prognosis is less favorable, and a more aggressive open approach is needed. A relative period of immobilization is also required in more severe cases. With more destructive articular surface changes, an arthrodesis may be inevitable (Fig. 6.6). Limited success with knee arthroplasty combined with chemotherapy has been described, although not without frequent morbidity, including possible reactivation of a quiescent infectious process. Zeng et al. reported successful total knee arthroplasty in nine patients with advanced tuberculous arthritis of the knee. Those with elevated inflammatory biomarkers had 3 months of antitubercular drug treatment followed by two-stage arthroplasty, whereas those with normal biomarkers had no preoperative drug therapy and one-stage arthroplasty. All patients received antitubercular therapy for 12 months after surgery, and there was no tuberculosis reactivation at an average 4-year follow-up.

Tuberculosis confined to the patella manifests with osteolytic changes radiographically and an accompanying sequestrum, which has a flaky appearance. Such a confined process may respond to a multiple-drug regimen. In refractory cases, a favorable functional outcome still can be salvaged with a patellectomy. An extraarticular abscess or lesion (bursal or cystic) requires excision and drainage. If the lesion involves the distal femur or proximal tibia, curettage of adjacent bone is required. Active early mobilization is allowed, unless the lesion is extensive.

Nag et al. reported tubercular infection after anterior cruciate ligament reconstruction with autograft in immunocompetent patients. Although still a rare complication, it should be considered in areas with high endemic rates of tuberculosis.

HIP

If tuberculosis of the hip is diagnosed early and the disease is limited to the synovium, rest and chemotherapy may be sufficient treatment. This situation is more common in children. Most hips (50%) appear normal on radiographs and usually respond well to chemotherapy. These patients usually tolerate early mobilization.

If the lesion extends to articular cartilage and bone and is not extensive, partial synovectomy and curettage often are

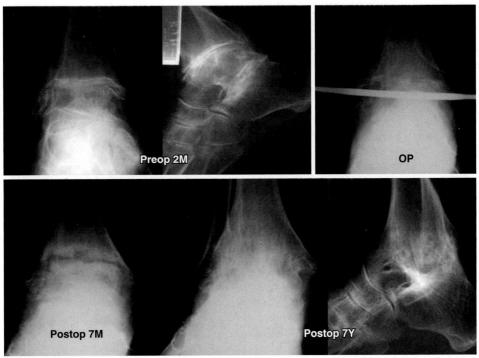

FIGURE 6.5 A 22-year-old man with tuberculous infection of the ankle. Seven years after arthrodesis, fusion was solid. (From Chen SH, Lee CH, Wong T, et al: Long-term retrospective analysis of surgical treatment for irretrievable tuberculosis of the ankle, *Foot Ankle Int* 34:372, 2013.)

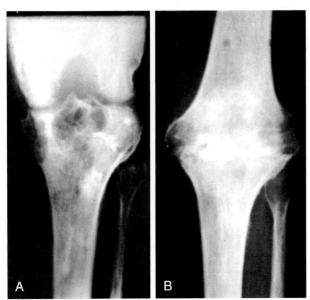

FIGURE 6.6 Tuberculosis of knee before **(A)** and 3.5 months after **(B)** arthrodesis.

successful (Fig. 6.7). Atrophic-appearing hips (<10%) and dislocating hips have a less favorable outcome. If articular cartilage and adjacent bone are extensively involved, arthrodesis is indicated. The greater trochanter may be involved in less than 1.8% of patients who have osseous tuberculosis. Abscess formation may also occur in the peritrochanteric and psoas regions. Operations such as drainage of an abscess near the joint, diagnostic biopsy, or removal of an extraarticular sequestrum may be needed. More novel approaches using streptomycin-loaded bone cement beads have been described in treating tuberculous bursitis and osteomyelitis.

PARTIAL SYNOVECTOMY AND CURETTAGE

TECHNIQUE 6.8

(WILKINSON)
- Expose the hip by an anterolateral approach (see Technique 1.64).
- Curet the lesions in the femoral neck or head or in the acetabulum.
- Excise the thickened capsule and perform a synovectomy, but do not dislocate the hip in an effort to remove all tuberculous tissue.
- Suture the wound in layers without drainage.

POSTOPERATIVE CARE Buck traction is used until irritability of the hip disappears. Active range-of-motion exercises are started. Unprotected weight bearing is not allowed for several months, or until radiographs show healing of the bone lesions.

Tuberculous foci in the ilium above the acetabulum may be curetted without arthrotomy if they are discovered before they spread into the joint.

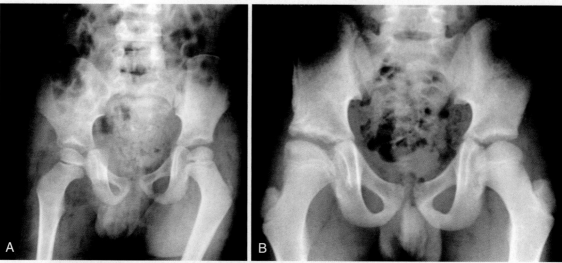

FIGURE 6.7 Tuberculosis of hip immediately before **(A)** and 7 years after **(B)** synovectomy, marsupialization, and antibacterial therapy. Disease is clinically cured; patient has no limp and only slight limitation of motion. Note distortion of femoral head and acetabulum.

LESIONS ABOVE ACETABULUM

TECHNIQUE 6.9

- Use an anterolateral approach (see Technique 1.64); keep the dissection extracapsular and locate the tuberculous lesion by radiographic imaging if necessary.
- Curet the lesion and, unless secondary infection is present, fill the cavity with autogenous cancellous grafts if desired.
- Close the incision in layers.

POSTOPERATIVE CARE Postoperative care is the same as for synovectomy and curettage, just as described in Technique 6.8.

Tuberculous foci confined to the femoral neck can be evacuated, preventing their spread into the hip joint.

LESIONS OF THE FEMORAL NECK

TECHNIQUE 6.10

- Use a lateral longitudinal incision and expose the subtrochanteric area of the femur.
- Remove a cortical window laterally and locate the lesion by radiographic imaging.
- Evacuate the focus with a curet, taking care not to enter the joint, and fill the cavity with autogenous cancellous grafts if necessary.
- Close the incision in layers.

POSTOPERATIVE CARE Postoperative care is the same as for synovectomy and curettage (see Technique 6.8).

Often, the trochanteric bursa and the underlying bone are involved in the infection. Excision of the bursa is then indicated.

LESIONS OF THE TROCHANTERIC AREA

TECHNIQUE 6.11

(AHERN)
- Expose the trochanteric bursa and greater trochanter through a lateral longitudinal incision.
- Excise the diseased bursa and curet any lesions found in the greater trochanter.
- Close the wound in layers.

POSTOPERATIVE CARE Protected weight bearing is begun when the patient's condition permits, progressing to full activity in 6 to 12 weeks.

▋ ARTHRODESIS
Patients with advanced tuberculosis of the hip involving articular cartilage and bone are best treated by arthrodesis. The techniques are described in other chapter.

▋ EVACUATION OF ABSCESSES
Tuberculous abscesses should usually be evacuated. Radiographs frequently show distention of the joint capsule. If the capsule ruptures, the abscess may point in the adductor region, in the anterior thigh 5.0 to 7.5 cm below the anterior superior iliac spine, over the greater trochanter, or in the buttock. Drainage by incision directly over the abscess, evacuation of the cavity, and primary closure usually promote prompt healing.

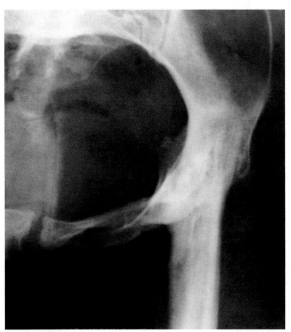

FIGURE 6.8 Osseous ankylosis after excision of hip for tuberculosis complicated by pyogenic infection.

Excision of the hip joint is indicated in adults with extensive involvement of the femoral head and neck and the acetabulum complicated by secondary infection (Fig. 6.8).

EXCISION OF THE HIP JOINT

TECHNIQUE 6.12

- Expose the hip through a lateral or posterolateral approach (see Techniques 1.67 and 1.72).
- Excise the capsule and remove the femoral head and neck and the diseased bone around the acetabulum.
- Place the greater trochanter in the acetabulum and close the wound loosely over large drains.

POSTOPERATIVE CARE A double spica cast, holding the involved hip in 45 degrees of abduction, is applied. Immobilization is continued for approximately 3 months. Proximal femoral osteotomy or arthrodesis may be indicated for any residual instability.

■ SACROILIAC JOINT

Symptoms of tuberculosis of the sacroiliac joint include buttock pain, reluctance to bear weight on the involved side, radicular complaints, and low back pain. Plain radiographs are usually abnormal, as are bone scans. Diagnosis can be confirmed by percutaneous transiliac biopsy. When the diagnosis of tuberculosis of the sacroiliac joint is made early, chemotherapy and rest are usually sufficient. When involvement is more extensive, partial synovectomy and curettage or arthrodesis may be indicated.

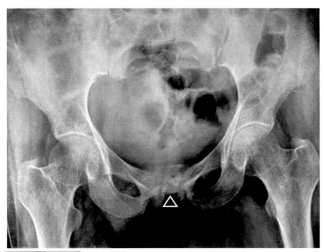

FIGURE 6.9 Erosion of the pubic rami with widening of the symphysis in a 49-year-old woman with tuberculosis. (From Lal H, Jain VK, Kannan S: Tuberculosis of the pubic symphysis: four unusual cases and literature review, *Clin Orthop Relat Res* 471:3372, 2013.)

■ PUBIS

Tuberculosis of the pubis may involve the symphysis (Fig. 6.9). Chemotherapy and curettage usually promote healing.

■ CLAVICLE

One end of the clavicle is usually infected by tuberculosis. Chemotherapy and curettage of the focus or excision of the involved end of the bone are recommended.

■ SHOULDER

Tuberculosis can involve all adjacent osseous structures of the shoulder, including the scapula, humerus, glenoid, clavicle, acromioclavicular, and sternoclavicular joints. Periarticular soft tissue or bursae may also be involved. Khan et al. described tubercular infection after arthroscopic rotator cuff repair in one patient. Although the infection was well controlled with medical treatment, function was poor. Tuberculosis of the shoulder that is diagnosed early and confined to the synovium is best treated by chemotherapy and rest. Extraarticular abscesses require evacuation. More extensive disease is treated by partial synovectomy and curettage. Rarely is arthrodesis required.

■ ELBOW

Although tuberculosis occurs more frequently in the elbow than in other upper extremity joints, the elbow is involved in only 5% of patients with osseous disease. The proximal segment of the ulna (olecranon) is more typically affected (Fig. 6.10), which can result in a progressive degenerative process and a significant elbow flexion contracture. Functional positioning becomes paramount in such cases. Tuberculosis of the elbow often can be treated satisfactorily by rest and chemotherapy. Aspiration of an abscess or evacuation of a lesion in the olecranon may be necessary. Occasionally, partial synovectomy and curettage, arthrodesis, or excision of the elbow joint may be indicated.

Excision of the elbow joint is indicated in adults when the disease is extensive and more conservative measures have failed. It usually results in less disability than does arthrodesis.

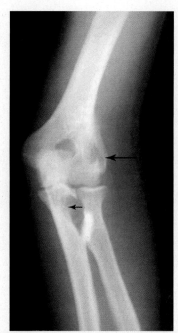

FIGURE 6.10   Plain radiograph of the elbow shows lytic lesion in the lateral condyle *(arrow)* and erosion of the radial aspect of the proximal ulnar shaft *(short arrow)*. (From Prakash M, Gupta P, Dhillon MS, et al: Magnetic resonance imaging findings in tubercular arthritis of the elbow, *Clin Imaging* 40:114, 2016.)

EXCISION OF ELBOW JOINT

TECHNIQUE 6.13

- Make a longitudinal incision over the posterolateral aspect of the elbow beginning 10 cm proximal and ending 5 cm distal to the joint.
- Incise the triceps muscle down to the humerus, parallel with the lateral border of the aponeurosis.
- Open the posterior capsule of the elbow joint and continue the incision of the deep structures to approximately 2.5 cm distal to the head of the radius.
- Subperiosteally dissect the distal end of the humerus and resect the bone just proximal to the condyle, leaving as much of the metaphysis as possible.
- Resect the ulna and radius just distal to the head of the radius; a more extensive resection would produce a flail joint.
- Remove the synovial membrane and all diseased tissues and close the wound.

POSTOPERATIVE CARE A long arm cast is applied with the elbow at 90 degrees of flexion. After 3 or 4 weeks, the cast is removed, and a sling is applied. Strengthening and active range-of-motion exercises are started. Muscular reeducation and active use usually result in a serviceable but unstable joint.

ARTHRODESIS

Arthrodesis may be required. This technique is discussed in other chapter.

WRIST AND HAND

The wrist may be involved in patients with skeletal tuberculosis. Tenosynovitis of the flexor and extensor tendons may result; consequently, carpal tunnel syndrome may occur. If the disease is limited to the synovium, synovectomy and chemotherapy constitute sufficient treatment. If involvement of cartilage and bone is moderate, synovectomy and curettage are indicated; if involvement is extensive, arthrodesis or, rarely, excision of the joint is needed.

Excision of the wrist joint is indicated if extensive destruction of the carpus precludes arthrodesis.

EXCISION OF WRIST JOINT

TECHNIQUE 6.14

- Make a dorsal longitudinal midline incision 7.5 cm long.
- Deepen the dissection between the extensor indicis proprius and extensor pollicis longus tendons down to the dorsal capsule of the wrist.
- Incise the capsule and expose the distal end of the radius and the metacarpal bones.
- Excise the carpus and remove the articular surfaces of the distal radius and ulna down to healthy bone.
- Close the wound in the usual manner.

POSTOPERATIVE CARE A long arm cast is applied with the elbow at 90 degrees of flexion, the forearm in neutral rotation, and the wrist dorsiflexed 25 degrees. Active range-of-motion exercises of the fingers and shoulder are started as soon as possible. After 3 months, the cast is removed, and a brace is applied that is periodically removed to permit active wrist exercises. If possible, the brace is discarded after 6 months.

TUBERCULOSIS OF LONG BONES

Metaphyseal and diaphyseal tuberculosis is rare. The diagnosis is usually established by biopsy and cultures (Fig. 6.11). The infection is often associated with active pulmonary tuberculosis. It may be localized to one area, usually near a joint, or may diffusely involve much of the bone. Radiographs may show a solitary irregular cavity, a series of confluent cavities or, occasionally, fusiform enlargement of the shaft. Multiple bones may be involved simultaneously.

Effective treatment requires chemotherapy plus evacuation of abscesses and sequestrectomies, an operative treatment similar to that for chronic pyogenic osteomyelitis. Wounds in tuberculous osteomyelitis can be closed primarily, however, unless secondary pyogenic infection is present.

AMPUTATION

Amputation is indicated when extensive tuberculous involvement renders less radical treatment unsuccessful, especially in

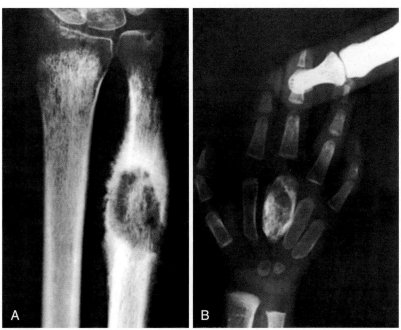

FIGURE 6.11 Tuberculosis of long bones. **A,** Atypical tuberculosis of ulna proved by biopsy. **B,** Typical spina ventosa. This patient had multiple cavities throughout the skeleton. First diagnosis was syphilis; Wassermann test was positive. No improvement occurred with antisyphilitic treatment. Biopsy revealed typical tuberculosis. Tuberculous otitis media developed later, and patient died 2 years after the first examination.

adults with extensive lower extremity involvement. Extensive amyloid disease adds to the desirability of amputation. The operation should be done proximal to an affected joint. In children, lower extremity amputation is also justifiable when tuberculous osteomyelitis results in marked shortening of the limb.

OTHER UNUSUAL INFECTIONS
NONTUBERCULOUS MYCOBACTERIAL INFECTIONS
Musculoskeletal infections caused by nontuberculous *Mycobacterium* species have increased since 1985, as have infections caused by *M. tuberculosis*. Incidence rates vary from 1.0 to 1.8 cases per 100,000 persons. The incidence of nontuberculous pulmonary disease is estimated to be at least 10 times more common than tuberculosis in the U.S., at 150,000 cases per year. A recently reported source of nontuberculous mycobacterial infections is medical tourism (i.e., travel to another country for health care services, particularly cosmetic surgery). Multiple case reports implicate at least 15 different species of *Mycobacterium* as causes of osteoarticular and tenosynovial infections. The most common causative organisms are *Mycobacterium avium* complex, *Mycobacterium marinum,* and *Mycobacterium kansasii.* In their study of over 29,000 patients with rheumatoid arthritis matched to a cohort without rheumatoid arthritis, Yeh et al. determined that those with rheumatoid arthritis were four times more likely to develop nontuberculosis mycobacterial disease.

The clinical, radiographic, and histopathologic manifestations of musculoskeletal nontuberculous *Mycobacterium* species may be indistinguishable from those in tuberculosis, often requiring an initial antibiotic regimen that covers *M. tuberculosis.* Nontuberculous *Mycobacterium* species have differing drug susceptibilities, however, and species identification is important for appropriate chemotherapy. Optimal culture requirements for some nontuberculous *Mycobacterium* species vary, such as for *M. marinum,* which grows best at 30°C to 33°C. Nonstandard chemotherapeutic agents have been developed, such as rifabutin and clarithromycin for treatment of *M. avium* complex, which tends to be resistant to the standard agents. The operative principles and techniques that apply to musculoskeletal tuberculosis also are appropriate for musculoskeletal infections caused by nontuberculous *Mycobacterium* species.

BRUCELLOSIS
Brucellosis, or undulant fever, is a zoonotic disease most commonly caused by the gram-negative coccobacillus *Brucella melitensis* and is usually found in goats. Almost all infections result from direct or indirect exposure to animals. The primary mode of transmission is the ingestion of unpasteurized milk or milk products. The disease is most commonly seen in the Mediterranean basin, the Arabian Peninsula, the Indian subcontinent, Mexico, and Central and South America. In the United States, the San Diego, California, region has the most frequently infected patient population. Occupations that place individuals at risk include farming, veterinary medicine, meat handling, and laboratory work. The annual occurrence rate worldwide is more than 500,000 cases.

The most common presentation for brucellosis is fever accompanied by osteoarticular involvement. The first symptoms of infection normally appear 2 to 4 weeks after inoculation. The worldwide literature indicates that the axial skeleton is the most likely site of osteoarticular involvement, normally occurring as sacroiliitis, spondylitis, or spondylodiscitis. Involvement of bone is noted in 20% to 50% of infected patients. In a prospective study in Turkey, 251 patients were identified over a 4-year period who were infected with *Brucella*. Sacroiliitis was confirmed in 71 patients (28%) who had low back pain and a positive flexion abduction external rotation (FABER) test. All of these patients had positive bone scans for sacroiliitis as well. Spondylodiscitis was seen in 26 patients with back pain. All of these patients had positive bone scans with increased uptake in the vertebral bodies and discs as well as positive spinal MRI. The frequency of a lumbar pathologic process was significantly higher than thoracic or cervical ones, with cervical disorders the least frequent. MRI findings included low signal intensity in the vertebral bodies on the sagittal T1-weighted images, high signal intensity in the vertebral bodies on the sagittal T2-weighted images, and high signal intensity in the involved vertebrae and discs after gadolinium administration on sagittal T1-weighted images. Eight patients in the study had paraspinal or epidural abscesses. Rarely, nonaxial bones, such as the tibia, humerus, and calcaneus, can be involved.

A diagnosis of brucellosis is best made with a combination of serology with a *Brucella* agglutinin titer greater than 1:160 and a positive blood culture. For patients with osteoarticular involvement, a bone scan is recommended. If there are axial symptoms, then spinal MRI is also appropriate. It is important to differentiate tuberculous spondylodiscitis from that of brucellosis—because it can appear similar on MRI and has similar patient profiles—for correct antibiotic treatment.

A 6-month three-drug course of rifampin, doxycycline, and streptomycin is recommended for patients with osteoarticular involvement. This regimen helps prevent a brucellosis relapse, which occurs in about 11% of patients with osteoarticular infection.

TYPHOID FEVER

Typhoid fever is caused by *Salmonella typhi,* a gram-negative anaerobic bacillus that is rarely seen in developed countries. Because the primary mode of transmission is oral-fecal, it occurs in individuals who have ingested contaminated food or fluids. Approximately 400 cases per year are reported in the U.S.

Symptoms include fever, abdominal pain with diarrhea, dehydration, weight loss, headaches, fatigue, and, at times, altered consciousness. Multiple systems may be affected, with cardiopulmonary involvement, hepatosplenomegaly, and gastrointestinal infiltration. Approximately 30% of patients with typhoid fever may have arthralgias and myalgias. Septic sacroiliitis and osteomyelitis of multiple regions have been described. More frequently, the thoracolumbar junction is affected, with accompanying disc involvement. Although rare, osteomyelitis is seen in isolated bones of the upper and lower extremities. There may be accompanying bone marrow infiltration with suppression and necrosis. Soft tissues, such as the greater trochanteric bursa, can also be involved.

Diagnosis is confirmed by isolating *S. typhi* from one of multiple sites (e.g., blood, fecal or intestinal samples, and bone marrow); measurement of agglutinating antibodies is also helpful. Traditional primary antibiotic treatment with chloramphenicol has been used, although third-generation cephalosporins may be as effective. Other pharmacologic approaches have included ampicillin and trimethoprim/sulfamethoxazole. Resistant cases may be more sensitive to the third-generation cephalosporins. Lynch et al. reported that of 2016 isolates they tested, 272 (13%) were resistant to ampicillin, chloramphenicol, and trimethoprim-sulfamethoxazole. Infection with antimicrobial-resistant *S. typhi* strains was associated with travel to the Indian sub-continent, and an increasing proportion of these infections were caused by bacterial strains with decreased susceptibility to fluoroquinolones.

SYPHILIS

According to the CDC, during 2000 and 2001, the national rate of reported primary and secondary syphilis was 2.1 cases per 100,000 population; however, the rate has increased almost every year since then. In 2016, the rate increased to 8.7 cases per 100,000 population, a 17.6% increase over 2013, and the highest rate reported since 1993.

Syphilis is caused by a spirochete, *Treponema pallidum,* that is transmitted transplacentally, by sexual contact, or through blood products. Bone can become involved at any stage of the disease or at any age. In congenital syphilis, periostitis of the temporal bone and palate and cortical thickening of the upper one half of the tibia ("saber shins") may be seen. Vascular extension to bone (e.g., sternum or vertebral body) has been described. Early osseous involvement may be noted on bone scans in relatively asymptomatic areas, such as the hands, feet, forearms, clavicle, or tibias. Spinal involvement has been reported and shows similarity with spinal tuberculosis or tumor. Chronic arthralgias may develop and, because of neuropathic or vascular involvement, may lead to the development of a "Charcot joint" (Fig. 6.12).

Diagnosis is made primarily by darkfield microscopy with identification of the pathogen from the sampled fluid. Antibody assays such as Venereal Disease Research Laboratory (VDRL), rapid plasma reagin (RPR), or the more specific tests, microhemagglutination *T. pallidum* and syphilis IgG antibody by electroimmune assay (EIA) are frequently included as part of the workup. Untreated disease has three stages. In primary syphilis, dark field microscopy will be positive, and screening reagin tests (VDRL and RPR) may be positive. This stage lasts 10 to 90 days and a canker sore may be present. Secondary syphilis lasts 6 weeks to 6 months and is characterized by multiple eruptions. All general screening and organism-specific tests will be positive. Tertiary syphilis also has a latency of 10 to 30 years after the primary phase. Untreated disease can have central nervous system involvement with impairment of dorsal-column function with loss of touch and position sense leading to severe lower extremity joint destruction (Fig. 6.13). General screening tests (VDRL and RPR) may become negative but more specific tests (MHA-TP and IgG-EIA) will be positive even in treated disease. Although treatment may vary depending on the stage of the disease, the mainstay of treatment is penicillin G benzathine.

ANAEROBIC INFECTIONS

Anaerobic infections are discussed in chapter 4.

VIRAL OSTEITIS AND ARTHRITIS

Viral infections of bone remain as a diverse group of diseases. Virus strains, such as varicella, rubella, and vaccinia, have

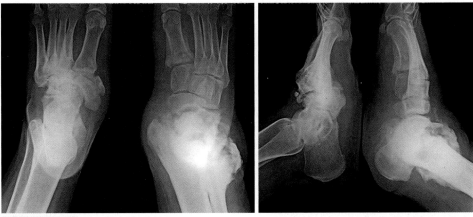

FIGURE 6.12 Neuroarthropathy of the ankle in a 48-year-old man with syphilis. He had painless swelling of the ankles for 3 years before seeking medical advice. (From Samia M, Ezzahara AF, Kahdija B, et al: Bilateral neuro-arthropathy of the ankle as a sequel of undiagnosed tabes dorsalis, *Joint Bone Spine* 80:664, 2013.)

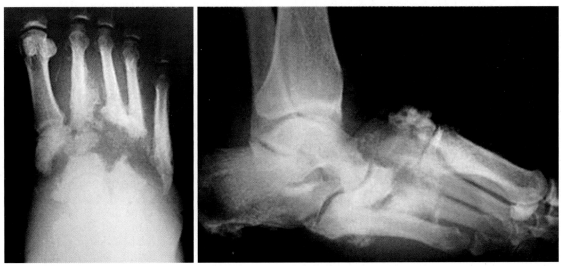

FIGURE 6.13 Right midfoot destruction secondary to syphilitic neuropathic arthropathy.

been isolated from synovitic joints. Osteomyelitis variolosa was recognized by joint swelling and lytic lesions before the suppression of smallpox. Paramyxovirus antigens have been detected in bone in patients with Paget disease, but a direct causal relationship has not been proven.

ACTINOMYCOSIS

Actinomycosis is a chronic granulomatous disease characterized by external sinuses. It is most commonly caused by *Actinomyces israelii. Actinomyces* are gram-positive anaerobic filamentous bacteria, not fungi. They are extremely fastidious and difficult to culture. Diagnosis is usually made by identifying sulfur granules or branching mycelia. Image-guided aspiration of infected regions is helpful in obtaining appropriate samples.

Actinomycotic osteomyelitis most typically affects the cervicofacial regions, particularly the mandible. Such osseous involvement is usually a secondary extension from a primary soft-tissue site. With spinal involvement there may be sclerotic changes; however, vertebral body height is usually preserved. Spinal involvement may resemble tuberculosis but usually does not affect the disc. Abscesses may extend to the skin, and paravertebral abscesses may be present. Rib lesions have been described with sinus tract extension to the skin. Osseous involvement of the pelvis may be associated with the use of intrauterine devices.

Diagnosis is made by identification of the pathogen from an image-guided aspirant of infected tissue. Penicillin typically is used for treatment, although tetracycline, erythromycin, and chloramphenicol can be used.

LYME DISEASE

Lyme disease is the most common tick-borne illness in the United States. The *Ixodes* tick family is the primary vector for the spirochete bacteria *Borrelia burgdorferi* that causes the disease. The *Ixodes* hosts, the white-footed mouse and white-tailed deer, are found in New England, the Mid-Atlantic states, and around the Great Lakes. Therefore most cases are discovered in these regions, primarily from April through November. More than 30,000 confirmed and probable cases are reported to the CDC yearly, nearly 300,000 presumed cases go unreported, and approximately 2.4 million specimens are submitted for Lyme disease testing with an associated cost of nearly $500 million. Two peak age groups that are more commonly affected with the disease include children aged 5 to 14 years and adults aged 55 to 70 years. Leisure activities such as hiking, fishing, hunting, and gardening, as well as outdoor employment, place individuals at higher risk for contracting the infection. Interestingly, only 50% to 70% of patients remember being bitten by a tick.

Most patients with Lyme disease present with a characteristic bull's-eye rash (erythema migrans) within 1 month of the tick bite (Fig. 6.14), although up to 20% of patients may not display this associated rash. Normally, the rash is accompanied by viral-like symptoms of fever, chills, fatigue, and headaches. Arthralgia, usually polyarthralgia involving both large and small joints and potentially the neck and back, typically accompanies the viral-like symptoms and characteristic bull's-eye rash.

A total of 60% of patients who are not treated appropriately initially will develop intermittent arthritis. Not having the prodromal polyarthralgias at symptom onset does not preclude patients from developing intermittent arthritis. Although the joint may appear extremely warm and swollen, usually with an effusion, patients normally note only mild pain. The knee is the most commonly involved joint, followed

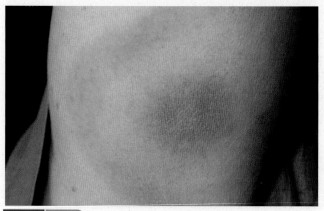

by the ankle and wrist. The arthritic attacks usually last about 2 weeks to a month. After the bouts resolve, patients normally do not complain of any joint symptoms. Because different joints may be involved with different flare-ups, the intermittent arthritis often is described as "migratory arthritis."

Chronic arthritis can develop in around 10% of patients with intermittent arthritis that is not properly treated. Having the alloantigen HLA-DR4 increases the risk of developing chronic arthritis. One to three joints are involved, with one or both knees almost always involved. The hip is the next most likely joint afflicted with this condition. Unlike patients with acute Lyme arthritis, patients with chronic arthritis usually have unrelenting joint swelling and pain for at least 1 year.

Patients with early disseminated Lyme disease may also develop neurologic and cardiac signs and symptoms. Fifteen percent of patients develop neurologic problems, including meningitis, Bell palsy, and radiculopathies. Eight percent develop cardiac complications such as an arteriovenous block.

The CDC recommends using enzyme-linked immunosorbent assay (ELISA) followed by the Western immunoblot test for diagnosis (Fig. 6.15). The Western immunoblot test will diagnose most patients with Lyme disease if performed at least 4 weeks after tick contact. Synovial fluid analysis is usually nonspecific with mildly elevated white blood cell count (normally <50,000 cells/mm^3). Genomic DNA of *B. burgdorferi* can be found in the synovial fluid by using polymerase chain reaction (PCR). Successful treatment with antibiotics for Lyme arthritis can be documented by the transformation of a positive PCR to a negative PCR. Currently, multiple assays have received FDA clearance for the detection of Lyme disease. However, the FDA warns that many of these can be easily misinterpreted and advises that assays for antibodies to *B. burgdorferi* should be used only to support a clinical diagnosis of Lyme disease. Dessau et al. reported the overuse of diagnostic testing for Lyme disease. Their recommendations based on the current European cases are as follows: typical erythema migrans should be diagnosed clinically and does not need laboratory testing. Diagnosis of Lyme neuroborreliosis requires spinal fluid testing for intrathecal antibody production. Polyarthralgias with viral-like symptoms require

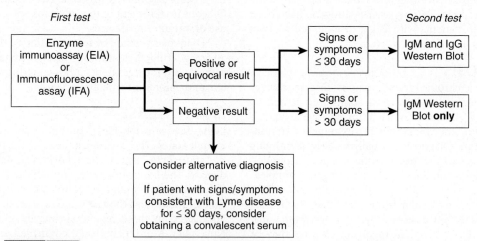

FIGURE 6.15   Two-tiered testing for Lyme disease as recommended by the CDC. (From CDC, www.cdc.gov/lyme/diagnosistesting/labtest/twostep/index.html.)

testing for antibodies to *B. burgdorferi.* Testing patients with nonspecific symptoms has a low positive predictive value.

First-line antibiotic therapy employs doxycycline orally for 30 to 60 days for Lyme disease–associated arthritis. Second-line antibiotic treatment uses amoxicillin for the same duration. Either one of these choices is effective in about 90% of patients. If a patient does not respond to a 30- to 60-day course of oral antibiotics, then a 30-day course of intravenous ceftriaxone is recommended. About 5% of patients with Lyme arthritis have antibiotic-refractory disease, however.

FUNGAL INFECTION

Fungal osteomyelitis generally develops slowly, and diagnosis and treatment may be delayed. Because diagnosis usually depends on specific stains and cultures, the diagnosis must be suspected before it can be established. These infections often imitate metastatic neoplasms, especially when spinal involvement is present. Immunocompromised individuals are more susceptible. Treatment plans for these unusual infections should be made in collaboration with an infectious disease consultant.

COCCIDIOIDOMYCOSIS

Coccidioidomycosis is endemic to Arizona, New Mexico, west Texas, and the San Joaquin Valley of California. Cases have also been described in Mexico and some regions of South America. The incidence of infection in long-time residents of these areas may be 80%. An estimated 150,000 new infections are reported each year, with 97% of them occurring in Arizona and California. Transmission primarily is by inhalation of airborne *Coccidioides immitis.* Most of these infections do not cause symptoms; infections that do usually are confined to the lungs. A more disseminated presentation can occur with kidney, liver, spleen, pericardium, and bone. A hypersensitivity arthritis, which is self-limited to 2 to 4 weeks, can occur.

Extrapulmonary or disseminated infections are rare and seen in fewer than 5% of patients. Immunocompromised individuals with HIV or who are taking the tumor necrosis factor-α inhibitor infliximab, individuals of Filipino or African-American ethnicity, and pregnant women are at higher risk for extrapulmonary infection.

Bone involvement is noted in 20% to 50% of extrapulmonary coccidioidal infections. The axial skeleton is more commonly affected than the appendicular skeleton, and the vertebral column is the most susceptible location of bony involvement for the disease. The infection can spread into adjacent soft tissues, causing paraspinal abscesses. Infections have also been seen in the skull and ribs. Joint infections are more likely to be seen in the lower extremities, especially the knee. Involvement of the metatarsals or metacarpals may be noted. Focal tendinitis or tenosynovitis can also occur. Ho et al. described 20 children with coccidioidomycosis, all of whom presented with bone and joint pain; only three patients had pulmonary symptoms, and none had cutaneous symptoms. The most common location of infection was the foot (28%), followed by the knee, spine, forearm, lower leg, and other sites.

Diagnosis of long-standing skeletal coccidioidomycosis can be assisted by radiographic evaluation. Normally, a chronic infection will display single or multiple lytic punched-out lesions with osteopenia and ill-defined borders. A moth-eaten appearance may be noted in small bones. Some studies have noted 100% sensitivity for identifying skeletal coccidioidomycosis using bone scans. Diagnostic confirmation depends on histopathologic examination of a bone culture specimen, which demonstrates granulomatous inflammation and often spherules.

Medical treatment is preferred but often is not sufficient. Itraconazole has been shown superior to fluconazole in treating skeletal coccidioidomycosis. Other newer triazole antifungals are now available, but randomized studies for skeletal coccidioidomycosis are not yet available. Intravenous amphotericin B was previously used for treatment, but it has many unwanted complications and, therefore, should not be used unless necessary. The most effective treatment duration with these antibiotics is not known. Additional surgical methods may be required for antibiotic refractory infections. This may include debridement and removal of infected bone or synovium. Relapses are also common.

BLASTOMYCOSIS

North American blastomycosis is rare. Infection usually occurs after the inhalation of the spores of *Blastomyces dermatitidis,* a dimorphic soil-dwelling fungus. This infection is frequently found in immunocompromised patients. Osseous involvement is the third most frequent form of primary blastomycosis. Pulmonary and cutaneous lesions are the most frequent sites of infection, although 10% of patients have skeletal involvement as the presenting symptom. This infection occurs in North America, extending throughout the Appalachian states and the watersheds of the Ohio, Mississippi, Missouri, and St. Lawrence rivers. Skeletal infection occurs by hematogenous spread from the lungs or by direct extension from a cutaneous infection. Osseous findings are nonspecific for blastomycosis and resemble other forms of osteomyelitis. Some asymptomatic regions may have osseous involvement with cortical erosions noted. The first sign of involvement may be a cutaneous sinus or abscess. In a long bone, the infection tends to localize in the epiphysis and extends into the adjacent joint. Lesions in vertebrae mimic tuberculosis. Definitive diagnosis is made by showing the characteristic broad-based budding yeast on microscopic examination of a joint or bone aspirate. Culture of the yeast or mold form establishes the diagnosis but may take 1 to 5 weeks to grow. Amphotericin B is the antibiotic of choice, with ketoconazole or itraconazole being effective alternative drugs.

HISTOPLASMOSIS

In the United States, histoplasmosis is caused by *Histoplasma capsulatum.* It is usually a mild pulmonary infection that occurs after inhalation of the infecting particle. The disease is usually self-limited, but it can become a progressive disseminated infection in immunocompromised patients. Although pulmonary involvement is most predominant, bone and soft tissues can be affected, usually manifesting as a self-limited hypersensitivity arthritis. Care and Lacey described a recurrent histoplasmosis in the wrist of a patient who was not immunocompromised and did not have pulmonary involvement (Fig. 6.16). Because of the prolonged period between initial infection and clinical recurrence in their patient, these authors suggest that *Histoplasma* can remain latent in the bone marrow for a decade. They recommend prolonged antibiotic treatment after debridement and resection of grossly involved tissue.

Antifungal agents, such as ketoconazole or itraconazole, are effective for the treatment of mild disseminated histoplasmosis involving bones or joints. For more resistant cases,

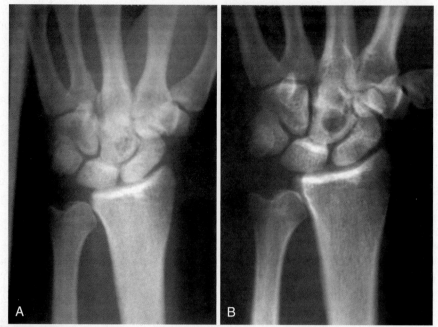

FIGURE 6.16   Histoplasmosis of wrist in patient without immunocompromise or pulmonary involvement. **A,** Wrist at initial presentation showing cystic lesions of capitate with sclerotic borders. **B,** Appearance at time of recurrence with progression of cystic changes in capitate. (From Care SB, Lacey SH: Recurrent histoplasmosis of the wrist: a case report, *J Hand Surg Am* 23:1112, 1998.)

especially in immunocompromised patients, amphotericin B is recommended.

CRYPTOCOCCOSIS

Cryptococcosis, caused by *Cryptococcus neoformans,* is a rare fungal disease that is being increasingly found in immunologically compromised patients. It usually produces asymptomatic pulmonary disease in immunologically competent hosts. In immunologically compromised patients, it is generally a widespread disseminated disease with prominent pulmonary involvement. Hematogenous dissemination results in metastatic foci, most commonly in the central nervous system; however, isolated bone lesions have been reported in 10% of patients. These may mimic primary bone neoplasms or have a presentation similar to other fungal bone lesions. The spine and long and flat bones also may be involved. The diagnosis is established by biopsy, and antigen titers are used. Treatment of the bone lesions consists of curettage. In the absence of neurologic involvement, ketoconazole can be effective. In more severe cases, amphotericin B should be used.

SPOROTRICHOSIS

Sporotrichosis is usually produced by inoculation of *Sporothrix schenckii* through a minor cut or abrasion. This fungus is found in many environments, but infection is rare. Although a suppurative granulomatous lesion with an ulcerated appearance develops on the skin, there may be lymph, hematogenous, or contiguous spread to other structures. This disease can affect the bones, joints, and periarticular soft tissues. Joint spaces may narrow, and eventual subchondral bone demise may occur. Serologic tests are useful, as are fungal cultures. The gold standard for diagnosis is isolation of the fungus in culture. The sporotrichin skin test relies on the serologic testing for sporotrichin, which is peptido-rhamnomannan antigen complex. Bonifaz et al. reported a sensitivity of 94.5% and a specificity of 95.2% when used along with positive cultures. Cultures can take 2 weeks to be positive. The sporotrichin skin test is rapid and results are readily available to guide earlier treatment.

Operative intervention may include debridement and chemotherapy with amphotericin. Other chemotherapeutic regimens, including ketoconazole, itraconazole, or fluconazole, have been used. Oral potassium iodide is used to treat skin lesions and, at times, osseous lesions.

ECHINOCOCCOSIS

Echinococcosis, also called unilocular or human hydatid disease, is caused by the larval stage of *Echinococcus granulosus,* which is found most frequently in cattle and sheep-raising areas of the United States (Arizona, Utah, New Mexico, Wyoming); similar diseases have been found in South America, Europe, and Australia. Canidae (domestic dogs, fox, and coyotes) serve as definitive hosts, whereas sheep act as intermediate hosts. Although the liver is the most frequently involved, other organ systems can be affected (e.g., kidneys, intestines, central nervous system, and bone). Bone involvement is usually seen in less than 1% of cases and is exhibited by cystic or lytic lesions in the trabecular bone that can extend into other subcortical areas. The most commonly affected areas in bone are the vertebrae, pelvis, and the skull. Long bones may also be affected. Progressive changes may resemble tumor formation with an expansile cystic appearance. In rare cases, extension to the spinal cord has been described. Antigen or antibody titers are helpful in making the diagnosis, and imaging studies (CT and ultrasonography) may delineate the characteristics of the cyst and guide treatment.

The best treatment for a bone infection resulting from echinococcosis is to resect the involved bone or to amputate. Erol et al. described successful treatment of 10 patients, eight with muscle involvement and two with bone involvement, with chemotherapy (albendazole) and wide resection. In their literature review, however, Steinmetz et al. found that of 721 reported patients, complete excision of the lesion was possible in only 16%. Curettage and instilling solutions, such as hypertonic saline, 1% formalin, or 0.5% silver nitrate, have been tried. In suspected cases of echinococcosis, diagnostic biopsy or aspiration is contraindicated. Operative management should include careful planning and meticulous technique to avoid spillage of the cyst contents, which may cause spread of the disease. If spillage occurs, application of cetyltrimethylammonium bromide (Cetrimide), 2% formalin, or 1% iodine can reduce the danger of spreading. Albendazole or mebendazole can also be used chemotherapeutically but resolution varies.

REFERENCES

TUBERCULOSIS

Ahsan MJ, Ansari MY, Yasmin S, et al.: Tuberculosis: current treatment, diagnostics, and newer antitubercular agents in clinical trials, *Infect Disord Drug Targets* 15(1):32–41, 2015.

Arathi N, Ahmad F, Huda N: Osteoarticular tuberculosis—a three years' retrospective study, *J Clin Diag Res* 7:2189, 2013.

Benator D, Ghattacharya M, Bozeman L, et al. Rifapentine and isoniazid once a week versus rifampicin and isoniazid twice a week for treatment of drug-susceptible pulmonary tuberculosis in HIV-negative patients: a randomized clinical trial. *Lancet* 360:528, 2002.

Cantini F, Nannini C, Niccoli L, et al.: Risk of tuberculosis reactivity in patients with rheumatoid arthritis, ankylosing spondylitis, and psoriatic arthritis receiving non-anti-TNF-targeted biologics, *Mediators Inflamm* 2017:89909834, 2017.

Carrega G, Bartolacci V, Burastero G, et al.: Prosthetic joint infections due to *Mycobacterium tuberculosis*: a report of 5 cases, *Int J Surg Case Rep* 4:178, 2013.

Centers for Disease Control and Prevention: Morbidity and mortality weekly report, *Weekly* 67(11), 2018.

Chang KC, Yew WW, Sotgiu G: Clinical research in the treatment of tuberculosis: current status and future prospects, *Int J Tuberc Lung Dis* 19:1417, 2015.

Chen SH, Lee CH, Wong T, Feng HS: Long-term retrospective analysis of surgical treatment for irretrievable tuberculosis of the ankle, *Foot Ankle Int* 34:372, 2013.

Chevannes W, Memarzadeh A, Pasapula C: Isolated tuberculous osteomyelitis of the talonavicular joint without pulmonary involvement—a rare case report, *Foot* 25:66, 2015.

Griffith DE, Aksamit T, Brown-Elliott B, et al.: American thoracic society guidelines: diagnosis, treatment and prevention of nontuberculous mycobacterial diseases, *Am J Respiratory and Critical Care Medicine* 175(4):367, 2007.

Khan PS, Thilak J, George MJ, Nair AV, Madanan A: Tubercular infection after arthroscopic rotator cuff repair, *Knee Surg Sports Traumatol Arthrosc* 25(7):2205, 2017.

Lee HJ, Kim KW, Kim KS, et al.: Primary musculoskeletal mycobacterium infection with large cystic masses after total hip arthroplasty, *J Arthroplasty* 28:374, 2013.

Jindani A, Harrison TS, Nunn AJ, et al.: High-dose rifapentine with moxifloxacin for pulmonary tuberculosis, *N Engl J Med* 371:1599, 2014.

Murray CJ, Ortblad KF, Guinovart C, et al.: Global, regional, and national incidence and mortality for HIV, tuberculosis, and malaria during 1990-2013: a systematic analysis for the Global Burden of Disease Study, 2013, *Lancet* 384:935, 2014.

Nahid P, Dorman SE, Alpanah N, et al: Official American Thoracic Society/Centers for Disease Control and Prvention/Infectious Diseases Society of America clinical practice guidelines: treatment of drug-susceptible tuberculosis, *Clin Infect Dis* 63(7):147, 2016.

Pattamapaspong N, Muttarak M, Sivasomboon C: Tuberculosis arthritis and tenosynovitis, *Semin Musculoskeletal Radiol* 15:459, 2011.

Prakash M, Gupta P, Dhillon MS, et al.: Magnetic resonance imaging findings in tubercular arthritis of the elbow, *Clin Imaging* 40:114, 2015.

Rauf F, Chaudhry UR, Atif M, et al.: Spinal tuberculosis: our experience and a review of imaging methods, *Neuroradiol J* 28:498, 2015.

Sait S, Mubashir M, Anwar R, Khan N: Poncet's disease (tubercular rheumatism) with primary involvement of the foot. a case report, *Foot Ankle Surg* 22(3):317, 2016.

Schaaf HS, Garcia-Prats AJ, Donald PR: Antituberculosis drugs in children, *Clin Pharmacol Ther* 98:252, 2015.

Sergeant A, Conaglen P, Laurenson IF, et al.: Mycobacterium chelonae infection: a complication of tattooing, *Clin Exp Dermatol* 38(2):140, 2012.

Sharma A, Pinto B, Dogra S, et al.: A case series and review of Poncet's disease, and the utility of current diagnostic criteria, *Int J Rheum Dis* 19(10):1010, 2016.

Sterling TR, Villarino ME, Borisov AS, et al.: Three months of rifapentine and isoniazid for latent tuberculosis infection, *N Engl J med* 365:2155, 2011.

Tang Y, Yin L, Tang S, et al.: Application of molecular, microbiological, and immunological tests for the diagnosis of bone and joint tuberculosis, *J Clin Lab Anal* 32:322260, 2018.

Walsh TP, Yates BJ: Calcanectomy: avoiding major amputation in the presence of calcaneal osteomyelitis—a case series, *Foot* 23:130, 2013.

Zou J, Shi Z, Mei G, et al.: Two-stage operation to treat destructive midfoot tuberculosis: 14 cases experience, *Orthop Traumatol Surg Res* 102(8):1075, 2016.

OTHER UNUSUAL INFECTIONS

Akrun R, Mete BD: Musculoskeletal brucellosis, *Semin Musculoskelet Radiol* 15:470, 2011.

Belthur MV, Blair JE, Shrader MW, Malone JB: Musculoskeletal coccidioidomycosis, *Current Orthopaedic Practice* 29(4):400, 2018.

Bibbo C, Spellman J: Successful salvage of complicated calcaneal blastomycosis in disseminated disease with staged surgical reconstruction and local-systemic antifungal therapy, *J Foot Ankle Surg* 53:472, 2014.

Biesiada C, Czepiel J, Lesniak MR, et al.: Lyme disease: review, *Arch Med Sci* 8:978, 2012.

Bonifaz A, Toriello C, Araiza J, et al.: Sporotrichin skin test for the diagnosis of sporotrichosis, *J Fungi* 4:55, 2018.

Bosilkovski M, Zezoski M, Siskova D, et al.: Clinical characteristics of human brucellosis in patients with various monoarticular involvements, *Clin Rheumatol*, 35(10):2579, 2016.

Bouaziz C, Ladeb MF, Chakroun M, Chaabane S: Spinal brucellosis: a review, *Skeletal Radiol* 37:785, 2008.

Dessau RB, van Dam AP, Fingerle V, et al.: To test or not to test? Laboratory support for the diagnosis of Lyme borreliosis: a position paper of ESGBOR, the ESCMID study group for lyme borreliosis, *Clin Microbiol Infect* 24(2):118, 2018.

Erol B, Onay T, Caliskan E, Okay E: Oncological approach with antihelminthic chemotherapy and wide resection in the treatment of musculoskeletal hyudatidosis. A review of 10 cases with mean follow-up of 64 months, *Acta Orthop Belg* 81(3):530, 2015.

Feder Jr HM: Lyme disease in children, *Infect Dis Clin North Am* 22:315, 2008.

Gomez JV, Molnar SL, Val SM, Arnal RG: Musculoskeletal involvement of syphilis—a forgotten lesson, *BMJ Case Rep*, 2012.

Green DA, Whittier S, Greendyke W, et al.: Outbreak of rapidly growing nontuberculous mycobacteria among patients undergoing cosmetic surgery in the dominican republic, *Ann Plast Surg*, 78(1):17, 2017.

Heidari B, Heidari P: Rheumatologic manifestations of brucellosis, *Rheumatol Int* 31:721, 2011.

Ho AK, Shrader MW, Falk MN, Segal LS: Diagnosis and initial management of musculoskeletal coccidioidomycosis in children, *J Pediatr Orthop* 34:571, 2014.

Kim CW, Lee CR: Multifocal neuropathic arthropathy in patient with undiagnosed neurosyphilis: a case report, *Int J STD AIDS* 28(7):729, 2017.

Kursun E, Turunc T, Demiroglu Y, Arsian H: Evaluation of four hundred and forty seven brucellosis cases, *Intern Med* 52:745, 2013.

Minozzi S, Bonovas S, Lytras T, et al.: Risk of infections using anti-TNF agents in rheumatoid arthritis, psoriatic arthritis, and ankylosing spondylitis: a systematic review and meta-analysis, *Expert Opin Rug Saf* 15(Suppl 1):11, 2016.

Monge-Maillo B, Chamorrow TS, López-Vélez R: Management of osseous cystic echinococcosis, *Expert Rev Anti Infect Ther* 15(12):1075, 2017.

Park JW, Kim YS, Yoon JO, et al.: Non-tuberculous mycobacterial infection of the musculoskeletal system: pattern of infection and efficacy of combined surgical/antimicrobial treatment, *Bone Joint J* 96-B:1561, 2014.

Sigal LH: Musculoskeletal features of lyme disease: understanding the pathogenesis of clinical findings helps make appropriate therapeutic choices, *J Clin Rheumatol* 17:256, 2011.

Smith BG, Cruz Jr AI, Milewski MD, Shapiro ED: Lyme disease and the orthopaedic implications of Lyme arthritis, *J Am Acad Orthop Surg* 19:91, 2011.

Steinmetz S, Racloz G, Stern R, et al.: Treatment challenges associated with bone echinococcosis, *J Antimicrob Chemother* 69:821, 2014.

Taljanovic MS, Adam RD: Musculoskeletal coccidioidomycosis, *Semin Musculoskelet Radiol* 15:511, 2011.

Theel ES: The past, present and (possible) future of serologic testing for lyme disease, *J Clin Microbiol* 54(5):1191–1196, 2016.

Wain J, Hendriksen RS, Mikoleit ML, et al.: Typhoid fever, *Lancet* 385:1136, 2015.

Yeh JJ, Wang YC, Sung FC, Kao CH: Rheumatoid arthritis increases the risk of nontuberculosis mycobacterial disease and active pulmonary tuberculosis, *PLoS ONE* 9:e110922, 2014.

Yin R, Wang L, Zhang T, Zhao B: Syphilis of the lumbar spine. A case report and review of literature, *Medicine* 96:50, 2017.

Zeng M, Xie J, Wang L, Hu Y: Total knee arthroplasty in advanced tuberculous arthritis of the knee, *Int Orthop* 40(7):1433, 2016.

The complete list of references is available online at Expert Consult.com.

TUMORS

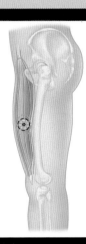

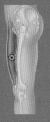

A team comprising an orthopaedic surgeon, radiologist, pathologist, radiation oncologist, and medical oncologist is necessary to treat the spectrum of musculoskeletal tumors. Other surgical specialists frequently are required, such as a vascular surgeon, thoracic surgeon, or plastic surgeon. The orthopaedic surgeon must be well versed in the principles of oncologic surgery, and the radiologist and pathologist should have a special interest in bone and soft-tissue tumors. The medical oncologist coordinates the adjuvant therapies and becomes the primary physician for a patient who has a metastatic tumor.

DIAGNOSTIC EVALUATION

GENERAL APPROACH TO MUSCULOSKELETAL NEOPLASMS

An adequate history and physical examination are the first steps in evaluating a patient with a musculoskeletal tumor. Patients may present to the orthopaedic oncologist with pain, a mass, or an abnormal radiographic finding detected during the evaluation of an unrelated problem. Patients with bone tumors most frequently present with pain. The pain initially may be activity related, but a patient with a malignancy of bone often complains of progressive pain at rest and at night. Patients with benign bone tumors also may have activity-related pain if the lesion is large enough to weaken the bone. Other benign lesions, most notably osteoid osteoma, may cause night pain initially. Conversely, patients with soft-tissue tumors rarely complain of pain but more often complain of a mass. Exceptions to this rule are patients with nerve sheath tumors who have pain or neurologic signs.

Although some tumors show a sex predilection (e.g., female predominance with giant cell tumors), this is rarely of diagnostic significance. Race likewise is of little significance, with the exception that Ewing sarcoma is exceedingly rare in individuals of African descent. Family history

occasionally can be helpful, as in cases of multiple hereditary exostosis (autosomal dominant inheritance) and neurofibromatosis (autosomal dominant inheritance). Age may be the most important information obtained in the history, however, because most benign and malignant musculoskeletal neoplasms occur within specific age ranges.

◼ PHYSICAL EXAMINATION

The physical examination should include evaluation of the patient's general health and a careful examination of the part in question. A mass should be measured, and its location, shape, consistency, mobility, tenderness, local temperature, and change with position should be noted. Atrophy of the surrounding musculature should be recorded, as should neurologic deficits and adequacy of circulation. *Café-au-lait* spots or cutaneous hemangiomas also may provide diagnostic clues. Potential sites of lymph node metastases should be palpated. Although lymph node metastases are rare with most sarcomas, they often are present with rhabdomyosarcomas, epithelioid sarcomas, and synovial sarcomas.

◼ RADIOGRAPHIC EXAMINATION

All suspected musculoskeletal neoplasms should be evaluated initially with plain biplanar radiographs. Compared with any other test, conventional radiography provides more useful diagnostic information for evaluation of bone lesions. Often, the patient's age and plain radiographic findings are sufficient to arrive at a specific diagnosis. Radiographic evaluation should begin by determining the site of the lesion because many bone tumors have specific site predilections (Boxes 7.1 to 7.4). An epiphyseal lesion in a skeletally mature patient is likely to be a giant cell tumor, whereas an epiphyseal lesion in a skeletally immature patient is likely to be a chondroblastoma. The differential diagnosis for diaphyseal lesions includes Ewing sarcoma, osteomyelitis, osteoid osteoma, osteoblastoma, histiocytosis, lymphoma, fibrous dysplasia,

Differential Diagnosis for Epiphyseal Lesions

- Chondroblastoma (ages 10-25)
- Giant cell tumor (ages 20-40)
- Clear chondrosarcoma (rare)

Differential Diagnosis for Diaphyseal Lesions

- Ewing sarcoma (ages 5-25)
- Lymphoma (adult)
- Fibrous dysplasia (ages 5-30)
- Adamantinoma (consider in the tibia)
- Histiocytosis (ages 5-30)

Differential Diagnosis for Lesions of the Spine

Older than 40 Years
- Metastases
- Multiple myeloma
- Hemangioma
- Chordoma (in sacrum)

Younger than 30 Years
- Vertebral body
  - Histiocytosis
  - Hemangioma
- Posterior elements
  - Osteoid osteoma
  - Osteoblastoma
  - Aneurysmal bone cyst

Differential Diagnosis for Multiple Lesions

- Histiocytosis
- Enchondroma
- Osteochondroma
- Fibrous dysplasia
- Multiple myeloma
- Metastases
- Hemangioma
- Infection
- Hyperparathyroidism

and adamantinoma (especially in the tibia). Most vertebral lesions in adult patients are metastases, myelomas, or hemangiomas. In the sacrum, chordoma and giant cell tumor are at the top of the list of differential diagnoses. In younger patients with a vertebral body lesion, the most likely diagnosis is histiocytosis; if the lesion is in the posterior elements, the differential diagnoses include aneurysmal bone cyst, osteoblastoma, and osteoid osteoma. Even if a specific diagnosis cannot be made, the aggressiveness of the lesion, and whether it is likely to be benign or malignant, usually can be determined by

careful evaluation of the plain films. Lesions of low biologic activity are usually well marginated, often with a surrounding rim of reactive bone formation. Aggressive lesions usually have a less well-defined zone of transition between the lesion and the host bone because the host response is slower than the progression of the tumor. Cortical expansion can be seen with aggressive benign lesions, but frank cortical destruction usually is a sign of malignancy. Periosteal reactive new bone formation results when the tumor destroys cortex and may take the form of Codman's triangle, "onion-skinning," or a "sunburst" pattern. It usually is a sign of malignancy but may be present with infection or histiocytosis. Often, bone lesions replace the normal trabecular pattern of bone with a characteristic matrix. Punctate, stippled calcification is suggestive of cartilage formation in bone lesions such as an enchondroma or chondrosarcoma. Matrix ossification combined with destructive features of host bone is a radiographic finding in a typical osteosarcoma. The irregular osteoid trabeculae in a collagenous stroma produce the classic radiographic "ground glass" appearance in fibrous dysplasia. Plain radiographs are less helpful for soft-tissue lesions but nevertheless should be obtained in all patients because some useful information can be acquired, such as the presence of myositis ossificans, phleboliths in a hemangioma, calcification in a synovial sarcoma, or a fat density with a lipoma.

◼ OTHER IMAGING EXAMINATIONS

The resolution of computed tomography (CT) is most helpful in assessing ossification and calcification and in evaluating the integrity of the cortex. It also is the best imaging study to localize the nidus of an osteoid osteoma, to detect a thin rim of reactive bone around an aneurysmal bone cyst, to evaluate calcification in a suspected cartilaginous lesion, and to evaluate endosteal cortical erosion in a suspected chondrosarcoma. Reconstructions in the sagittal and coronal planes may provide useful information with regard to surgical planning. CT of the lungs also is the most effective study to detect pulmonary metastases. In patients in whom magnetic resonance imaging (MRI) is prohibited (e.g., pacemaker), CT with intravenous contrast is useful in differentiating cystic lesions from vascular lesions in soft-tissue tumors.

Technetium bone scans are used to determine the activity of a lesion and to determine the presence of multiple lesions or skeletal metastases. Bone scans frequently are falsely negative in multiple myeloma and some cases of renal cell carcinoma. Excluding these exceptions, however, most other malignant neoplasms of bone show increased uptake on technetium bone scans. A normal bone scan is reassuring; however, the converse statement is not true because benign active lesions of bone also show increased uptake.

Positron emission tomography (PET) records the whole-body distribution of positron-emitting radioisotopes linked to biologically active molecules. This modality provides a noninvasive three-dimensional visualization and quantitative assessment of in vivo physiologic and biochemical processes. PET is proving to be useful in staging, planning the biopsy, evaluating the response to chemotherapy, and helping to direct subsequent treatment. Fluorine-18 (^{18}F)-fluorodeoxyglucose-labeled positron emission tomography (FDG-PET) has a growing role as an imaging modality in the detection, staging, and management of sarcomas. FDG is an analogue of glucose that becomes trapped in malignant cells in proportion to their respective rate of glycolysis. When used in conjunction with other imaging modalities (e.g., CT and MRI), it can be useful with post-treatment surveillance, helping to differentiate viable tumor cells from postoperative changes. Early results in its application have been encouraging, but the number of published studies is limited.

MRI has replaced CT as the study of choice to determine the size, extent, and anatomic relationships of bone and soft-tissue tumors. It is the most accurate technique for determining the extent of intramedullary and extraosseous disease and the relationship to neurovascular structures. MRI may yield a specific diagnosis with tumors such as lipoma, hemangioma, hematoma, or pigmented villonodular synovitis, all of which have characteristic appearances. With regard to most neoplasms, however, the MRI appearance is nonspecific. Likewise, MRI frequently cannot differentiate benign from malignant lesions. A study at our institution found substantial differences between MRI-based opinions given by specialized musculoskeletal radiologists and those given by outside radiologists: only about half of the outside reports listed the most likely diagnosis as such, and only 60% listed it at all. In general, any soft-tissue neoplasm deep to the fascia or larger than 5 cm in its greatest dimension should be considered highly likely to be a sarcoma.

Ultrasonography is useful for distinguishing cystic from solid soft-tissue lesions but otherwise offers little information. Angiography, which previously was used to determine the relationship of a neoplasm to the vessels, has been supplanted by MRI. Angiography still is useful, however, to rule out nonneoplastic conditions, such as pseudoaneurysms or arteriovenous malformations, and for preoperative embolization of highly vascular lesions, such as renal cell carcinoma and aneurysmal bone cysts.

■ LABORATORY TESTS

Blood and urine tests rarely lead to a diagnosis but can be useful in selected situations. A basic metabolic panel may be indicated to evaluate the overall health of a patient. Risks of wound healing problems and infection have been shown to be significantly greater in patients whose serum albumin value is less than 3.5 g/dL or whose total lymphocyte count is less than 1500/mL. A complete blood cell count may be helpful to rule out infection and leukemia. The erythrocyte sedimentation rate usually is elevated in infection, metastatic carcinoma, and small "blue cell" tumors, such as Ewing sarcoma, lymphoma, leukemia, and histiocytosis. Serum protein electrophoresis should be ordered if multiple myeloma is part of the differential diagnosis. Likewise, a prostate-specific antigen test should be ordered if prostate carcinoma is a possibility. Hypercalcemia may be present with metastatic disease, multiple myeloma, and hyperparathyroidism. Alkaline phosphatase may be elevated in metabolic bone disease, metastatic disease, osteosarcoma, Ewing sarcoma, or lymphoma. Blood urea nitrogen and creatinine may be elevated with renal tumors, and a urinalysis may reveal hematuria in this setting. Brown tumors of hyperparathyroidism sometimes can look like giant cell tumors and can be evaluated with serum calcium and parathyroid hormone levels. Finally, Paget disease may be in the differential diagnosis and can be evaluated by serum alkaline phosphatase and urinary pyridinium cross-links.

Musculoskeletal neoplasms should be evaluated completely before biopsy is done. The differential diagnosis, extent of the lesion, and potential resectability of the lesion can affect the type of biopsy, the placement of the biopsy incision, and the pathologic management of the tissue obtained. A complete workup helps to narrow the differential diagnosis and to bring about a more accurate pathologic diagnosis. Finally, tests, such as MRI or bone scanning, can be adversely affected by postoperative changes in the tissues. Bone and soft-tissue neoplasms suspected of being malignant should be evaluated with radiographs of the involved limb and a chest radiograph to evaluate possible metastases. MRI of the lesion delineates the extent of the lesion in the bone and soft-tissue involvement and the relationship to other anatomic structures. A bone scan should be obtained to detect any other areas of skeletal involvement, and a CT scan of the chest should be obtained to rule out pulmonary metastases. Other tests may be added to this minimal basic workup as indicated.

METASTASES OF UNKNOWN ORIGIN

In a patient older than age 40 with a new, painful bone lesion, multiple myeloma and metastatic carcinoma are the most likely diagnoses even if the patient has no known history of carcinoma. Prostate cancer and breast cancer are the two most common primary sources for bone metastases. If a patient has no known primary tumor, however, the most likely sources are lung cancer and renal cell carcinoma. Rougraff et al. described the proper evaluation of a patient with suspected metastases of unknown origin. The evaluation begins with a history focusing on any previous malignancies, even in the remote past, followed by a physical examination that includes not only the involved extremity but also the thyroid, lungs, abdomen, prostate in men, and breasts in women. Laboratory analysis should include complete blood cell count, erythrocyte sedimentation rate, electrolytes, liver enzymes, alkaline phosphatase, serum protein electrophoresis, and possibly prostate-specific antigen. Plain radiographs of the involved bone and the chest should be obtained. A whole-body bone scan should be ordered to evaluate other possible areas of skeletal involvement, and a CT scan of the chest, abdomen, and pelvis should be obtained (Fig. 7.1). A mammogram is not routinely indicated as an initial procedure because breast cancer is a rare source of metastases without a known primary lesion. The authors were able to identify the primary lesion in 85% of patients with skeletal metastases of unknown origin using this simple approach. They listed six reasons why the biopsy should not be done until the evaluation is complete: (1) The lesion may be a primary sarcoma of bone that may require a biopsy technique that allows for future limb salvage surgery; (2) another, more accessible lesion may be found; (3) if renal cell carcinoma is considered likely, the surgeon may wish to consider preoperative embolization to avoid excessive bleeding; (4) if the diagnosis of multiple myeloma is made by laboratory studies, an unnecessary biopsy can be avoided; (5) the pathologic diagnosis is more accurate if aided by appropriate imaging studies; and (6) the pathologist and surgeon may be more assured of a diagnosis of metastasis made on frozen section analysis if supported by the preoperative evaluation. This is important if stabilization of an impending fracture is planned for the same procedure.

STAGING

Enneking and others have shown the desirability of staging benign and malignant musculoskeletal tumors to aid in

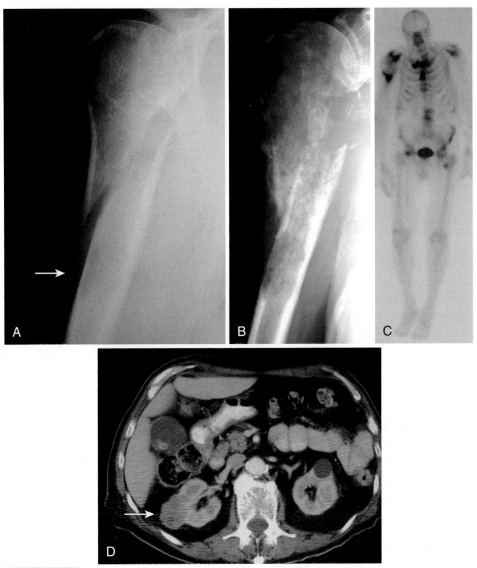

FIGURE 7.1 Humeral fracture after minimal trauma in 81-year-old man with no known history of malignancy. **A,** Lesion *(arrow)* was not identified initially, and patient was treated conservatively at another institution. **B,** Radiograph 10 weeks after injury shows progression of malignant process. Patient was referred to orthopaedic oncology center, where most likely diagnosis was thought to be either multiple myeloma or metastatic carcinoma. **C,** Bone scan reveals multiple sites of disease. **D,** CT of abdomen reveals lesion in the right kidney, which proved to be primary lesion *(arrow).*

treatment decision making, provide some determination of prognosis, and allow meaningful comparisons of treatment methods. Benign and malignant tumors of bone and soft tissue can be staged according to the Enneking staging system (Table 7.1). The stages of benign tumors are designated by Arabic numbers, and malignant tumors are designated by Roman numerals.

Benign tumors are staged as follows: stage 1, latent; stage 2, active; and stage 3, aggressive. Stage 1 lesions are intracapsular, usually asymptomatic, and frequently incidental findings. Radiographic features include a well-defined margin with a thick rim of reactive bone. There is no cortical destruction or expansion. These lesions do not require treatment because they do not compromise the strength of the bone and usually resolve spontaneously. An example is a small asymptomatic nonossifying fibroma

discovered incidentally on radiographs taken to evaluate an unrelated injury (Fig. 7.2). Stage 2 lesions also are intracapsular but are actively growing and can cause symptoms or lead to pathologic fracture. They have well-defined margins on radiographs but may expand and thin the cortex. Usually they have only a thin rim of reactive bone. Treatment usually consists of extended curettage (Fig. 7.3). Stage 3 lesions are extracapsular. Their aggressive nature is apparent clinically and radiographically. They do not respect natural anatomic barriers and usually have broken through the reactive bone and possibly the cortex (Fig. 7.4). MRI may show a soft-tissue mass, and metastases may be present in 1% to 5% of patients with these lesions (e.g., giant cell tumor). Treatment consists of extended curettage, marginal resection, or possibly wide resection, and local recurrences are common.

TABLE 7.1

Enneking System for Staging Benign and Malignant Musculoskeletal Tumors

BENIGN

1. Latent—low biologic activity; well marginated; often incidental findings (e.g., nonossifying fibroma)
2. Active—symptomatic; limited bone destruction; may present with pathologic fracture (e.g., aneurysmal bone cyst)
3. Aggressive—aggressive; bone destruction/soft-tissue extension; do not respect natural barriers (e.g., giant cell tumor)

MALIGNANT			
STAGE	GRADE	SITE	METASTASES
IA	Low	Intracompartmental	None
IB	Low	Extracompartmental	None
IIA	High	Intracompartmental	None
IIB	High	Extracompartmental	None
III	Any	Any	Regional or distant metastases

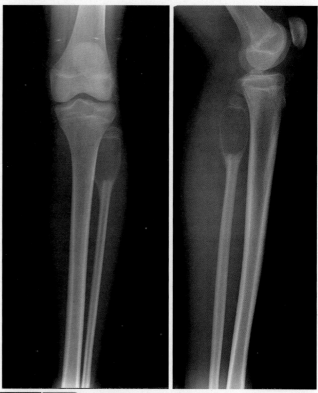

FIGURE 7.3   Stage II benign lesion: aneurysmal bone cyst of the proximal fibula.

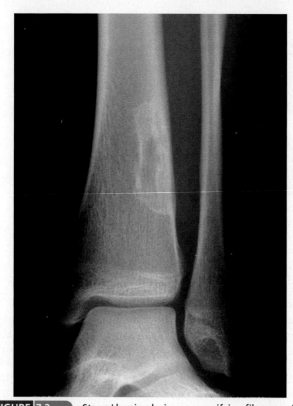

FIGURE 7.2   Stage I benign lesion: nonossifying fibroma of the distal tibia.

Reconstruction may sometimes prove difficult. Some interobserver discrepancy may be present when trying to assign a bone lesion to a particular stage.

Musculoskeletal sarcomas also can be staged according to the surgical staging system as described by Enneking et al. This system was designed to incorporate the most significant prognostic factors into a system of progressive stages that helps to guide surgical and adjuvant treatments. The system is based on the histologic grade of the tumor, its local extent, and the presence or absence of metastases. Low-grade lesions are designated as stage I. These lesions are well-differentiated, have few mitoses, and exhibit only moderate cytologic atypia. The risk for metastases is low (<25%). High-grade lesions are designated as stage II. They are poorly differentiated with a high mitotic rate and a high cell-to-matrix ratio. Stage I and II lesions are subdivided according to the extent of local growth. Stage IA and IIA lesions are contained within well-defined anatomic compartments (Fig. 7.5). Anatomic compartments are determined by the natural anatomic barriers to tumor growth, such as cortical bone, articular cartilage, fascial septa, or joint capsules. Stage IB and IIB lesions extend beyond the compartment of origin (Fig. 7.6). Stage III refers to any lesion that has metastasized regardless of the size or grade of the primary tumor. No distinction is made between lymph node metastases or distant metastases because both circumstances are associated with a poor prognosis.

Alternatively, many orthopaedic oncologists stage musculoskeletal malignancies according to the American Joint Committee on Cancer (AJCC) system. The AJCC staging system for soft-tissue sarcomas (Table 7.2) is based on prognostic variables, including tumor grade (low or high), size (≤5 cm or >5 cm in greatest dimension), depth (superficial or deep to the fascia), and presence of metastases. Stage I tumors are low grade regardless of size or depth. Stage II tumors are high grade; they may be small and any depth or large and superficial. Stage III tumors are high grade, large, and deep. Stage IV tumors are tumors associated with metastases (including local lymph nodes) regardless of grade, size, or depth.

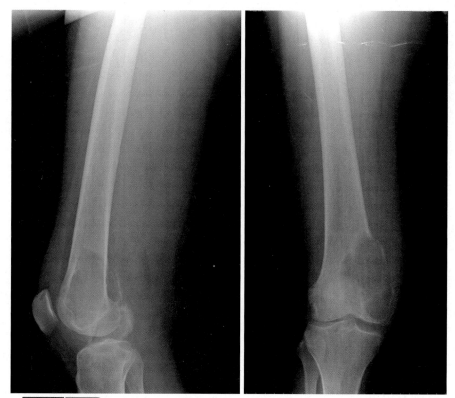

FIGURE 7.4   Stage III benign lesion: giant cell tumor of the distal femur.

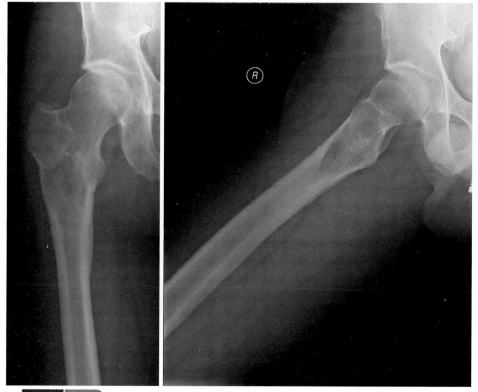

FIGURE 7.5   Stage IA malignant lesion: chondrosarcoma of the proximal femur.

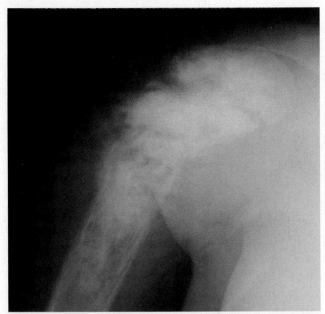

FIGURE 7.6 Stage IIB malignant lesion: osteosarcoma of the proximal humerus.

TABLE 7.2

American Joint Committee on Cancer System for Staging Soft-Tissue Sarcomas

STAGE	GRADE	SIZE	DEPTH	METASTASES
I	Low	Any	Any	None
II	High	≤5 cm	Any	None
	High	>5 cm	Superficial	None
III	High	>5 cm	Deep	None
IV	Any	Any	Any	Regional or distant

TABLE 7.3

American Joint Committee on Cancer System for Staging Bone Sarcomas

STAGE	GRADE	SIZE	METASTASES
I-A	Low	≤8 cm	None
I-B	Low	>8 cm	None
II-A	High	≤8 cm	None
II-B	High	>8 cm	None
III	Any	Any	Skip metastasis
IV-A	Any	Any	Pulmonary metastases
IV-B	Any	Any	Nonpulmonary metastases

The AJCC system for bone sarcomas (Table 7.3) is based on tumor grade, size, and presence and location of metastases. Stage I tumors, which are low grade, and stage II tumors, which are high grade, are subdivided based on tumor size. Stage I-A and II-A tumors are 8 cm or less in their greatest linear measurement; stage I-B and II-B tumors are larger than 8 cm. Stage III tumors have "skip metastases," which are defined as discontinuous lesions within the same bone. Stage IV-A involves pulmonary metastases, whereas stage IV-B involves nonpulmonary metastases. The subdivision of stage IV was made because it has been shown that patients with nonpulmonary metastases from osteosarcoma and Ewing sarcoma have worse prognoses than patients with only pulmonary metastases.

BIOPSY

In 1982, Mankin et al. reported 18.2% major errors in diagnosis, 10.3% nonrepresentative or technically poor biopsy specimens, and 17.3% wound complications associated with biopsy of musculoskeletal sarcomas. As a result of these complications, the optimal treatment plan had to be altered in 18.2%, including unnecessary amputations in 4.5%. These complications occurred three to five times more frequently when the biopsy was done by a surgeon at a referring institution, rather than by a member of the Musculoskeletal Tumor Society. A series of recommendations were made regarding the technical aspects of the biopsy, stating that whenever possible a patient with a suspected primary musculoskeletal malignancy should be referred before biopsy to the institution where definitive treatment will take place. The study was repeated 10 years later, and the results were essentially unchanged.

A biopsy should be planned as carefully as the definitive procedure. Biopsy should be done only after clinical, laboratory, and radiographic examinations are complete. As stated previously, completion of the evaluation before biopsy aids in planning the placement of the biopsy incision, helps provide more information leading to a more accurate pathologic diagnosis, and avoids artifacts on imaging studies. If the results of the evaluation suggest that a primary malignancy is in the differential diagnosis, the patient should be referred to a musculoskeletal oncologist before biopsy.

Regardless of whether a needle biopsy or an open biopsy is done, the biopsy track should be considered contaminated with tumor cells. Placement of the biopsy is a crucial decision because the biopsy track needs to be excised en bloc with the tumor. The surgeon performing the biopsy should be familiar with incisions for limb salvage surgery and standard and nonstandard amputation flaps. If a tourniquet is used, the limb can be elevated before inflation but should not be exsanguinated by compression to prevent "squeezing" the tumor's cells into the systemic circulation. Care should be taken to contaminate as little tissue as possible. Transverse incisions should be avoided because they are extremely difficult or impossible to excise with the specimen (Fig. 7.7). The deep incision should go through a single muscle compartment rather than contaminating an intermuscular plane. Major neurovascular structures should be avoided. Soft-tissue extension of a bone lesion should be sampled because this leading edge contains the most viable tumor for making the diagnosis. Care should be taken, however, to sample more than just the pseudocapsule surrounding the lesion. A frozen section should be sent intraoperatively to ensure that diagnostic tissue has been obtained. If a hole must be made in the bone, it should be round or oval to minimize stress concentration and prevent a subsequent fracture, which could preclude limb salvage surgery (Fig. 7.8). The hole should be plugged with methacrylate to limit hematoma formation. Only the minimal amount of methacrylate needed to plug the hole should be used because excessive amounts push the tumor up and down the bone. If a tourniquet has been used, it should be deflated and meticulous hemostasis ensured before closure, because a hematoma would be contaminated with tumor cells. If a drain is used, it should exit

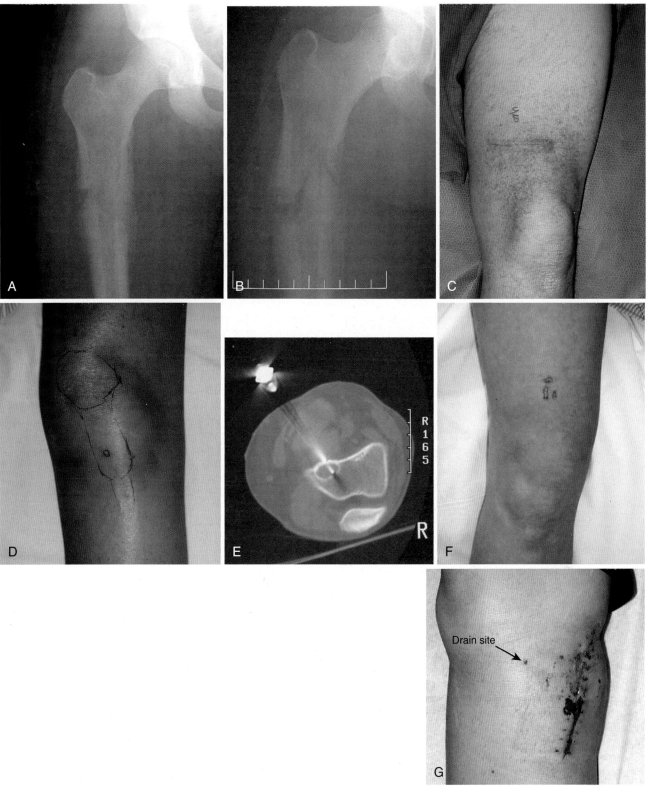

FIGURE 7.7 Examples of poorly performed biopsies. **A and B,** Biopsy resulted in irregular defect in bone, which led to pathologic fracture. **C,** Transverse incisions should not be used. **D,** Needle biopsy track contaminated patellar tendon. **E,** Needle track placed posteriorly, a location that would be extremely difficult to resect en bloc with tumor if it had proved to be sarcoma. **F,** Multiple needle tracks contaminate quadriceps tendon. **G,** Drain site was not placed in line with incision.

TABLE 7.4

Types of Biopsy

BIOPSY TYPE	TISSUE OBTAINED	ADVANTAGES	DISADVANTAGES
Fine-needle aspiration	Cells	Cost effective Fewer complications Good for obese patient or tumor near neurovascular structure	Small sample size Need expert pathologist
Core needle	Small tissue core	Cost effective More tissue than fine-needle aspiration	More complications* than fine-needle aspiration
Incisional biopsy	Adequate sample of mass/lesion	Adequate tissue sample (gold standard)	Increased complications* May compromise definitive resection
Excisional biopsy	Entire lesion removed	Removes entire lesion Indicated for small lesion or expendable bone	Increased complications*

*Complications include infection, bleeding/hematoma, pathologic fracture, tumor contamination/seeding.

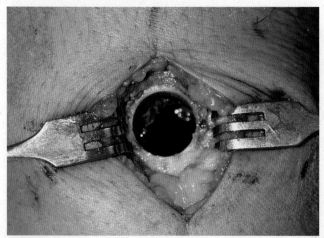

FIGURE 7.8 If hole must be made in bone during biopsy, defect should be round to minimize stress concentration, which otherwise could lead to pathologic fracture.

in line with the incision so that the drain track also can be easily excised en bloc with the tumor. The wound should be closed tightly in layers. Wide retention sutures should not be used.

A biopsy can be done by fine-needle aspiration, core needle biopsy, or an open incisional procedure (Table 7.4). Most musculoskeletal neoplasms can be diagnosed with a well-done needle biopsy. Fine-needle aspiration may be 90% accurate at determining malignancy; however, its accuracy at determining specific tumor type is much lower because only cells rather than tissue architecture are evaluated. This technique may be best applied when there is a high probability that the diagnosis is known such as metastases or infection and when evaluating lymph nodes. An experienced pathologist is helpful in determining the diagnosis because of the limited sample size obtained. A core needle biopsy uses a larger-gauge needle than a fine-needle aspiration, providing for tissue and preservation of the tissue architecture. The limited amount of tissue obtained may not be adequate, however, for accurate grading or for any additional studies that may dictate subsequent treatment. The few dedicated series that have analyzed outpatient core needle

biopsies have reported an overall diagnostic accuracy ranging from 84% to 98%. A study of 252 outpatient core needle biopsies of malignant bone and soft-tissue neoplasms reported an accuracy rate of 97% for determining whether or not a lesion is malignant; core needle biopsy was accurate for a specific histopathologic diagnosis and grade in 81%.

Open biopsy is the gold standard for biopsy of bone and soft-tissue tumors, but complications are greater with incisional biopsy when compared with needle biopsy (e.g., bleeding, infection, tissue contamination). However, this procedure is least likely to be associated with a sampling error, and it provides the most tissue for additional diagnostic studies, such as cytogenetics and flow cytometry. If the administration of chemotherapy is anticipated before further surgery, a central venous access catheter may be placed at the same setting as the biopsy if the frozen section is confirmatory. The definitive procedure can be done immediately after biopsy only if the frozen section diagnosis confirms the clinical and radiographic diagnosis. In cases of discrepancy or doubt, the definitive procedure should be delayed until a firm diagnosis is established. If a giant cell tumor is suspected on clinical and radiographic grounds, definitive curettage can proceed immediately after confirmation of the diagnosis on frozen section. Likewise, if the suspicion of an impending fracture from metastatic carcinoma is confirmed on frozen section, prophylactic fixation can be applied immediately. Conversely, if the frozen section in either of these scenarios exhibited any atypical cells that might represent a sarcoma, definitive surgery should be delayed until the final pathologic evaluation is complete.

Rarely, a primary resection (i.e., excisional biopsy) should be done instead of a biopsy. A small (<3 cm) subcutaneous mass that is unlikely to be malignant may be marginally resected primarily. In the rare circumstance that the lesion turns out to be malignant, the tumor bed can be reexcised with wide margins without adversely affecting the outcome. Primary resection should not be done on larger soft-tissue lesions or lesions deep to the fascia unless the MRI appearance is diagnostic of a benign lesion, such as a lipoma. Some benign bone lesions, such as osteoid osteoma and osteochondroma, have a characteristic radiographic appearance and can be primarily resected, if indicated, without biopsy. A final relative indication for primary resection is a painful lesion in an expendable bone, such

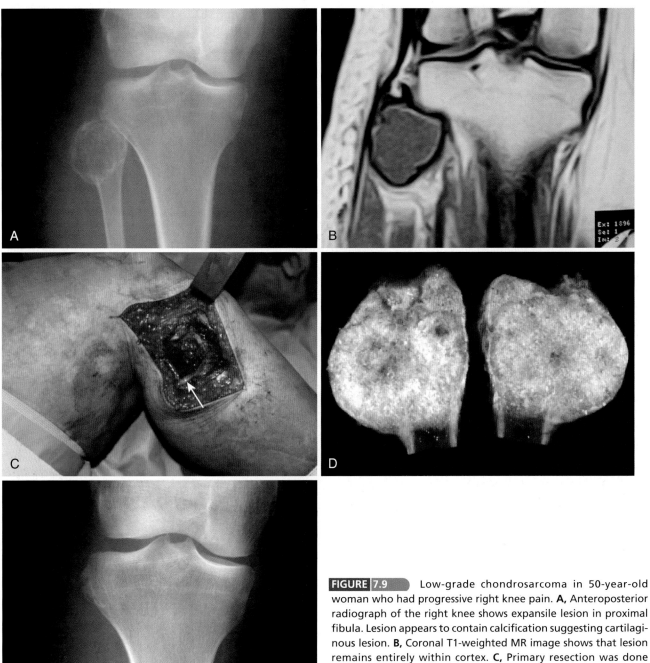

FIGURE 7.9 Low-grade chondrosarcoma in 50-year-old woman who had progressive right knee pain. **A,** Anteroposterior radiograph of the right knee shows expansile lesion in proximal fibula. Lesion appears to contain calcification suggesting cartilaginous lesion. **B,** Coronal T1-weighted MR image shows that lesion remains entirely within cortex. **C,** Primary resection was done without biopsy. This treatment strategy allowed for wide margins without contamination of common peroneal nerve *(arrow).* **D,** Lesion proved to be low-grade chondrosarcoma. **E,** Radiograph after primary resection of proximal fibula.

as the proximal fibula or distal ulna. If a symptomatic lesion in one of these locations is confined within the cortex and would be resected regardless of a benign or malignant tissue diagnosis, it can be resected without biopsy (Fig. 7.9).

ADJUVANT TREATMENT

The primary goal of treatment in a patient with a primary malignancy of the musculoskeletal system is to make the patient disease free. The goal of treatment of a patient with metastatic carcinoma to bone is to minimize pain and to preserve function. The optimal treatment of the tumor often requires a combination of radiation therapy, chemotherapy, and surgery.

RADIATION THERAPY

Radiation causes cell death by inducing the formation of intracellular free radicals that subsequently cause DNA damage. The sensitivity of a cell to radiation depends on several factors, including (1) the cell's position in the cell cycle (actively mitotic cells are most sensitive), (2) tissue oxygenation (local hypoxia provides a protective effect because oxygen-free radicals cannot be formed in hypoxic tissue), and (3) the cell's ability to repair DNA damage or its inability to undergo apoptosis (programmed cell death) in response to this damage.

The dose of radiation is measured in Gray (Gy): 1 Gy is equal to 1 joule of absorbed energy per kilogram; 1 rad is equal to 1 centigray (cGy). The goal of radiation treatment is to deliver the highest possible dose of radiation to the tumor cells while minimizing toxicity to normal tissues. This is accomplished by using linear accelerators that deliver a high dose to the target tissues with sharp lateral field edges that limit the dose to nontarget tissues. Therapeutic advantage also is gained by fractionation of the dose. After a single treatment of 200 cGy, all cells in the most sensitive phase of the cell cycle are killed. Delivering another dose at a specified interval allows additional cells to enter this phase of the cell cycle. In addition, with progressive tumor cell death, previously hypoxic areas of the tumor may become reoxygenated and may become more sensitive to radiation. The interval also allows time for normal cells to repair damage. Most radiation treatment protocols deliver 150 to 200 cGy/day until the target dose is achieved. This dose ranges from 30 to 40 Gy for myeloma to 60 Gy for treatment of a soft-tissue sarcoma.

Most primary bone malignancies are relatively radioresistant. Exceptions are the small blue cell tumors, including multiple myeloma, lymphoma, and Ewing sarcoma, which are each exquisitely sensitive. Carcinomas metastatic to bone, with the exception of renal cell carcinoma, also frequently are sensitive to radiation treatment. For most other bone tumors, radiation has a limited role because local control is achieved better with surgery. Advances in spinal surgery have diminished the frequency of use of radiotherapy for tumors that were previously surgically inaccessible. Radiation therapy can be used to reduce the incidence of local recurrence of malignant soft-tissue tumors treated with marginal resection when the alternative would be a more mutilating resection or amputation. Radiation also can be used for preoperative treatment of soft-tissue sarcomas in the hopes of reducing the tumor volume and making the resection easier.

Radiation therapy is associated with significant acute and long-term complications. Acutely, the most common complication is skin irritation. Initial erythema may progress later to desquamation, especially in patients who also are being treated with cytotoxic drugs. Other common acute side effects include gastrointestinal upset, urinary frequency, fatigue, anorexia, and extremity edema. Late effects include chronic edema, fibrosis, osteonecrosis, and pathologic fracture. Malignant transformation of irradiated tissues (i.e., radiation sarcoma) is being reported with increasing frequency in survivors of childhood and adolescent cancers. These secondary sarcomas occur with a mean lag time of approximately 10 years and often are associated with a poor prognosis. Radiation-induced pathologic fractures also are becoming more common and can be extremely difficult to treat. In a study by Lin et al., the incidence of pathologic fracture was 29% at 5 years after treatment of a soft-tissue sarcoma of the thigh if treatment included radiation therapy and wide resection with periosteal stripping. This risk increased to 47% in female patients and to 66% in female patients who received chemotherapy. Radiation therapy in children has several adverse sequelae, such as scoliosis, kyphosis, chest wall deformities, hypoplasia of the ilium, and limb-length discrepancy, as a result of radiation-induced growth arrest. Radiotherapy is

rarely used for benign conditions; possible exceptions include an extensive pigmented villonodular synovitis that cannot be controlled by surgery or a large spinal giant cell tumor.

In addition to conventional external beam radiation, radiation can be delivered by brachytherapy (from the Greek, *brachys,* meaning "close"). By this method, hollow catheters are implanted in the tumor bed at the time of resection (Fig. 7.10). These catheters exit through the skin. Postoperative radiographic evaluation and computer calculations determine the optimal loading of the catheters with radioisotopes. This technique allows for high doses to be delivered to the target tissues. The radiation levels fall off rapidly at the edges of the field, sparing normal tissues.

CHEMOTHERAPY

Before the routine use of chemotherapy for osteosarcoma, patients usually were treated with immediate wide or radical amputation on diagnosis. This approach usually treated the local disease adequately. Nevertheless, 80% of patients eventually died of metastatic disease even if metastasis was not evident at presentation. From this, it can be deduced that 80% of patients with apparently localized osteosarcoma actually have undetectable metastases, or micrometastases, on presentation. With the use of modern chemotherapy protocols, the current 5-year survival rate for osteosarcoma is approximately 70%. Similar numbers are available regarding the treatment of Ewing sarcoma. Similarly, chemotherapy has a well-defined role in the treatment of other high-grade malignancies of bone, such as malignant fibrous histiocytoma, and high-grade soft-tissue malignancies of childhood, such as rhabdomyosarcoma. The role of chemotherapy is less well defined for adult soft-tissue malignancies, with most investigations showing modest improvements in outcome. In general, chemotherapy is not useful for cartilaginous lesions and most low-grade malignancies.

Adjuvant chemotherapy refers to chemotherapy administered postoperatively to treat presumed micrometastases. Neoadjuvant chemotherapy refers to chemotherapy administered before surgical resection of the primary tumor. No study has proved a survival advantage with regard to the timing of chemotherapy; however, multiple authors have cited several theoretical advantages of neoadjuvant chemotherapy over adjuvant chemotherapy. Preoperative chemotherapy frequently causes regression of the primary tumor, making a successful limb salvage operation easier. In a study by Malawar et al., 9 of 12 lesions that initially were deemed unresectable were treated later with limb salvage surgery after chemotherapy-induced tumor regression. Neoadjuvant chemotherapy followed by surgical resection allows for histologic evaluation of the effectiveness of treatment. This is one of the most valuable prognostic indicators (i.e., percent tumor necrosis) of successful long-term outcome. In addition, histologic evaluation may lead to alteration of further chemotherapy in poor responders. Preoperative chemotherapy theoretically may decrease the spread of tumor cells at the time of surgery, and neoadjuvant chemotherapy usually can be started immediately, effectively treating micrometastases at the earliest time possible and avoiding tumor progression, which may occur during any delay before surgery. This allows time to plan the operation properly, including the possible manufacturing of a custom implant. It also allows time for the patient and the family to consider fully the options of limb salvage

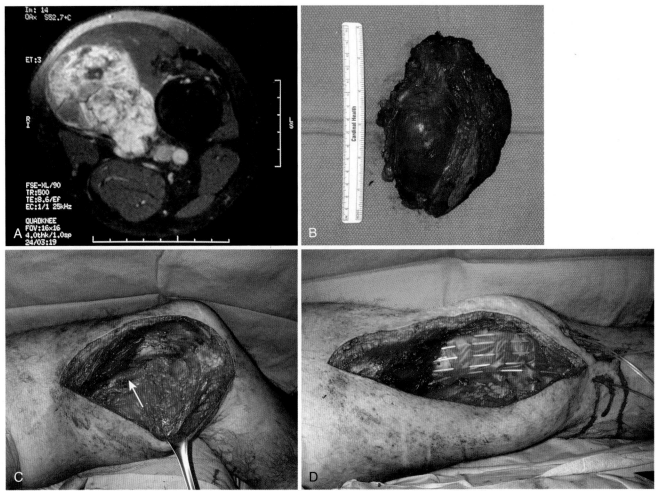

FIGURE 7.10 **A,** MR image of soft-tissue sarcoma in 85-year-old man shows tumor adjacent to distal femur and femoral vessels. **B,** Resected specimen. **C,** Tumor cavity with exposed distal femur and femoral vessels *(arrow).* **D,** Brachytherapy catheters woven through polyglactin 910 (Vicryl) mesh to help maintain proper spacing. Catheters placed along vessels and bone (where margins were close) exiting through separate stab wounds. Wound was closed over catheters.

surgery versus amputation. It has been suggested, however, that neoadjuvant chemotherapy may increase significantly the risks of perioperative complications, especially delayed wound healing and infection. Others have not found this to be true, and currently most orthopaedic oncologists favor preoperative chemotherapy with the definitive procedure performed 3 to 4 weeks after the last dose has been administered. Chemotherapy is restarted 2 weeks postoperatively if the wound has healed.

Although it is presumed that most malignancies arise from a single cell, the actual tumor is composed of a heterogeneous population of cells. This is the result of rapid turnover and genetic lability of these cells. As a result, various cells within the same tumor evolve different mechanisms of chemoresistance. To combat this diversity in resistance, most chemotherapy regimens involve combinations of toxic drugs. Table 7.5 lists the most common agents used in the treatment of bone and soft-tissue sarcomas and their most common dose-limiting side effects. This field is rapidly changing, but certain general statements can be made. These drugs are most effective when the tumor against which they are directed is small. Combinations of

these drugs are more effective than single agents. Dosage, sequence of drugs, and schedule seem to be important in achieving the maximal response. All have toxicity for normal tissues and should be given in a controlled setting by someone skilled in their use.

PRINCIPLES OF SURGERY
AMPUTATION VERSUS LIMB SALVAGE

Advances in diagnostic imaging, chemotherapy, radiation therapy, and surgical technique for resection and reconstruction now allow limb salvage to be a reasonable option for most patients with bone or soft-tissue sarcomas. Specifically, preoperative radiation therapy for soft-tissue sarcomas and neoadjuvant chemotherapy for bone sarcomas have helped surgeons to successfully resect some tumors that in the past would have been deemed unresectable. Rarely, involvement of neurovascular structures, a displaced pathologic fracture, or complications secondary to a poorly performed biopsy preclude the possibility of limb salvage. More often, however, the choice between limb salvage and amputation must be made on the basis of the expectations and desires of the individual

TABLE 7.5

Chemotherapeutic Agents Commonly Used for Treatment of Bone and Soft-Tissue Tumors

AGENT	SIDE EFFECTS
ALKYLATING AGENTS	
Mustards	
Cyclophosphamide	Myelosuppression (leukopenia), hemorrhagic cystitis, alopecia, nausea and vomiting
Ifosfamide	Hemorrhagic cystitis, myelosuppression, nausea and vomiting, nephrotoxicity, neurotoxicity
Platinum Compounds	
Cisplatin	Nausea and vomiting, nephrotoxicity (cumulative and irreversible), ototoxicity (cumulative and irreversible), peripheral neuropathy (reversible)
Carboplatin	Myelosuppression, nausea and vomiting, alopecia, hepatotoxicity, nephrotoxicity
Antimetabolites	
Methotrexate	Myelosuppression, mucositis, nephrotoxicity, hepatotoxicity, pneumonitis, neurotoxicity
Topoisomerase	
INTERACTIVE AGENTS	
Antitumor Antibiotics	
Doxorubicin	Myelosuppression (neutrophils), nausea and vomiting, mucositis, alopecia, severe tissue necrosis (with extravasation), acute and chronic cardiotoxicity
Dactinomycin	Myelosuppression (platelets and neutrophils), nausea and vomiting, diarrhea, tissue necrosis (with extravasation), myelosuppression
Epipodophyllotoxins	
Etoposide (VP-16)	Mucositis, nausea and vomiting
Antimicrotubule Agents	
***Vinca* Alkaloids**	
Vincristine	Peripheral neuropathy (irreversible), tissue necrosis (with extravasation), seizures, alopecia

patient and the family. Simon described four issues that must be considered whenever contemplating limb salvage instead of an amputation:

1. Would survival be affected by the treatment choice?
2. How do the short-term and long-term morbidity compare?
3. How would the function of a salvaged limb compare with that of a prosthesis?
4. Are there any psychosocial consequences?

Several studies have shown the effect of treatment choice on survival in patients with osteosarcoma. With the use of multimodal treatment including surgery and chemotherapy, long-term survival for patients with osteosarcoma has improved from approximately 20% to approximately 70% in most series. For osteosarcoma of the distal femur, the rate of local recurrence after wide resection and limb salvage is 5% to 10%. This is equivalent to the rate of local recurrence after a transfemoral amputation in this setting. Although hip disarticulation is associated with an extremely low rate of local recurrence, no study has shown a survival advantage for this technique. Although local recurrence is associated with an extremely poor prognosis, no study has proved any one of these surgical techniques (i.e., limb salvage, transfemoral amputation, hip disarticulation) to be superior in terms of survival, provided that wide surgical margins are obtained. From these data it

can be hypothesized that patients with a local recurrence despite wide margins may represent a subset of patients with especially aggressive disease or chemotherapy-resistant disease who would do poorly regardless of the surgical procedure. With regard to overall patient survival, the most important technical aspect of the surgical procedure is the attainment of a wide margin regardless of whether this is achieved by amputation or local resection.

Amputation for malignancy can be technically demanding, often requiring nonstandard flaps for closure or bone graft augmentation to obtain a more functional residual limb. Complications include infection, wound dehiscence, a chronically painful limb, phantom limb pain, and appositional bone overgrowth requiring revision surgery. Limb salvage is associated, however, with greater perioperative and long-term morbidity compared with amputation. Limb salvage requires a much more extensive surgical procedure with greater risks for infection, wound dehiscence, flap necrosis, blood loss, and deep venous thrombosis. Long-term complications of limb salvage vary depending on the type of reconstruction. These include periprosthetic fractures, prosthetic loosening or dislocation, nonunion of the graft-host junction, allograft fracture, leg-length discrepancy, and late infection. A patient with a salvaged limb is much more likely to need multiple future operations for treatment of complications. After initially successful limb salvage surgery, one third of long-term survivors ultimately may require an amputation depending on the location of the tumor and the type of reconstruction.

With regard to function, location of the tumor is the most important issue. Resection of an upper extremity lesion with limb salvage, even with the sacrifice of one or two major nerves, generally provides better function than amputation and subsequent prosthetic fitting. Similarly, resection of a proximal femoral or pelvic lesion with local reconstruction generally provides better function than would be possible after a hip disarticulation or hemipelvectomy. Around the ankle and foot, however, large sarcomas frequently are treated with amputation followed by prosthetic fitting. Treatment of sarcomas around the knee must be individualized.

Most patients with osteosarcomas around the knee are treated with wide resection with prosthetic knee replacement or transfemoral amputation. Less commonly performed operations include osteoarticular allograft reconstruction, allograft arthrodesis, and rotationplasty. In a study of patients with osteosarcoma, Otis, Lane, and Kroll showed that, compared with transfemoral amputees, patients who had undergone resection and prosthetic knee replacement showed higher self-selected walking velocities and a more efficient gait with regard to oxygen consumption. Many of the transfemoral amputees were functioning at greater than 50% of their maximal aerobic capacity at free walking speeds. At greater than 50% of the maximal aerobic capacity, anaerobic mechanisms are required to sustain muscle metabolism, and endurance is greatly decreased. The problem is compounded by the decreased cardiac function in many of these patients as a result of doxorubicin-induced cardiomyopathy.

Harris et al. compared the long-term function of amputation, arthrodesis, and arthroplasty for tumors around the knee. They showed that patients who had amputations had difficulty walking on steep, rough, or slippery surfaces but were active and were the least worried about damaging the affected limb. Patients with an arthrodesis performed the most demanding physical work and recreational activities but had difficulty with sitting, especially in the back seats of cars, theaters, or sports arenas. Patients who had an arthroplasty generally led more sedentary lives and were more protective of the limb but had little difficulty with activities of daily living. These patients also were the least self-conscious about the limb.

In patients who are long-term survivors after resection of an extremity sarcoma, the probability of limb survival is associated with the type of reconstruction and the location of the tumor. A successful arthrodesis is more durable in the long term than a mobile joint reconstruction. Regarding prosthetic or allograft-prosthetic composite reconstructions, location is the most important issue, with proximal reconstructions generally outlasting more distal reconstructions. (This is the inverse of the prognosis for overall patient survival, with distal sarcomas having a better prognosis than proximal sarcomas.) Proximal femoral reconstructions generally outlast distal femoral reconstructions, which generally outlast proximal tibial reconstructions.

No study has shown a significant difference between amputation and limb salvage with regard to psychologic outcome or quality of life in long-term survivors of sarcoma. The choice of limb salvage or amputation involves more than the question of whether the lesion can be resected with wide margins. The patient ultimately must make the final decision in light of long-term goals and lifestyle decisions.

MARGINS

When describing an oncologic surgical procedure, it is imperative that the surgical margin be appropriately defined. The terms *amputation* and *resection* mean little without a modifier describing the margin. This is especially important when evaluating surgical procedures and outcomes in the literature. In orthopaedic oncology, the surgical margin is described by one of four terms: *intralesional, marginal, wide,* or *radical.* Amputations and limb-sparing resections may be associated with any of the four types of margins, and the margin must be specifically defined with each procedure (Figs. 7.11 and 7.12).

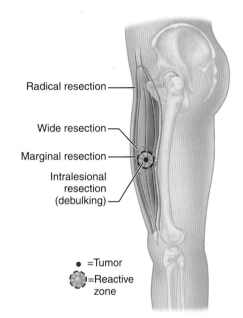

Radical resection

Wide resection

Marginal resection

Intralesional resection (debulking)

● =Tumor

⬤ =Reactive zone

FIGURE 7.11 Enneking classification of local procedures. (From Enneking WF: *Musculoskeletal tumor surgery,* vol 1, New York, 1983, Churchill Livingstone.)

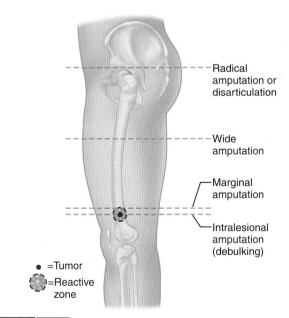

Radical amputation or disarticulation

Wide amputation

Marginal amputation

Intralesional amputation (debulking)

● =Tumor

⬤ =Reactive zone

FIGURE 7.12 Enneking classification of amputations. (From Enneking WF: *Musculoskeletal tumor surgery,* vol 1, New York, 1983, Churchill Livingstone.)

An intralesional margin is one in which the plane of surgical dissection is within the tumor. This type of procedure is often described as "debulking" because it leaves behind gross residual tumor. This procedure may be appropriate for symptomatic benign lesions when the only surgical alternative would be to sacrifice important anatomic structures. This also may be appropriate as a palliative procedure in the setting of metastatic disease.

As musculoskeletal tumors grow, they compress the surrounding tissues and appear to become encapsulated. This surrounding reactive tissue often is referred to as the *pseudocapsule*. A marginal margin is achieved when the closest plane of dissection passes through the pseudocapsule. This type of margin usually is adequate to treat most benign lesions and some low-grade malignancies. In high-grade malignancy, however, the pseudocapsule often contains microscopic foci of disease, or "satellite" lesions. A marginal resection often leaves behind microscopic disease that may lead to local recurrence if the remaining tumor cells do not respond to adjuvant chemotherapy or radiation therapy. Despite an increased risk of local recurrence, a marginal resection may be preferable if the alternative is a more mutilating procedure. Improvements in preoperative radiation therapy and neoadjuvant chemotherapy have made marginal resections an acceptable alternative to amputation in some selective circumstances.

Wide margins are achieved when the plane of dissection is in normal tissue. Although no specific distance is defined, the entire tumor remains completely surrounded by a cuff of normal tissue. The quality of a margin is more important than the quantity (thickness) of the margin. For instance, a fascial margin provides a better plane for containing tumor spread than does a similar or thicker plane of subcutaneous tissue. If the plane of dissection touches the pseudocapsule at any point, the margin should be defined as being marginal and not wide. Although sometimes impossible to achieve, wide margins are the goal of most procedures for high-grade malignancies.

Radical margins are achieved when all the compartments that contain tumor are removed en bloc. For deep soft-tissue tumors, this involves removing the entire compartment (or multiple compartments) of any involved muscles. For bone tumors, this involves removing the entire bone and the compartments of any involved muscles. Radical operations were previously the procedures of choice for most high-grade neoplasms; however, with improvements in imaging studies, radical procedures now are rarely performed because equivalent oncologic results usually can be obtained with wide margins.

From an oncologic standpoint, there are eight different surgical procedures because resections and amputations may be defined further by any of the four margins. Amputations usually achieve wide margins (e.g., a high transfemoral amputation for an osteosarcoma of the distal femur) or radical margins (e.g., a hip disarticulation for a femoral lesion), but this is not always the case. A hemipelvectomy for a large intrapelvic tumor may allow only marginal margins to be obtained and would be referred to as a *marginal amputation*. Rarely, a palliative procedure or an inappropriate amputation level leaves behind gross residual disease. These procedures would be referred to as *intralesional amputations*. Likewise, limb-sparing resections of bone or soft-tissue tumors can be categorized by any one of the types of margins, although radical resections of bone tumors are extremely rare.

CURETTAGE

Many benign bone tumors are treated adequately by curettage. Compared with resection, curettage is associated with a higher rate of local recurrence; however, curettage often allows for a better functional result. Although this is not a technically difficult procedure, the surgeon should adhere strictly to several principles to avoid an unacceptably high rate of local recurrence, especially with more aggressive benign tumors.

Curettage is done by first making a large cortical window over the lesion. This window must be at least as large as the lesion itself. If the window is smaller than the lesion, the surgeon inevitably leaves residual tumor on the undersurface of the near cortex. The bulk of the tumor is scooped out with large curets. Next, the cavity is enlarged back to normal host bone in each direction with a power burr. (Use of a power burr is mandatory for curettage of bone tumors.) Finally, the cavity and the wound should be copiously irrigated to remove any debris and tumor cells. These are the minimal requirements for a "simple" curettage.

"Extended" curettage includes the use of adjuvants, such as liquid nitrogen, phenol, polymethyl methacrylate, or thermal cautery (Fig. 7.13) to extend destruction of tumor cells. Several authors have reported greatly reduced recurrence rates of aggressive tumors with the use of adjuvants. The recurrence rate after extended curettage for giant cell tumors is now approximately 10%. Although not proved in randomized trials, this seems to be a great improvement compared with the 25% to 50% recurrence rate in historic controls reported before the routine use of adjuvants.

Although each adjuvant treatment has its proponents, no study has proved that any one is superior, with each having advantages and disadvantages. Cryosurgery with liquid nitrogen is effective at extending the tumor kill. Studies have shown it to be superior to phenol and methacrylate at creating a rim of necrotic bone (≤14 mm) around experimental cavities in animal and cadaver models. Liquid nitrogen usually is applied by the "direct pour" technique and may be associated with greater complications, including pathologic fracture and nerve injury. Phenol, conversely, has relatively poor penetration into bone (<1 mm). Although it is relatively easy to use, serious complications have been reported when phenol was inadvertently applied to the surrounding normal tissues. Adjuvant treatment also can be accomplished through thermal cautery, such as with an argon beam coagulator. Studies have shown the depth of necrosis in cancellous bone treated with argon beam coagulation to be approximately 4 mm. We have extensive experience with the use of argon beam coagulation and have noted no complications that can be attributed directly to its use. Finally, despite some disagreement in the literature, polymethyl methacrylate bone cement may act as an adjuvant through its heat of polymerization or through direct toxicity of the monomer. It is easily applied and can be used as a filling agent in conjunction with other adjuvants.

The final issue that must be considered involves filling the cavity left after curettage. Options include autogenous bone graft, allograft, demineralized bone matrix, artificial bone graft substitutes, and bone cement. Autogenous bone graft provides the most rapid and most reliable healing rate because it is osteogenic, osteoinductive, and osteoconductive, but it is associated with additional morbidity at the harvest site, and it may not be available in sufficient quantity to fill a large cavity. Autogenous bone graft must be harvested using a different set of instruments

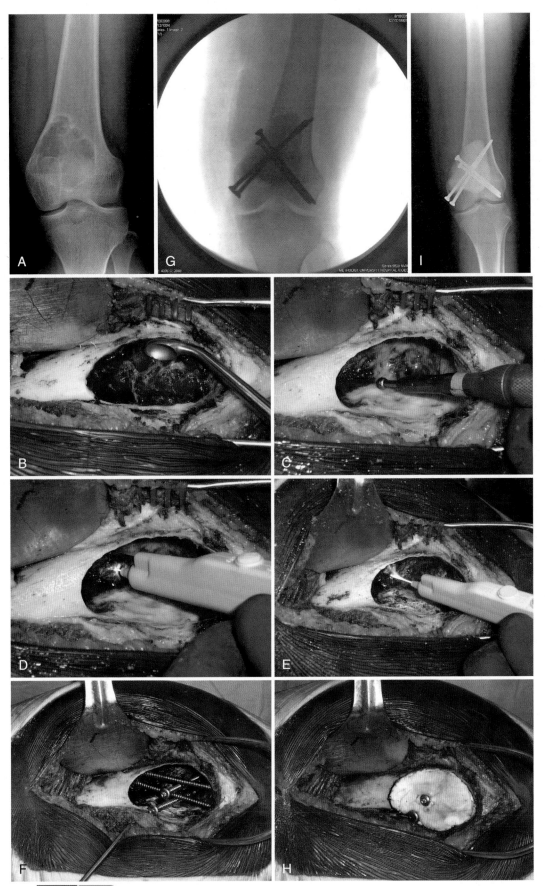

FIGURE 7.13 Curettage. **A,** Giant cell tumor of the distal femur. **B,** After pathologic diagnosis is confirmed, the cortical window is made larger than the tumor to allow adequate exposure. **C,** After gross tumor is removed with large curets, the entire tumor cavity is enlarged in all directions with a high-speed burr. **D and E,** Tumor cavity is treated with argon beam coagulation. **F,** Screws are placed to augment strength of reconstruction. **G,** Fluoroscopy is used to confirm screw position. **H,** Bone cement is used to fill cavity. **I,** Postoperative view.

to prevent contamination of the donor site. Even though it is only osteoconductive, cancellous allograft is reliably incorporated. It is readily available in large quantities and does not involve any further operative morbidity. Although allograft is associated with the theoretical risk of disease transmission, we are not aware of any reported cases of hepatitis or human immunodeficiency virus transmission through the use of freeze-dried cancellous allograft. Another alternative is demineralized bone matrix. The material is osteoconductive, but in contrast to cancellous allograft, demineralized bone matrix also is osteoinductive. Artificial bone graft substitutes (e.g., calcium sulfate, calcium phosphate) are osteoconductive, are easy to use, and are readily available. They can be used alone or in combination with autogenous bone graft, bone marrow aspirates, or demineralized bone matrix. Early reports have shown their efficacy with regard to filling relatively large defects. Finally, bone cement can be used as a filling agent. In addition to its use as an adjuvant, it has the advantage of providing immediate stability, which makes rehabilitation easier and lessens the risk of pathologic fracture. Another advantage of bone cement is associated with the detection of local recurrence. Although tumor recurrences are difficult to recognize after a tumor cavity has been filled with bone graft or bone graft substitutes, recurrent tumor is easily recognized as an expanding lucency adjacent to bone cement. One potential disadvantage of bone cement (although not proved) is that it may lead to early joint degeneration secondary to biomechanical alteration of the subchondral bone. Adding a layer of bone graft to the subchondral bone before cement may help minimize the suggested biomechanical alteration. Some authors subsequently have recommended routine removal of the cement at a later date and replacement with bone graft.

We currently use argon beam coagulation as adjuvant treatment after curettage. For most benign lesions, the defects are filled with freeze-dried cancellous allograft chips or with a calcium sulfate/calcium phosphate bone graft substitute. For more aggressive benign lesions, such as giant cell tumors, we usually use bone cement to fill the defect and consider adjuvant fixation if the defect is thought to need additional structural support. We do not routinely remove the cement at a later date to decrease the theoretical risk of degenerative joint disease.

RESECTION AND RECONSTRUCTION

Currently, most musculoskeletal malignancies are treated with local resection and reconstruction. Aggressive benign neoplasms also can be treated in this manner. The goal of resection of a malignancy is to achieve wide surgical margins if possible. If this is impossible because of anatomic constraints, a marginal resection combined with adjuvant or neoadjuvant treatment (e.g., radiation for a soft-tissue sarcoma) may be preferable to an amputation, although this decision must be made on an individual basis in conjunction with the patient and family. A marginal resection usually is adequate for most benign neoplasms. Specific techniques for resection are discussed later in this chapter.

Although allograft arthrodesis still has a role in some circumstances, most reconstructions involve preserving a mobile joint, for which three general options are available: osteoarticular allograft reconstruction, endoprosthetic reconstruction, and allograft-prosthesis composite reconstruction. (An additional option, rotationplasty, is discussed later in the chapter.) In general, oncologic reconstructions involve higher complication rates than do standard total joint arthroplasties because of the extensive nature of the operation, the extensive tissue loss, and the

compromising effects of associated radiation and chemotherapy. In addition, these reconstructions often are done on young patients who are extremely active. Some complications, such as wound necrosis and infection, are universal to all types of reconstructions. Other complications are more specific to the method of reconstruction. Although each method has proponents, we have made the most extensive use of endoprosthetic reconstruction, reserving other methods for specific indications.

Osteoarticular allografts offer several attractive advantages, including the ability to replace ligaments, tendons, and intraarticular structures. Several authors have reported success with this method of reconstruction; however, other authors have reported high rates of complications, including nonunion at the graft-host junction, fatigue fracture, infection, articular collapse, dislocation, degenerative joint disease, and failure of ligament and tendon attachments. Osteoarticular allografts may have a role as a temporary measure to preserve an adjacent physis in an immature patient when the alternatives include amputation or sacrifice of both physes. A proximal tibial osteoarticular allograft could be used in an immature patient in an attempt to preserve the distal femoral physis until skeletal maturity. This could be converted later to an endoprosthetic reconstruction when it becomes necessary.

Allograft-prosthesis composites may provide a long-term solution for some patients. They avoid the complications of degenerative joint disease and articular collapse while still preserving the ability to attach soft-tissue structures directly, such as the patellar tendon or the hip abductors. They are associated, however, with fatigue fracture, infection, and nonunion at the graft-host junction. Although many surgeons use allograft-prosthesis composite as their primary method of reconstruction, our main indication is an inadequate length of remaining host bone to secure the stem of an endoprosthesis. We still use a tumor prosthesis for reconstruction with allograft for fixation to the remaining host bone (Fig. 7.14).

Endoprosthetic reconstruction also may provide long-term function for some patients and is associated with its own complications. Endoprosthetic reconstruction provides the advantage of predictable immediate stability that allows for quicker rehabilitation with immediate full weight bearing. Most endoprostheses are modular, allowing for incremental limb lengthening as an immature patient grows. Improvements in implant materials have greatly increased the durability of modern endoprostheses; however, all are associated with long-term complications if a patient is cured of disease. Polyethylene wear is still a limiting factor for articulating surfaces, but the inserts are easily replaceable in most prostheses. Fatigue fracture can occur at the rotating hinge, but this, too, is easily replaceable. Fatigue fracture at the base of the intramedullary stem where it attaches to the body of the prosthesis is more problematic. In this location, extraction of the remaining stem can be extremely difficult.

Segmental bone and joint prostheses are most commonly secured through composite fixation. An intramedullary stem is fixed with cement, and the shoulder region of the prosthesis is constructed with a porous coating with the goal of promoting late extramedullary cortical bridging (Fig. 7.15).

Initial fixation with cement provides immediate stability for quick rehabilitation. The purpose of the extramedullary cortical bridging is to serve as a purse string to protect the cement-bone interface from particulate debris generated at the articulating surface and to provide additional structural

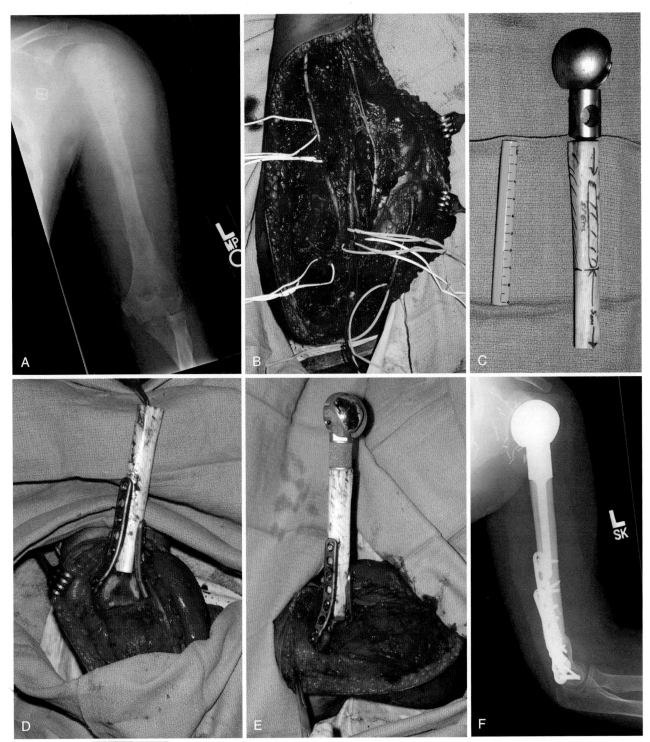

FIGURE 7.14 Ten-year-old girl with osteosarcoma of humerus. **A,** Anteroposterior radiograph of left humerus shows tumor extending down to distal diaphysis. **B,** Intraoperative photograph after wide resection of tumor. **C,** Humeral allograft is prepared to accept stem of tumor prosthesis. **D,** Allograft is fixed to remaining bone with medial and lateral plates. **E,** Prosthesis is cemented into allograft. **F,** Postoperative radiograph.

support protecting the junction of the base of the stem with the body of the prosthesis. This area is otherwise susceptible to fatigue fracture as a result of stress concentration. Although its benefit has not been established, bone grafting the shoulder region of the prosthesis to promote extracortical bridging has been advocated by several authors.

CONSIDERATIONS FOR PEDIATRIC PATIENTS

For pediatric patients, future limb-length inequality must be considered. For patients who are near skeletal maturity, the reconstructed limb can be lengthened 1 cm at the initial procedure. Also, epiphysiodesis of the contralateral limb can be

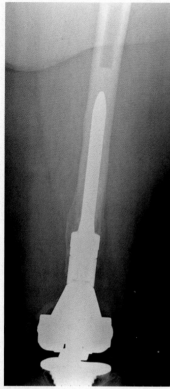

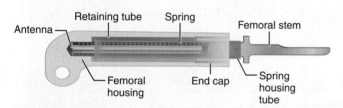

done at the appropriate age to preserve limb-length equality or minimize inequality. For younger patients, however, other options should be considered. Although amputation and rotationplasty were previously considered the only reasonable treatments for very young patients with bone sarcomas, use of expandable prostheses currently is gaining support.

We have gained considerable experience with use of the Repiphysis Expandable Prosthesis (Wright Medical Technology, Arlington, TN) (Fig. 7.16). The surgical technique for implantation of this device is similar to that of other endoprostheses (Fig. 7.17). The postoperative course, rehabilitation, function, and complications likewise are similar. The device is unique, however, in that it uses energy stored in a compressed spring to allow for future expansion of the prosthesis as the child grows. When a leg-length discrepancy develops, the child is scheduled for an expansion (Fig. 7.18). The procedure is done in the fluoroscopy suite with the patient under light sedation. The locking mechanism on the prosthesis is identified using fluoroscopy, and an electromagnetic coil is placed over the patient's leg at that level. The electromagnetic coil is activated for 20 seconds, which heats

an element in the prosthesis, melting a small segment of polyethylene and allowing controlled expansion of the spring. The leg lengths are reevaluated under fluoroscopy, and the procedure is repeated one or two times as necessary. We have been able to gain 0.5 to 1.5 cm during each scheduled expansion session. Expansion sessions can be scheduled 4 weeks apart if needed to allow the operated leg to "catch up." After the expansion sessions, patients usually are able to ambulate immediately without an assistive device. Although this device is not as durable and mechanical problems are common, complications are usually relatively easy to address. Moreover, skeletally immature patients treated for bone sarcomas are allowed to maintain limb-length equality at the completion of growth.

SURGICAL TECHNIQUES
UPPER EXTREMITY

In contrast to the lower extremity, even the best artificial limb fails to provide comparable function in the upper extremity. Modern imaging and surgical techniques allow for limb salvage in most circumstances. Resections of the proximal humerus frequently require sacrifice of the axillary nerve, and resections of the humeral shaft frequently require sacrifice of the radial nerve. Even with sacrifice of three major nerves, limb salvage usually provides better function than an artificial limb. If the median or ulnar nerve must be sacrificed, limb salvage still may be worthwhile if functioning muscles are available for transfers. One indication for amputation is extensive neurovascular involvement. A displaced pathologic fracture may be a relative indication.

■ RESECTION OF THE SHOULDER GIRDLE

Tumors of the scapula frequently are complicated by extension into the glenohumeral joint, requiring extraarticular resection of the humeral head en bloc with the scapula. Likewise, the biceps tendon provides a passageway for tumors of the proximal humerus to extend into the joint, and resection often requires extraarticular partial scapulectomy. To create a standard terminology for various surgical procedures for shoulder girdle resection and to allow meaningful comparison of results, Malawer et al. proposed a classification of these procedures. They noted that previous concepts have not adequately described surgical margins, the relationship of the tumor to anatomic compartments, the status of the glenohumeral joint, the magnitude of the surgical procedure, or the status of the abductor mechanism.

The proposed system is based solely on the structures removed, reflecting the type of resection and its relationship to the glenohumeral joint, and indicates a progressive increase in the magnitude of the surgical procedure. Additionally, it indicates the status of the abductor mechanism. Procedures are divided into six types: type I, intraarticular proximal humeral resection; type II, partial scapular resection; type III, intraarticular total scapulectomy; type IV, extraarticular total scapulectomy and humeral head resection; type V, extraarticular humeral head resection; and type VI, extraarticular humeral and total scapular resection. Each type is subdivided according to the status of the abductor mechanism: A, intact, or B, partial or complete resection (Fig. 7.19).

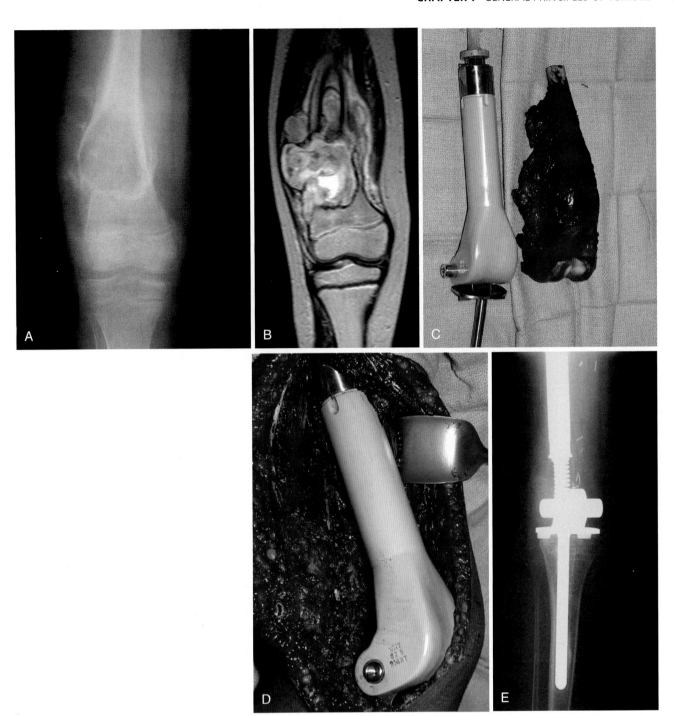

FIGURE 7.17 **A,** Anteroposterior radiograph of distal femur of 7-year-old girl with telangiectatic osteosarcoma. **B,** Coronal MR image. **C,** Intraoperative photograph of resected specimen and custom Repiphysis prosthesis. **D,** Intraoperative photograph after placement of prosthesis. **E,** Anteroposterior radiograph.

RESECTION OF THE SHOULDER GIRDLE

The Tikhoff-Linberg procedure for resection of the shoulder girdle consists of total scapulectomy, partial or complete excision of the clavicle, and excision of the proximal humerus. This procedure is useful in treating malignant tumors around the shoulder in which there exists a sufficient margin of normal tissue to clear the neurovascular structures.

TECHNIQUE 7.1

(MARCOVE, LEWIS, AND HUVOS)

- Place the patient in a loose lateral position that allows access to both the anterior and posterior portions of the shoulder. Prepare the entire extremity, the neck up to the ear, and the midline of the torso both anteriorly and posteriorly down to the iliac crest within the sterile field.

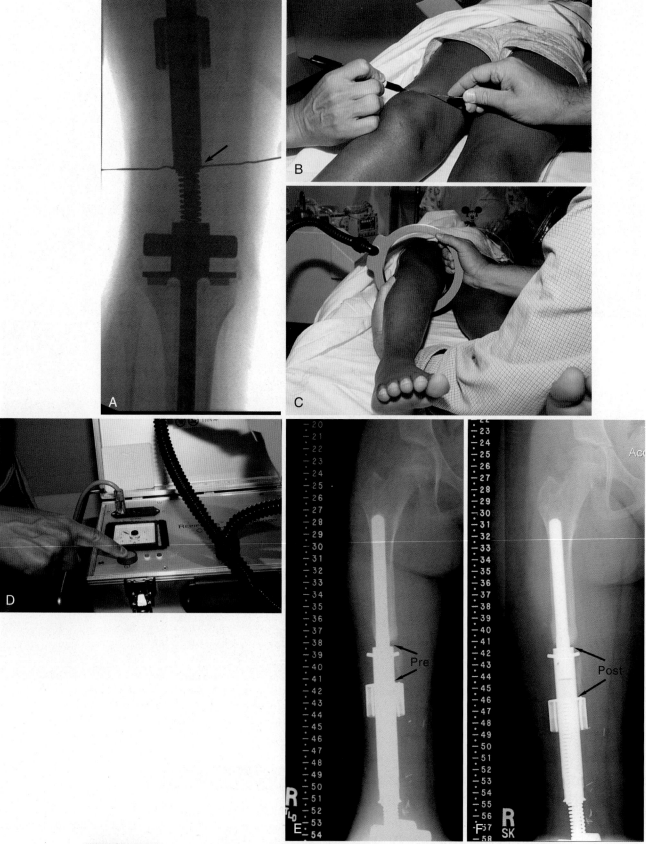

FIGURE 7.18   Lengthening procedure with Repiphysis expandable prosthesis. **A,** Locking mechanism *(arrow)* located. **B,** The patient's leg is marked at this site. **C,** Electromagnetic coil is placed around the patient's leg at the level of the locking mechanism. **D,** Device activated. **E and F,** Preexpansion and postexpansion radiographs.

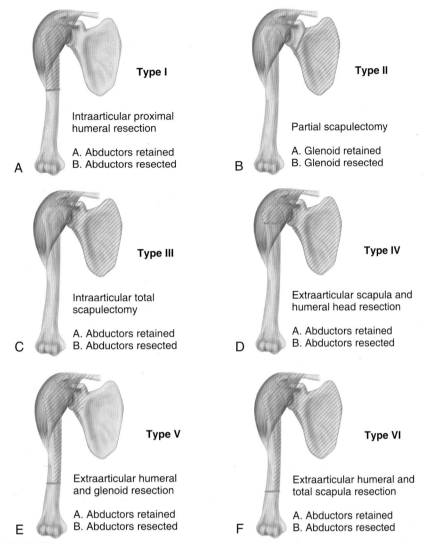

Type I

Intraarticular proximal
humeral resection

A. Abductors retained
B. Abductors resected

A

Type II

Partial scapulectomy

A. Glenoid retained
B. Glenoid resected

B

Type III

Intraarticular total
scapulectomy

A. Abductors retained
B. Abductors resected

C

Type IV

Extraarticular scapula and
humeral head resection

A. Abductors retained
B. Abductors resected

D

Type V

Extraarticular humeral
and glenoid resection

A. Abductors retained
B. Abductors resected

E

Type VI

Extraarticular humeral and
total scapula resection

A. Abductors retained
B. Abductors resected

F

FIGURE 7.19 Surgical classification of shoulder girdle resections. **A,** Type I: intraarticular proximal humeral resection. **B,** Type II: partial scapulectomy. **C,** Type III: intraarticular total scapulectomy. **D,** Type IV: extraarticular scapular and humeral head resection. **E,** Type V: extraarticular humeral and glenoid resection. **F,** Type VI: extraarticular humeral head and total scapular resection.

■ Make an incision beginning from the medial end of the clavicle and extend it laterally along the medial two thirds of the bone. Curve the incision is inferiorly over the coracoid process and continued along the medial aspect of the arm (Fig. 7.20A). From the middle of this incision, make a posterior longitudinal extension along the middle of the scapula to its inferior angle. Incise the deltoid and pectoralis major inferior to the clavicle and medial to the coracoid (Fig. 7.20B). Access to the neurovascular structures is facilitated by dividing and reflecting the pectoralis minor and the conjoined tendon at the insertion into the coracoid process. A gloved finger or instrument can be passed deep to these tendons to protect the deep structures during their division.

■ Ligate the cephalic vein and expose the axillary vessels and brachial plexus. Determine that the neurovascular bundle is not involved by tumor. Gentle medial traction of the neurovascular structures aids in identifying the anterior and posterior humeral circumflex vessels, which are then ligated. Protect the axillary vessels through the remainder of the case by medial retraction. If necessary, sacrifice the radial and musculocutaneous nerves.

■ Divide the biceps, triceps, teres major, and latissimus dorsi muscles away from the tumor (Fig. 7.20C).

■ Osteotomize the medial end of the clavicle.

■ Develop the posterior extension of the just-described incision. Maintain skin flaps as thick as possible and expose the medial and lateral borders of the scapula. Mobilize the inferior angle and vertebral border of the scapula by dividing the latissimus dorsi, trapezius, rhomboids, and levator scapulae muscles (Fig. 7.20D).

■ Take care to maintain wide soft-tissue margins in scapular lesions. If the lesion is in the proximal humerus, a scapular osteotomy can be made at the level of the coracoid; then the body of the scapula is spared.

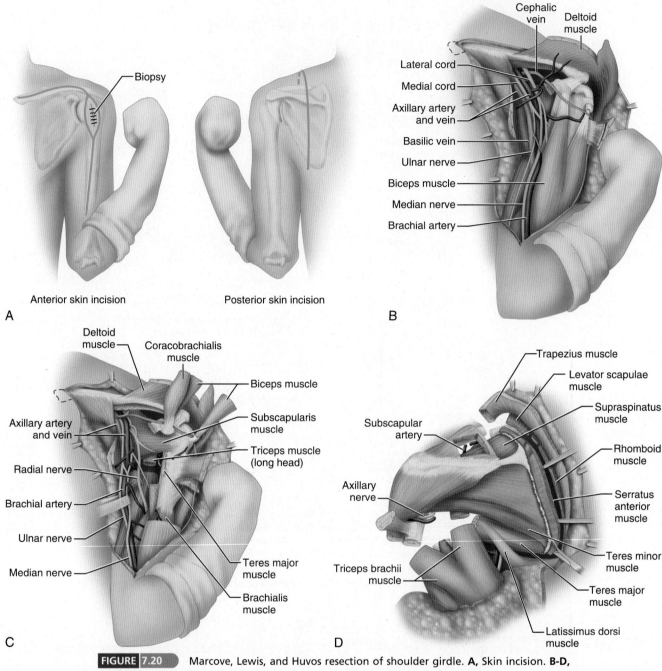

FIGURE 7.20 Marcove, Lewis, and Huvos resection of shoulder girdle. **A,** Skin incision. **B-D,** Surgical anatomy of resection (see text). (From Marcove RC, Lewis MM, Huvos AG: En bloc upper humeral interscapulothoracic resection: the Tikhoff-Linberg procedure, *Clin Orthop Relat Res* 124:219, 1977.) **SEE TECHNIQUE 7.1.**

- Raise a lateral skin flap over the upper arm, leaving the deltoid with the specimen.
- Complete the mobilization of the scapula by dividing the omohyoid and serratus anterior muscles and dividing and ligating the suprascapular, subscapular, and transverse cervical vessels.
- Divide the biceps and brachialis muscles at the intended site of the humeral osteotomy as determined from the preoperative imaging. Osteotomize the humerus at that

level and remove the specimen. Confirm adequate margins by biopsy and frozen sections.
- Reattach the biceps and triceps to the trapezius, pectoralis major, and latissimus dorsi.
- Insert a humeral prosthesis into the remaining humerus and attach the upper end to the second rib or remaining clavicle.
- Close the wound over drains and apply a shoulder immobilizer.

■ RESECTION OF THE CLAVICLE

Because the clavicle is subcutaneous, lesions in it usually are discovered early. Either end can be resected, or even the entire bone can be excised with little loss of function. Techniques of resecting the medial or lateral end of the clavicle are discussed in other chapter.

■ RESECTION OF THE SCAPULA

Parts of the scapula, varying from a small segment to the entire body of the bone, can be resected for benign or malignant tumors and infection. The subscapularis muscle often provides a good margin, protecting tumors of the scapula from direct chest wall invasion until late. Extension of the tumor into the chest wall or involvement with the neurovascular structures in the axilla would preclude consideration for scapular resection alone. After the scapular body or spine has been resected, the shoulder is fairly stable and functional because the acromion, the glenoid, and the coracoid are not disturbed and the humerus remains in a nearly normal position (Figs. 7.21 to 7.23). However, resection of the glenoid requires repair of the remaining soft tissues about the proximal humerus to provide some element of stability. Stability and functionality are less predictable in this situation.

RESECTION OF THE SCAPULA

TECHNIQUE 7.2

(DAS GUPTA)
- Place the patient in a loose lateral position. Drape the arm free so that an assistant can move the arm as required during the procedure (Fig. 7.23A).
- Make an elliptical skin incision encompassing the tumor and extending from the tip of the acromion superolaterally to the paravertebral region inferomedially (Fig. 7.23A).
- Raise the medial and lateral skin flaps on the investing fascia. Divide the attachment of the trapezius muscle to the scapular spine and retract the muscles superomedially, exposing the supraspinatus muscle (Fig. 7.23B).
- Divide the attachment of the deltoid muscle to the acromion. Divide the attachment of the latissimus dorsi to the inferior angle of the scapula and retract the muscle inferiorly.
- Apply traction to the inferior angle of the scapula with a towel clip and divide the muscles attached to the verte-

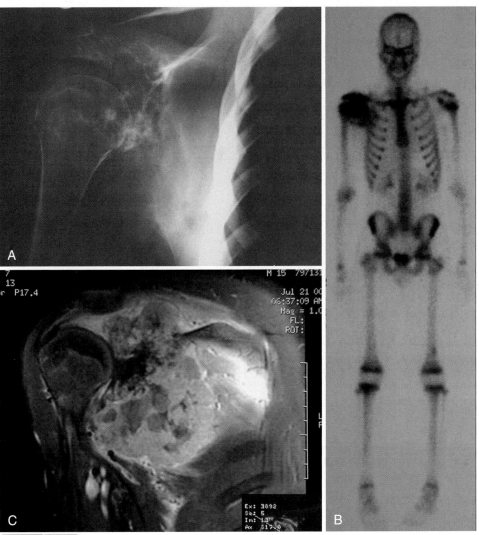

FIGURE 7.21 Scapulectomy in a 15-year-old boy with osteosarcoma of right scapula. **A,** Anteroposterior radiograph. **B,** Bone scan. **C,** MR image.

Continued

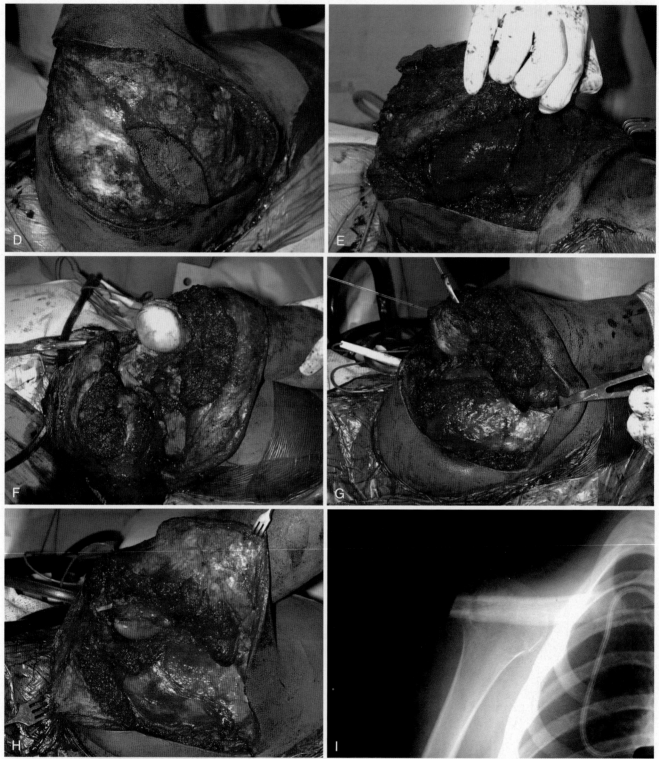

FIGURE 7.21, Cont'd   **D,** Medial and lateral flaps are raised. **E,** Deltoid, trapezius, rhomboids, and levator scapulae have been released from their insertions on the scapula. **F,** Scapula has been removed. **G,** Sutures are placed into tendon of long head of biceps and conjoined tendon. **H,** Tendons repaired through drill hole in clavicle. Deltoid is repaired to trapezius muscle. **I,** Postoperative radiograph.

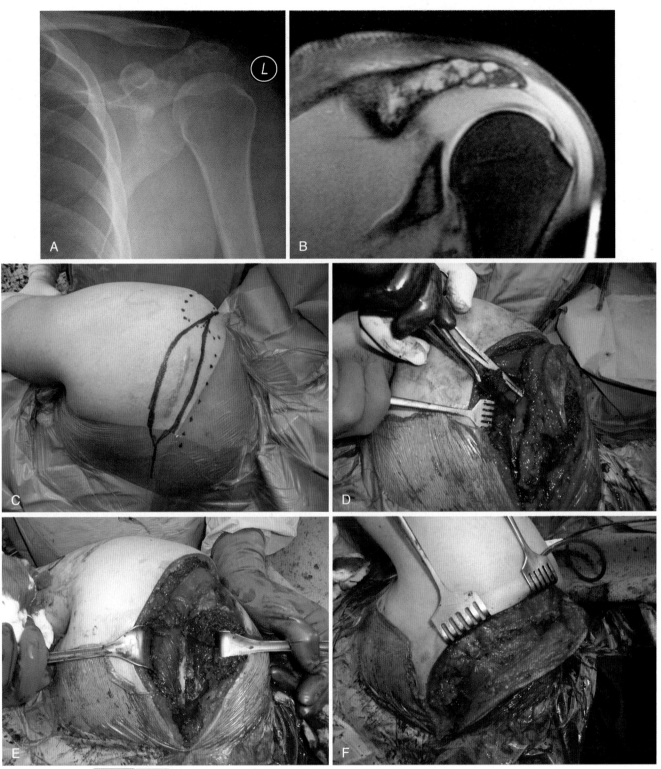

FIGURE 7.22 Chondrosarcoma of scapular spine and acromion. **A,** Anteroposterior radiograph. **B,** MR image shows extent of tumor. **C,** Incision ellipses around biopsy track. **D,** Osteotomy at base of scapular spine. **E,** Spine and acromion have been resected. **F,** Deltoid repaired to trapezius muscle.

Continued

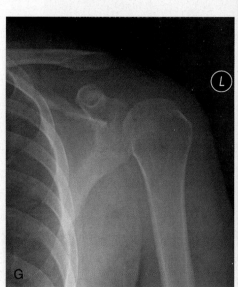
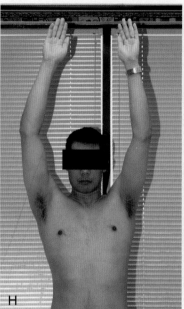
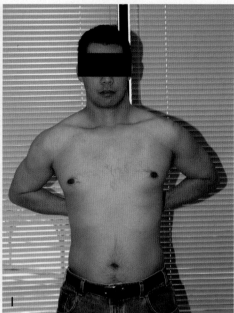

FIGURE 7.22, Cont'd   **G,** Postoperative radiograph. **H and I,** Clinical photographs show good shoulder function.

bral border of the scapula and the levator scapulae at the superior angle of the scapula (Fig. 7.23C).

- Rotate the scapula and abduct the arm, permitting the axillary contents to be retracted out of the operative field (Fig. 7.23D).
- Divide the teres major and minor and the long head of the triceps, followed by the supraspinatus and infraspinatus tendons and the attachment of the serratus anterior.
- Expose the shoulder joint and divide the scapular spine near the acromion using an osteotome or sagittal saw (Fig. 7.23E).
- Divide the subscapularis and pass a Gigli saw around the neck of the scapula, avoiding the glenohumeral joint, and divide the scapular neck to remove the specimen.
- Obtain hemostasis and approximate the trapezius and deltoid muscles (Fig. 7.23F). Suture the teres major and minor muscles to the chest wall, insert suction drains, and close the wound. Apply a shoulder immobilizer.

POSTOPERATIVE CARE   The immobilizer is removed after 48 hours, and a simple sling is applied. Active and active-assisted exercises of the shoulder are begun as soon as symptoms permit.

RESECTION OF THE PROXIMAL HUMERUS

Biopsy of a proximal humeral lesion should be done through the anterior third of the deltoid, taking care not to contaminate the deltopectoral interval. Contamination of this interval potentially could allow tumor cells to spread over a greater distance and would make a successful resection more difficult. Resection of the proximal humerus, with contiguous soft tissues, usually achieves satisfactory margins

for the treatment of sarcomas. We also have used this technique for treatment of aggressive benign neoplasms and metastatic carcinoma of the proximal humerus. Reconstructive alternatives after resection include flail shoulder, passive spacer, arthroplasty (implant or allograft), and arthrodesis. Allograft arthrodesis has been reported to be the most stable reconstruction for young patients who wish to pursue more vigorous activities; however, we have no experience with this procedure and use an endoprosthesis more frequently even if it serves only as a passive spacer.

TECHNIQUE 7.3

- Place the patient supine with a bolster under the scapula to elevate the shoulder from the table.
- Make an incision from the acromioclavicular joint along the deltopectoral groove and the lateral border of the biceps muscle to an appropriate level in the arm. The incision should form an ellipse around the biopsy track in the anterior third of the deltoid.
- Preoperative consideration must be given to the extraosseous extent of the tumor because this portion must also be resected with a wide margin.
- Divide the pectoralis major near its insertion into the proximal humerus leaving a margin of tissue. This allows good exposure of the neurovascular structures.
- Develop the interval between the neurovascular structures and the proximal humerus and dissect circumferentially around the proximal humerus leaving a cuff of normal muscle over the tumor. The conjoined tendon may be preserved and serves as a landmark for identifying the neurovascular structures, which are just medial. The musculocutaneous nerve is found within the substance of the conjoined tendon, and care must be exercised during retraction.
- Reflect the pectoralis muscle medially exposing the subscapularis muscle. Detach the muscles that insert on the

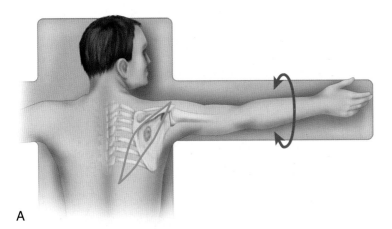

A

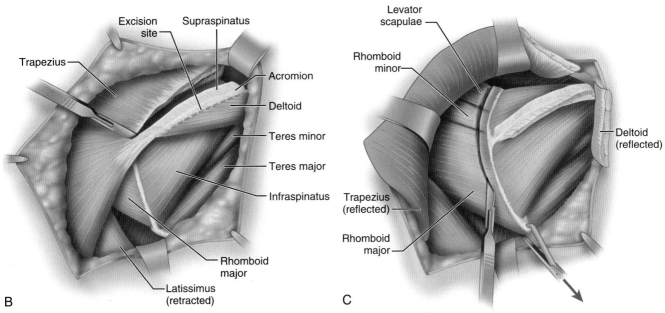

B   C

FIGURE 7.23   Scapulectomy for tumor. **A,** Position of patient and incision for surgery for tumor located in center of scapula *(dark spot).* Arm should be draped completely free so that it can be mobile to facilitate excision of muscular attachments. **B,** Scapular muscles exposed after raising skin flaps. Trapezius muscle is resected at scapular spine as shown. *Green dashed line* indicates site of excision of deltoid muscle. **C,** Trapezius and deltoid muscles have been reflected, and latissimus dorsi muscle has been retracted distally. Assistant is pulling tip of scapula laterally *(arrow).* This maneuver facilitates resection of muscles attached to vertebral border of scapula.

Continued

tuberosities and proximal humerus, preserving the radial and axillary nerves if possible.
■ Incise the capsule circumferentially. Lift the biceps tendon from its groove, retract it laterally, and then divide the humerus at a level distal to the tumor as determined by preoperative imaging (i.e., MRI).
■ After the osteotomy the specimen may be manipulated to facilitate release of any remaining soft-tissue attachments. With bone-holding forceps, grasp the distal end of the proximal fragment, detach any remaining soft tissues, and remove the specimen.

RECONSTRUCTION WITH FLAIL SHOULDER
■ The wound is closed over suction drains, and a shoulder immobilizer is applied. After 2 to 5 days, an arm sling is applied and active exercises are encouraged.

RECONSTRUCTION WITH PASSIVE SPACER
■ If sufficient soft tissue remains to provide adequate stability, a passive spacer yields better cosmesis and slightly better function than a flail shoulder. Allograft, autograft fibula, or prosthetic implant can be used (Fig. 7.24).

RECONSTRUCTION WITH ARTHROPLASTY
■ If the tumor resection permits sparing of the rotator cuff and deltoid muscle, reconstruction with arthroplasty is feasible using an osteoarticular allograft, allograft-prosthetic composite, or tumor prosthesis (Fig. 7.25).

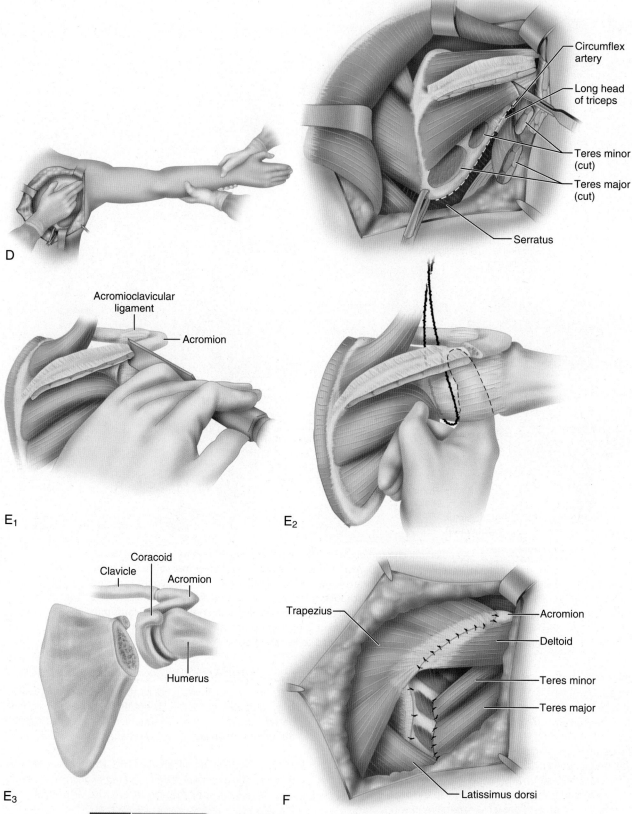

D

E₁

Acromioclavicular ligament

Acromion

E₂

E₃

Clavicle

Coracoid

Acromion

Humerus

F

Trapezius

Acromion

Deltoid

Teres minor

Teres major

Latissimus dorsi

Circumflex artery

Long head of triceps

Teres minor (cut)

Teres major (cut)

Serratus

FIGURE 7.23, Cont'd   **D,** *Inset,* Palpation of axillary contents, which need to be retracted out of operative field. Main illustration shows tip of scapula pulled inferomedially and muscles detached as shown. *Green broken line* indicates line of section of supraspinatus, infraspinatus, and serratus anterior muscles. **E₁,** Section of scapular spine at base of acromion with osteotome. After subscapularis muscle is cut under guidance of operator's finger, Gigli saw is passed around neck of scapula, which is sectioned (**E₂**). **E₃,** Excised scapula with intact shoulder joint. **F,** Closure and reattachment of muscles. Deltoid and trapezius are sutured to each other and to acromion process. Teres major and minor muscles are attached to thoracic wall. (Redrawn from Das Gupta TK: Scapulectomy: indications and technique, *Surgery* 67:601, 1970.) **SEE TECHNIQUE 7.2.**

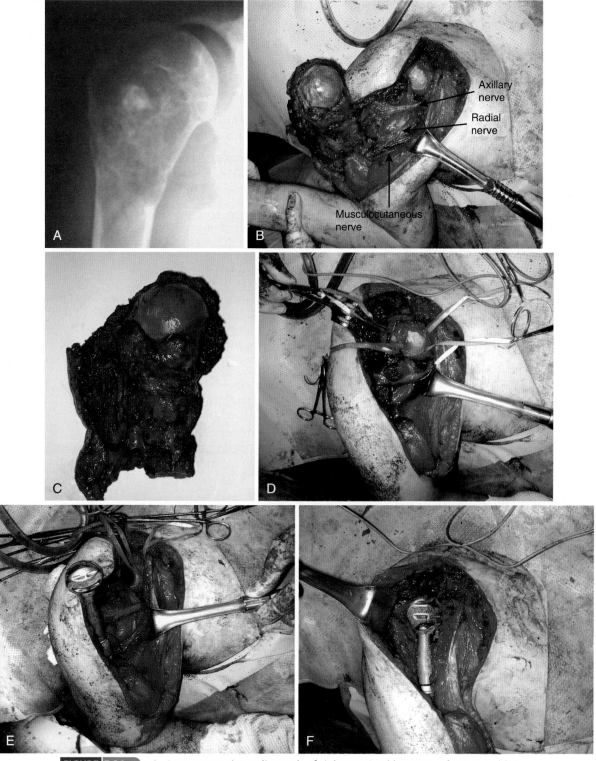

FIGURE 7.24   **A,** Anteroposterior radiograph of right proximal humerus of 47-year-old man with chondrosarcoma. **B,** Intraoperative photograph during wide resection of tumor. **C,** Resected specimen. **D,** Mersilene tapes placed through glenoid labrum. **E,** Prosthesis cemented into distal humerus. **F,** Humeral head secured by Mersilene tape. **SEE TECHNIQUE 7.3.**

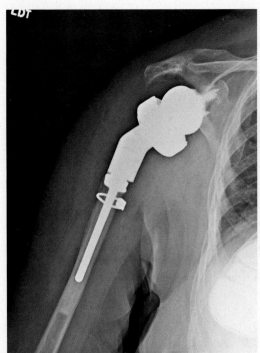

FIGURE 7.25   If deltoid function can be preserved, reconstruction can consist of a tumor prosthesis with reverse total shoulder arthroplasty.

INTERCALARY RESECTION OF THE HUMERAL SHAFT

Tumors of the humeral diaphysis can be treated with an intercalary resection, preserving the patient's own shoulder and elbow. Reconstruction is achieved by allograft, autograft (vascularized or not), or intercalary prosthetic replacement (Fig. 7.26).

TECHNIQUE 7.4

(LEWIS)
- Use the Henry extensile exposure to the humerus.
- Detach the pectoralis major insertion and retract the long head of the biceps laterally and the short head of the biceps and coracobrachialis medially.
- Identify the neurovascular bundle and mobilize it medially. Identify and protect the musculocutaneous, axillary, and radial nerves.
- Detach the latissimus dorsi, teres major, coracobrachialis, and triceps brachii muscles from the humerus. Make the proximal humeral osteotomy at an appropriate level. Elevate the humerus anteriorly from the wound, detach the remaining soft tissues, make the distal osteotomy, and remove the specimen from the wound. Reconstruct the skeleton with bone graft or prosthesis and close the wound over suction drains.

POSTOPERATIVE CARE A shoulder immobilizer is applied and worn for several days. An arm sling is then substituted, and gentle active exercises are begun.

RESECTION OF THE DISTAL HUMERUS

Bone sarcomas around the elbow suitable for limb-sparing resection are rare. Patients with metastatic carcinomas, multiple myeloma, or aggressive benign lesions, such as chondroblastoma or giant cell tumor, may be best treated with such surgery (Fig. 7.27). Reconstruction options include flail elbow, osteoarticular allograft, implant arthroplasty, and arthrodesis.

TECHNIQUE 7.5

- Use the Henry extensile approach to the humerus (see chapter 1).
- Identify and mobilize the radial and median nerves and the brachial vessels. (Alternatively, approach the distal humerus through a posterior approach after isolating and protecting the ulnar nerve.)
- Osteotomize the humerus at an appropriate level.
- Attach a bone-holding forceps and draw the bone anteriorly from the wound.
- Detach all muscle attachments extraperiosteally by sharp dissection and remove the specimen.
- Reconstruct the elbow and close the wound over suction drains.

POSTOPERATIVE CARE A bulky Jones-type dressing is applied with the elbow at 90 degrees and the forearm in midrotation. The extremity is supported with a sling.

RESECTION OF THE PROXIMAL RADIUS

Considerable portions of the proximal radius can be resected without reconstruction (Fig. 7.28).

TECHNIQUE 7.6

- Either the dorsal (Thompson) or anterior (Henry) approach can be used (see chapter 1).
- Identify and protect the radial vessels and deep branch of the radial nerve.
- Divide the bone at an appropriate level, elevate it from the wound with bone-holding forceps, detach the muscles extraperiosteally by sharp dissection, and remove the specimen.
- Close the wound over suction drains and apply a posterior plaster splint with the elbow at 90 degrees and the forearm in neutral rotation. Active exercises are begun at about 2 weeks.

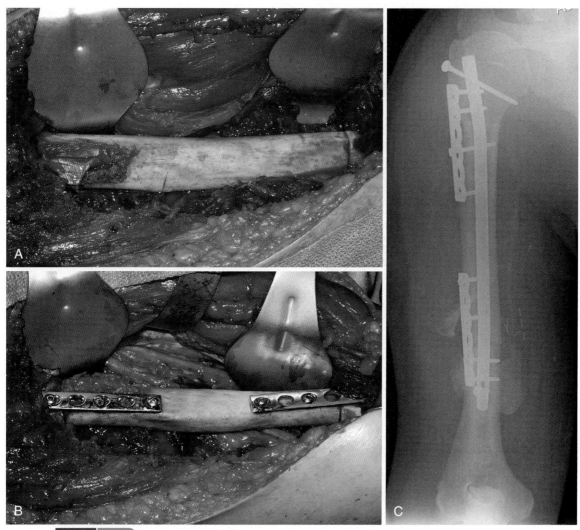

FIGURE 7.26 Intercalary humeral allograft in 19-year-old man with Ewing sarcoma. **A,** Allograft is fashioned to fit defect and is fixed with intramedullary nail. **B,** Compression plates used to fix proximal and distal junctions. **C,** Postoperative radiograph. **SEE TECHNIQUE 7.4.**

RESECTION OF THE PROXIMAL ULNA

TECHNIQUE 7.7

- Make a longitudinal posterior approach to the proximal ulna. Detach the triceps mechanism and make the osteotomy in the ulna at an appropriate level.
- Elevate the bone from the wound with bone-holding forceps and sharply detach any remaining soft tissues extraperiosteally.
- A size-matched osteoarticular allograft reconstruction can be performed (Fig. 7.29). The allograft should come with triceps tendon as well as medial and lateral ligaments, which can be repaired to host structures.
- Close the wound over suction drains and apply a posterior splint with the elbow at 90 degrees and the forearm in midrotation. Active exercises are begun at 4 to 6 weeks.

RESECTION OF THE DISTAL RADIUS

Resection of the distal radius has been particularly useful in treating patients with giant cell tumor. Reconstruction can be accomplished by arthroplasty or arthrodesis using allograft or autograft bone. We prefer resection followed by proximal fibular autograft reconstruction arthroplasty for patients who wish to maintain motion and perform light activities and arthrodesis for patients who wish to sacrifice motion in exchange for a more stable reconstruction (Fig. 7.30).

TECHNIQUE 7.8

- Use the dorsal approach to the radius (see chapter 1).
- Divide the extensor retinaculum and develop an interval between the third and fourth extensor compartments.

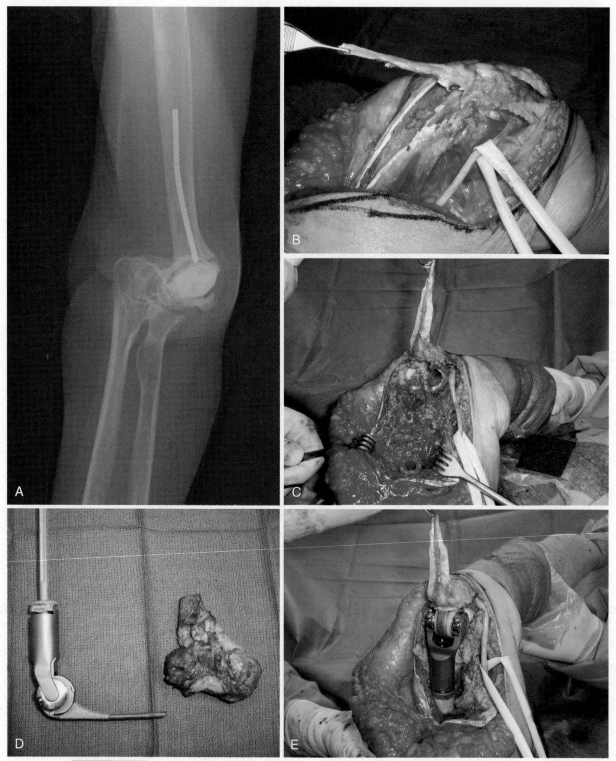

FIGURE 7.27   Fifty-nine-year-old woman with isolated metastasis from renal cell carcinoma was treated initially at outside facility with radiation, curettage, and cementation for pathologic distal humeral fracture. **A,** Anteroposterior radiograph shows failure of construct. **B,** Tongue of triceps tendon is reflected distally. **C,** Distal humerus is resected, and ulna is prepared to receive prosthesis. **D,** Resected distal humerus and prosthesis. **E,** Prosthesis cemented into humerus and ulna.

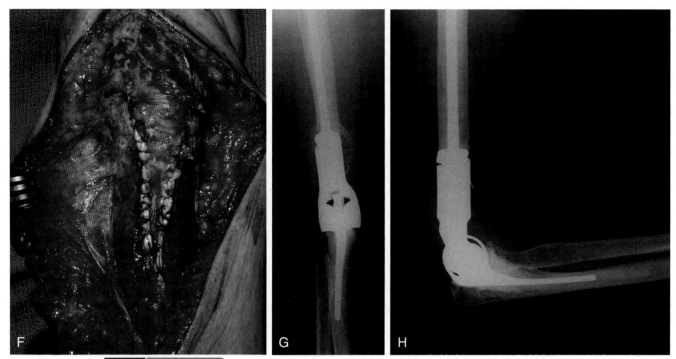

FIGURE 7.27, Cont'd · **F,** Triceps repaired. **G and H,** Anteroposterior and lateral postoperative radiographs.

Retract the extensor tendons to allow full exposure of the distal radius.

- Use a power saw to divide the radius proximal to the tumor at a level determined from preoperative imaging.
- Grasp the proximal end of the distal fragment with bone-holding forceps and draw it gently forward from the wound. Using sharp extraperiosteal dissection, remove bone and tumor.
- Change gown and gloves and use separate instruments to remove an appropriate length (the length of the resected radius) of the ipsilateral proximal fibula.
- As an alternative, use a size-matched distal radial allograft to replace the resected portion.
- Insert the transplant so that the apex of its head replaces the radial styloid and its articular cartilage on the anteromedial aspect of its head articulates with the scaphoid.
- Fix the fibular graft to the radius with a plate and screws. Stabilize the carpus on the distal end of the fibular transplant with one or two Kirschner wires.

PROXIMAL FIBULAR AUTOGRAFT FUSION

- With rongeurs and curets, remove the cartilage from the proximal ends of the carpus (i.e., scaphoid and lunate) and the distal radial allograft. Use a power burr if needed to obtain congruency between the two surfaces. Fashion the cortical ends of the host radius and the proximal allograft to achieve maximal contact.
- Contour a 3.5-mm plate with the wrist in slight dorsiflexion and fixed dorsally. The plate extends distally from the radial diaphysis and is centered over the third metacarpal. Compression at the allograft-host junction can be achieved using the plate (Fig. 7.30).

POSTOPERATIVE CARE The upper extremity is splinted from above the elbow to the proximal palmar crease with the elbow at 90 degrees, the forearm in neutral rotation, and the wrist in 20 degrees of dorsiflexion. At 6 weeks, the splint and wires are removed and gentle active exercises are begun.

RESECTION OF THE DISTAL ULNA

We have used resection of the distal ulna for a giant cell tumor; no graft is used (Fig. 7.31). The operation is similar to that of Darrach, but the periosteum is excised along with the tumor.

RESECTION OF THE HAND

Resection of tumors of the hand is discussed in other chapter.

PELVIS

Local resections of the pelvis often can be performed with the same surgical margins obtainable by amputation. Amputation is associated with fewer complications, quicker recovery, a more predictable outcome, and a lower incidence of local recurrence. Amputation may be indicated if the internal or external iliac vessels are involved. Resection is technically more demanding than amputation, but function usually is better if the limb can be preserved even without a functioning sciatic or femoral nerve. Preoperative planning is crucial. Imaging modalities are utilized to determine the osseous and extraosseous extent of tumor and their respective relationships to neurovascular structures and pelvic viscera. We have begun performing computer-assisted surgery in selected cases (Fig. 7.32). Resections of the pelvis are classified as

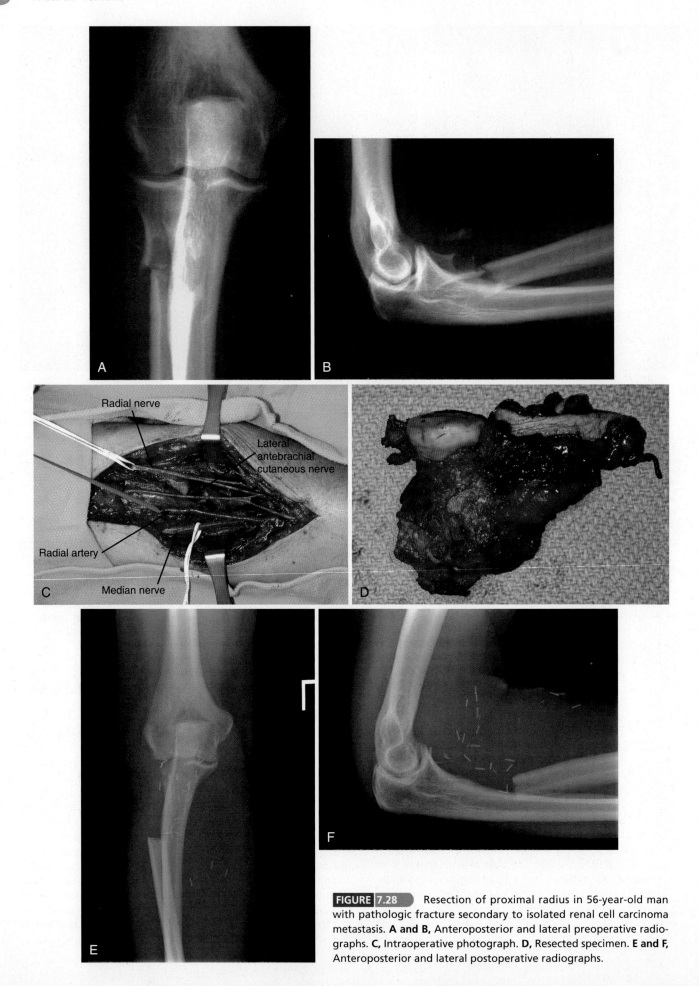

Resection of proximal radius in 56-year-old man with pathologic fracture secondary to isolated renal cell carcinoma metastasis. **A and B,** Anteroposterior and lateral preoperative radiographs. **C,** Intraoperative photograph. **D,** Resected specimen. **E and F,** Anteroposterior and lateral postoperative radiographs.

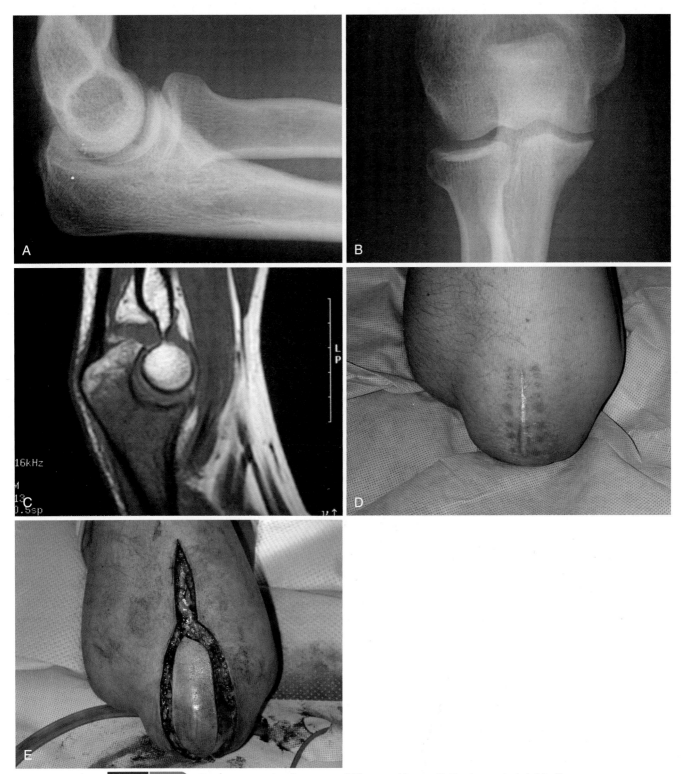

FIGURE 7.29 Osteosarcoma in olecranon of 20-year-old man. Patient reported right elbow pain 3 years after resection of femoral osteosarcoma. **A and B,** Lateral and anteroposterior radiographs of right elbow appear normal. **C,** MR image clearly shows lesion in olecranon. Incisional biopsy revealed osteosarcoma. **D,** Biopsy scar. **E,** Incision was made over subcutaneous border of proximal ulna, leaving biopsy track intact.

Continued

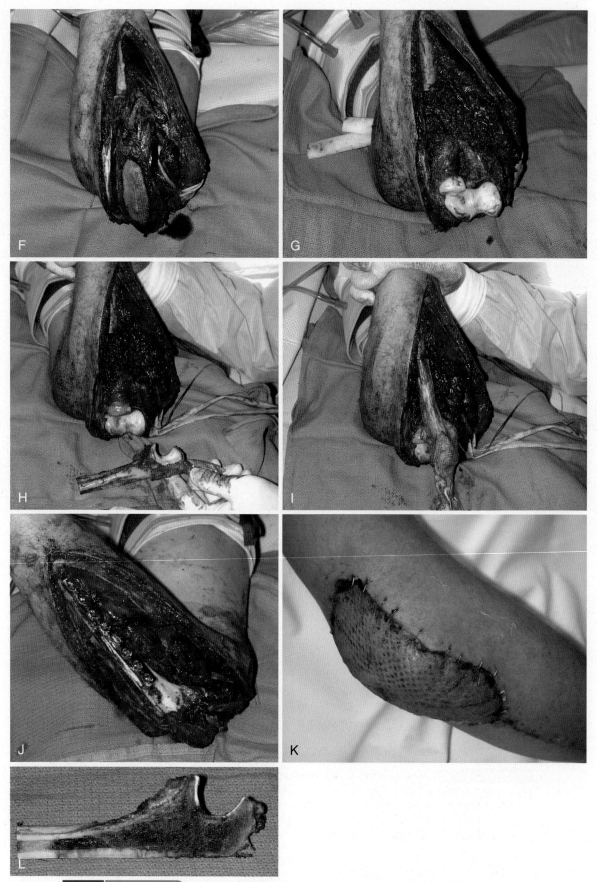

FIGURE 7.29, Cont'd   **F,** Ulnar osteotomy was performed distally to ensure wide margin. Ulnar nerve isolated and protected while proximal ulna was resected with wide margins. **G,** Specimen removed from field. **H and I,** Allograft of proximal ulna with triceps tendon cut and placed in defect. **J,** Allograft was fixed to distal ulna using 3.5-mm dynamic compression plate. Triceps tendon and elbow joint capsule are repaired. **K,** Wound was covered with free gracilis flap and split-thickness skin graft. **L,** Photograph of cut specimen after removal of soft tissue. **SEE TECHNIQUE 7.7.**

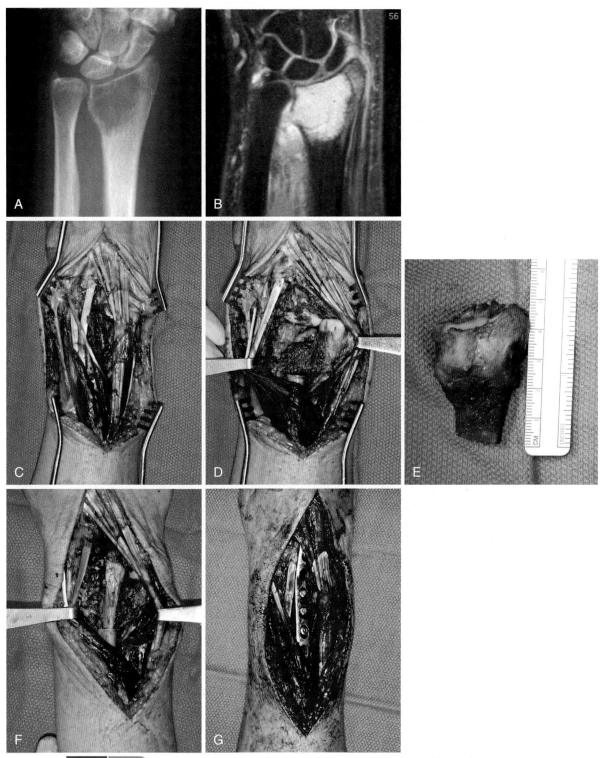

FIGURE 7.30   **A,** Anteroposterior radiograph of 56-year-old woman with giant cell tumor of distal radius. **B,** MR image shows extent of tumor and soft-tissue mass. **C,** Distal radius approached dorsally. **D,** Tumor was resected. **E,** Resected specimen. **F,** Proximal fibular autograft fashioned to fit defect. **G,** Wrist fusion with contoured 3.5-mm plate extending from radial diaphysis to third metacarpal. **SEE TECHNIQUE 7.8.**

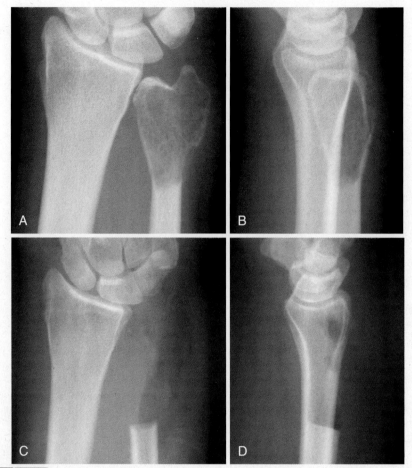

FIGURE 7.31 Resection of distal ulna. **A and B,** Anteroposterior and lateral radiographs of giant cell tumor of distal ulna. **C and D,** Postoperative radiographs.

type I, iliac; type II, periacetabular; type III, obturator; and type IV, sacral (Fig. 7.33). Resections involving more than one area are described by combining the numbers. A resection that involves the acetabulum and the iliac wing would be described as a type I, II pelvic resection. The letter *H* is added as a suffix if the femoral head is resected with the specimen.

All pelvic resections can be done through all or part of a standard utilitarian incision (Fig. 7.34). The incision begins at the anterior superior iliac spine and courses parallel to the inguinal ligament to the pubic tubercle medially. For posterior exposure along the ilium, the incision can be curved posteriorly along the iliac brim to the posterior superior iliac spine. Exposure of the femoral vessels anteriorly, the posterior acetabulum, the proximal femur, and ischium can be accomplished by a T-shaped extension incision beginning at the anterior superior iliac spine and coursing distally and posteriorly over the greater trochanter. A similar T-shaped incision can be made medially to expose the obturator foramen and ischial tuberosity.

Type I resections do not require reconstruction. A 1- to 2-cm leg-length discrepancy may result if the entire ilium is resected because there is no osseous bridge between the acetabulum and sacrum; however, this usually is not problematic because an ipsilateral shoe lift can be used. Alternatively, an allograft strut can be used to bridge the gap between the acetabulum and the sacrum to prevent the superior migration of the lower extremity and subsequent development of a limb-length discrepancy (Fig. 7.35). Type II resections can be

reconstructed with an iliofemoral or an ischiofemoral arthrodesis with an allograft-prosthesis composite, or with a saddle prosthesis (Fig. 7.36). Alternatively, type II resections can be treated simply by repairing the remaining soft tissues. Patients treated in this manner experience significant shortening of the limb but ambulate remarkably well with a shoe lift (Fig. 7.37). Type III resections do not require reconstruction because the pubis does not bear weight. Additionally, pelvic stability is maintained by the intact sacroiliac joints posteriorly.

RESECTION OF THE PUBIS AND ISCHIUM

Partial or complete resection of the pubis or ischium or both may be indicated for tumor or infection (Fig. 7.38 and Fig. 7.39). The surgical approach is a modification of that described by Milch.

TECHNIQUE 7.9

(RADLEY, LIEBIG, AND BROWN)

- Position the patient as for a lithotomy and elevate the buttocks.

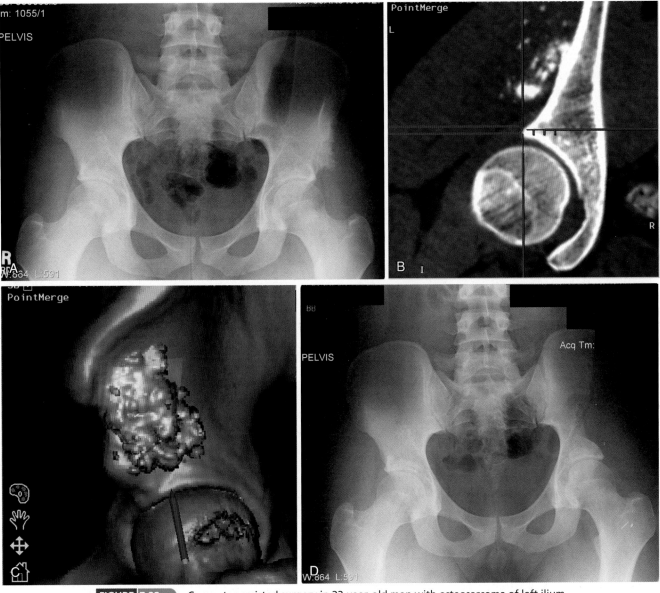

FIGURE 7.32 Computer-assisted surgery in 22-year-old man with osteosarcoma of left ilium. **A,** Anteroposterior radiograph. **B and C,** Intraoperative computer-assisted guidance allowed resection of tumor with preservation of hip joint. **D,** Postoperative anteroposterior radiograph.

- Palpate the tuberosity of the ischium, the inferior border of the pubis, and the connecting ramus. Make an incision through the skin and subcutaneous tissues, beginning at a point 0.6 cm distal to the middle of the inguinal ligament and proceeding medially and parallel to it (Fig. 7.38A). At the lateral aspect of the base of the penis or mons pubis, curve the incision distalward lateral to the scrotum or labium majus pudenda and continue it along the inferior ramus of the ischium to the ischial tuberosity.
- Detach the adductor and obturator externus muscles subperiosteally from the pubis and ischium and expose a part of the body of the pubis, the lateral border of the inferior ramus of the pubis, the inferior ramus of the ischium, and the ischial tuberosity.
- To expose the pubis and ischium more completely, retract or incise the distal edge of the gluteus maximus muscle in

line with the skin incision. Dissect the hamstring muscles and the quadratus femoris from the lateral aspect of the ischial tuberosity; free the sacrotuberous ligament from its attachment to the medial surface of the tuberosity.
- Protect the pudendal vessels and nerve that emerge from the pelvis through the greater sciatic foramen, cross the spine of the ischium and the sacrotuberous ligament, enter the lesser sciatic foramen, and proceed anteriorly in the Alcock canal within the fascia of the obturator internus muscle. To avoid damaging this canal and its contents, elevate subperiosteally the ischiocavernosus and obturator internus muscles.
- Subperiosteally free the deep and superficial transverse perineal muscles, the crus penis, and the constrictor urethrae from the medial borders of the inferior ischial and pubic rami.

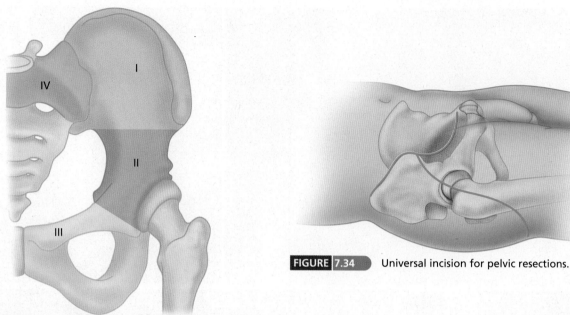

FIGURE 7.34   Universal incision for pelvic resections.

FIGURE 7.33   Types of pelvic resections: type I, iliac; type II, periacetabular; type III, obturator; type IV, sacral.

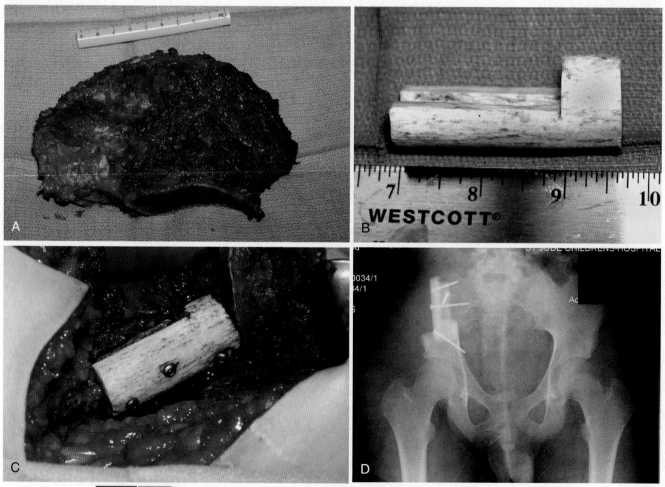

FIGURE 7.35   Femoral allograft for type I pelvic resection in 16-year-old boy with Ewing sarcoma. **A,** Resected ilium. **B,** Femoral allograft fashioned to fit between acetabulum and sacrum. **C,** Multiple screws used to secure allograft. **D,** Postoperative radiograph.

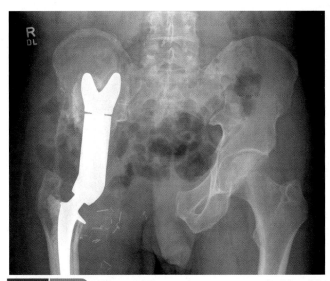

FIGURE 7.36 Type II pelvic resection reconstructed with saddle prosthesis.

- Dissect the urogenital diaphragm from the inferior border of the symphysis pubis but avoid injuring the urethra and the deep dorsal vein, dorsal artery, and nerve of the penis.
- Free the rectus abdominis and pyramidalis muscles from the pubis.
- Divide the inguinal ligament at its pubic end and free the pectineus muscle from its origin along the pectineal line of the superior ramus of the pubis (Fig. 7.38B).
- Mobilize the pectineus muscle but avoid injuring the femoral sheath and its contents that lie on the lateral part of the muscle.
- Dissect the obturator internus and externus muscles subperiosteally and, if possible, preserve the obturator nerves and vessels that may be encountered.
- Divide the bone superiorly and inferiorly with an osteotome or Gigli saw (Fig. 7.38C).
- If the wound is to be closed primarily, suture the deep fascia; if not, omit suturing the fascia and allow the muscles to fall into position.

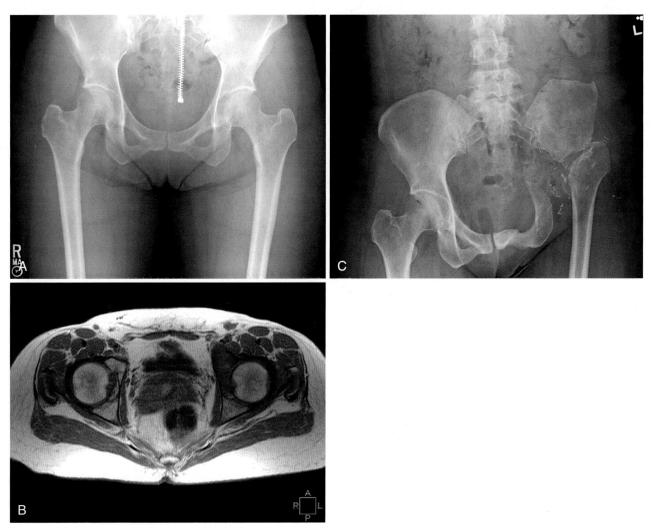

FIGURE 7.37 A 42-year-old female with complaints of left groin pain. Although the anteroposterior pelvic radiograph **(A)** was unremarkable, axial T-1 weighted magnetic resonance imaging **(B)** demonstrated a lesion involving the left acetabulum; biopsy revealed conventional chondrosarcoma. **C,** Ten years after resection and soft-tissue reconstruction, the patient has no pain and ambulated well with a shoe lift with only a mild Trendelenburg gait.

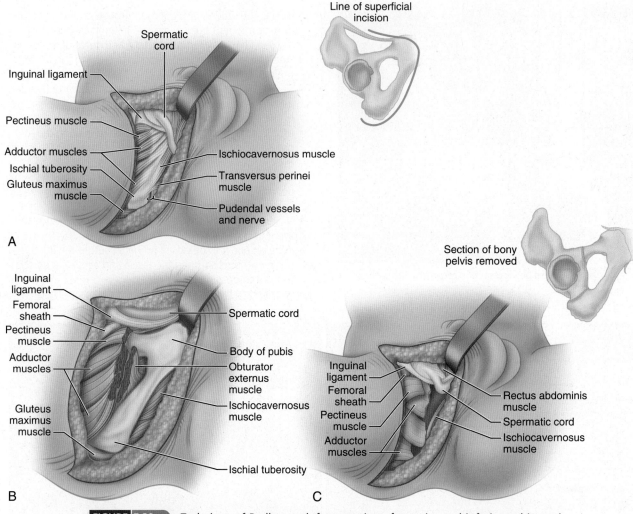

FIGURE 7.38 Technique of Radley et al. for resection of superior and inferior pubic rami and body of pubis, inferior ischial ramus, and tuberosity of ischium. *Inset,* Incision. **A,** Superficial approach. **B,** Further exposure. Note amount of bony pelvis resectable through this approach. **C,** Appearance after resection of pubis and ischium (see text for method of closure). (Modified from Radley TJ, Liebig CA, Brown JR: Resection of the body of the pubic bone, the superior and inferior pubic rami, the inferior ischial ramus, and the ischial tuberosity: a surgical approach, *J Bone Joint Surg* 36A:855, 1954.) **SEE TECHNIQUE 7.9.**

RESECTION OF THE ACETABULUM

Resection of the acetabulum with preservation of the limb is indicated for lesions that can be treated satisfactorily by wide resection of the mid and anterior hemipelvis. Careful staging is required, and any biopsy track must be excised en bloc with the resection.

TECHNIQUE 7.10

- Place the patient in the lateral decubitus position and strapped to the table so that the table can be tilted to either side. Prepare and drape the involved limb and pelvis from toes to rib cage.

- Make an incision extending from the posterior crest of the ilium coursing over the anterior superior iliac spine to the symphysis pubis. Make a vertical T-shaped extension from this incision over the greater trochanter and extending into the proximal thigh. Divide the middle of the inguinal ligament and retract the peritoneum superiorly.
- Mobilize and medially retract the femoral artery and vein and the femoral nerve. The femoral nerve is found within the iliopsoas sheath and may be left in continuity.
- Divide the iliacus and pectineus muscles.
- Expose the innominate bone from the symphysis pubis to the anterior superior iliac spine and both surfaces of the bones posteriorly to the sciatic notch. A renal pedicle clamp can be used to pass a Gigli saw through the sciatic notch.

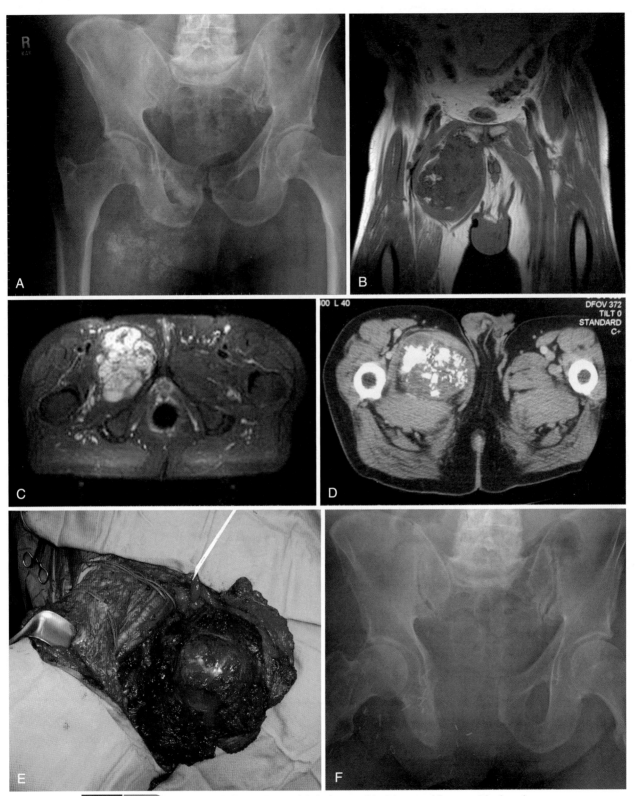

FIGURE 7.39 Resection of superior and inferior rami in 79-year-old man with chondrosarcoma. **A,** Anteroposterior radiograph. **B and C,** MR images. **D,** CT scan shows extent of lesion. **E,** Intraoperative photograph of wide resection. Femoral vessels and nerve have been dissected away from tumor. **F,** Postoperative radiograph.

The clamp must stay in contact with the bone as it is advanced within the sciatic notch to avoid entrapment of the sciatic nerve or other neurovascular structures beneath the Gigli saw. With a Gigli saw, divide the bone along a line extending from the sciatic notch to a point inferior to the anterior superior iliac spine.

- After the osteotomy, the bone may be mobilized enough to help determine remaining soft-tissue attachments that need to be detached. Divide the sacrotuberous and sacrospinous ligaments and release the hamstrings.
- Anteriorly, divide the pubic bone or symphysis pubis and rotate the segment of bone in various directions to release the remaining soft tissues.
- Release the piriformis from the greater trochanter, divide the femoral neck at its base, and remove the resected part of the pelvis and the femoral head and neck.
- Fix the proximal femur to the remaining ilium with heavy nonabsorbable suture. Reattach the inguinal ligament to the iliopsoas tendon to prevent a hernia.
- Close the wound over suction drains.

POSTOPERATIVE CARE Protected ambulation in a hip abduction brace with crutches is begun postoperatively.

RESECTION OF THE INNOMINATE BONE (INTERNAL HEMIPELVECTOMY)

Numerous surgeons have described methods of pelvic resection, including Karakousis and Vezeridis; Eilber et al.; Steel; Enneking and Dunham; Braund and Pigott; and others. The technique of Karakousis and Vezeridis is described here (Figs. 7.40 and 7.41). This procedure is indicated in patients who are willing to undergo the vigorous rehabilitation necessary and in whom appropriate margins can be obtained by pelvic resection.

TECHNIQUE 7.11

(KARAKOUSIS AND VEZERIDIS)
- Place the patient in a loose lateral position to allow both anterior and posterior rotation of the patient. Begin with the involved hemipelvis elevated 45 degrees. Extend the incision from the posterior superior iliac spine along the iliac crest and inguinal ligament to the symphysis pubis. Make a vertical limb from this incision passing just posterior to the greater trochanter and extending into the upper thigh.
- Detach the abdominal muscles from the iliac crest and displace the peritoneum medially to expose the external iliac vessels.
- Divide the inguinal ligament near the anterior superior iliac spine and divide and ligate the inferior epigastric vessels (Fig. 7.40A).
- Detach the inguinal ligament from the pubic tubercle and the rectus abdominis from the pubic crest. Clear the pubic symphysis of soft tissue and divide it with a Gigli saw (Fig.

7.40B). A malleable retractor can be placed posterior to the pubic symphysis to protect the bladder during this portion of the operation.
- Expose the common iliac vessels and the femoral nerve.
- Preserve the iliopsoas muscle unless involved by tumor. Next, pass an umbilical tape around the psoas muscle and iliac vessels (Fig. 7.40C).
- Divide the iliacus muscle at the level of the sacroiliac joint and sever the adductor muscles from the pubis. Divide the obturator nerve and vessels.
- Divide the origins of the sartorius, tensor fascia lata, and rectus femoris. The origins of the gluteus medius and minimus can be removed from the ilium leaving a small cuff of tissue.
- Incise the hip joint capsule and divide the femoral neck with a power saw.
- Incise the gluteus maximus muscle inferior and posterior to the greater trochanter, exposing the sciatic nerve. Divide the external rotators at the greater trochanter, expose the sacroiliac joint, and divide it with an osteotome (Fig. 7.40D). If tumor involves the joint, osteotomize the sacrum while retracting the lumbosacral nerve trunk medially (Fig. 7.40E).
- Divide the levator ani muscle and the sacrospinous and sacrotuberous ligaments.
- Release the hamstring origins from the ischial tuberosity.
- Retract the hemipelvis laterally and release the remaining attachments of the adductor magnus from the ischial ramus, allowing removal of the specimen (Fig. 7.40F).
- The procedure can be modified so that uninvolved portions of the innominate bone are spared.
- Cover the exposed femoral neck with one of the adjacent divided muscles. Close the wound in layers.

POSTOPERATIVE CARE The patient is placed in a hip abduction brace. Non-weight-bearing ambulation is continued for 6 weeks. The abduction brace is then discontinued, and the patient may progress weight bearing as tolerated. After several months, walking with the aid of a single cane may be possible.

RESECTION OF THE SACROILIAC JOINT

The sacroiliac joint can be resected using a combined posterior and anterior approach. The surgical team includes a general surgeon, a neurosurgeon, and an orthopaedic surgeon.

TECHNIQUE 7.12

- Place the patient in the lateral decubitus position with the affected side uppermost. Prepare and drape the trunk and affected extremity to below the knee.
- Make an L-shaped incision with the vertical portion along the lumbar spinous processes and the transverse portion extending from the distal end of the vertical incision along the iliac crest and onto the lower abdomen.

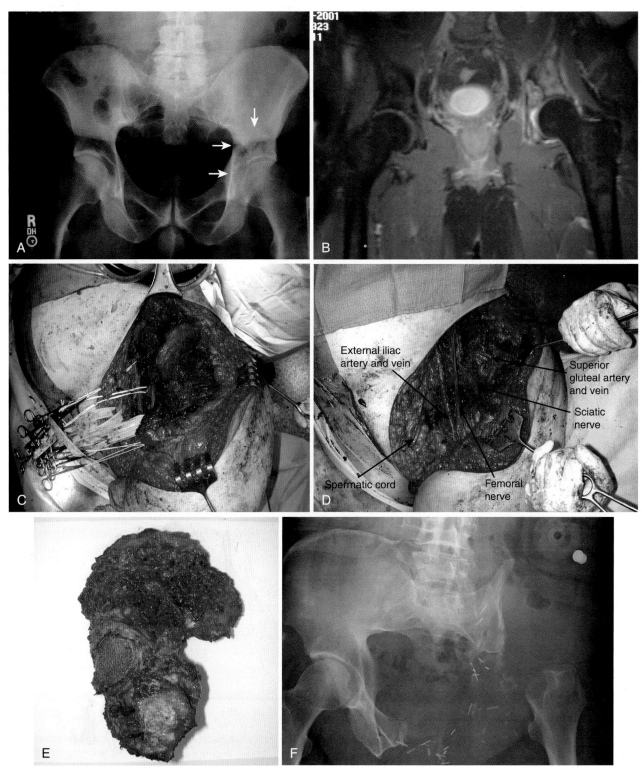

FIGURE 7.40   Internal hemipelvectomy. **A,** Anteroposterior radiograph. *Arrows* point to lytic lesion. **B,** MR image shows osteosarcoma in 57-year-old man. **C,** Extensile approach is used, and external iliac vessels, femoral nerve, and spermatic cord are isolated. **D,** Hemipelvis has been removed. All major neurovascular structures were protected. **E,** Resected specimen. **F,** Postoperative anteroposterior radiograph. **SEE TECHNIQUE 7.11.**

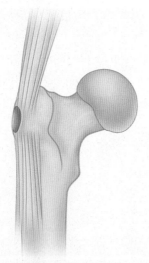

FIGURE 7.41   Proximal femoral biopsy site.

- Dissect subperiosteally the sacrospinalis along the side of the lesion and divide it at its sacroiliac origin.
- Identify the L4, L5, and S1 nerve roots and dissect them laterally to the region of the sacroiliac joint.
- Dissect the gluteal musculature from the external surface of the ilium subperiosteally and dissect the anterior abdominal wall musculature and iliacus from the inner surface of the ilium.
- Push the ureter and great vessels anteriorly by blunt retroperitoneal dissection.
- Divide the ilium and sacrum with a Gigli saw and osteotome, carefully protecting the L4, L5, and S1 nerve roots. Remove the lesion and the contiguous sacrum and ilium.
- Insert suction drains and approximate the sacrospinalis and iliacus muscles, the abdominal wall musculature, and the gluteal musculature.

POSTOPERATIVE CARE Non–weight-bearing ambulation is permitted with a walker for 6 weeks and then gradually increased weight bearing as tolerated is allowed over the next several weeks.

RESECTION OF THE SACRUM

Sacral tumors, such as giant cell tumor or chordoma, are probably best resected using a combined anterior and posterior (abdominosacral) exposure. A team consisting of a general surgeon, a neurosurgeon, and an orthopaedic surgeon makes the operation easier and safer. A preoperative bowel preparation is recommended.

Stener and Gunterberg described a technique for near-total resection of the sacrum. Combined anterior and posterior exposures are required. If the rectum must be sacrificed, the operation starts anteriorly, continues posteriorly, and finishes anteriorly; if the rectum can be saved, the operation starts anteriorly and finishes posteriorly. The anterior exposure is performed with the patient in the lithotomy position; the posterior exposure is accomplished with the patient prone.

TECHNIQUE 7.13

(STENER AND GUNTERBERG)

- Close the anus (temporarily if the rectum is to be preserved) by suture. Make an incision across the lower abdomen. Divide the rectus abdominis bilaterally 1 cm above the pubis and cut through the remainder of the abdominal wall musculature bilaterally along the lateral borders of the rectus sheath. Push the peritoneum aside to expose the common iliac vessels. Continue the subperitoneal dissection bilaterally until the right and left dissections meet under the rectum, exposing the sacral promontory.
- If the rectum is to be resected, incise the peritoneum in the midline and divide and ligate the superior rectal vessels.
- Divide the bowel at the rectosigmoid junction and close both ends by invagination.
- Divide and ligate the middle rectal vessels and incise the inferior peritoneal reflection.
- Dissect the rectum from above as far distally as possible; make an inverted-U incision around the anus and dissect from below the anal canal and rectum anteriorly and on each side as far proximally as possible.
- Divide and ligate the internal iliac artery and vein and the lateral and middle sacral vessels. If the resection is to be carried out above the level of the S1 roots, also ligate and divide the iliolumbar vessels.
- Strip the periosteum from the most proximal portions of the sacrum and distally to the level of osteotomy.
- Locate the sympathetic trunk and divide it where it passes anterior to S1. Laterally identify the lumbosacral trunk so that it can be protected at the time of osteotomy. If the S1 roots are to be saved, expose them where they emerge from the first anterior sacral foramina.
- Osteotomize the anterior sacral cortex at the appropriate level and carry the osteotomy laterally past the sacroiliac joint on each side.
- Close the anterior wound (temporarily if the rectum was resected) and turn the patient prone.
- Make a vertical elliptical incision including any biopsy site and the skin and subcutaneous tissue overlying the sacral hiatus through which tumor might have penetrated. If the rectum has been resected, the incision joins the previously made inverted-U incision around the anus. Superior to the skin to be removed, extend a midline incision proximally far enough to expose the posterior elements of L5.
- Raise skin flaps bilaterally and transect the gluteus maximus well away from the sacrum.
- Divide the piriformis muscle at its musculotendinous junction. Ligate and divide the superior and inferior gluteal vessels.
- Preserve the superior gluteal nerve.
- Divide the sacrotuberous ligament at the ischial tuberosity and release the sacrospinous ligament and coccygeus muscle by osteotomizing the ischial spine.
- If the rectum is to be spared, release the bands attaching the anal canal to the coccyx. If the rectum is resected, divide the levator ani bilaterally.
- Divide the sacrospinalis muscles transversely at the lumbosacral level.

- If the S1 nerves are to be preserved, perform a partial laminectomy at the L5-S1 level. If the S1 nerves are to be sacrificed, perform a complete laminectomy at L5 and remove the lumbosacral ligamentum flavum.
- At the appropriate level, ligate and divide the dural sac.
- If the S1 nerves are preserved, make the sacral osteotomy between S1 and S2 with the inferior half of the canals of the S1 roots included in the specimen. Guide the osteotomy from a posterior direction by palpating the line of osteotomy previously made in the anterior sacral cortex. A probe also can be introduced into the S1 canal starting posteriorly.
- Divide the remaining sacral nerves where they converge to form the sciatic nerve and remove the specimen.
- If the S1 nerves are sacrificed, make the osteotomy through S1 above the S1 root canals. It is helpful to make a deep notch in the iliac crest at the level of the L5 transverse process so that the anterosuperior surface of the sacral wing and the sacroiliac joint can be palpated from behind.
- Make the osteotomy 1 cm posteroinferior to this surface in a plane parallel to it. Palpating the previously made osteotomy in the anterior cortex of the sacrum and ilium also guides the plane of osteotomy.
- Divide the sacral nerves and remove the specimen.
- Close the posterior wound over drains.
- If the rectum has been resected, turn the patient supine and reopen the anterior wound. Close the pelvic portion of the peritoneum and perform a sigmoid colostomy. The sigmoid mesentery can be used to repair the peritoneal defect in the lesser pelvis.
- Close the abdominal wound.

RESECTION OF THE SACRUM

TECHNIQUE 7.14

(LOCALIO, FRANCIS, AND ROSSANO)
- Expose the abdominal cavity through a left paramedian incision.
- Incise the peritoneum of the left lumbar gutter; mobilize the colon, identifying the left ureter, and expose the peritoneum of the cul-de-sac and reflect the rectosigmoid colon anteriorly at the level of the L5-S1 junction.
- Expose the upper limits of the tumor distal to the level of the levators and identify the lateral extension of the tumor.
- Ligate the middle sacral vessels and lateral sacral veins. Replace the colon in its original position and close the abdomen.
- Turn the patient prone and make a transverse incision across the buttocks at the level of the S4 vertebra. Raise the lower flap to below the coccyx and the upper flap to L5.
- Divide the rectococcygeal ligament, reflect the rectum anteriorly, and enter the previously opened presacral space.
- Identify the lower limit of the tumor and then proceed with sacral resection, dividing the lateral sacral ligaments. Using an osteotome, divide the sacroiliac articulations at a

level previously determined by the abdominal exploration. Transect the sacrum and remove it from the field. Make no attempt to preserve the sacral nerves below the level of transection.
- Close the posterior wound over suction drains.

Localio et al. subsequently pointed out that simultaneous anterior and posterior exposure of the sacrum by two teams with the patient in the lateral decubitus position may be feasible and has the added advantages of less blood loss and not having to turn the patient.

RESECTION OF THE SACRUM THROUGH POSTERIOR APPROACH

TECHNIQUE 7.15

(MACCARTY ET AL.)
- Place the patient prone and raise the buttocks on a kidney elevator (Kraske position).
- Make a posterior longitudinal incision in the midline over the sacrum and coccyx.
- Remove the coccyx and carefully dissect the rectum from any presacral tumor mass.
- Detach the gluteus maximus, the piriformis, and the coccygeus muscles and the sacrotuberous and sacrospinous ligaments.
- Divide the fourth and fifth sacral nerves bilaterally and identify and preserve the pudendal nerves. Split the third sacral foramen anteriorly and posteriorly; this usually makes resecting the distal three sacral segments possible without sacrificing the pudendal nerves or either of their two components (the second and third sacral nerves).
- Divide the arch and body of the sacrum between the second and third sacral segments, cut the filum terminale, and remove the distal part of the sacrum and the tumor.
- When the tumor and consequently the resection extend into the proximal sacral segment or the lumbar canal or into the sacroiliac joints and ilium, there may be residual neurologic deficits.
- Repair any perforation of the rectal wall or any defect in the caudal sac that may have been made if the sac extends farther distally than normal.
- Drain the large dead space that remains; suture the gluteal muscles as snugly as possible and close the subcutaneous tissues and the skin.

RESECTION OF VERTEBRAE

Surgical treatment of tumors of the spine is discussed in other chapter.

LOWER EXTREMITY

RESECTION OF THE PROXIMAL FEMUR

Most tumors of the proximal femur can be resected with adequate margins, and the reconstruction usually provides better function than would be possible after a hip disarticulation. Indications for amputation include recurrent tumor, displaced pathologic fracture, or complications from the biopsy. Biopsy of the proximal femur should be performed through a round or oval hole placed laterally at the junction between the insertion of the abductors and the origin of the vastus lateralis (Fig. 7.42). This location minimizes the amount of contaminated tissue and the risk of pathologic fracture. Although some authors have recommended reconstruction with an osteoarticular allograft, allograft-prosthesis composite, or allograft arthrodesis, we routinely use an endoprosthetic reconstruction. Endoprosthetic reconstruction provides immediate stability and quicker rehabilitation. Whenever possible, we use a bipolar cup to improve stability (see Fig. 7.42). Some of the function of the abductor mechanism may be preserved by maintaining the continuity of the fascia between the abductors and the vastus lateralis. If margins will allow a trochanteric osteotomy, a thin sleeve of bone in continuity with the fascia proximally and distally may be reattached to the prosthesis. If an osteotomy is not possible, the sleeve of continuous fascia can be sutured to the prosthesis, allowing for easier abductor reattachment and function (Fig. 7.43).

TECHNIQUE 7.16

(LEWIS AND CHEKOFSKY)
- Place the patient in the lateral decubitus position.
- Make a posterolateral hip incision.
- Separate the gluteus maximus at the junction of its proximal 20% and distal 80%, dividing its femoral attachment 2 cm from the linea aspera. Also divide the external rotators and the proximal portion of the adductor magnus 2 cm from the femur.
- Identify and protect the sciatic nerve.
- Divide the gluteus medius and minimus near their attachments to the greater trochanter and the reflected head of the rectus femoris. If possible, maintain the continuity between the fascia of the abductors and vastus lateralis.
- Incise the hip joint capsule.
- At the predetermined level of femoral osteotomy, expose the bone through the vastus lateralis and divide the femur with a power saw. Surrounding soft tissues can be protected with Bennett retractors. Dislocate the hip and divide the iliopsoas tendon, removing the specimen.
- Reconstruct the hip using a modular proximal femoral endoprosthesis. Reconstruct the abductor mechanism by reattaching the remaining gluteus medius and minimus tendons through holes in the trochanteric area of the prosthesis. The abductors also should be sutured to the iliotibial tract if this attachment has been disrupted during the resection. This may require proximal release of the muscles from the ilium or lengthening by multiple relaxing

incisions. The abductors are best placed in the neutral axis of the femur.
- Insert suction drains.

POSTOPERATIVE CARE The reconstructed abductor mechanism is protected by an abduction brace for 6 weeks. Immediate ambulation is allowed with crutches, and later a cane is used in the opposite hand indefinitely.

RESECTION OF THE ENTIRE FEMUR

Lewis described a technique for resection of the entire femur and reconstruction using hip and knee replacement arthroplasty.

TECHNIQUE 7.17

(LEWIS)
- Make a lateral incision extending from 10 cm proximal to the greater trochanter along the lateral aspect of the femur and curving anteriorly to end just distal to the tibial tuberosity (Fig. 7.44).
- Divide the fascia in line with the skin incision, flex the knee, and identify the common peroneal nerve posterior to the biceps femoris tendon.
- Incise the lateral head of the gastrocnemius and identify the popliteal artery and vein. Divide the geniculate branches, allowing the popliteal vessels to fall away from the femur. Dissect the vascular bundle to the adductor hiatus and incise it. Dissect the peroneal nerve to its junction with the sciatic nerve.
- Detach the gluteus maximus from its femoral insertion, detach the external rotators from the femur, and identify the proximal portion of the sciatic nerve.
- Detach the gluteus medius and minimus near the greater trochanter. Maintain continuity of the fascia between the abductors and the vastus lateralis.
- Ligate the branches of the medial femoral circumflex artery and vein and detach the adductor muscles from the femur.
- Enter the knee joint through a lateral parapatellar capsular incision. Leave the articularis genu and vastus intermedius attached to the femur. Resect the other portions of the quadriceps as appropriate.
- Dislocate the patella medially and incise the iliotibial band, lateral collateral ligament, and lateral capsule.
- Detach the cruciate ligaments, popliteus and plantaris tendons, medial capsule, medial collateral ligaments, and medial head of the gastrocnemius.
- Elevate the distal femur and incise the remaining muscle attachments from distal to proximal.
- Ligate the perforating vessels.
- Detach the iliopsoas, incise the hip joint capsule, and remove the specimen.
- Implant a custom-designed total femur and close the wound over suction drains. Depending on the nature of the soft-tissue resection, gastrocnemius or free vascularized muscle flaps may be required.

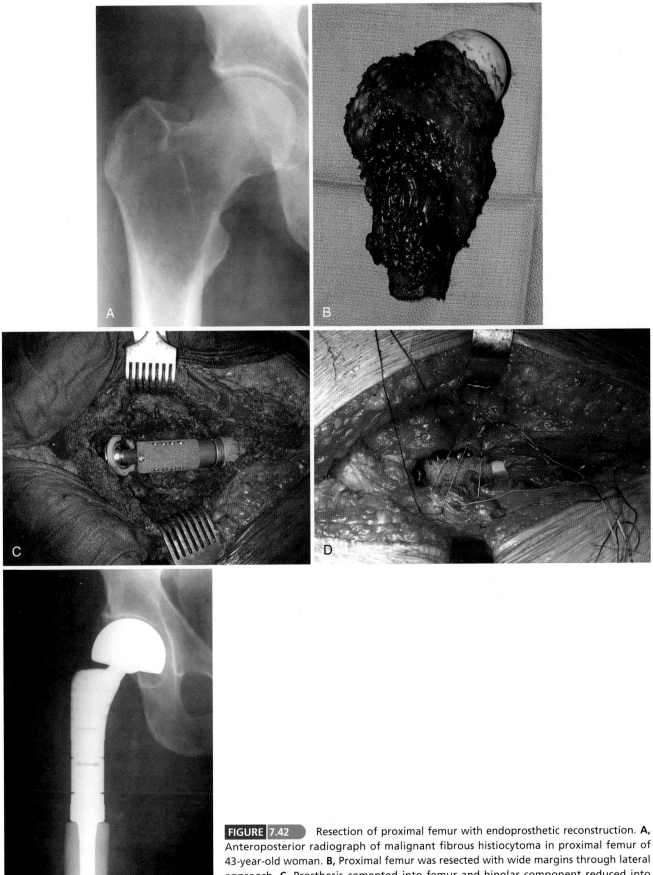

FIGURE 7.42 Resection of proximal femur with endoprosthetic reconstruction. **A,** Anteroposterior radiograph of malignant fibrous histiocytoma in proximal femur of 43-year-old woman. **B,** Proximal femur was resected with wide margins through lateral approach. **C,** Prosthesis cemented into femur and bipolar component reduced into acetabulum. **D,** Abductors and vastus lateralis repaired through holes in prosthesis. **E,** Postoperative anteroposterior radiograph.

■ Proximally suture the iliotibial band to the vastus lateralis and gluteal musculature.

POSTOPERATIVE CARE The hip is protected with an abduction brace for 6 weeks. Protected ambulation is begun immediately. Knee range of motion is begun as soon as the wound seems stable.

■ RESECTION OF THE DISTAL FEMUR

The distal femur is the most common location of primary malignancies of bone. Tumors in this location rarely involve the joint or neurovascular structures. Biopsy specimens of distal femoral lesions can be obtained through an anteromedial or anterolateral approach. Dissection should proceed directly through the vastus medialis or vastus lateralis, taking care not to raise flaps, not to contaminate the joint space, and not to contaminate the popliteal space. A tourniquet should be used during the biopsy, and strict hemostasis should be obtained before closing to decrease the potential of hematoma formation. The soft-tissue component of the lesion should be sampled, if possible. If a hole must be made in the bone, it should be circular to minimize stress concentration, reducing the risk of a pathologic fracture.

Reconstruction options include arthrodesis, osteoarticular allograft, allograft-prosthesis reconstruction, and endoprosthetic reconstruction. We use endoprosthetic reconstructions most often (Fig. 7.45), although arthrodesis is a reasonable option in a young person who wishes to perform heavy labor. If the knee joint is involved with tumor, consideration should be given to a primary transfemoral amputation or extraarticular resection. In young children in whom leg-length discrepancy would be a difficult problem, we most commonly use an expandable prosthesis.

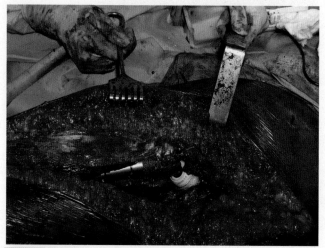

FIGURE 7.43 The continuity of the fascia between the abductors and the vastus lateralis has been maintained to allow easier reattachment of the abductors and better function.

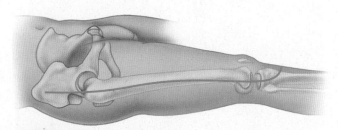

FIGURE 7.44 Lateral incision for resection of the entire femur. **SEE TECHNIQUE 7.17.**

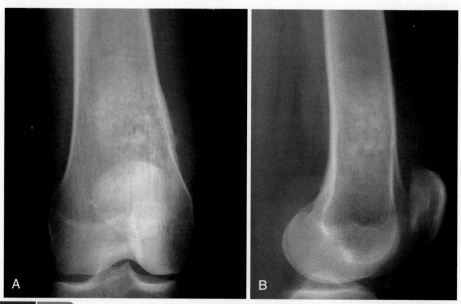

FIGURE 7.45 Resection of distal femur and endoprosthetic reconstruction in 36-year-old woman with osteosarcoma. **A and B,** Anteroposterior and lateral radiographs show osteosarcoma of distal femur.

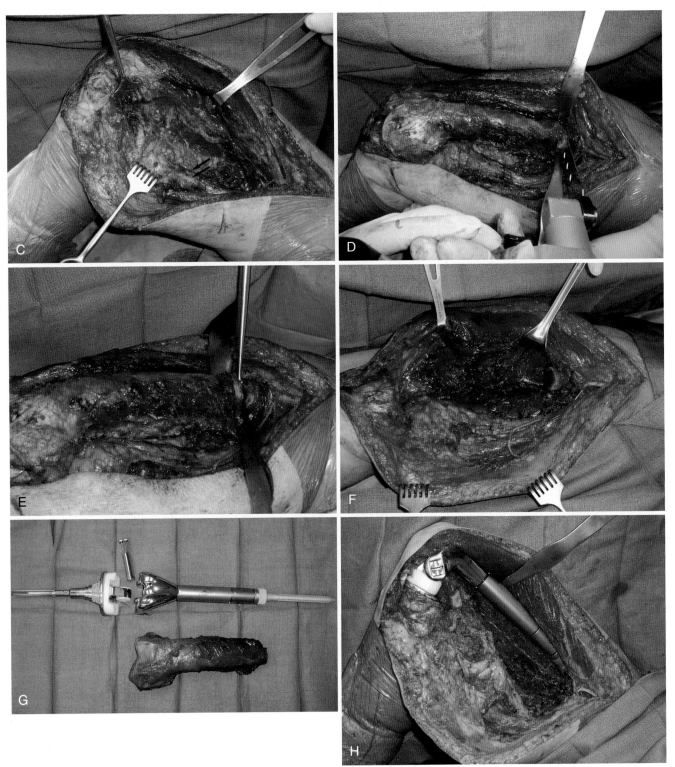

FIGURE 7.45, Cont'd **C,** Plane between femoral vessels *(arrows)* and tumor is developed. **D,** Osteotomy performed with oscillating saw. **E,** Curet used to obtain specimen for frozen section to check marrow margin. **F,** Distal femur resected. **G,** Resected specimen and prosthesis. **H,** Prosthesis cemented into femur and tibia.

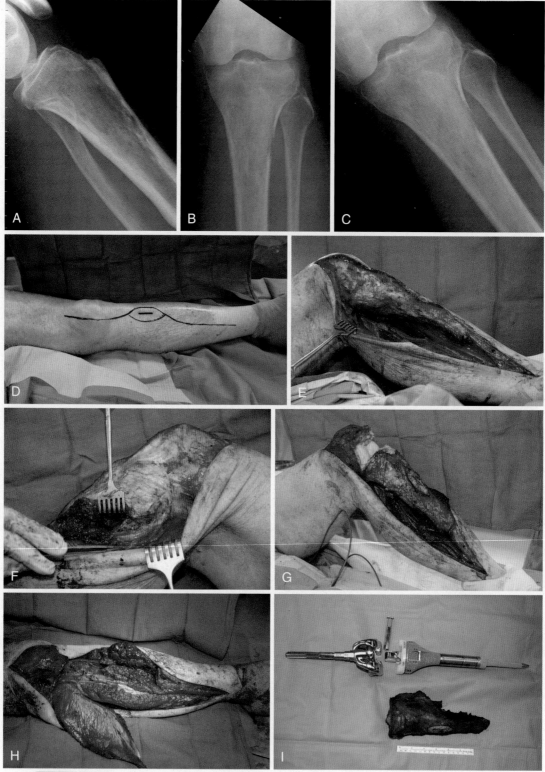

FIGURE 7.46   **A-C,** Radiographs of a 58-year-old man show malignant fibrous histiocytoma in proximal tibia. **D,** Incision as outlined includes resection of the biopsy track. **E,** Medial flap is raised to expose vascular structures posteriorly. **F,** On the lateral side, the peroneal nerve is dissected and isolated from tumor. **G,** Intraarticular resection is done because joint is not involved. **H,** Proximal tibia has been removed, and medial head of gastrocnemius has been harvested for extensor mechanism reconstruction and coverage. **I,** Proximal tibial endoprosthesis.

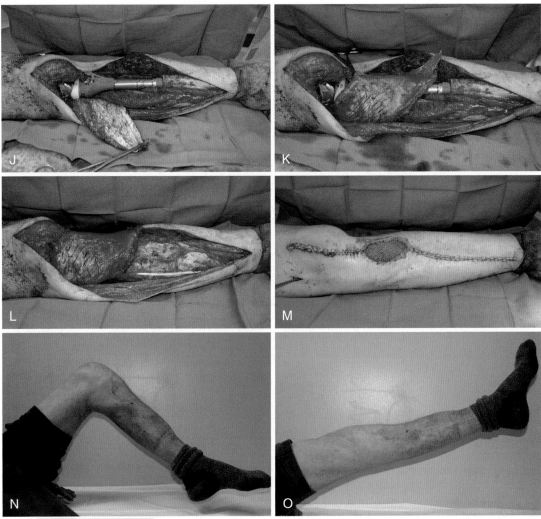

FIGURE 7.46, Cont'd **J,** Patellar tendon is attached to the prosthesis. **K,** Medial gastrocnemius is rotated anteriorly and sutured to lateral fascia. **L,** Prosthesis is completely covered with soft tissue. **M,** Skin graft is required to complete closure. **N and O,** At one year after surgery, the patient has good range of motion and no extensor lag.

INTRAARTICULAR RESECTION OF THE DISTAL FEMUR WITH ENDOPROSTHETIC RECONSTRUCTION

TECHNIQUE 7.18

- Resect the distal femur through a medial or a lateral incision, depending on where the biopsy was done. Make a longitudinal incision, incorporating an ellipse around the biopsy scar. Resect the biopsy track en bloc with the specimen.
- If an intraarticular resection is to be done, inspect the joint early to confirm that it is not contaminated with tumor. (If the joint is unexpectedly involved with tumor, the wound should be closed in layers and definitive treatment should be delayed until options can be discussed again with the patient and family.)
- Raise large medial and lateral flaps. Make these flaps as thick as possible to preserve the blood supply to the skin.

- Dissect deep to the rectus femoris, quadriceps tendon, and patella. The vastus intermedius may be left intact with the portion of distal femur to be removed. Flex the knee to take tension off the posterior tissues.
- Dissect the popliteal vessels, taking care to ligate any branches to the tumor.
- Isolate and protect the tibial and common peroneal nerves.
- Incise the knee joint capsule and ligaments to allow better exposure for dissection around the distal femur.
- Leave a cuff of normal muscle over the tumor. Divide remaining muscles just off their respective origins and insertions into the femur.
- Before the femoral osteotomy, mark the anterior aspect of the femoral shaft proximal to the osteotomy site to help with rotational alignment for the reconstruction. Make an osteotomy of the femur with a wide margin proximal to the most proximal extent of marrow involvement as determined by preoperative MRI.
- Remove the tumor from the operative field.

ENDOPROSTHETIC RECONSTRUCTION WITH ROTATING HINGE

- If the anterior aspect of the femoral shaft has not already been marked, do so at this time using the specimen to help with orientation. (The linea aspera should not be used as a reference point because its rotational orientation varies.) Before removing the resected specimen from the operative field, measure its length. In an adult, this length should be restored by the prosthesis. In a skeletally immature patient, the prosthesis may be 1 cm longer than the resected specimen to help compensate for future growth.
- Use alignment guides to make the proximal tibial cut perpendicular to the tibial shaft and prepare the proximal tibia using the provided instrumentation.
- Ream the femoral canal to accept the largest stem possible. The stem should be at least 12 cm long. (If the length of proximal femur remaining is less than this, consideration should be given to using a prosthesis that gains fixation in the femoral head or using an allograft-prosthesis composite reconstruction.)
- Place the trial components and move the knee through a full range of motion. Cement the femoral and tibial components into place in the proper orientation, specifically avoiding internal rotation of the femoral component that could result in patellar maltracking. Close the wound over drains. Local or free flaps may be necessary for closure.
- Dress the wound with a bulky dressing and apply a knee immobilizer.

POSTOPERATIVE CARE Protected ambulation with crutches and a knee immobilizer is begun on the first postoperative day. Drains are left in place until output is minimal. Range-of-motion and strengthening exercises are begun immediately. Antibiotics are continued until the drains are removed and the wound is dry. The knee immobilizer is worn for ambulation until adequate strength has returned.

RESECTION OF THE PROXIMAL TIBIA

The proximal tibia is the second most common location for primary malignancies of bone. Tumors in this area are typically smaller at presentation than tumors in more proximal locations. Overall survival for these patients subsequently has been better than for patients with more proximal tumors. Historically, skeletally immature patients with proximal tibial tumors have been treated with knee disarticulation to preserve the distal femoral physis and to prevent the complication of appositional bone overgrowth. Skeletally mature patients have been treated with a long transfemoral amputation. The overall good function after amputation, along with the potential difficulty of reconstructing the extensor mechanism, had dampened the enthusiasm for proximal tibial resection and reconstruction. Currently, however, with routine use of a gastrocnemius flap to assist with soft-tissue coverage and to help reconstruct the extensor mechanism, surgeons are reporting good results after limb salvage surgery. A mobile knee joint with active extension is now a reasonable goal for patients who are willing to accept the activity restrictions that are mandatory after this reconstruction. Patients who wish to be involved in sports or heavy labor should strongly consider an arthrodesis or an amputation.

Wide surgical margins usually are obtainable for tumors in the proximal tibia because the popliteus muscle and the muscles of the deep posterior compartment usually protect the posterior tibial artery and the tibial nerve. Biopsy of the proximal tibia should be done along the medial subcutaneous surface, taking care not to contaminate the joint space, the patellar tendon, or the popliteal space. Contraindications to limb salvage include involvement of the popliteal vessels, displaced pathologic fracture, recurrent tumor, and complications (e.g., infection, hematoma, poorly placed incision, or joint contamination) resulting from the biopsy. A relative contraindication is a very young patient who would subsequently develop a leg-length discrepancy; however, with the use of modern expandable prostheses, we have had success with limb salvage surgery even in these patients.

TECHNIQUE 7.19 *Figure 7.46*

(MALAWER)

- Make an anteromedial incision starting proximally at the distal third of the femur and extend it distally to the lower third of the tibia. Excise any biopsy site with a 2-cm margin.
- Develop medial and lateral flaps beneath the investing fascia. Divide the medial hamstrings proximal to their insertions. Mobilize the medial head of the gastrocnemius muscle and split the soleus muscle to expose the popliteal vessels.
- Preserve the medial sural artery, the principal blood supply of the medial gastrocnemius. Apply posterior traction to the popliteal artery and identify and divide the anterior tibial vessels at the inferior border of the popliteus muscle. With a large tumor, the peroneal vessels also may require division and ligation.
- If the knee joint is free of tumor, divide the patellar ligament 1 to 2 cm proximal to its insertion. When possible, maintain continuity of the fascia between the patellar tendon and the anterolateral fascia of the proximal leg.
- Mobilize the popliteal vessels by dividing the inferior geniculate vessels; then circumferentially incise the capsule of the knee 1 to 2 cm from its tibial insertion.
- Divide the cruciate ligaments at the femur. Keep a portion of the anterior tibial muscle on the specimen as well as the popliteus and a portion of the soleus muscle.
- Identify and protect the peroneal nerve and divide the biceps tendon near its insertion, leaving a cuff of normal tissue. Osteotomize the fibula if the extraosseous component of the tumor dictates. Leave a sleeve of muscle on the proximal tibiofibular joint. If the proximal fibula is not involved, preservation of the lateral collateral ligament and its attachment to the fibular head provides some stability to the reconstructed joint.
- Osteotomize the tibia distal to the lesion at a level determined by preoperative imaging; divide the intermuscular septum and remove the specimen.

- If an extraarticular resection is required, the technique is similar except that the femur is osteotomized above the capsule of the knee and the patella is split coronally, dissecting the patellar ligament from the underlying fat pad.
- Reconstruct the extremity by osteoarticular allograft, arthrodesis, or prosthetic implantation. Advance the extensor mechanism and attach the remaining patellar tendon to the allograft or endoprosthesis. Transpose the medial head of the gastrocnemius anteriorly and suture it to the remaining anterior muscles as well as the soft tissues of the extensor mechanism. A split-thickness skin graft is often required because of the bulk of the gastrocnemius flap and the loss of tissue coverage from biopsy track excision.

POSTOPERATIVE CARE Drains are left in place until the output is minimal. Antibiotics are continued until the drain is out and the wound is dry. Protected ambulation is begun on the first postoperative day. We routinely keep the knee in full extension for 6 weeks to allow the reconstructed knee extensor mechanism to heal. Range-of-motion exercises are then begun.

RESECTION OF THE DISTAL FEMUR OR PROXIMAL TIBIA WITH ALLOGRAFT ARTHRODESIS

An arthrodesis can be done using an intercalary allograft to replace the resected segment. This usually is done with an intramedullary nail along with plates at the proximal and distal allograft-host junctions. This technique potentially provides a stable limb; however, reported complication rates are high.

RESECTION OF THE PROXIMAL FIBULA

Malawer described a technique for local wide resection of proximal fibular lesions.

TECHNIQUE 7.20

(MALAWER)
- Place the patient semisupine and prepare and drape the entire lower extremity from the toes to above the hip so that if a local procedure is found to be inappropriate, above-knee amputation is possible without redraping. Use a sterile rubber tourniquet at midthigh.
- Begin the incision posteriorly 8 cm proximal to the middle of the popliteal crease and curve it anteriorly and distally across the fibula, ending 5 cm distal to the planned osteotomy. Modify the incision appropriately to incorporate any previous biopsy site.
- Raise a large lateral flap based in the midline posteriorly and make a smaller medial flap to expose the tibial crest.

- Expose and divide the common peroneal nerve at the biceps femoris tendon. Its branches are sacrificed distally when the anterior and peroneal compartment muscles are resected.
- Find the popliteal vessels and their trifurcation by detaching the lateral gastrocnemius and soleus through their substances near the fibula. If necessary, the proximal origin of the lateral gastrocnemius on the femur can be released as well.
- Find and divide the anterior tibial vessels 2 to 3 cm distal to the inferior border of the popliteus. Apply traction to the popliteal artery, allowing the vessels to fall away from the posterior surface of the mass.
- Incise the anterior and peroneal compartment muscles proximally at their origins and distally at their musculotendinous junctions. Release the interosseous membrane.
- Divide the fibular collateral ligament and biceps femoris tendon 2.5 cm proximal to their fibular insertions.
- Resect the proximal tibiofibular joint through the tibia. Posteriorly, this requires incision of the popliteus muscle.
- Repair any resulting defect of the posterior capsule of the knee. Reattach the biceps femoris tendon and the fibular collateral ligament to the lateral condyle of the tibia.
- Rotate the lateral gastrocnemius anteriorly by releasing it in the midline posteriorly and distally where it joins the soleus. This permits coverage of the exposed popliteal and posterior tibial vessels and the bared tibia. The lateral sural vessels providing vascular supply to the lateral gastrocnemius should be carefully preserved.
- Use suction drainage for 3 to 5 days.

POSTOPERATIVE CARE Ambulation is begun on the first postoperative day with weight bearing as tolerated. A hinged knee brace is used for 6 weeks. An ankle-foot orthosis is required if the peroneal nerve has been resected.

RESECTION OF THE TIBIAL DIAPHYSIS

If the extent of a tibial tumor is such that the knee and ankle joints can be preserved, an intercalary resection should be done with allograft or vascularized autograft fibular reconstruction (Fig. 7.47).

RESECTION OF THE DISTAL THIRD OF THE FIBULA

The distal third of the fibula can be resected without reconstruction and without creating significant instability or valgus deformity (Figs. 7.48 and 7.49).

TECHNIQUE 7.21

- Place the patient supine with a nonsterile tourniquet on the ipsilateral thigh. A sandbag can be placed under the

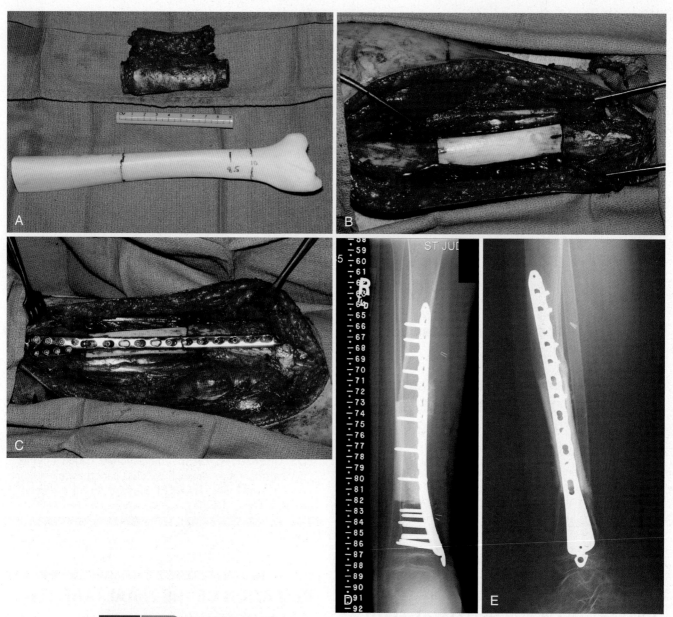

FIGURE 7.47 Intercalary tibial allograft in 11-year-old boy with Ewing sarcoma. **A,** Allograft fashioned to match resected specimen. **B and C,** Allograft placed in defect and fixed with distal tibial locking plate. **D and E,** Postoperative anteroposterior and lateral radiographs.

buttock to aid in exposure by allowing internal rotation of the extremity during the procedure.

■ After gravity exsanguination, make a direct lateral incision spanning the extent of bone to be resected. Any biopsy site should be incorporated and maintained with the resected specimen throughout the entire case.

■ Raise anterior and posterior flaps to expose the bone and any soft-tissue component associated with the tumor.

■ Identify any sensory branches of the superficial peroneal nerve in the proximal aspect of the wound coursing anteriorly and preserve them if they are not involved in the tumor.

■ Retract the peroneus longus and brevis tendons posteriorly and dissect around the lateral malleolus leaving a cuff of normal tissue.

■ Make the fibular osteotomy proximally at a level determined by preoperative imaging (i.e., MRI) and retract the cut end out of the wound.

■ Dissect distally to excise the remaining soft-tissue attachments between the distal tibia and lateral malleolus. Divide the ankle ligaments.

■ Deliver the specimen from the wound and release the tourniquet. After achieving hemostasis, close the wound over suction drainage in a standard fashion.

■ Apply a short leg posterior splint.

■ RESECTION-ARTHRODESIS OF THE ANKLE

Rarely in our experience is a lesion in the distal tibia best treated by wide resection arthrodesis of the ankle. The

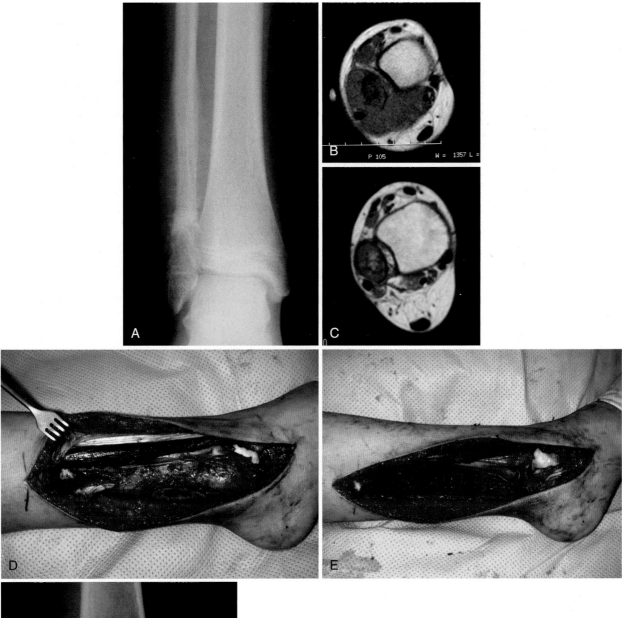

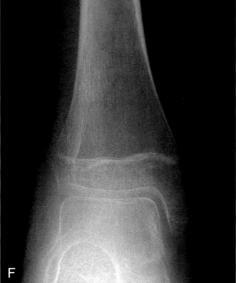

FIGURE 7.48 Resection of distal fibula in 13-year-old girl with Ewing sarcoma. **A,** Anteroposterior radiograph shows tumor of distal fibula. **B,** Initial MR image. **C,** MR image after neoadjuvant chemotherapy shows decrease in size of tumor. **D,** Distal fibula resected with wide margins. **E,** Distal fibula has been removed. **F,** Anteroposterior radiograph at 6 months after surgery. Patient is pain free and walks with ankle brace.

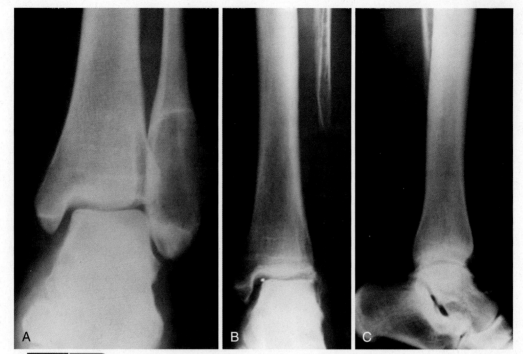

FIGURE 7.49 Long-term follow-up (40 years) of patient with resection of the distal fibula for osteosarcoma. No recurrence, deformity, instability, or metastasis occurred. **A,** Preoperative radiograph. **B and C,** Anteroposterior and lateral radiographs 39 years later.

morbidity and prolonged recovery must be balanced against the almost certain satisfactory function of below-knee amputation and prosthetic fitting. Lewis advocated a longitudinal anterior approach; Enneking recommended parallel medial and lateral incisions. Reconstruction after resection of the distal tibia is accomplished by autograft or allograft arthrodesis.

■ RESECTION OF THE TALUS

In our experience, resection of the talus is rarely necessary. Wide resection of the talus can be accomplished through an extended anterolateral approach to the ankle and hindfoot (see chapter 1). If a portion of the head and neck can be spared, a Blair fusion provides a good reconstruction. If total resection is necessary, calcaneotibial fusion is advisable.

ROTATIONPLASTY

In 1975, Kristen, Knahr, and Salzer first reported using the Borggreve rotationplasty in the treatment of distal femoral osteosarcoma as an alternative to amputation. The technique subsequently has been modified so that lesions in various parts of the femur and proximal tibia can be treated by rotationplasty.

Winkelmann classified rotationplasty into five groups, as follows:

Group AI—Lesion in distal femur. The distal femur, knee joint, and proximal tibia are resected; the lower leg is rotated 180 degrees, and the tibia is joined to the remaining femur (Fig. 7.50).

Group AII—Lesion in the proximal tibia. The distalmost femur, knee joint, and proximal tibia are resected. After rotation of 180 degrees, the distal tibia is joined to the distal femur (Fig. 7.51).

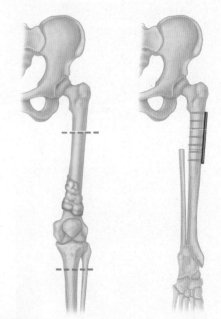

FIGURE 7.50 Rotationplasty type AI for a lesion in the distal femur. (Redrawn from Winkelmann WW: Rotationplasty in the local treatment of osteosarcoma, *Semin Orthop* 3:40, 1988.)

Group BI—Lesion in the proximal femur sparing the hip joint and gluteal muscles. The upper femur and hip joint are resected, and the leg is rotated 180 degrees. The distal femur is joined to the pelvis so that the knee functions as the hip and the ankle functions as the knee (Fig. 7.52).

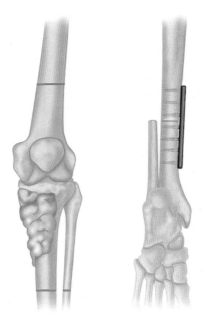

FIGURE 7.51 Rotationplasty type AII for a lesion in the proximal tibia. (Redrawn from Winkelmann WW: Rotationplasty in the local treatment of osteosarcoma, *Semin Orthop* 3:40, 1988.)

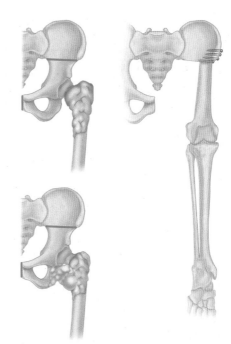

FIGURE 7.53 Rotationplasty type BII for lesion in proximal femur with involvement of hip joint and contiguous soft tissue. (Redrawn from Winkelmann WW: Rotationplasty in the local treatment of osteosarcoma, *Semin Orthop* 3:40, 1988.)

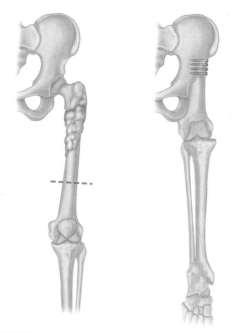

FIGURE 7.52 Rotationplasty type BI for lesion in proximal femur. (Redrawn from Winkelmann WW: Rotationplasty in the local treatment of osteosarcoma, *Semin Orthop* 3:40, 1988.)

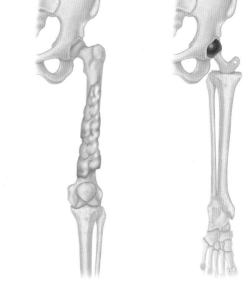

FIGURE 7.54 Rotationplasty type BIII for malignant lesion in femur. (Redrawn from Winkelmann WW: Rotationplasty in the local treatment of osteosarcoma, *Semin Orthop* 3:40, 1988.)

Group BII—Lesion in the proximal femur with involvement of hip joint and contiguous soft tissue. The upper femur, hip joint, and lower hemipelvis are resected, and the leg is rotated 180 degrees. The remaining femur is joined to the remnant of the ilium so that the knee functions as a hinged hip joint and the ankle functions as the knee (Fig. 7.53).

Group BIII—Lesion in the midfemur. The entire femur is resected. The tibia is attached to the pelvis using an endoprosthesis (Fig. 7.54).

ROTATIONPLASTY FOR A LESION IN THE DISTAL FEMUR

TECHNIQUE 7.22

(KOTZ AND SALZER)

- Make a skin incision in the shape of a large rhombus with its long axis on the anterior surface and its two lateral points meeting on the posterior surface of the lower limb (Fig. 7.55A). Any biopsy track must be entirely within the rhombus-shaped area of skin and must be excised en bloc with the tumor. The long axis of the rhombus is 5 to 10 cm longer than the intended length of bone resection.
- Incise the fascia at the level of skin incision.
- Identify and dissect the common peroneal, tibial, and sciatic nerves. Next, identify the femoral vessels proximally in the adductor canal and dissect them distally, ligating branches as necessary. Resect the vessels with the tumor if involved and subsequently reconstruct them.
- Expose the femur and transect it 5 cm or more proximal to the proximal margin of the lesion.
- Expose the proximal part of the tibia just distal to the knee joint capsule and proximal to the anterior tibial artery and divide the tibia distal to the proximal physis.
- Remove the specimen from the operative field and have it immediately inspected by the pathologist to ensure adequate margins.
- Externally rotate the leg 180 degrees to situate the tibial and peroneal nerves on the medial side of the femur.
- Join the femur and tibia with a compression plate. Before osteosynthesis, consider limb length and placement of the ankle joint. Because of faster growth of the femur compared with the externally rotated distal tibia, the ankle joint (which now serves as the knee joint) should be no more than 4 to 6 cm distal to the contralateral normal knee. More exact predictions of length and normal growth can be made by using the Green-Anderson tables. In an adult, the ankle and knee joint should be at the same level.
- If sacrifice of the femoral vessels is necessary, reconstruction should be accomplished within 2 hours, but after osteosynthesis is completed. If the vessels are preserved, place them in loops between muscles to avoid kinking.
- Suture the muscles of the thigh to the fascia of the leg.
- During skin closure, redundant skin from the proximal portion of the wound can be removed to allow for differences in the circumference of the thigh and leg. Gebhart et al. suggested modifying the skin incision so that circumferential thigh and fish-mouth leg incisions are used to equalize the circumferences of the incisions in the thigh and leg and decrease skin length disproportion (Fig. 7.55B).

POSTOPERATIVE CARE Non–weight-bearing ambulation is begun initially. At 6 weeks, a temporary prosthesis is fitted and progressive weight bearing is allowed.

ROTATIONPLASTY FOR A LESION OF THE PROXIMAL FEMUR WITHOUT INVOLVEMENT OF THE HIP JOINT

TECHNIQUE 7.23   Figure 7.56A

(WINKELMANN)

- Begin the proximal skin incision medially at the inguinal crease and continue it anteriorly over the thigh two fingerbreadths distal and parallel to the inguinal ligament. Curve it upward just distal to the anterior superior iliac spine onto the lateral aspect of the thigh. Follow the lateral border of the thigh and gluteal fold to join the start of the incision medially (Fig. 7.56B).
- Measure the distance between the superior border of the anterior superior iliac spine and the inferior border of the ischium on the anteroposterior radiograph of the pelvis. This distance is measured proximally from the medial joint line on the medial aspect of the thigh. This marks the superior extent of the distal skin incision. The distal extent of the distal skin incision, which forms an elongated oval, is on the lateral aspect of the thigh 6 to 8 cm above the lateral joint line. The anterior connecting skin incision follows the course of the femoral artery and vein, and the posterior connecting skin incision follows the course of the sciatic nerve. The track of any previous biopsy must be in the resected part of the lower limb.
- Incise the fascia of the thigh in line with the skin incision and detach the sartorius muscle from its origin.
- Expose the femoral neurovascular bundle at the junction of the saphenous and femoral veins. Divide the femoral nerve just distal to the inguinal ligament and ligate the saphenous vein near its junction with the femoral vein.

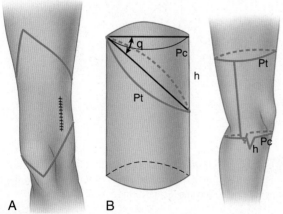

A   B

FIGURE 7.55   **A,** Rhomboid-shaped incision for type AI rotationplasty. **B,** Alternative circumferential thigh incision and fish-mouth leg incision. (**A** redrawn from Kotz R, Salzer M: Rotationplasty for childhood osteosarcoma of the distal part of the femur, *J Bone Joint Surg* 64A:959, 1982; **B** redrawn from Gebhart MJ, McCormack RR Jr, Healey JH, et al: Modification of the skin incision for the Van Nes limb rotationplasty, *Clin Orthop Relat Res* 216:179, 1987.) **SEE TECHNIQUE 7.22.**

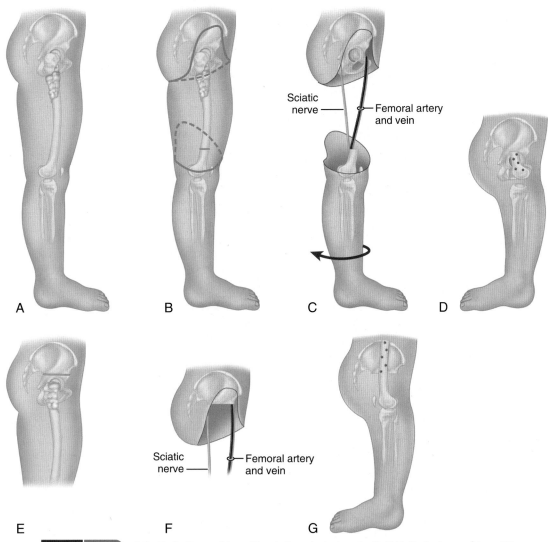

FIGURE 7.56   A-D, Technique of type BI rotationplasty (see text). **E-G,** Technique of type BII rotationplasty (see text). (Redrawn from Winkelmann WW: Hip rotationplasty for malignant tumors of the proximal part of the femur, *J Bone Joint Surg* 68A:362, 1986.) **SEE TECHNIQUES 7.23 AND 7.24.**

Dissect the vascular bundle distal to the Hunter canal, dividing all branching vessels as necessary (Fig. 7.56C). If the femoral artery and vein are involved with tumor, sacrifice and reconstruct them.

■ Detach the tensor fasciae latae, rectus femoris, and adductor muscles from their origins.

■ Ligate the obturator nerve, artery, and vein.

■ Divide the obturator externus near its origin and divide the iliopsoas muscle deep to the inguinal ligament.

■ Posteriorly, detach the gluteus maximus from the femur 3 cm from its insertion and reflect it proximally.

■ Dissect the sciatic nerve distally as far as the inferior line of resection.

■ Preserve the gluteus medius and minimus muscles if possible. Incise the hip joint capsule circumferentially close to the pelvis.

■ Distally, create a musculotendinous flap of the quadriceps mechanism for later suture to the gluteal muscles. Divide the hamstring tendons at a point distal enough to allow later suture to the iliopsoas.

■ Determine the length of the distal part of the femur to be retained by using the anteroposterior radiograph of the pelvis. In adults, the inferior border of the femoral condyles should be slightly above the distal border of the ischium (Fig. 7.56D). In children, the inferior border of the femoral condyle is positioned 1 to 2 cm below the distal border of the ischium. Leave the shaft of the femur only as long as is needed to fix it to the lateral surface of the ilium with at least four screws.

■ After removal of the lesion and proximal femur, carefully support the remaining limb because it is attached only by the neurovascular bundle.

■ Expose subperiosteally the lateral aspect of the wing of the ilium.

■ Rotate the extremity 180 degrees so that the foot faces posteriorly. Shape the lateral aspect of the cortex of the distal femur so that the lower limb is in neutral in the coronal plane and in 10 degrees of external rotation with the knee in full extension when it is apposed to the iliac wing.

- Fix the femoral shaft to the ilium with at least four screws or bolts.
- Suture the muscles with the knee flexed 70 degrees. Posteriorly, suture the gluteal muscles to the quadriceps, and anteriorly, suture the hamstring tendons to the iliopsoas. Position the sciatic nerve and femoral vessels in loops in the subcutaneous space to prevent kinking. Excise any redundant skin on the thigh.

ROTATIONPLASTY FOR A LESION OF THE PROXIMAL FEMUR INVOLVING THE HIP JOINT

TECHNIQUE 7.24

(WINKELMANN)

- The proximal extent of resection is determined by the size and location of the tumor (Fig. 7.56E). When necessary, remove all the posterior musculature of the hip and the sacrospinous and sacrotuberous ligaments from their origins and transect the iliopsoas muscle within the pelvis.
- Divide the ilium as far proximally as necessary, leaving enough to allow fixation of the femur to the pelvis with at least four screws (Fig. 7.56F and G).
- Anteriorly, resect the hemipelvis to the symphysis pubis if necessary.
- If the gluteal muscles are resected, spare the femoral nerve and vessels because the distal and middle parts of the quadriceps muscle are used as the hip (knee) extensors.
- Depending on the level of transection of the iliopsoas muscle, leave the flexor tendons of the knee longer or shorter as needed.

POSTOPERATIVE CARE A single spica cast is applied with the anterior half made removable so that passive hip exercises can be started soon after surgery. Active exercises of the ankle also are begun soon after surgery, and active hip exercises are started after 3 weeks.

REFERENCES

GENERAL

Abdel MP, Papagelopoulos PJ, Morrey ME, et al.: Malignant proximal fibular tumors: surgical management of 112 cases, *J Bone Joint Surg Am* 94:e165, 2012.

Aggerholm-Pedersen N, Maretty-Nielsen K, Keller J, et al.: The importance of standardized treatment in high-grade osteosarcoma: 30 years of experience from a hospital-based database, *Acta Oncol* 54:17, 2015.

Ahmad I, Ahmed MM, Ahsraf MF, et al.: Pain management in metastatic bone disease: a literature review, *Cureus* 10:e3286, 2018.

Angelini A, Pala E, Calabro T, et al.: Prognostic factors in surgical resection of sacral chordoma, *J Surg Oncol* 112:334, 2015.

Biermann JS, Holt GE, Lewis VO, et al.: Metastatic bone disease: diagnosis, evaluation, and treatment, *Instr Course Lect* 59:593, 2010.

Bosma SE, Ayu O, Fiocco M, et al.: Prognostic factors for survival in Ewing sarcoma: a systematic review, *Surg Oncol* 27:603, 2018.

Brennan MF, Antonescu CR, Moraco N, Singer S: Lessons learned from the study of 10,000 patients with soft tissue sarcoma, *Ann Surg* 260:416, 2014.

Colding-Rasmussen T, Thorn AP, Horstmann P, et al.: Survival and prognostic factors at time of diagnosis in high-grade appendicular osteosarcoma: a 21 year single institution evaluation from east Denmark, *Acta Oncol* 57:420, 2018.

Corradi D, Wenger DE, Bertoni F, et al.: Multicentric osteosarcoma: clinicopathologic and radiographic study of 56 cases, *Am J Clin Pathol* 136:799, 2011.

Czajka CM, DiCaprio MR: What is the proportion of patients with multiple hereditary exostoses who undergo malignant degeneration? *Clin Orthop Relat Res* 473:2355, 2015.

Enneking WF: History of orthopedic oncology in the United States: progress from the past, prospects for the future, *Cancer Treat Res* 152:529, 2010.

Friedman DN, Chastain K, Chou JF, et al: Morbidity and mortality after treatment of Ewing sarcoma: a single-institution experience, *Pediatr Blood Cancer* 64. doi: 10.1002/pbc.26562. [Epub Apr 18, 2017]

Gaston CL, Bhumbra R, Watanuki M, et al.: Does the addition of cement improve the rate of local recurrence after curettage of giant cell tumors in bone? *J Bone Joint Surg Br* 93:1665, 2011.

Houdek MT, Sherman CE, Inwards CY, et al.: Adamantinoma of bone: longterm follow-up of 46 consecutive patients, *J Surg Oncol* 118:1150, 2018.

Kimura T: Multidisciplinary approach for bone metastasis: a review, *Cancers (Basel)* 10:E156, 2018.

Lawrenz JM, Styron JF, Parry M, et al.: Longer duration of symptoms at the time of presentation is not associated with worse survival in primary bone sarcoma, *Bone Joint J* 100-B:652, 2018.

Li J, Wang Z, Ji C, et al.: What are the oncologic and functional outcomes after joint salvage resections for juxtaarticular osteosarcoma about the knee? *Clin Orthop Relat Res* 475:2095, 2017.

Liu YP, Li KH, Sun BH: Which treatment is the best for giant cell tumors of the distal radius? A meta-analysis, *Clin Orthop Relat Res* 470:2886, 2012.

Malagelada F, Tarrago LT, Tibrewal S, et al.: Pathological fracture in osteosarcoma: is it always an indication for amputation? *Ortop Traumatol Rehabil* 16:67, 2014.

Özger H, Alpan B, Aycan OE, et al.: Management of primary malignant bone and soft tissue tumors of the foot and ankle: is it worth salvaging? *J Surg Oncol* 117:307, 2018.

Park KJ, Menendez ME, Mears SC, et al.: Patients with multiple myeloma have more complications after hip fracture, *Geriatr Orthop Surg Rehabil* 7:158, 2016.

Parry MC, Laitinen M, Albergo J, et al.: Osteosarcoma of the pelvis, *Bone Joint J* 98-B:555, 2016.

Pendharkar AV, Ho AL, Sussman ES, et al.: Surgical management of sacral chordomas: illustrative cases and current management paradigms, *Cureus* 7:e301, 2015.

Piccioli A, Maccauro G, Spinelli MS, et al.: Bone metastases of unknown origin: epidemiology and principles of management, *J Orthop Traumatol* 16:81, 2015.

Ramu EM, Houdek MT, Isaac CE, et al.: Management of soft-tissue sarcomas: treatment strategies, staging, and outcomes, *SICOT J* 3:20, 2017.

Raskin KA, Schwab JH, Manking HJ, et al.: Giant cell tumor of bone, *J Am Acad Orthop Surg* 21:118, 2013.

Ruosi C, Colella G, Di Donato SL, et al.: Surgical treatment of sacral chordoma: survival and prognostic factors, *Eur Spine J* 24(Suppl 7):912, 2015.

Schwab JH, Springfield DS, Raskin KA, et al.: What's new in primary malignant musculoskeletal tumors, *J Bone Joint Surg Am* 95:2240, 2013.

Steffner RJ, Jang ES, Danford NC: Lymphoma of bone, *JBJS Rev* 6:e1, 2018.

Takeucki A, Lewis VO, Satcher RL, et al.: What are the factors that affect survival and relapse after local recurrence of osteosarcoma? *Clin Orthop Relat Res* 472:3188, 2014.

Terrando S, Sambri A, Bianchi G, et al.: Angiosarcoma around total hip arthroplasty: case series and review of the literature, *Musculoskelet Surg* 102:21, 2018.

Weber KL, Peabody T, Frassica FJ, et al.: Tumors for the general orthopedist: how to save your patients and practice, *Instr Course Lect* 59:579, 2010.

Worch J, Matthew KK, Neuhaus J, et al.: Ethnic and racial differences in patients with Ewing sarcoma, *Cancer* 116:983, 2010.

Zhao Z, Yan T, Guo W, et al.: Surgical outcomes and reconstruction strategies for primary bone tumors of distal tibia: a systematic review of complications and functional outcome, *J Bone Oncol* 14:100209, 2018.

RADIOGRAPHIC EVALUATION

Araz M, Aras G, Kücük ÖN: The role of 18F-NaF PETCT in metastatic bone disease, *J Bone Oncol* 4:92, 2015.

Balily C, Leforestier R, Campion L, et al.: Prognostic value of FDG-PET indices for the assessment of histological response to neoadjuvant chemotherapy and outcome in pediatric patients with Ewing sarcoma and osteosarcoma, *PLoS One* 12:e0183841, 2017.

Behzadi AH, Raza SI, Carrino JA, et al.: Applications of PET/CT and PET/MRI imaging in primary bone malignancies, *PET Clin* 13:623, 2018.

Douis H, Parry M, Vaiyapuri S, et al.: What are the differentiating clinical and MRI- features of enchondromas from low-grade chondrosarcomas? *Eur Radiol* 28:398, 2018.

Fisher SM, Joodi R, Madhurantrhakam AJ, et al.: Current utilities of imaging in grading musculoskeletal soft tissue sarcomas, *Eur J Radiol* 85:1336, 2016.

George A, Grimer RJ, J James SL: Could routine magnetic resonance imaging detect local recurrence of musculoskeletal sarcomas earlier? A cost-effectiveness study, *Indian J Orthop* 52:81, 2018.

Gersing AS, Pfeiffer D, Kopp FK, et al.: Evaluation of MR-derived CT-like images and simulated radiographs compared to conventional radiography in patients with benign and malignant bone tumors, *Eur Radiol* 29:13, 2019.

Huang T, Li F, Yan Z, et al.: Effectiveness of 18-FDG PET/CT in the diagnosis, staging and recurrence monitoring of Ewing sarcoma family of tumors: a meta-analysis of 23 studies, *Medicine (Baltimore)* 97:e13457, 2018.

Kasalak Ö, Gludemans AWJM, Overbosch J, et al.: Can FDG-PET/CT replace blind marrow biopsy of the posterior iliac crest in Ewing sarcoma? *Skeletal Radiol* 47:363, 2018.

Katal S, Gholamrezanezhad A, Kessler M, et al.: PET in the diagnostic management of soft tissue sarcomas of musculoskeletal origin, *PET Clin* 13:609, 2018.

Kransdorf MJ, Murphey MD: Imaging of soft-tissue musculoskeletal masses: fundamental concepts, *Radiographics* 36:1931, 2016.

Madej T, Flak-Nurzynska J, Dutkiewicz E, et al.: Ultrasound image of malignant bone tumors in children: an analysis of nine patients diagnosed in 2011-2016, *J Untrason* 18:103, 2018.

Palmerini E, Colangeli M, Nanni C, et al.: The role of FDG PET/CT in patients treated with neoadjuvant chemotherapy for localized bone sarcomas, *Eur J Nucl Med Mol Imaging* 44:215, 2017.

Parghane RV, Basu S: Dual-time point 18F-FDG-PET and ET/CT for differentiating benign from malignant musculoskeletal lesions: opportunities and limitations, *Semin Nucl Med* 47:373, 2017.

Sharma P, Kahngembam BC, Suman KC, et al.: Diagnostic accuracy of 18F-FDG PET/CT for detecting recurrence in patients with primary skeletal Ewing sarcoma, *Eur J Nucl Med Mol Imaging* 40:1036, 2013.

Wang L, Pretell-Massini J, Kerf DA, et al.: MRI findings associated with microscopic residual tumor following unplanned excision of soft tissue sarcomas in the extremities, *Skeletal Radiol* 47:181, 2018.

Wang LJ, Wu HB, Wang M, et al.: Utility of F-18 FDG PET/CT on the evaluation of primary bone lymphoma, *Eur J Radiol* 84:2275, 2015.

STAGING

Cates JM: Comparison of the AJCC, MSTS, and modified Spanier systems for clinical and pathological staging of osteosarcoma, *Am J Surg Pathol* 41:405, 2017.

Cates JMM: Simple staging system for osteosarcoma performs equivalently to the AJCC and MSTS systems, *J Orthop Res* 36:2802, 2018.

Doyle LA: Sarcoma classification: an update based on the 2013 World Health Organization Classification of Tumors of Soft Tissue and Bone, *Cancer* 120:1763, 2014.

Jeys LM, Thorne CJ, Parry M, et al.: A novel system for the surgical staging of primary high-grade osteosarcoma: the Birmingham classification, *Clin Orthop Relat Res* 475:842, 2017.

Jones NB, Iwenofu H, Scharschmidt T, Kraybill S: Prognostic factors and staging for soft tissue sarcomas: an update, *Surg Oncol Clin N Am* 21:187, 2012.

Maki RG, Moraco N, Antonescu CR, et al.: Toward better soft tissue sarcoma staging: building on American Joint Committee on Cancer staging systems versions 6 and 7, *Ann Surg Oncol* 20:3377, 2013.

Mansour 3rd AA, Kelley MC, Hatmaker AR, et al.: Verification of musculoskeletal FDG-PET-CT findings performed for melanoma staging, *Ann Surg Oncol* 17:1144, 2010.

O'Donnell PW, Griffin AM, Eward WC, et al.: Can experienced observers differentiate between lipoma and well-differentiated liposarcoma using only MRI? *Sarcoma* 982784, 2013.

Steffner RJ, Jang ES: Staging of bone and soft-tissue sarcomas, *J Am Acad Orthop Surg* 26:e269, 2018.

BIOPSY

Adams SC, Potter BK, Pitcher DJ, et al.: Office-based core needle biopsy of bone and soft tissue malignancies: an accurate alternative to open biopsy with infrequent complications, *Clin Orthop Relat Res* 468:2774, 2010.

Barrientos-Ruiz I, Ortiz-Cruz EJ, Serrano-Montilla J, et al.: Are biopsy tracts a concern for seeding an local recurrence in sarcomas? *Clin Orthop Relat Res* 475:511, 2017.

Ceraulo A, Ouziel A, Lavergne E, et al.: Percutaneous guided biopsy for diagnosing suspected primary malignant bone tumors in pediatric patients: a safe, accurate, and cost-saving procedure, *Pediatr Radiol* 47:235, 2017.

Das S, Dalai BS, Mukhopadhyay D, et al.: Fine needle aspiration cytology aided diagnosis of chordoma at an unusual site, *Cytopathology* 27:503, 2016.

Hedge V, Burke ZDC, Park HY, et al.: Is core needle biopsy reliable in differentiating between aggressive benign and malignant radiolucent tumors? *Clin Orthop Relat Res* 476:568, 2018.

Hodel S, Laux C, Farei-Campagna J, et al.: The impact of biopsy sampling errors and the quality of surgical margins on local recurrence and survival in chondrosarcoma, *Cancer Manag Res* 10:402, 2018.

Kaur I, Handa U, Kundu R, et al.: Role of fine-needle aspiration cytology and core needle biopsy in diagnosing musculoskeletal neoplasms, *J Cytol* 33:7, 2016.

Kubo T, Furuta T, Johan MP, et al.: A meta-analysis supports core needle biopsy by radiologists for better histological diagnosis in soft tissue and bone sarcomas, *Medicine (Baltimore)* 97:e11567, 2018.

Matti A, Farfolfi, Frisoni T, et al.: FDG-PET/CT guided biopsy in angiosarcoma of bone: diagnosis, staging and beyond, *Clin Nucl Med* 43:e48, 2018.

Ng VY, Thomas K, Crist M, et al.: Fine needle aspiration for clinical triage of extremity soft tissue masses, *Clin Orthop Relat Res* 468:1120, 2010.

Pohlig F, Kirchoff C, Lenze U, et al.: Percutaneous needle core biopsy versus open biopsy in diagnostics of bone and soft tissue sarcoma: a retrospective study, *Eur J Med Res* 17:29, 2012.

Rimondi E, Rosse G, Bartalena T, et al.: Percutaneous CT-guide biopsy of the musculoskeletal system: results of 2027 cases, *Eur J Radiol* 77:34, 2011.

Roitman PD, Farfalli GL, Ayerza MA, et al.: Is needle biopsy clinically useful in preoperative grading of central chondrosarcoma of the pelvic an long bones? *Clin Orthop Relat Res* 475:808, 2017.

Trieu J, Schlicht SM, Choong PF: Diagnosing musculoskeletal tumours: how accurate is CT-guided core needle biopsy? *Eur J Surg Oncol* 42:1049, 2016.

Wu JS, McMahon CJ, Lozano-Caleron S, et al.: JOURNAL CLUB: utility of repeat core needle biopsy of musculoskeletal lesions with initially nondiagnostic findings, *AJR Am J Roentgenol* 609:208, 2017.

Yang J, Frassica FJ, Fayad L, et al.: Analysis of nondiagnostic results after image-guided needle biopsies of musculoskeletal lesions, *Clin Orthop Relat Res* 468:3103, 2010.

Yu GH, Maisel J, Frank R, et al.: Diagnostic utility of fine-needle aspiration cytology of lesions involving bone, *Diagn Cytopathol* 45:608, 2017.

ADJUVANT TREATMENT

Albergo JI, Gaston CCL, Parry MC, et al.: Risk analysis factors for recurrence in Ewing's sarcoma: when should adjuvant radiotherapy be administered? *Bone Joint J* 100-B:247, 2018.

Albergo JI, Gaston CL, Laitinen M, et al.: Ewing's sarcoma: only patients with 100% of necrosis after chemotherapy should be classified as having a good response, *Bone Joint J* 98-B:1138, 2016.

Caracciolo JT, Letson GD: Radiologic approach to bone and soft tissue sarcomas, *Surg Clin North Am* 96:963, 2016.

Colangelo S, Parchi P, Andreani L, et al.: Cryotherapy efficacy and safety as local chondrosarcoma therapy in surgical treatment of musculoskeletal tumours. A retrospective case series of 143 patients, *J Biol Regul Homeost Agents* 32(6 Suppl 1):65, 2018.

De Felice F, Piccioli A, Musio D, et al.: The role of radiation therapy in bone metastases management, *Oncotarget* 8:25691, 2017.

Groenen KH, Pouw MH, Hannick G, et al.: The effect of radiotherapy, and radiotherapy combimed with bisphosphonates or RANK ligand inibitors on bone quality in bone metastases. A systematic review, *Radiother Oncol* 119:194, 2016.

Himelstein AL, Foster JC, Khatcheressian LJ, et al.: Effect of longer-interval vs standard dosing of zolendronic acid on skeletal events in patients with bone metastases: a randomized clinical trial, *JAMA* 317:48, 2017.

Mhaskar R, Djulbegovic B: Bisphosphonates for patients diagnosed with multiple myeloma, *JAMA* 320:1463, 2018.

Mhaskar R, Kumar A, Miladinovic B, et al.: Bisphosphonates in multiple myeloma: an updated network meta-analysis, *Cochrane Database Syst Rev* 12:CD003188, 2017.

Miller BJ, Gao Y, Duchman KR: Does surgery or radiation provide the best overall survival in Ewing's sarcoma? A review of the National Cancer Data Base, *J Surg Oncol* 116:384, 2017.

Traub F, Singh J, Dickson BC, et al.: Efficacy of denosumab in joint preservation for patients with giant cell tumour of bone, *Eur J Cancer* 59:1, 2016.

Tsang RW, Campbell RW, Goda JS, et al.: Radiation therapy for solitary plasmacytoma and multiple myeloma: guidelines from the International Lympoma Radiation Oncology Group, *Int Radiol Oncol Biol Phys* 101:794, 2018.

Wolaczyk MJ, Fakhrian K, Adamietz IA: Radiotherapy, bisphosphonates and surgical stabilization of complete or impending pathologic fractures in patients with metastatic bone disease, *J Cancer* 7:121, 2016.

Wu PK, Chen CF, Wang JY, et al.: Freezing nitrogen ethanol composite may be a viable approach for cryotherapy of human giant cell tumor of bone, *Clin Orthop Relat Res* 475:1650, 2017.

PRINCIPLES OF SURGERY

Angelini A, Drago G, Trovarelli G, et al.: Infection after surgical resection for pelvic bone tumors: an analysis of 270 patients from one institution, *Clin Orthop Relat Res* 472:349, 2014.

Asavamongkolkul A, Waikakul S: Wide resection of sacral chordoma via a posterior approach, *Int Orthop* 36:607, 2012.

Avedian RS, Haydon RC, Peabody TD: Multiplanar osteotomy with limited wide margins: a tissue preserving surgical technique for high-grade bone sarcomas, *Clin Orthop Relat Res* 468:2754, 2010.

Benevenia J, Rivero SM, Moore J, et al.: Supplemental bone grafting in giant cell tumor of the extremity reduces nononcologic complications, *Clin Orthop Relat Res* 475:776, 2017.

Blank A, Riesgo A, Gitelis S, et al.: Bone grafts, substitutes, and augments in benign orthopaedic conditions: current concepts, *Bull Hosp Jt Dis* 75:119, 2017.

Chen X, Yu LJ, Peng HM, et al.: Is intralesional resection suitable for central grade 1 chondrosarcoma: a systematic review and updated meta-analysis, *Eur J Surg Oncol* 43:1718, 2017.

Chen YC, Wu PK, Chen CF, et al.: Intralesional curettage of central low-grade chondrosarcoma: a midterm follow-up study, *J Chin Med Assoc* 80:178, 2017.

Chung SW, Han I, Oh JH, et al.: Prognostic effect of erroneous surgical procedures in patients with osteosarcoma: evaluation using propensity score matching, *J Bone Joint Surg Am* 96:e60, 2014.

Clarkson PW, Sandford K, Phillips AE, et al.: Functional results following vascularized versus nonvascularized bone grafts for wrist arthrodesis following excision of giant cell tumors, *J Hand Surg [Am]* 38:935, 2013.

Colangeli S, Muratori F, Bettini L, et al.: Surgical treatment of sacral chordoma: en bloc resection with negative margins is a determinant of the long-term outcome, *Surg Technol Int* 33:343, 2018.

Denaro L, Berton A, Ciuffreda M, et al.: Surgical management of chordoma: a systematic review, *J Spinal Cord Med* 1–16, 2018, [Epub ahead of print].

Dagan R, Indelicato DJ, McGee L, et al.: The significance of a marginal excision after preoperative radiation therapy for soft tissue sarcoma of the extremity, *Cancer* 118:3199, 2012.

Errani C, Tsukamoto S, Leone G, et al.: Higher local recurrence rates after intralesional surgery for giant cell tumor of the proximal femur compared to other sites, *Eur J Orthop Surg Traumatol* 27:813, 2017.

Ferrone ML, Raut CP: Modern surgical therapy: limb salvage and the role of amputation for extremity soft-tissue sarcomas, *Surg Oncol Clin N Am* 21:201, 2012.

Gronchi A, Colombo C, Raut CP: Surgical management of localized soft tissue tumors, *Cancer* 120:2638, 2014.

Groot OQ, Ogink PT, Janssen SJ, et al.: High risk of venous thromboembolism after surgery for long bone metastases: a retrospective study of 682 patients, *Clin Orthop Relat Res* 476:2052, 2018.

Guo W, Li D, Tang X, Ji T: Surgical treatment of pelvic chondrosarcoma involving periacetabulum, *J Surg Oncol* 101:160, 2010.

Guo W, Sun X, Ji T, Tang X: Outcome of surgical treatment of pelvic osteosarcoma, *J Surg Oncol* 106:406, 2012.

Guo W, Tang X, Zang J, Ji T: One-stage total en bloc sacrectomy: a novel technique and report of nine cases, *Spine (Phila Pa 1976)* 38:E626, 2013.

Han G, Bi WZ, Xu M, et al.: Amputation versus limb-salvage surgery in patients with osteosarcoma: a meta-analysis, *World J Surg* 40:2016, 2016.

Huang J, Bi W, Han G, et al.: The multidisciplinary treatment of osteosarcoma of the proximal tibia: a retrospective study, *BMC Musculoskelet Disord* 19:315, 2018.

Jeys L, Matharu GS, Nandra RS, Grimer RJ: Can computer navigation-assisted surgery reduce the risk of an intralesional margin and reduce the rate of local recurrence in patients with a tumour of the pelvis or sacrum? *Bone Joint J* 95:1417, 2013.

Kamal AF, Simbolon EL, Prabowo Y, et al.: Wide resection versus curettage with adjuvant therapy for giant cell tumour of bone, *J Orthop Surg (Hong Kong)* 24:228, 2016.

Kennedy S, Mayo Z, Gao Y, et al.: What are the results of surgical treatment of postoperative wound complications in soft tissue sarcoma? A retrospective, multi-center case series, *Iowa Orthop J* 38:131, 2018.

Kim JH, Kang HG, Kim HS: MRI-guided navigation surgery with temporary implantable bone markers in limb salvage for sarcoma, *Clin Orthop Relat Res* 468:2211, 2010.

King DM, Hackbarth DA, Kirkpatrick A: Extremity soft-tissue sarcoma resections: how wide do you need to be? *Clin Orthop Relat Res* 470:692, 2012.

Meftah M, Schult P, Henshaw RM: Long-term results of intralesional curettage and cryosurgery for treatment of low-grade chondrosarcoma, *J Bone Joint Surg Am* 95:1358, 2013.

Mei J, Zhu XZ, Wang ZY, Cai XS: Functional outcomes and quality of life in patients with osteosarcoma treated with amputation versus limb-salvage surgery: a systematic review and meta-analysis, *Arch Orthop Trauma Surg* 134:1507, 2014.

Mashhour MA, Abdel Rahman M: Lower recurrence rate in chondroblastoma using extended curettage and cryosurgery, *Int Orthop* 38:1019, 2014.

Mavrogenis AF, Abati CN, Romagnoli C, Ruggieri P: Similar survival but better function for patients after limb salvage versus amputation for distal tibia osteosarcoma, *Clin Orthop Relat Res* 470:1735, 2012.

Nota SP, Russchen MJ, Raskin KA, et al.: Functional and oncological outcome after surgical resection of the scapular and clavicle for primary chondrosarcoma, *Musculoskelet Surg* 101:67, 2017.

Omlor GW, Lohnherr V, Lange J, et al.: Endhoncromas and atypical cartilaginous tumors at the proximal humerus treated with intralesional resection and bone cement filling with or without osteosynthesis: retrospective analysis of 42 cases with 6 years mean follow-up, *World J Surg Oncol* 16:139, 2018.

Potter BK, Hwang PF, Forsberg JA, et al.: Impact of margin status and local recurrence on soft-tissue sarcoma outcomes, *J Bone Joint Surg Am* 95:e151, 2013.

Puri A, Pruthi M, Gulia A: Outcomes after limb sparing resection in primary malignant pelvic tumors, *Eur J Surg Oncol* 40:27, 2014.

Reddy KI, Wafa H, Gaston CL, et al.: Does amputation offer any survival benefit over limb salvage in osteosarcoma patients with poor chemonecrosis and close margins? *Bone J Journal* 97-B:115, 2015.

Sherman CE, O'Connor MI, Sim FH: Survival, local recurrence, and function after pelvic limb salvage at 23 to 38 years of follow-up, *Clin Orthop Relat Res* 470:712, 2012.

Souna BS, Belot N, Duval H, et al.: No recurrences in selected patients after curettage with cryotherapy for grade I chondrosarcomas, *Clin Orthop Relat Res* 468:1956, 2010.

Stihsen C, Panotopoulos J, Puchner SE, et al.: The outcome of the surgical treatment of pelvic chondrosarcomas: a competing risk analysis of 58 tumours from a single center, *Bone Joint J* 99-B:686, 2017.

Takeuchi A, Suwanpramote P, Yamamoto N, et al.: Mid- to long-term clinical outcome of giant cell tumor of bone treated with calcium phosphate cement following thorough curettage and phenolization, *J Surg Oncol* 117:1232, 2018.

van Houdt WJ, Griffin AM, Wunder JS, et al.: Oncologic outcome and quality of life after hindquarter amputation for sarcoma: is it worth it? *Ann Surg Oncol* 25:378, 2018.

Wang Y, Guo W, Shen D, et al.: Surgical treatment of primary chondrosarcoma of the sacrum: a case series of 26 patients, *Spine (Phila Pa 1976)* 42:1207, 2017.

Wong JC, Abraham JA: Upper extremity considerations for oncologic surgery, *Orthop Clin North Am* 45:541, 2014.

Xie L, Guo W, Li Y, et al.: Pathologic fracture does not influence local recurrence and survival in high-grade extremity osteosarcoma with adequate surgical margins, *J Surg Oncol* 106:820, 2012.

Yacob O, Umer M, Gul M, et al.: Segmental excision versus intralesional curettage with adjuvant therapy for giant cell tumour of bone, *J Orthop Surg (Hong Kong)* 24:88, 2016.

Yang Y, Han L, He Z, et al.: Advances in limb salvage treatment of osteosarcoma, *J Bone Oncol* 10:36, 2017.

Zhang Y, He Z, Li Y, et al.: Selection of surgical methods in the treatment of upper tibia osteosarcoma and prognostic analysis, *Oncol Res Treat* 40:528, 2017.

Zhao Z, Yan T, Guo W, et al.: Surgical treatment of primary malignant tumours of the distal tibia, *Bone Joint J* 100-B:1633, 2018.

RESECTION AND RECONSTRUCTION

Abdel MP, von Roth P, Perry KI, et al.: Early results of acetabular reconstruction after wide periacetabular oncologic resection, *J Bone Joint Surg Am* 99:e9, 2017.

Albergo JI, Gaston CL, Aponte-Tinao LA, et al.: Proximal tibia reconstruction after bone tumor resection: are survivorship and outcomes of endoprosthetic replacement and osteoarticular allograft similar? *Clin Orthop Relat Res* 475:676, 2017.

Bernthal NM, Schwartz AJ, Oakes DA, et al.: How long do endoprosthetic reconstructions for proximal femoral tumors last? *Clin Orthop Relat Res* 468:2867, 2010.

Biau DJ, Larousserie F, Thévenin F, et al.: Results of 32 allograft-prosthesis composite reconstructions of the proximal femur, *Clin Orthop Relat Res* 468:834, 2010.

Böhler C, Brönimann S, Kaider A, et al.: Surgical and functional outcome after endoprosthetic reconstruction in patients with osteosarcoma of the humerus, *Sci Rep* 8:16148, 2018.

Bus MP, Dijkstra PD, van de Sande MA, et al.: Intercalary allograft reconstructions following resection of primary bone tumors: a nationwide multicenter study, *J Bone Joint Surg Am* 96:e26, 2014.

Bus MP, van de Sande MA, Taminiau AH, et al.: Is there still a role for osteoarticular allograft reconstruction in musculoskeletal tumour surgery? A long-term follow-up study of 38 patients and systematic review of the literature, *Bone Joint J* 99-B:522, 2017.

Campanacci L, Ali N, Casanova JM, et al.: Resurfaced allograft prosthetic composite for proximal tibial reconstruction in children: intermediate-term results of an original technique, *J Bone Joint Surg Am* 97:241, 2015.

Campanacci D, Chacon S, Mondanelli N, et al.: Pelvic massive allograft reconstruction after bone tumour resection, *Int Orthop* 36:2529, 2012.

Guo Z, Li J, Pei GX, et al.: Pelvic reconstruction with a combined hemipelvic prosthesis after resection of primary malignant tumor, *Surg Oncol* 19:95, 2010.

Goulding KA, Schwartz A, Hattrup SJ, et al.: Use of compressive osseointegration endoprostheses for massive bone loss from tumor and failed arthroplasty: a viable option in the upper extremity, *Clin Orthop Relat Res* 475:1702, 2017.

Grimer RJ, Aydin BK, Xu M, et al.: Very long-term outcomes after endoprosthetic replacement for malignant tumours of bone, *Bone Joint J* 98-B:875, 2016.

Holm CE, Bardram C, Riecke AF, et al.: Implant and limb survival after resection of primary bone tumors of the lower extremities and reconstruction with mega-prosthesis: fifty patients followed for a mean of fourteen years, *Int Orthop* 42:1175, 2018.

Horstmann PF, Hettwer WN, Petersen MM: Treatment of benign and borderline bone tumors with combined curettage and bone defect reconstruction, *J Orthop Surg (Hong Kong)* 26:2309, 2018.

Li J, Wang Z, Guo Z, et al.: Precise resection and biological reconstruction under navigation guidance for young patients with juxta-articular bone sarcoma in lower extremity: preliminary report, *J Pediatr Orthop* 34:101, 2014.

Li J, Wang Z, Guo Z, et al.: The use of massive allograft with intramedullary fibular graft for intercalary reconstruction after resection of tibial malignancy, *J Reconstr Microsurg* 27:37, 2011.

Li X, Moretti VM, Ashana AO, Lackman RD: Perioperative infection rate in patients with osteosarcomas treated with resection and prosthetic reconstruction, *Clin Orthop Relat Res* 469:2889, 2011.

Lozano-Calderón SA, Swaim SO, Federico A, et al.: Predictors of soft-tissue complications and deep infection in allograft reconstruction of the proximal tibia, *J Surg Oncol* 113:811, 2016.

Lu C, Tu C, Min L, Duan H: Allograft arthrodesis of the knee for giant cell tumors, *Orthopedics* 35:e397, 2012.

Muscolo DL, Ayerza MA, Farfalli G, et al.: Proximal tibia osteoarticular allografts in limb-salvage surgery, *Clin Orthop Relat Res* 468:1396, 2010.

Pala E, Henderson ER, Calabro T, et al.: Survival of current production tumor endoprostheses: complications, functional results, and a comparative statistical analysis, *J Surg Oncol* 108:403, 2013.

Pradhan A, Reddy KI, Grimer RJ, et al.: Resurfaced allograt-prosthetic composite for proximal tibial reconstruction in children: intermediate-term results of an original technique, *J Bone Joint Surg Am* 97:241, 2015.

Puri A, Gulia A: The results of total humeral replacement following excision for primary bone tumour, *J Bone Joint Surg Br* 94:1277, 2012.

Schwartz AJ, Kabo JM, Eilber FC, et al.: Cemented distal femoral endoprostheses for musculoskeletal tumor: improved survival of modular versus custom implants, *Clin Orthop Relat Res* 468:2198, 2010.

Schwartz AJ, Kabo JM, Eilber FC, et al.: Cemented endoprosthetic reconstruction of the proximal tibia: how long do they last? *Clin Orthop Relat Res* 468:2875, 2010.

Ruggieri P, Mavrogenis AF, Pala E, et al.: Outcome of expandable prostheses in children, *J Pediatr Orthop* 33:244, 2013.

Wafa H, Reddy K, Grimer R, et al.: Does total humeral endoprosthetic replacement provide reliable reconstruction with preservation of a useful extremity? *Clin Orthop Relat Res* 473:917, 2015.

Wong KC, Kumta SM: Joint-preserving tumor resection and reconstruction using image-guided computer navigation, *Clin Orthop Relat Res* 471:762, 2013.

CONSIDERATIONS FOR PEDIATRIC PATIENTS

Aporte-Tinao LA, Albergo JI, Ayerza MA, et al.: What are the complications of allograft reconstructions for sarcoma resection in children younger than 10 years at long-term followup? *Clin Orthop Relat Res* 476:548, 2018.

Arkader A, Yang CH, Tolo VT: High long-term local control with sacretomy for primary high-grade bone sarcoma in children, *Clin Orthop Relat Res* 470:1491, 2012.

Beneditti MG, Okita Y, Recubini E, et al.: How much clinical and functional impairment do children treated with knee rotationplasty experience in adulthood? *Clin Orthop Relat Res* 474:1004, 2016.

Decilveo AP, Szczech BW, Topfer J, et al.: Reconstruction using expandable endoprostheses for skeletally immature patients with sarcoma, *Orthopedics* 40:e157, 2017.

Dotan A, Dadia S, Bickels J, et al.: Expandable endoprosthesis for limb-sparing surgery in children: long-term results, *J Child Orthop* 4:391, 2010.

Erol B, Topkar MO, Aydemir AN, et al.: A treatment strategy for proximal femoral benign bone lesions in children and recommended surgical procedures: retrospective analysis of 62 patients, *Arch Orthop Trauma Surg* 136:1051, 2016.

Fan H, Guo Z, Fu J, et al.: Surgical management of pelvic Ewing's sarcoma in children and adolescents, *Oncol Lett* 14:3917, 2017.

Farfalli GL, Slullitel PA, Muscolo DL, et al.: What happens to the articular surface after curettage for epiphyseal chondroblastoma? A report on functional results, arthritis, and arthroplasty, *Clin Orthop Relat Res* 475:760, 2017.

Groundland JS, Ambler SB, Houskamp LD, et al.: Surgical and functional outcomes after limb-preservation surgery for tumor in pediatric patients: a systematic review, *JBJS Rev* 4 pii: 01874474-201602000-00002, 2016.

Haddox CL, Han G, Anijar L, et al.: Osteosarcoma in pediatric patients and young adults: a single institution retrospective review of presentation, therapy, and outcome, *Sarcoma* 2014:402, 2014.

Harris JD, Trinh TQ, Scharschmidt TJ, Mayerson JL: Exceptional functional recovery and return to high-impact sports after Van Nes rotationplasty, *Orthopedics* 36:e126, 2013.

Isakoff MS, Barkauskas DA, Ebb D, et al.: Poor survival for osteosarcoma of the pelvis: a report from the Children's Oncology Group, *Clin Orthop Relat Res* 470:2012, 2007.

Jamshidi K, Bahrabadi M, Mirzaei A: Long-term results of osteoarticular allograft reconstruction in children with distal femoral bone tumors, *Arch Bone Jt Surg* 5:296, 2017.

Kaim M, Womer RB, Dormans JP: Surgical treatment of pelvic sarcoma in children: outcomes for twenty-six patients, *Int Orthop* 41:2149, 2017.

Kang S, Lee JS, Park J, et al.: Staged lengthening and reconstruction for children with a leg-length discrepancy after excision of an osteosarcoma around the knee, *Bone Joint J* 99-B:401, 2017.

Laitinen M, Parry M, Albergo JI, et al.: Outcome of pelvic bone sarcomas in children, *J Pediatr Orthop* 38:537, 2016.

Leary SE, Wozniak AW, Billups CA, et al.: Survival of pediatric patients after relapsed osteosarcoma: the St. Jude Children's Research Hospital experience, *Cancer* 119:2645, 2013.

Levin AS, Arkader A, Morris CD: Reconstruction following tumor resections in skeletally immature patients, *J Am Acad Orthop Surg* 25:204, 2017.

Madej T, Flak-Nurzynska J, Dutkiewicz E, Ciechomska A, et al.: Ultrasound image of malignant bone tumors in children. An analysis of nine patients diagnosed in 2011-2016, *J Ultrason* 18:103, 2018.

Ottaviani G, Robert RS, Huh WW, et al.: Sociooccupational and physical outcomes more than 20 years after the diagnosis of osteosarcoma in children and adolescents: limb salvage versus amputation, *Cancer* 119:3727, 2013.

Schinhan M, Tiefenboeck T, Funovics P, et al.: Extendible prostheses for children after resection of primary malignant bone tumor: twenty-seven years of experience, *J Bone Joint Surg Am* 97:1585, 2015.

Thacker MM: Malignant soft tissue tumors in children, *Orthop Clin North Am* 44:657, 2013.

Torner F, Segur JM, Ullot R, et al.: Non-invasive expandable prosthesis in musculoskeletal oncology paediatric patients for the distal and proximal femur. First results, *Int Orthop* 40:1683, 2016.

Tsagozis P, Parry M, Grimer R: High complication rate after extendible endoprosthetic replacement of the proximal tibia: a retrospective study of 42 consecutive children, *Acta Orthop* 89:678, 2018.

Xiong Y, Lang Y, Yu Z, et al.: The effects of surgical treatment with chondroblastoma in children and adolescents in open epiphyseal plate of long bones, *World J Surg Oncol* 16:14, 2018.

ROTATIONPLASTY

Benedetti MG, Coli M, Campanacci L, et al.: Postural control skills, proprioception, and risk of fall in long-term survivor patients treated with knee arthroplasty, *Int J Rehabil Res* 42:68, 2019.

Benedetti MG, Okita Y, Recubini E, et al.: How much clinical and functional impairment do children treated with knee rotationplasty experience in adulthood, *Clin Orthop Relat Res* 474:995, 2016.

Gradl G, Postl LK, Lenze U, et al.: Long-term functional outcome and quality of life following rotationplasty for treatment of malignant tumors, *BMC Musculoskelet Disrod* 16:262, 2015.

Morri M, Forni C: Rotationplasty in adult cancer patients: what is the rehab strategy and what results can be expected? A case study, *Prosthet Orthot Int* 41:517, 2017.

Sakkers R, van Wijk I: Amputation and rotationplasty in children with limb deficiencies: current concepts, *J Child Orthop* 10:619, 2016.

Sawamura C, Matsumoto S, Shimoji T, et al.: Indications for and complications of rotationplasty, *J Orthop Sci* 17:775, 2012.

The complete list of references is available online at Expert Consult.com.

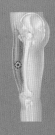

CHAPTER 8

BENIGN BONE TUMORS AND NONNEOPLASTIC CONDITIONS SIMULATING BONE TUMORS

Patrick C. Toy, Robert K. Heck Jr.

This chapter discusses bony lesions that do not usually behave aggressively locally and that have never been shown to metastasize. Most are either asymptomatic or minimally symptomatic except when complications, such as a pathologic fracture, occur. Many are discovered incidentally (Table 8.1).

BONE-FORMING TUMORS
OSTEOID OSTEOMA

Osteoid osteoma is a benign neoplasm most often seen in young men. Most osteoid osteomas are found in the second or third decades of life, but an occasional lesion has been reported in older patients. Almost any bone can be involved, although there is a predilection for the lower extremity, with half the cases involving the femur or tibia. The tumor may be found in cortical or cancellous bone. Multicentric lesions have been reported. No malignant change has ever been documented. The typical patient with an osteoid osteoma has pain that is worse at night and is relieved by aspirin or other nonsteroidal antiinflammatory medications. Increased levels of cyclooxygenases and prostaglandins have been demonstrated in the lesions. This fact explains the cause of the intense pain as well as the dramatic pain relief that results from treatment with nonsteroidal antiinflammatory medication. When the lesion is near a joint, swelling, stiffness, and contracture may occur. When the lesion is in a vertebra, scoliosis may occur. Imaging studies are usually diagnostic. Biopsy is rarely required to confirm the diagnosis. The lesion consists of a small (<1.5 cm), central radiolucent nidus with surrounding bony sclerosis. Plain radiographs are often sufficient to make the diagnosis. Computed tomography (CT) is the best technique to identify the nidus and confirm the diagnosis. The lesions demonstrate marked increased uptake on technetium bone scans. Magnetic resonance imaging (MRI) studies usually demonstrate extensive surrounding edema.

The microscopic appearance consists of fibrovascular tissue with immature bony trabeculae that are rimmed by prominent osteoblasts. The histologic appearance is similar to that of an osteoblastoma, with the exception that osteoblastomas are larger. The lesion is usually surrounded by a sclerotic rim. There is no nuclear atypia. Osteoclasts and occasional giant cells can be seen. There are no aggressive features.

Multiple treatment options are available, including medical treatment, percutaneous radiofrequency ablation, and open surgical procedures. If the patient's symptoms are adequately controlled and the patient is willing to undergo long-term medical management, antiinflammatory medication can be used as the definitive treatment. Patients treated in this manner usually experience spontaneous healing of the lesion within 3 to 4 years.

Most patients with lesions of the pelvis or long bones of the extremities can be treated with percutaneous radiofrequency ablation (Fig. 8.1). This technique involves a CT-guided core needle biopsy after which a radiofrequency electrode is inserted through the cannula of the biopsy needle. The temperature at the tip is increased to 90°C for 6 minutes. Multiple authors have reported excellent results with this procedure. It is usually done as an outpatient procedure, and patients can usually return immediately to full activity. Recurrence rates are less than 10%. Great care must be exercised when performing radiofrequency ablation on vertebral lesions because of the risk of injury to the spinal cord or nerve roots. The procedure may not be indicated for lesions of the small bones of the hands or feet because of the risk of thermal injury to the skin.

Surgical management involves removal of the entire nidus. This can be accomplished by curettage or en bloc resection. The latter is associated with a low recurrence rate but is rarely indicated for lesions in the long bones because of an increased risk of postoperative pathologic fracture. More often, removal is done using the burr-down technique (Fig. 8.2). This method consists of identifying the nidus intraoperatively with fluoroscopy and using a power burr to remove the sclerotic bone directly over the nidus. The nidus is removed

Text continued on page 348

343

TABLE 8.1

Lesions of Bone

TUMOR	AGE	DEMOGRAPHICS	SITE	PRESENTATION	IMAGING	HISTOLOGY	TREATMENT	COMMENTS
BONE-FORMING								
Osteoid osteoma	2nd-3rd decades	Male:female 3:1	Lower extremity long bones Posterior elements spine Diaphyseal/metaphyseal	Pain; worse at night Frequently responds to NSAIDs	Cortical radiolucent nidus <1.5 cm with marked cortical thickening	Trabeculae surrounded by loose fibrovascular tissue	NSAIDs Burr down technique Radiofrequency ablation	High levels of cyclooxygenases and prostaglandins in the lesion
Bone island	Adults	Male = female	Pelvis Femur	Usually asymptomatic	Small round area of increased density in cancellous bone with radiating spicules at periphery	Mature bone with thickened trabeculae that merge with normal bone at the periphery	Observation	Osteopoikilosis—multiple bone islands
CARTILAGE LESIONS								
Chondroma	Adults	Male = female	Hand Proximal humerus Distal femur Proximal tibia	Usually asymptomatic	Lobulated areas of stippled calcification Minimal cortical erosion (except in hand)	Benign-appearing hyaline cartilage	Observation Curettage if symptomatic	Ollier disease—multiple enchondromas (malignant transformation common) Maffucci syndrome—multiple enchondromas with soft-tissue hemangiomas (malignant transformation common)
Osteochondroma	2nd-3rd decades	Slight male predominance	Metaphysis of long bones	Mass; may be painful secondary to irritation of soft-tissue structures, fracture, or overlying bursa	Pedunculated or sessile bone lesion that communicates with intra-medullary canal of host bone. Lesion has overlying cartilage cap	Similar to epiphysis that undergoes endochondral ossification	Observation if asymptomatic Resection if symptomatic; cartilage cap must be removed entirely	Malignant transformation to chondrosarcoma is rare Multiple hereditary exostoses (MHE) is autosomal dominant with incomplete penetrance MHE—mutation of *EXT1* or *EXT2*

FIBROUS LESIONS

Lesion	Age	Sex	Location	Clinical Features	Radiographic Findings	Histology	Treatment	Notes
Nonossifying fibroma (NOF)	1st–2nd decades	Male=female	Metaphysis of long bones	Asymptomatic; usually discovered incidentally on plain radiographs unless pathologic fracture	Geographic, eccentric lesion located in metaphysis of long bones. Multilobulated appearance with well-defined sclerotic margins	Bland-appearing spindle cells arranged in a storiform pattern in a collagenous matrix	Observation. Curettage if large. Fractures usually treated nonoperatively	Jaffe-Campanacci syndrome—multiple NOFs with *café-au-lait* spots
Cortical desmoid	2nd decade	Male	Posteromedial distal femoral metaphysis	Usually asymptomatic	Erosion of the posteromedial distal femoral cortex with a sclerotic base	Fibrous tissue with collagenous stroma. Bland-appearing spindle cells arranged in a storiform pattern in a collagenous matrix (similar to NOF)	Observation	Possibly a reaction to pull of adductor magnus
Benign fibrous histiocytoma	4th–5th decades	Male=female	Pelvis Femur	Progressive pain	Lobulated, centrally located, radiolucent with sclerotic rim		Curettage	
Fibrous dysplasia	1st–3rd decades	Male=female	Femur Tibia	Pain Deformity Cutaneous pigmentation Endocrine abnormalities	Ground-glass appearance with well-defined sclerotic rim	Irregular woven bone spicules with a fibrous stroma	Prophylactic fixation of impending fractures. Correction of deformity. Bisphosphonates for severe cases	McCune-Albright syndrome—polyostotic fibrous dysplasia, cutaneous pigmentation, endocrine abnormalities. Mazabraud syndrome—polyostotic fibrous dysplasia, intramuscular myxomas

Continued

TABLE 8.1

Lesions of Bone—cont,d

TUMOR	AGE	DEMOGRAPHICS	SITE	PRESENTATION	IMAGING	HISTOLOGY	TREATMENT	COMMENTS
Osteofibrous dysplasia	1st-2nd decades	Male=female	Tibia (diaphysis)	Asymptomatic unless pathologic fracture Anterior bowing	Multicentric radiolucent lesions in the cortex of the tibia	Irregular trabeculae with prominent osteoblastic rimming Loose fibrous stroma	Observation Fractures usually treated nonoperatively Surgery for correction of deformity	
Desmoplastic fibroma	2nd-3rd decades	Male:female 2:1	Any	Pain Pathologic fracture	Radiolucent lesion with cortical erosion Frequently with septations May have soft-tissue mass	Hypocellular fibrous tissue with abundant collagen	Extended curettage vs. wide resection	
CYSTIC LESIONS								
Unicameral bone cyst	1st-2nd decades	Male:female 2:1	Proximal humerus Proximal femur	Asymptomatic unless pathologic fracture	Centrally located, purely radiolucent lesion Concentrically expands cortex No cortical destruction	Cyst filled with straw-colored fluid Thin fibrovascular lining	Observation Aspiration/ injection (steroids, bone marrow, bone graft substitute) Curettage	
Aneurysmal bone cyst	1st-2nd decades	Slight female predominance	Proximal humerus Distal femur Proximal tibia Spine (posterior elements)	Pain	Eccentric expansile radiolucent lesion Thin cortical shell Fluid/fluid levels on MRI	Hemorrhagic cavernous spaces Septae of fibroblasts, histiocytes, hemosiderin-laden macrophages, and giant cells	Extended curettage Consider preoperative embolization for pelvic lesions	
FATTY TUMORS								
Lipoma	Adults	Male=female	Any	Asymptomatic	Well-defined radiolucent lesions frequently with matrix calcification Normal fat signal on MRI	Fatty tissue with focal areas of necrosis	Observation	

VASCULAR TUMORS

	Age	Sex	Location	Symptoms	Imaging	Histology	Treatment	Comments
Hemangioma	Adults	Male:female 1:2	Vertebral body	Asymptomatic	Thickened vertically oriented trabeculae ("jailhouse" appearance on radiographs, "polka dot" appearance on CT) MRI bright on T1- and T2-weighted images	Proliferation of blood vessels	None	

OTHER NONNEOPLASTIC LESIONS

	Age	Sex	Location	Symptoms	Imaging	Histology	Treatment	Comments
Paget disease	5th-8th decades	Slight male predominance	Vertebral body Pelvis Proximal femur	Pain	Early lytic phase Late—thickened cortex, coarse trabeculae Bone scan—hot MRI—normal marrow signal	Woven bone Irregular cement lines Fibrovascular stroma	Bisphosphonates NSAIDs Calcitonin	Virus-like inclusion bodies suggest viral etiology Common in people of Anglo-Saxon descent, rare in others Disorder of unregulated bone turnover
Brown tumor	Adults	Male=female	Any	Bone lesions frequently asymptomatic unless pathologic fracture Symptoms of hypercalcemia (nausea, weakness, headaches, generalized bone pain)	Diffuse osteopenia Multifocal radiolucent lesions with surrounding reactive bone	Giant cells, increased osteoclastic activity, marrow fibrosis Diagnosis usually made by serum hypercalcemia and hypophosphatemia	Medical management by endocrinologist Surgery for actual or impending pathologic fractures	Primary hyperparathyroidism usually caused by parathyroid adenoma Secondary hyperparathyroidism usually caused by chronic renal failure

CT, Computed tomography; MRI, magnetic resonance imaging; NSAIDs, nonsteroidal antiinflammatory drugs.

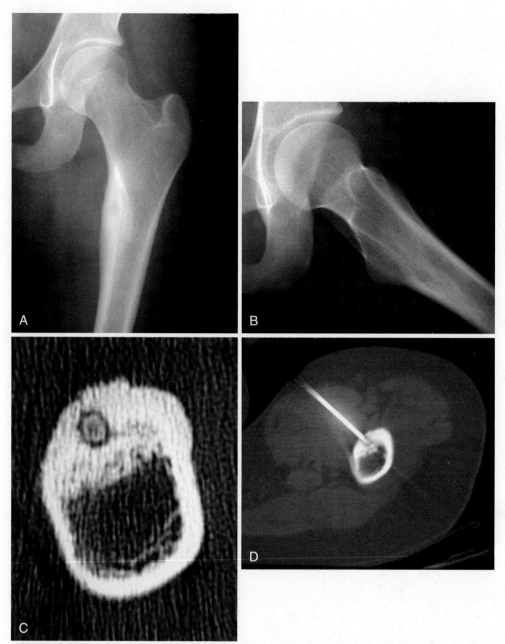

FIGURE 8.1   Imaging studies in 17-year-old girl who complained of left thigh pain for several months. Anteroposterior **(A)** and lateral **(B)** radiographs of left hip show small radiolucent lesion with thick sclerotic rim of reactive bone, suggestive of osteoid osteoma. **C,** Computed tomography clearly shows nidus and confirms diagnosis. **D,** Radiofrequency ablation probe placed into nidus under CT guidance.

using curets and sent for pathologic examination. The cavity is treated again with the power burr to ensure that the entire nidus has been removed. In this manner, only a minimal amount of surrounding reactive bone is removed, minimizing the risk of subsequent fracture. Recurrence rates with this technique are less than 10%.

A new noninvasive and radiation-free method of treatment is currently under investigation. Magnetic resonance–guided focused ultrasound (MRgFUS) ablation is a technique in which ultrasound waves are focused on the osteoid osteoma. When high-intensity waves are focused

on a single point, considerable heat can be generated. MRI is used for both lesion localization and temperature monitoring. Preliminary studies have shown this technique to be safe and effective. Larger studies are needed to confirm preliminary findings.

BONE ISLAND

Bone islands, also called enostoses, are benign lesions of cancellous bone. They are usually asymptomatic and are discovered incidentally. Almost any bone can be involved, but the

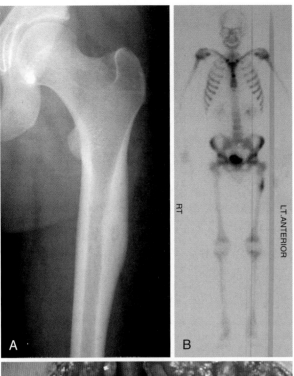

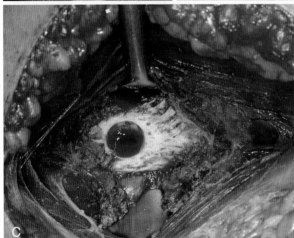

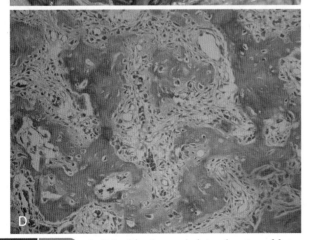

FIGURE 8.2 **A,** Osteoid osteoma in lateral cortex of femoral diaphysis of 16-year-old boy. **B,** Technetium bone scan shows increased uptake in area of lesion. **C,** Intraoperative photograph after burr-down procedure. **D,** Typical microscopic appearance of osteoid osteoma.

pelvis and the femur are the most common sites. It is unclear whether they represent a developmental abnormality or neoplastic process. Regardless, most remain quiescent. They are of interest primarily because other, more aggressive, lesions are occasionally in the differential diagnosis for patients with bone islands. Osteopoikilosis is a rare condition consisting of multiple small bone islands throughout the skeleton. Autosomal dominant and sporadic forms of the syndrome have been identified.

Bone islands can usually be diagnosed by plain radiographs. They are typically small, round or oval areas of homogeneous-increased density within the cancellous bone (Fig. 8.3A). Radiating spicules on the periphery of the bone islands merge with the native bone creating a brush-like border. No bony destruction or periosteal reaction is noted. They may show mildly increased uptake on bone scans; however, markedly positive scans should raise suspicion of more aggressive lesions. CT scans show thickened trabeculae, which merge with the surrounding bone. MRI usually shows well-defined lesions that are isointense to cortical bone and thus dark on T1- and T2-weighted images (Fig. 8.3B and C) with no surrounding edema. There are no aggressive imaging features.

The microscopic appearance reflects the imaging characteristics. Bone islands consist of mature bone with thickened trabeculae. At the periphery of the lesion, the lesional trabeculae merge with the normal bone. There is no sclerotic rim. Occasionally, woven bone is a minor part of the lesion.

Most patients with bone islands can be treated with observation with serial plain radiographs. As long as the lesions remain asymptomatic and do not grow, no further intervention is indicated. If a patient experiences pain, or if the lesion grows, biopsy is indicated to rule out more aggressive lesions, such as a sclerosing osteosarcoma, blastic metastasis, or sclerotic myeloma.

CARTILAGE LESIONS
CHONDROMA

Chondromas are benign lesions of hyaline cartilage. They are common, and all age groups are affected. Although any bone can be involved, the phalanges of the hand are the most common location. They are the most common tumor of the small bones of the hands and feet. Chondromas are usually asymptomatic and are frequently discovered incidentally during an unrelated radiographic examination. They can also be discovered after a pathologic fracture. They usually arise in the medullary canal, where they are referred to as *enchondromas*. Rarely, they arise on the surface of the bone, where they are referred to as *periosteal chondromas* or *juxtacortical chondromas*.

Multiple enchondromatosis, also known as Ollier disease, is a rare condition in which many cartilaginous tumors appear in the large and small tubular bones and in the flat bones. It is caused by failure of normal endochondral ossification. The tumors are located in the epiphysis and the adjacent parts of the metaphysis and shaft, and many bones may be affected. Deformities resulting from the tumors include shortening caused by lack of epiphyseal growth, broadening of the metaphyses, and bowing of the long bones. Multiple lesions of the small bones of the hand may cause considerable disability. When associated with hemangiomas of the overlying soft

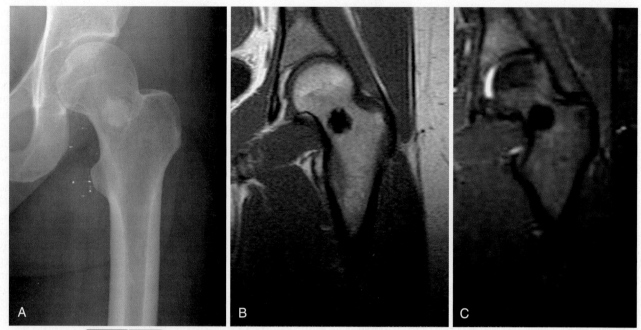

FIGURE 8.3   **A,** Bone island in femoral neck of 30-year-old woman. **B** and **C,** Lesion is dark on T1- and T2-weighted MR images.

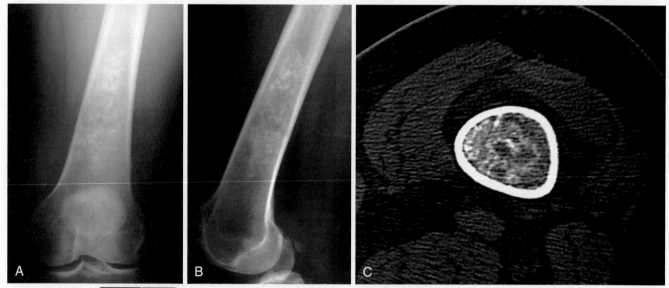

FIGURE 8.4   **A** and **B,** Anteroposterior and lateral radiographs of distal femur of 55-year-old woman show calcified lesion without cortical destruction most consistent with enchondroma. **C,** CT is best imaging study to confirm that there is no cortical destruction that might suggest chondrosarcoma.

tissues, the disease is known as Maffucci syndrome. The individual lesions are similar to solitary enchondromas but they have a definite tendency to become malignant. Approximately 25% of patients with Ollier disease are diagnosed with sarcomas by 40 years of age.

Radiographically, enchondromas are benign-appearing tumors with intralesional calcification (Fig. 8.4A and B). The calcification is irregular and has been described as "stippled," "punctate," or "popcorn." In the small bones of the hands and feet there may be considerable erosion and expansion of the overlying cortex. In more proximal locations (e.g., the pelvis, proximal humerus, or proximal femur), deep endosteal erosion (two thirds of the thickness of the cortex) frequently indicates a chondrosarcoma. An associated soft-tissue mass is never present with an enchondroma and always indicates a chondrosarcoma. Juxtacortical chondromas are usually small (<3 cm), well-defined lesions that frequently appear to fit in a saucer-shaped defect on the surface of the bone (Fig. 8.5). The underlying cortex appears sclerotic and the edges of the lesion appear to be buttressed by a thick rind of cortical bone. Plain radiographs are usually sufficient to diagnose a chondroma. If the diagnosis is in question, CT is best to evaluate endosteal erosion that could indicate a chondrosarcoma (Fig. 8.4C).

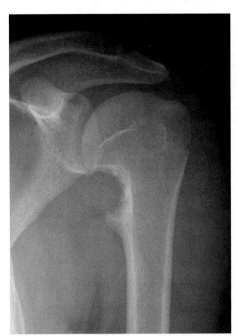

FIGURE 8.5   Anteroposterior radiograph of left proximal humerus of 18-year-old man with a juxtacortical chondroma.

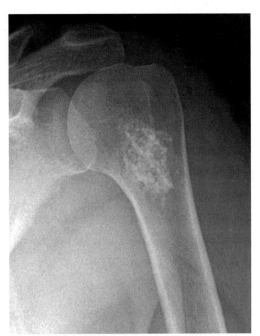

FIGURE 8.6   Anteroposterior radiograph of left shoulder of 41-year-old woman with proximal humeral enchondroma who complained of left shoulder pain with overhead activity. It was determined that her symptoms were caused by her rotator cuff. She responded well to physical therapy, and lesion remained radiographically stable.

The microscopic appearance of a chondroma is that of mature hyaline cartilage. Proximally located enchondromas should appear bland and hypocellular. Any degree of hypercellularity or atypia in a proximally located cartilage tumor should raise suspicion of a chondrosarcoma. Enchondromas of the hand, juxtacortical chondromas, and lesions associated with multiple enchondromatosis may be relatively hypercellular with mild atypia, and still be benign. The differentiation of benign from malignant cartilaginous tumors is one of the most difficult problems in bone pathology. All available tissue must be examined, and even then the diagnosis may depend more on the clinical and radiographic features than on the microscopic changes.

Treatment of patients with solitary enchondromas usually consists of observation with serial radiographs. If the lesion remains radiographically stable and asymptomatic, no further intervention is indicated. If a lesion grows or if it becomes symptomatic, extended curettage is usually curative. Before recommending surgery for a symptomatic lesion, however, all efforts should be made to rule out other possible sources of the patient's pain (e.g., rotator cuff tear in a patient with a proximal humeral enchondroma) (Fig. 8.6). Recurrence rates are low. Treatment of patients with multiple enchondromatosis can be more difficult. Although the individual lesions are usually not treated, the more obvious deformities can be corrected by osteotomy. These patients must also be monitored indefinitely for malignant change.

OSTEOCHONDROMA

Osteochondromas are common benign bone tumors. They are probably developmental malformations rather than true neoplasms and are thought to originate within the periosteum as small cartilaginous nodules. The lesions consist of a bony mass, often in the form of a stalk, produced by progressive endochondral ossification of a growing cartilaginous cap. In contrast to true neoplasms, their growth usually parallels that of the patient and usually ceases when skeletal maturity is reached. Most lesions are found during the period of rapid skeletal growth. Approximately 90% of patients only have a single lesion. Osteochondromas may occur on any bone preformed in cartilage but are usually found on the metaphysis of a long bone near the physis (Fig. 8.7). They are seen most often on the distal femur, the proximal tibia, and the proximal humerus. They rarely develop in a joint. Trevor disease (dysplasia epiphysealis hemimelica) refers to an intra-articular epiphyseal osteochondroma. When multiple joints are involved, it is usually unilateral (hemimelica).

Many of these lesions cause no symptoms and are discovered incidentally. Some cause mechanical symptoms by irritating the surrounding structures and, rarely, one becomes painful due to a fracture. False aneurysms of major lower extremity vessels caused by pressure from osteochondromas have been reported. Also, neuropathies caused by pressure from contiguous osteochondromas have occurred; the physical finding is usually a palpable mass.

Multiple hereditary exostoses is an autosomal-dominant condition with variable penetrance. Most patients with this disorder have a mutation in one of two genes: *EXT1*, which is located on chromosome 8q24.11-q24.13, or *EXT2*, which is located on chromosome 11p11-12. In this disease, osteochondromas of many bones are caused by an anomaly of skeletal development. The most striking feature is the presence of many exostoses (Fig. 8.8), but disturbances in growth also occur, such as abnormal tubulation of bones, producing broad and blunt metaphyses, and sometimes bowing of

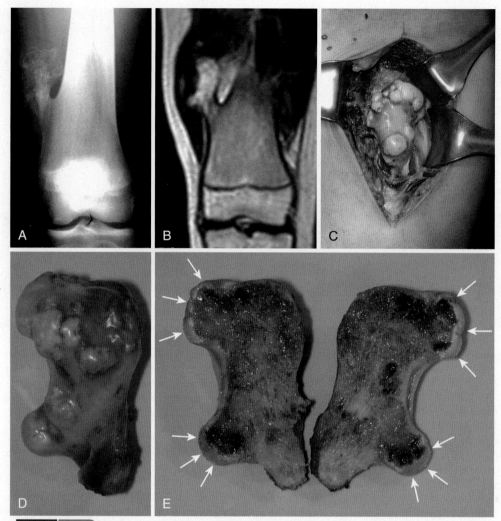

FIGURE 8.7   **A** and **B,** Radiograph and MR image of osteochondroma on distal femur of 15-year-old girl. **C,** Intraoperative photograph of lesion. **D,** Photograph of specimen. **E,** Photograph of bisected specimen. Cartilage caps are only 3 to 4 mm thick *(arrows).*

the radius and shortening of the ulna, producing ulnar deviation of the hand. The disease only occurs 5% to 10% as often as solitary osteochondroma and is more common in males. It is usually discovered at approximately the same age as the solitary lesion, but closer examination of children in families with the disease might lead to earlier discovery.

Osteochondromas are of two types: pedunculated and broad based or sessile. All gradations between these types also occur. Pedunculated tumors are more common, and any definite stalk is directed away from the physis adjacent to which it takes its origin. The projecting part of the lesion has cortical and cancellous components, both of which are continuous with corresponding components of the parent bone. The lesion is covered by a cartilaginous cap that is often irregular and cannot usually be seen on radiographs; occasionally, calcification within the cap may be seen. Typically, the cap is only a few millimeters thick in adults, although it may be 2 cm thick in a child. A bursa frequently overlies the tumor and may contain osteocartilaginous loose bodies. Plain radiographs are usually sufficient to make a diagnosis. Occasionally, a CT or MRI scan is needed to confirm the diagnosis.

Malignant degeneration is extremely rare. Large series have estimated the incidence of malignant degeneration to be approximately 1% for patients with a solitary osteochondroma and 5% for patients with multiple hereditary exostoses. However, these percentages were derived from pathologic data and thus there is inherent bias toward large, symptomatic lesions that subsequently underwent resection at a referral center. The true incidence of malignant degeneration is much lower than these figures suggest because the true prevalence of osteochondromas is unknown. Most patients are asymptomatic and never seek medical attention. Malignant transformation should be suspected when a previously quiescent lesion in an adult grows rapidly; it usually takes the form of a low-grade chondrosarcoma. In these cases, the cartilage cap is usually more than 2 cm thick. Malignant transformation is best evaluated by CT or MRI.

Surgery (en bloc resection) is indicated when the lesion is large enough to be unsightly or produces symptoms from pressure on surrounding structures or when imaging features suggest malignancy. On rare occasions, the diagnosis of a sessile lesion cannot be established by studying the radiographs, and biopsy is indicated. Recurrence is rare and is probably caused by failure to remove the entire cartilaginous cap. Patients with multiple hereditary exostoses may require osteotomies to correct deformity.

A similar lesion, subungual exostosis, may develop on a distal phalanx, especially of the great toe. Often there is a definite history of trauma. Excision is indicated when elevation of the nail produces pain. The history and location of the lesion distinguish it from a true osteochondroma.

FIBROUS LESIONS
NONOSSIFYING FIBROMA

Nonossifying fibromas (also known as metaphyseal fibrous defects, fibrous cortical defects, and fibroxanthomas) are common developmental abnormalities and are believed to occur in 35% of children. Usually, they are found incidentally. Generally, these lesions occur in the metaphyseal region of long bones in individuals 2 to 20 years old. Although any bone may be involved, approximately 40% of these lesions are found in the distal femur, 40% in the tibia, and 10% in the fibula. On plain radiographs, a nonossifying fibroma appears as a well-defined lobulated lesion located eccentrically in the metaphysis (Fig. 8.9). Multilocular appearance or ridges in the bony wall, sclerotic scalloped borders, and erosion of the cortex are frequent findings. There is no periosteal reaction in the absence of a pathologic fracture.

Histologically, the defect is filled with spindle-shaped cells distributed in a whorled or storiform pattern. There is fibroblastic proliferation with high cellularity. Giant cells and foam cells are almost always apparent.

Most nonossifying fibromas are asymptomatic and regress spontaneously in adulthood. Most pathologic fractures can be treated nonoperatively. Lesions may become symptomatic and require treatment if they become large or if they are subjected to repeated trauma. Some authors have recommended treatment for lesions that are larger than 50% of the diameter of the bone because of a theoretical increased risk of pathologic fracture, although this parameter is not universally accepted as an indication for surgery. Recurrence after curettage is rare (Fig. 8.10).

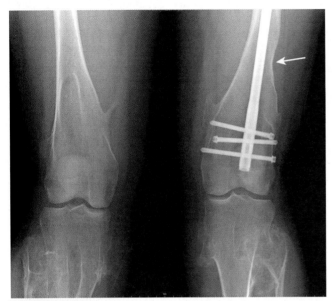

FIGURE 8.8 Knees of 22-year-old woman with multiple hereditary exostoses. *Arrow* marks healed femoral fracture sustained in postoperative period after resection of one of the lesions. Note tibial angulation.

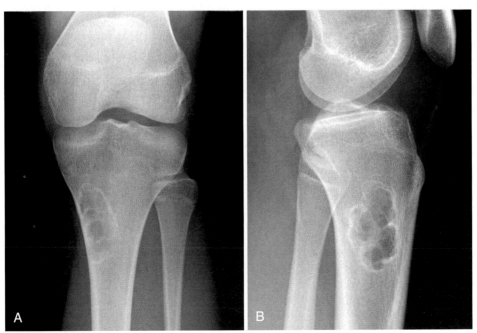

FIGURE 8.9 **A** and **B**, Anteroposterior and lateral radiographs of nonossifying fibroma of proximal tibia in a 15-year-old patient.

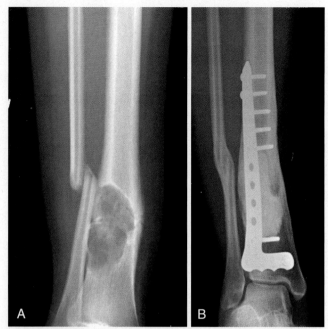

FIGURE 8.10 A 14-year-old adolescent sustained a pathologic fracture through distal tibial nonossifying fibroma after minimal trauma. **A,** Valgus malunion of distal tibia. **B,** Two years after osteotomy, curettage, and bone grafting (calcium phosphate/calcium sulfate bone graft substitute), patient was asymptomatic and had normal function.

CORTICAL DESMOID

A cortical desmoid is an irregularity in the posteromedial aspect of the distal femoral metaphysis and is usually seen in boys 10 to 15 years old. It may be a reaction to muscle stress exerted by the adductor magnus. The lesion is best seen on an oblique radiograph made with the lower extremity externally rotated 20 to 45 degrees. Clinical symptoms, if any, include soft-tissue swelling and pain. Radiographs and MRI reveal erosion of the cortex with a sclerotic base (Fig. 8.11). A biopsy is not warranted. Treatment usually consists of observation.

BENIGN FIBROUS HISTIOCYTOMA

Benign fibrous histiocytoma is a rare entity that was first described by Dahlin in 1978. This lesion occurs most frequently in the soft tissues and is less common in bone. Although it is histologically similar to nonossifying fibroma, it is a much more aggressive tumor in its biologic behavior and radiographic characteristics (Fig. 8.12). In contrast to nonossifying fibroma, which is usually an eccentric metaphyseal lesion, benign fibrous histiocytoma may occur in the diaphysis or epiphysis of long bones or in the pelvis. It is distinguished further by its occurrence in older patients between the ages of 30 and 40 years. Radiographically, benign fibrous histiocytoma is a well-defined, lytic, expanding lesion with little periosteal reaction. Bone scans are usually mildly positive. In contrast to nonossifying fibroma, this lesion is considered a true neoplasm. Because of its tendency for local recurrence, extended curettage or wide resection is recommended.

FIBROUS DYSPLASIA

Fibrous dysplasia is a developmental anomaly of bone formation that may exist in a monostotic or polyostotic form. The hallmark is replacement of normal bone and marrow by fibrous tissue and small, woven spicules of bone. Fibrous dysplasia can occur in the epiphysis, metaphysis, or diaphysis. Associated abnormalities, such as sexual precocity, abnormal skin pigmentation, intramuscular myxoma, and thyroid disease, may be present. McCune-Albright syndrome refers to polyostotic fibrous dysplasia, cutaneous pigmentation, and endocrine abnormalities. Mazabraud syndrome is polyostotic fibrous dysplasia with intramuscular myxomas. Malignant change is extremely rare but has been reported occasionally with and without prior radiotherapy.

The radiographic appearance is characteristic, with the lucent area having a granular, ground-glass appearance with a well-defined sclerotic rim (Fig. 8.13). Occasionally, biopsy is necessary to establish the diagnosis. The histopathologic appearance is that of irregular woven bone spicules with a fibrous stroma. Small areas of cartilaginous metaplasia and cystic changes may be present (Fig. 8.14). Surgical treatment is indicated when significant deformity or pathologic fracture occurs or when significant pain exists. Actual and impending pathologic fractures are best treated with intramedullary fixation when possible. Deformities are corrected by osteotomy with internal fixation. Because recurrence rates are high after curettage and bone grafting, cortical bone grafts are preferred over cancellous grafts or bone graft substitutes because of their slower resorption. Studies suggest that treatment with bisphosphonates is likely to be beneficial for patients with extensive disease.

OSTEOFIBROUS DYSPLASIA

Osteofibrous dysplasia (ossifying fibroma of long bones, also known as Campanacci disease) is a rare lesion usually affecting the tibia and fibula. Patients are usually in the first two decades of life. The middle third of the tibia is the most frequently affected location, and although the lesion usually is diaphyseal, it may encroach on the metaphysis. The tibia is enlarged and often bowed anterolaterally. Pain is usually absent unless pathologic fracture has occurred. The radiographs show eccentric intracortical osteolysis with expansion of the cortex (Fig. 8.15). Histologic studies reveal zonal architecture with loose fibrous tissue in the center of the lesion and a band of bony trabeculae rimmed by active osteoblasts at the periphery. The lesion must be distinguished from adamantinoma and monostotic fibrous dysplasia. The natural course of the lesion is unpredictable. Some lesions regress spontaneously during childhood; most progress during childhood, but not after puberty. Recurrence rates are high after curettage or marginal resection in children. Conversely, recurrence rates are low after surgery in skeletally mature patients. Pathologic fractures can be treated nonoperatively. Surgical management is aimed at preventing or correcting deformity.

DESMOPLASTIC FIBROMA

Desmoplastic fibroma is an extremely rare, locally aggressive benign bone tumor. It is similar to, and can be considered the bony counterpart of, the much more common desmoid tumor of soft tissue. It has been reported in all age groups but is more common in the second and third decades. The long tubular bones are involved most often, but involvement of the

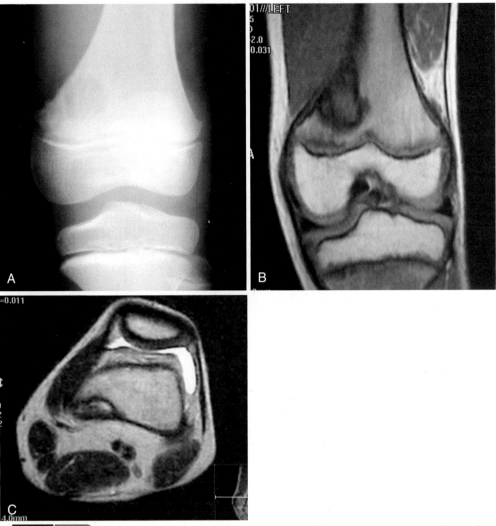

FIGURE 8.11   Cortical desmoid of left femur in 8-year-old boy. Anteroposterior radiograph **(A)** and coronal **(B)** and axial **(C)** MR images.

skull, mandible, pelvis, and spine has been reported. Pain is typically the chief complaint.

Radiographs typically reveal a well-circumscribed lytic lesion with a narrow zone of transition and, frequently, a thin rim of reactive bone (Fig. 8.16A and B). Cortical destruction may be present. The lesion sometimes appears septate. On MRI, desmoplastic fibroma, similar to other fibrous tumors, may show low signal intensity on T1- and T2-weighted images (Fig. 8.16C and D). Grossly, the lesional tissue is dense and tough, resembling the soft-tissue desmoid lesions. It also resembles these lesions microscopically; it is hypocellular and fibroblastic and contains much collagen and few mitoses (Fig. 8.16E).

This tumor does not metastasize, but local recurrence is common after simple curettage. Wide resection is generally recommended. Aggressive extended curettage may be a reasonable option in selected patients to try to preserve better function. Adjuvant treatments that have been shown to be effective for treating soft-tissue desmoid tumors (e.g., radiation, antiinflammatory agents, tamoxifen, and cytotoxic agents) may have a role in treating patients with desmoplastic fibromas; however, few data support this approach.

CYSTIC LESIONS
UNICAMERAL BONE CYST

Unicameral bone cysts are common lesions of childhood more consistent with a developmental or reactive lesion than a true tumor. Eighty-five percent occur in the first two decades with a 2:1 male predominance. Any bone of the extremities can be affected, but unicameral bone cysts are most common in the proximal humerus and femur. In adults, the ilium and calcaneus are more common locations. The lesions are most active during skeletal growth and usually heal spontaneously at maturity. Unicameral bone cysts are often asymptomatic unless a pathologic fracture has occurred. Two thirds of patients present with fractures that can stimulate the cyst to heal. Unicameral bone cysts in the flat bones are usually asymptomatic, found incidentally, and rarely fracture.

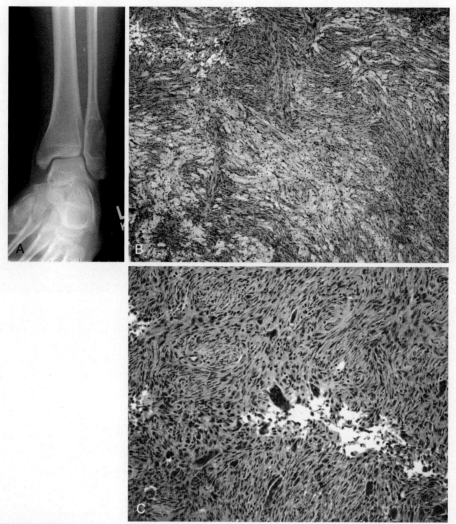

FIGURE 8.12 **A,** Radiograph of a benign fibrous histiocytoma of lateral malleolus. Low-power **(B)** and high-power **(C)** photomicrographs demonstrate typical histologic appearance of benign fibrous histiocytoma.

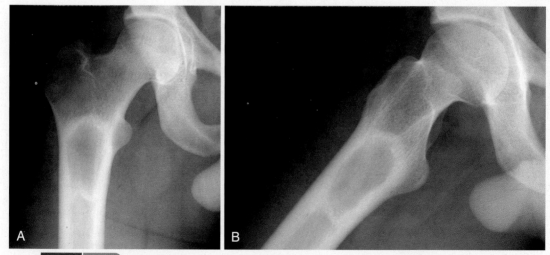

FIGURE 8.13 **A** and **B,** Anteroposterior and lateral radiographs of right hip of 22-year-old man with fibrous dysplasia of right proximal femur who complained of pain after water-skiing injury. He had no pain before injury. Symptoms resolved with conservative treatment, and lesion remained radiographically stable.

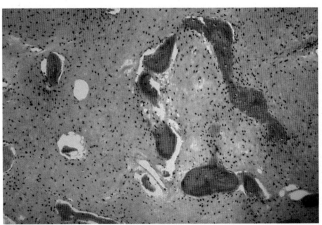

FIGURE 8.14 Typical histologic appearance of fibrous dysplasia.

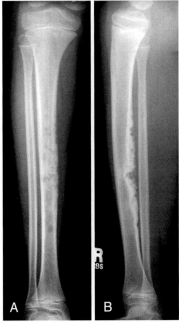

FIGURE 8.15 A and B, Anteroposterior and lateral radiographs of 10-year-old boy with osteofibrous dysplasia of the right tibia.

Plain radiographs reveal a centrally located, purely lytic lesion with a well-marginated outline and are usually diagnostic for a unicameral bone cyst. The cyst may expand concentrically but never penetrates the cortex. Prominent osseous ridges on the inner cortical wall may give it a multiloculated appearance. No periosteal reaction is present unless there has been a fracture. Occasionally (20%), a thinned cortical fragment fractures and falls into the base of the lesion, confirming its empty cystic nature. This "fallen fragment" sign is pathognomonic of a unicameral bone cyst with a fracture. Unicameral bone cysts start as metaphyseal lesions that abut the physis in growing children. With time, they appear to move into the diaphysis as the physis grows away from the cyst. Unicameral bone cysts are classified as active when they are within 1 cm of the physis and latent when they are closer to the diaphysis.

The exact pathogenesis of these cystic lesions is unclear. The most widely accepted theory is that a focal defect in metaphyseal remodeling blocks interstitial fluid drainage. This leads to increased pressure, which leads to focal bone necrosis and accumulation of fluid.

Investigations have shown that the cyst fluid contains prostaglandins, oxygen-free radicals, interleukins, cytokines, and metalloproteinases, all of which may contribute to bone resorption. Unicameral bone cysts are filled with a clear yellow, serous fluid unless a pathologic fracture has caused bleeding into the cavity. A fibrous membrane, usually less than 1 mm thick, lines the cyst wall. The lining of a unicameral bone cyst is composed of fibroblasts, rather than endothelial cells. Deep to this membrane lining, the cyst wall consists of fibrovascular tissue with fragments of immature bone, osteoclast-like giant cells, mesenchymal cells, and occasional lymphocytes.

Small, asymptomatic lesions in the upper extremities can be treated with observation with serial plain radiographs. Larger lesions (lesions at risk of pathologic fracture), symptomatic lesions, and lesions in the lower extremities are usually treated with curettage (with or without bone grafting or internal fixation) or aspiration and injection (often using corticosteroids, bone marrow aspirate, demineralized bone matrix, or other materials). Pathologic fractures in the upper extremity can be treated conservatively because the fracture may initiate cyst "healing." Fractures through unicameral bone cysts in the proximal femur should be treated with curettage, bone grafting, and internal fixation. Flexible intramedullary nailing has been used in the femur and humerus and provides early stability, often obviating the need for a cast, and decreases the risk of further pathologic fracture.

Corticosteroid injection was introduced as a treatment option for unicameral bone cysts in the mid-1970s because the recurrence rate after curettage and bone grafting was approximately 50%. Corticosteroid injection was described as an effective new treatment option that was inexpensive and involved less morbidity. The procedure is done with the patient heavily sedated or anesthetized. Fluoroscopic guidance is used to observe an 18-gauge spinal needle as it penetrates the cortex overlying the lesion at one end of the cyst; a second needle is placed at the opposite end. The diagnosis of a unicameral bone cyst is confirmed through the efflux of straw-colored cyst fluid. Many authors recommend that a cystogram be done using radiopaque dye and injecting each separate cavity if possible. Generally, 80 to 200 mg of methylprednisolone (Depo-Medrol) is used, depending on the size and age of the patient and the size of the lesion. This technique is believed to work either by an antiprostaglandin effect or by decreasing the pressure of the cyst. If the lesion does not show radiographic signs of healing in 2 months, repeat injections should be considered. More than 90% of patients can be treated successfully in this manner.

Other materials used for percutaneous treatment of unicameral bone cysts include autogenous bone marrow mixed with allograft demineralized bone matrix, high-porosity hydroxyapatite, calcium sulfate, calcium phosphate bone graft substitutes (Fig. 8.17), and cancellous allograft. No study has shown the superiority of one type of injection over another. Poor prognosis factors for successful percutaneous treatment of a unicameral bone cyst include

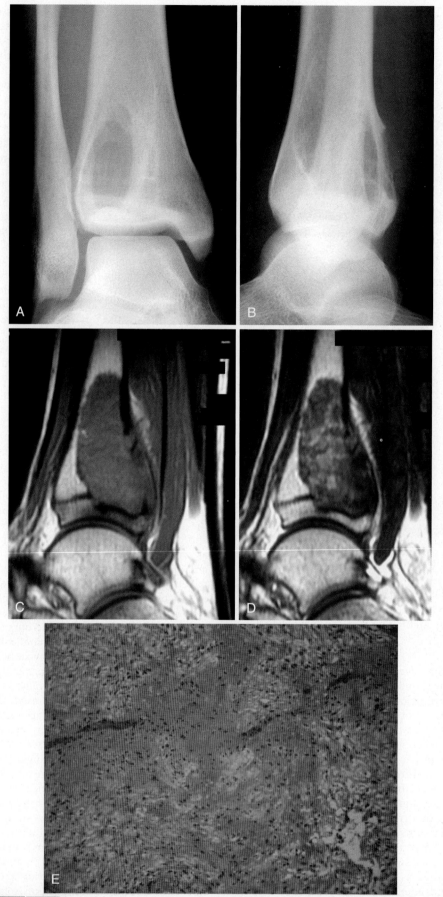

FIGURE 8.16 **A** and **B,** Anteroposterior and lateral radiographs of 19-year-old man with desmoplastic fibroma of right distal tibia. **C** and **D,** Note dark signal on T1- and T2-weighted MR images. **E,** Histologic appearance.

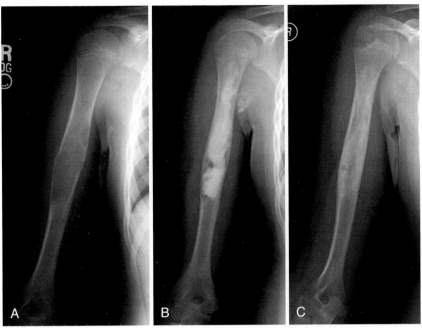

FIGURE 8.17 **A,** Anteroposterior radiograph of 8-year-old girl with pathologic fracture through unicameral bone cyst of the right humerus. **B,** Immediate postoperative radiograph after aspiration and injection using a calcium sulfate/calcium phosphate bone graft substitute. **C,** Radiograph at 1 year demonstrating remodeling of bone graft with no sign of cyst recurrence.

a multiloculated appearance, large size, radiographically active lesions, and patient age younger than 10 years. After three injections without healing, curettage and bone grafting should be considered.

Curettage, bone grafting, and internal fixation should be considered for large painful lesions in areas such as the proximal femur that are at high risk for fracture. Allograft bone or one of the many commercially available bone graft substitutes can provide excellent healing without the morbidity of autograft harvest.

ANEURYSMAL BONE CYST

Aneurysmal bone cysts are locally destructive, blood-filled reactive lesions of bone and are not considered to be true neoplasms. Any bone may be involved, but the most common locations include the proximal humerus, distal femur, proximal tibia, and spine. Vertebral lesions, accounting for 15% to 20% of these entities, are located in the posterior elements, with frequent extension into the vertebral body or to adjacent levels. Most occur in patients younger than 20-years old, and there is a slight female predominance. Most patients with aneurysmal bone cysts complain of mild-to-moderate pain that has been present for weeks to several months. Rapid growth can occur and clinically may mimic a malignancy. Spinal lesions may cause neurologic deficits or radicular pain.

Radiographs reveal an expansile lytic lesion that elevates the periosteum but remains contained by a thin shell of cortical bone. An aneurysmal bone cyst can have well-defined margins or a permeative appearance that mimics a malignancy. It is most often eccentrically located in the metaphysis. A bone scan shows diffuse or peripheral tracer uptake with a central area of decreased uptake. CT is

particularly helpful in delineating the cyst in areas of complex anatomy, such as the spine or pelvis. In addition, the thin rim of bone surrounding the cyst can be identified. MRI shows the multiloculated cavities and fluid levels. When differentiating between a unicameral and aneurysmal bone cyst using MRI, the presence of a double-density fluid level and intralesional septations usually indicates an aneurysmal bone cyst.

An aneurysmal bone cyst can arise de novo, but areas similar to an aneurysmal bone cyst are found in various other lesions, such as giant cell tumors, chondroblastomas, osteoblastomas, fibrous dysplasia, nonossifying fibromas, and chondromyxoid fibromas. Although the pathogenesis is uncertain, it is likely that aneurysmal bone cysts result from local circulatory disturbance leading to increased venous pressure and production of local hemorrhage. Grossly, an aneurysmal bone cyst is a cavitary lesion with blood-filled septate spaces. It is surrounded by a thin layer of bone covered by a raised periosteum. The microscopic appearance is of hemorrhagic tissue with cavernous spaces separated by a cellular stroma. The lining of the cavitary spaces consists of compressed fibroblasts and histiocytes (Fig. 8.18). Hemosiderin-laden macrophages, chronic inflammatory cells, and multinucleated giant cells are also present. A solid variant of aneurysmal bone cyst has been described and is frequently referred to as giant cell reparative granuloma.

We treat most aneurysmal bone cysts with extended curettage and grafting with a bone graft substitute (Figs. 8.19 and 8.20). Because the lesion may produce heavy bleeding, tourniquet control is advised. Marginal resection is sometimes indicated for lesions in expendable bones. Lesions in the spine or pelvis can be treated with preoperative

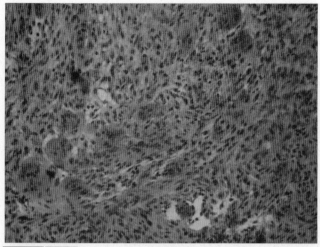

Histologic appearance of aneurysmal bone cyst.

embolization to minimize surgical blood loss (Fig. 8.21). Arterial embolization has been used as definitive treatment of aneurysmal bone cysts in locations where curettage would be extremely difficult. Low-dose radiation has been reported to be an effective method of treatment, often associated with rapid ossification; however, it is not used routinely because of the potential for malignant transformation. Studies have shown a possible role for denosumab in the treatment of aneurysmal bone cysts when surgery would be associated with unacceptable morbidity. Denosumab is a monoclonal antibody targeted against RANKL and has been shown to be useful in the treatment of giant cell tumors.

The recurrence rate after curettage of an aneurysmal bone cyst is 10% to 20%. Recurrence has been correlated with age younger than 15 years, centrally located cysts, and incomplete removal of the cystic cavity contents. Recurrent cysts can be treated with the same approach as the primary lesion.

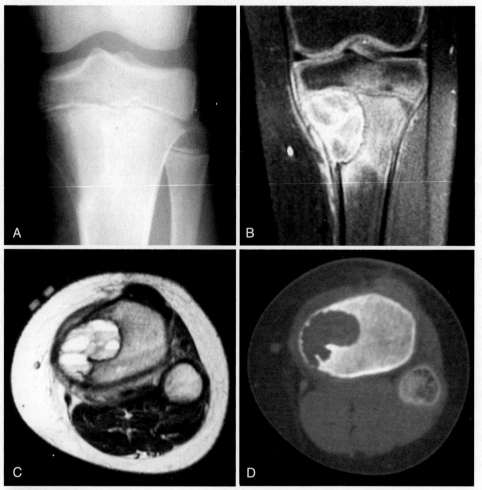

FIGURE 8.19 **A,** Radiolucent aneurysmal bone cyst of left proximal tibial metaphysis in 10-year-old boy. **B** and **C,** Coronal and axial MR images show multiloculated lesion with multiple fluid-fluid levels consistent with aneurysmal bone cyst. **D,** CT shows thin rim of remaining cortex over lesion. Biopsy confirmed diagnosis.

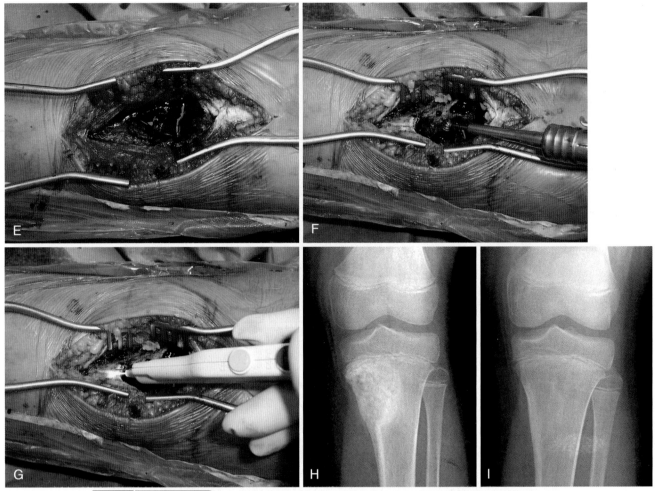

FIGURE 8.19, Cont'd **E,** Intraoperative photograph of multiloculated blood-filled cavity. **F,** After removal of cyst lining with large curets, tumor cavity is enlarged with power bur. **G,** Tumor cavity is treated with argon beam coagulation. Cavity was packed with freeze-dried cancellous bone chips and demineralized bone matrix. **H,** Postoperative anteroposterior radiograph. **I,** Radiograph 1 year later shows complete remodeling with no evidence of recurrence.

INTRAOSSEOUS GANGLION CYST

Ganglion cysts of bone typically occur in the ends of the long bones of middle-aged men, particularly the distal tibia, although the knee and shoulder are other common areas. These cysts are thought to be intraosseous extensions of ganglia of local soft tissues. Subperiosteal ganglia have also been reported. On radiographs and MRI they appear as uniloculated or multiloculated, well-demarcated, lytic defects with a thin rim of sclerotic bone (Fig. 8.22). Treatment of symptomatic lesions is by local excision of overlying soft tissues and curettage of the involved bone. Recurrence is uncommon.

EPIDERMOID CYST

Cysts filled with keratinous material and lined with a flattened squamous epithelium are occasionally seen in bone. Microscopically, they resemble epidermal inclusion cysts of the skin. In bone, these lesions are known as epidermoid cysts and are found most often in the skull. Radiographically, they appear as rarefied defects surrounded by sclerotic bone.

Epidermoid cysts may also be found in the phalanges of the fingers and are usually considered traumatic.

FATTY TUMORS
LIPOMA

Intraosseous lipoma is a relatively rare lesion in contrast to its soft-tissue counterpart. The true incidence is unknown because most are asymptomatic and never come to medical attention. Most intraosseous lipomas are discovered as incidental findings. The radiographic appearance varies but is generally benign. They usually appear as well-defined lucencies, possibly with a thin rim of reactive bone (Fig. 8.23A). CT and MRI show well-defined lesions with the same signal characteristics as fat (Fig. 8.23B and C). Central necrosis or calcification is sometimes evident. Biopsy is rarely necessary because imaging is usually diagnostic. Surgery is indicated only for the rare symptomatic lesion. In these cases, simple curettage is usually curative.

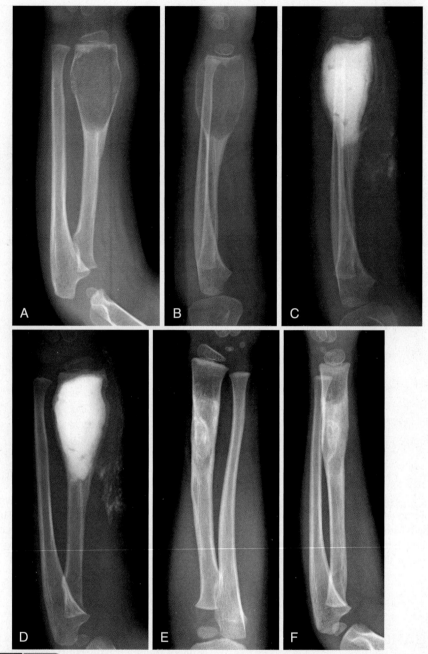

FIGURE 8.20 Anteroposterior **(A)** and lateral **(B)** radiographs of forearm in 2-year-old boy demonstrate an aneurysmal bone cyst. Anteroposterior **(C)** and lateral **(D)** radiographs after extended curettage and grafting with a calcium sulfate/calcium phosphate bone graft substitute. Anteroposterior **(E)** and lateral **(F)** radiographs 1 year later demonstrate remodeling of the graft material with no sign of cyst recurrence.

VASCULAR TUMORS
HEMANGIOMA

Hemangioma is a common benign bone lesion. It is estimated that 10% of the population has asymptomatic lesions of the vertebral bodies. Hemangiomas are also common in the skull. Hemangiomas of the long bones of the extremities are relatively uncommon. They are usually discovered as incidental findings. Spinal lesions are rarely symptomatic unless there is vertebral collapse or,

in rare cases with soft-tissue extension, nerve root or cord compression.

The radiographic appearance in the spine is usually characteristic, with thickened, vertically oriented trabeculae giving the classic "jailhouse" appearance (Fig. 8.24). In cross-section, these thickened trabeculae have a "polka dot" pattern on CT. On MRI, the lesions are usually bright on T1- and T2-weighted images. Biopsy is rarely required to make the diagnosis. When performed, however, histologic analysis reveals a proliferation of normal-appearing blood vessels.

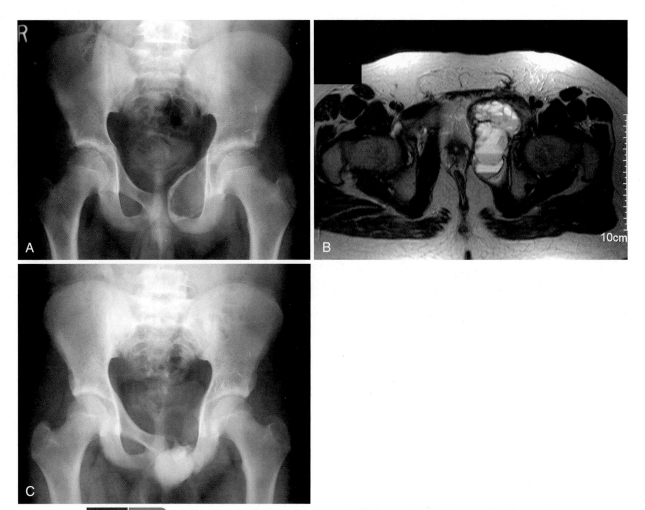

FIGURE 8.21   **A,** Recurrent aneurysmal bone cyst of left superior pubic ramus in 14-year-old boy. **B,** Axial MRI shows multiple fluid-fluid levels. **C,** Appearance 2 years after resection; the patient is doing well with no evidence of recurrence.

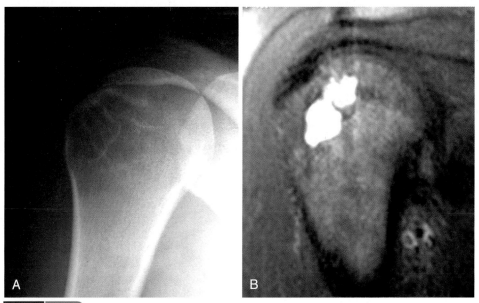

FIGURE 8.22   **A** and **B,** Radiograph and coronal MR image show intraosseous ganglion in right proximal humerus of 31-year-old woman.

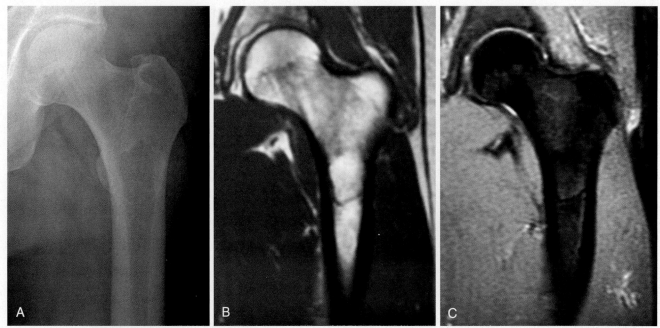

FIGURE 8.23 **A,** Intraosseous lipoma in left proximal femur of 51-year-old man. **B,** Lesion shows same signal as normal fat on T1- and T2-weighted **(C)** MR images.

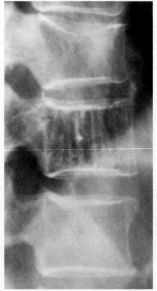

FIGURE 8.24 Lateral radiograph of lumbar spine shows typical "jailhouse" appearance of hemangioma.

Treatment is not usually necessary but multiple options exist for symptomatic lesions. Nerve root or cord decompression with spinal stabilization is required for rare cases of vertebral collapse with neurologic compromise. Most lesions of the long bones can be treated adequately with extended curettage. Preoperative embolization can help minimize intraoperative blood loss, which otherwise could be massive. Selective arterial embolization can also be used as definitive treatment for symptomatic lesions in surgically inaccessible locations. Low-dose radiation is also an option for inoperable lesions but carries the risk of malignant degeneration.

OTHER NONNEOPLASTIC LESIONS
PAGET DISEASE

Paget disease is a disorder of uncertain origin. The presence of virus-like inclusion bodies in the osteoclasts of affected bone has led to the theory that it may be of viral origin but this has not yet been proved. Paget disease may affect 4% of people of Anglo-Saxon descent who are older than 55 years, but it is rare in most other populations. It is a disorder of unregulated bone turnover. Excessive osteoclastic resorption is followed by increased osteoblastic activity. An early lytic phase is followed by excessive bone production with cortical and trabecular thickening.

Radiographic findings depend on the stage of the disease. In the lytic phase, bone resorption can take on a "blade of grass" or "flame" appearance beginning at the end of the bone and extending toward the diaphysis. Later, the radiographs show bony sclerosis, thickened cortices, and thickened trabeculae (Figs. 8.25A). Bone scans are usually "hot" (Fig. 8.25B). Sometimes, plain radiographs along with a positive bone scan suggest malignancy. MRI is helpful in this circumstance because the marrow signal in patients with Paget disease usually remains normal (Fig. 8.25C and D). Biopsy usually reveals a characteristic "mosaic" pattern with widened lamellae, irregular cement lines, and fibrovascular connective tissue.

Medical management of Paget disease consists of nonsteroidal antiinflammatory drugs, calcitonin, or bisphosphonates. Serum alkaline phosphatase levels and urine pyridinium crosslinks can be used to monitor the activity of

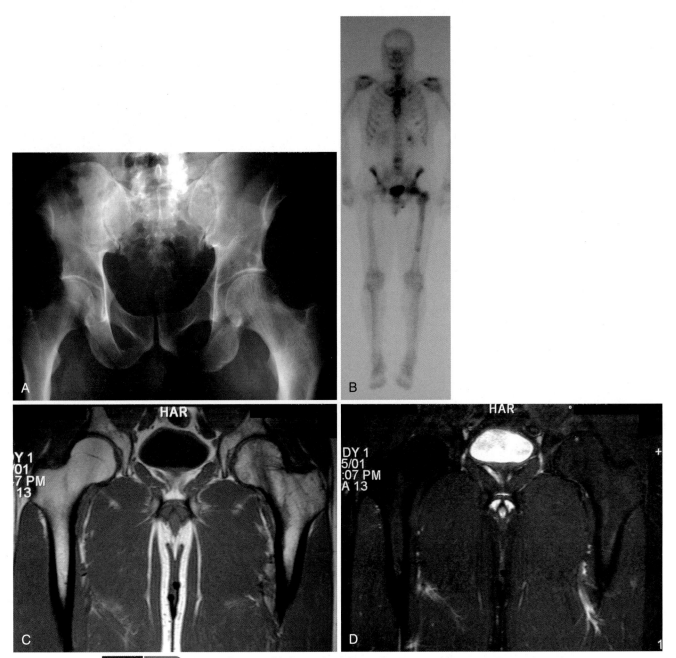

FIGURE 8.25 Paget disease of left proximal femur in 45-year-old man. **A,** Anteroposterior radiograph shows coarsened trabeculae. **B,** Bone scan shows increased uptake in left proximal femur. Note normal marrow signal on T1- **(C)** and T2-weighted **(D)** MR images.

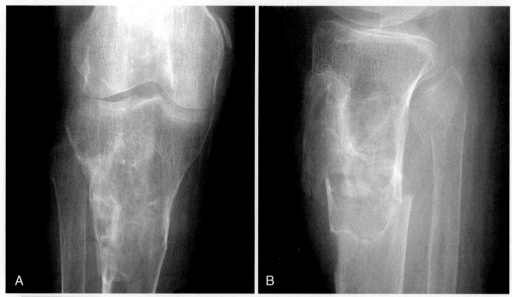

FIGURE 8.26 **A** and **B,** Pathologic fracture of right proximal tibia through "brown tumor" of hyperparathyroidism in 55-year-old woman.

the disease. Orthopaedic management consists of correcting the deformity and treating pathologic fractures. During periods of active disease, intraoperative bleeding from affected bones can be massive. Approximately 1% of patients with Paget disease develop a secondary bone sarcoma, usually an osteosarcoma. This risk is probably higher for patients with polyostotic disease.

"BROWN TUMOR" OF HYPERPARATHYROIDISM

Primary hyperparathyroidism is usually caused by an adenoma of the parathyroid glands. Secondary hyperparathyroidism can occur in patients with chronic renal failure. When the disease is discovered early, the skeletal change is usually limited to diffuse demineralization. Only rarely does the change become markedly focal and produce a "brown tumor," which resembles a giant cell tumor and is difficult to distinguish from one. The diagnosis of hyperparathyroidism should be established by determining the serum calcium, phosphorus, alkaline phosphatase, and parathyroid hormone levels, rather than by histologic examination of a focal lesion. Some microscopic features suggest hyperparathyroidism, however, rather than giant cell tumor. In hyperparathyroidism (1) the giant cells are a little smaller, often occurring in a nodular arrangement, especially around areas of hemorrhage; (2) the stromal cells are more spindle-shaped and delicate; and (3) evidence of osseous metaplasia within the stroma is prominent. The bone surrounding the lesion should also be examined; in hyperparathyroidism, it may show intense osteoclastic and osteoblastic activity associated with peritrabecular fibrosis. Patients with hyperparathyroidism are usually treated by an endocrinologist. Orthopaedic management consists of treating actual or impending pathologic fractures (Fig. 8.26).

BONE INFARCT

Bone infarcts are frequently seen in patients with a history of corticosteroid use, alcoholism, sickle cell anemia, Gaucher disease, or dysbaric conditions (Fig. 8.27); however, they can also occur in patients with no other apparent underlying disorder. The diagnosis is usually made from plain radiographs. Bone infarcts are usually well-defined metaphyseal lesions with irregular borders. The periphery of the lesion is calcified, in contrast to chondroid lesions, which are usually calcified throughout. Biopsy (usually unnecessary) shows mineralization of necrotic marrow elements. Bone infarcts are usually asymptomatic and no treatment is required. If a patient presents with pain, another etiology should be sought. Rarely, malignancy, such as a malignant fibrous histiocytoma, can occur at the site of a bone infarct.

OSTEOMYELITIS

Osteomyelitis of all stages, but especially subacute infection, can simulate tumors. Mistakes have been made in differentiating infection and Ewing sarcoma, osteogenic sarcoma, osteoid osteoma, and eosinophilic granuloma. Occasionally, an inflammatory response causes such an abundance of plasma cells that multiple myeloma is suspected. As a general rule, whenever biopsy of a suspected musculoskeletal neoplasm is done, tissue should routinely be sent for cultures and histology. Malignant change occasionally occurs in chronically draining osteomyelitic sinuses of long duration; squamous cell carcinoma and fibrosarcoma have been reported.

STRESS FRACTURE

Occasionally, fatigue fractures or stress fractures, particularly in the proximal tibial metaphysis, may simulate osteogenic sarcoma. If a biopsy is done, the microscopic picture may be difficult for an inexperienced pathologist to distinguish from sarcoma. The florid fracture callus seen in osteogenesis imperfecta may also simulate osteogenic sarcoma. If the diagnosis is uncertain, an experienced bone pathologist should be consulted.

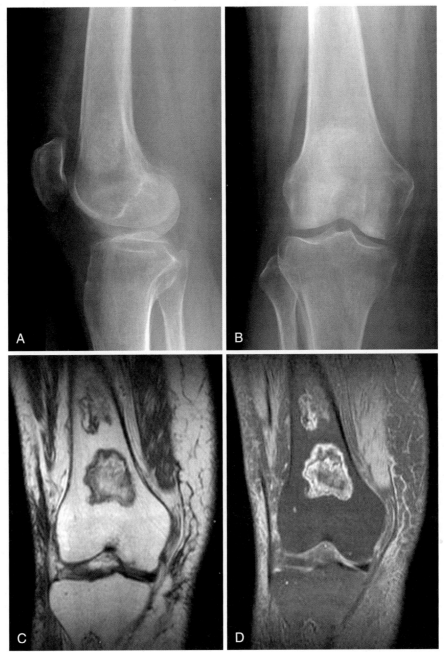

FIGURE 8.27 **A** and **B,** Irregular calcification in metaphysis of distal femur of 50-year-old woman with history of corticosteroid use. T1- **(C)** and T2-weighted **(D)** MR images show multiple bone infarcts.

POSTTRAUMATIC OSTEOLYSIS

Posttraumatic osteolysis has been described in the pubis of elderly osteopenic women and in the distal clavicle of athletes, particularly weightlifters. The radiographic appearance in both circumstances may simulate a malignant bone tumor.

REFERENCES

Aich RK, Deb AR, Banerjee A, et al.: Symptomatic vertebral hemangioma: treatment with radiotherapy, *J Cancer Res Ther* 6:199, 2010.

Akhlaghpoor S, Azoiz Ahari A, Arjmand Shabestari A, Alinaghizadeh MR: Radiofrequency ablation of osteoid osteoma in atypical locations: a case series, *Clin Orthop Relat Res* 468:1963, 2010.

Albisinni U, Facchini G, Spinnato P, et al.: Spinal osteoid osteoma: efficacy and safety of radiofrequency ablation, *Skeletal Radiol* 46(8):1087, 2017.

Alexander J, Meir A, Vrodos N, Yau YH: Vertebral hemangioma: an important differential in the evaluation of locally aggressive spinal lesions, *Spine* 35:E917, 2010.

Alhumaid I, Abu-Zaid A: Denosumab therapy in the management of aneurysmal bone cysts: a comprehensive literature review, *Cureus* 11(1):e3989, 2019.

Al-Rashid M, Ramkumar DB, Raskin K, et al.: Paget disease of bone, *Orthop Clin North Am* 46(4):577, 2015.

Andreacchio A, Alberghina F, Giacometti V, et al.: Single-stage surgery using calcium sulfate pellets in association with tumor resection as treatment for intraosseous hemangioma of the radius shaft in a 2-year-old boy, *J Hand Microsurg* 9(3):154, 2017.

Atesok KI, Alman BA, Schemitsch EH, et al.: Osteoid osteoma and osteoblastoma, *J Am Acad Orthop Surg* 19:678, 2011.

Aycan OE, Camurcu IY, Özer D, et al.: Unusual localizations of unicameral bone cysts and aneurysmal bone cysts: a retrospective review of 451 cases, *Acta Orthop Belg* 81(2):209, 2015.

Aycan OE, Keskin A, Sökücü S, et al.: Surgical treatment of confirmed intraosseous lipoma of the calcaneus: a case series, *J Foot Ankle Surg* 56(6):1205, 2017.

Bandeira F, Cusano NE, Silva BC, et al.: Bone disease in primary hyperparathyroidism, *Arq Bras Endocrinol Metabol* 58:553, 2014.

Beebe KS, Ippolito JA: Desmoplastic fibroma of the distal radius: an interesting case and a review of the literature and therapeutic implications, *J Surg Case Rep* 2016(1): pii:rjv171, 2016.

Benedetti Valentini M, Ippolito E, Catellani F, Farsetti P: Internal fixation after fracture or osteotomy of the femur in young children with polyostotic fibrous dysplasia, *J Pediatr Orthop B* 24(4):291, 2015.

Benhamou J, Gensburger D, Chapuralt R: Transient improvement of severe pain from fibrous dysplasia of bone with denosumab treatment, *Joint Bone Spine* 81:549, 2014.

Bierry G, Kerr DA, Nielsen GO, et al.: Enchondromas in children: imaging appearance with pathological correlation, *Skeletal Radiol* 41:1223, 2012.

Bolland MJ, Cundy T: Paget's disease of bone: clinical review and update, *J Clin Pathol* 66:924, 2013.

Boyce AM, Kelly MH, Brillanta BA, et al.: A randomized, double blind, placebo-controlled trial of alendronate treatment for fibrous dysplasia of bone, *J Clin Endocrinol Metab* 99:4133, 2014.

Brosjö O, Pechon P, Hesla A, et al.: Sclerotherapy with polidocanol treatment of aneurysmal bone cysts, *Acta Orthop* 84:502, 2013.

Butler BA, Lawton CD, Harold RE, et al.: Valgus osteotomy with plate-and-nail fixation for the treatment of proximal femoral deformities due to fibrous dysplasia: a report of two cases, *JBJS Case Connect* 8(3):e71, 2018.

Camacho J, Gutierrez LD, Rubio C, et al.: Multiple hereditary exostoses: report of an EXT2 gene mutation in a Colombian family, *J Pediatr Genet* 7(3):122, 2018.

Canavese F, Wright JG, Cole WG, Hopyan S: Unicameral bone cysts: comparison of percutaneous curettage, steroid, and autologous bone marrow injections, *J Pediatr Orthop* 31:50, 2011.

Carvallo PI, Griffin AM, Ferguson PC, Wunder JS: Response to letter to the editor re Carvallo et al: Salvage of the proximal femur following pathological fracture involving benign bone tumors, *J Surg Oncol* 114(2):255, 2016.

Carvallo PI, Griffin AM, Ferguson PC, Wunder JS: Salvage of the proximal femur following pathological fractures involving benign bone tumors, *J Surg Oncol* 112(8):846, 2015.

Chai JW, Hong SH, Choi JY, et al.: Radiologic diagnosis of osteoid osteoma: from simple to challenging findings, *Radiographics* 30:737, 2010.

Charest-Morin R, Boriani S, Fisher CG, et al.: Benign tumors of the spine: has new chemotherapy and interventional radiology changed the treatment paradigm? *Spine (Phila Pa 1976)* 41(Suppl 20):S178, 2016.

Cho HS, Han I, Kim HS: Secondary chondrosarcoma from an osteochondroma of the proximal tibia involving the fibula, *Clin Orthop Surg* 9(2):249, 2017.

Clement ND, Porter DE: Forearm deformity in patients with hereditary multiple exostoses: factors associated with range of motion and radial head dislocation, *J Bone Joint Surg* 95A:1586, 2013.

Corsi A, Ippolito E, Robey PG, et al.: Bisphosphonate-induced zebra lines in fibrous dysplasia of bone: histo-radiographic correlation in a case of McCune-Albright syndrome, *Skel Radiol* 46(10):1435, 2017.

Crim J, Schmidt R, Layfield L, et al.: Can imaging criteria distinguish enchondroma from grade 1 chondrosarcoma? *Eur J Radiol* 84(11):2222, 2015.

Cummings JE, Smith RA, Heck Jr RK: Argon beam coagulation as adjuvant treatment after curettage of aneurismal bone cysts: a preliminary study, *Clin Orthop Relat Res* 4687:231, 2010.

Cundy T, Bolland M: Paget disease of bone, *Trends Endocrinol Metab* 19:246, 2008.

Czajka CM, DiCaprio MR: What is the proportion of patients with multiple hereditary exostoses who undergo malignant degeneration? *Clin Orthop Relat Res* 473(7):2355, 2015.

Deckers C, Schreuder BH, Hannink G, et al.: Radiologic follow-up of untreated enchondroma and atypical cartilaginous tumors in the long bones, *J Surg Oncol* 114(8):987, 2016.

De Palma L, Candelari R, Antico E, et al.: Treatment of osteoid osteoma with CT-guided percutaneous radiofrequency thermoablation, *Orthopedics* 36:e581, 2013.

DiBella C, Dozza B, Frisoni T, et al.: Injection of demineralized bone matrix with bone marrow concentrate improves healing in unicameral bone cyst, *Clin Orthop Relat Res* 468:3047, 2010.

Dohan A, Parlier-Cuau C, Kaci R, et al.: Vertebral involvement in Paget's disease: morphological classification of CT and MR appearances, *Joint Bone Spine* 82:18, 2015.

Donati F, Proietti L, Burrofato A, et al.: Intraspinal extradural benign fibrous histiocytoma of the lumbar spine in a pediatric patient: case report and literature review, *Childs Nerv Syst* 32(8):1549, 2016.

Douis H, Parry M, Vaiyapuri S, Davies AM: What are the differentiating clinical and MRI-features of enchondromas from low-grade chondrosarcomas? *Eur Radiol* 28(1):398, 2018.

Douis H, Saifuddin A: The imaging of cartilaginous bone tumours. I. Benign lesions, *Skeletal Radiol* 41:1195, 2012.

Ebaş G, Şendur HN, Kiliç HK, et al.: Treatment-related alterations of imaging findings on osteoid osteoma after percutaneous radiofrequency ablation, *Skeletal Radiol*, 2019, https://doi.org/10.1007/s00256-019-03185-1.

Ebeid WA, Hasan BZ, Mesregah MK: Management of fibrous dysplasia of proximal femur by internal fixation without grafting: a retrospective study of 19 patients, *J Am Acad Orthop Surg Glob Res Rev* 2(1):e057, 2018.

Erol B, Topkar MO, Aydemir AN, et al.: A treatment strategy for proximal femoral benign bone lesions in children and recommended surgical procedures: retrospective analysis of 62 patients, *Arch Orthop Trauma Surg* 136(8):1051, 2016.

Fang X, Liu H, Lang Y, et al.: Fibrous dysplasia of bone: surgical management options and outcomes of 22 cases, *Mol Clin Oncol* 9(1):98, 2018.

Farr S, Balacó IMS, Martinez-Alvarez S, et al.: Current trends and variations in the treatment of unicameral bone cysts of the humerus: a survey of EPOS and POSNA members, *J Pediatr Orthop*, 2019, https://doi.org/10.1097/BPO.0000000000001376.

Ferrer-Santacreu EM, Ortiz-Cruz EJ, Diaz-Almirón M, Pozo Kreilinger JJ: Enchondroma versus chondrosarcoma in long bones of appendicular skeleton: clinical and radiological criteria - a follow-up, *J Oncol* 2016:8262079, 2016, Epub 2016 Feb 23.

Galant C, Docquier PL, Ameye G, et al.: Aneurysmal bone cyst lesions: value of genomic studies, *Acta Orthop Belg* 82(4):768, 2016.

Gallardo-Molina N: Some alternative treatments for aneurysmal bone cysts, *World Neurosurg* 127:658, 2019.

Gasbarrini A, Cappuccio M, Bandiera S, et al.: Osteoid osteoma of the mobile spine: surgical outcomes in 81 patients, *Spine* 36:2089, 2011.

Geiger D, Napoli A, Conchiglia A, et al.: MR-guided focused ultrasound (MRgFUS) ablation for the treatment of nonspinal osteoid osteoma: a prospective multicenter evaluation, *J Bone Joint Surg* 96A:743, 2014.

Gentile JV, Weinert CR, Schlecter JA: Treatment of unicameral bone cysts in pediatric patients with an injectable regenerative graft: a preliminary report, *J Pediatr Orthop* 33:254, 2013.

Gahier Penhoat M, Drui D, Ansquer C, et al.: Contribution of 18-FDG PET/CT to brown tumor detection in a patient with primary hyperparathyroidism, *Joint Bone Spine* 84(2):209, 2017.

Georgiannos D, Lampridis V, Bisbinas I: Phenolization and coralline hydroxyapatite grafting following meticulous curettage for the treatment of enchondroma of the hand. A case series of 82 patients with 5-year follow-up, *Hand (NY)* 10(1):111, 2015.

Ghanem I, Nicolas N, Rizkallah M, Slaba S: Sclerotherapy using Surgiflow and alcohol: a new alternative for the treatment of aneurysmal bone cysts, *J Child Orthop* 11(6):448, 2017.

Gholamrezanezhad A, Basques K, Kosmas C: Peering beneath the surface: juxtacortical tumors of bone (part I), *Clin Imaging* 51:1, 2018.

Gholamrezanezhad A, Basques K, Kosmas C: Peering beneath the surface: juxtacortical tumors of bone (part II), *Clin Imaging* 50:113, 2018.

Glushko T, Banjar SS, Nahal A, Colmegna I: Brown tumor of the pelvis, *Cleve Clin J Med* 82912:799, 2015.

Gong YB, Zu LM, Qi X, Liu JG: Desmoplastic fibroma in the proximal femur: a case report with long-term follow-up, *Oncol Lett* 10(4):24645, 2015.

Goto T, Shinoda Y, Okuma T, et al.: Administration of nonsteroidal anti-inflammatory drugs accelerates spontaneous healing of osteoid osteoma, *Arch Orthop Trauma Surg* 131:619, 2011.

Goud AL, Wuyts W, Bessems J, et al.: Intraosseous atypical chondroid tumor or chondrosarcoma grade 1 in patients with multiple osteochondromas, *J Bone Joint Surg Am* 97(1):24, 2015.

Grewal R, Natter P, Makary R, Silliman J: Desmoplastic fibroblastoma of the left upper arm, *BMJ Case Rep* 2018, pii: bcr-2017-221738.

Hakim DN, Pelly T, Kulendran M, Caris JA: Benign tumours of the bone: a review, *J Bone Oncol* 4(2):37–41, 2015.

Hasan K, Nguyen DM, Conway SA: Benign bone tumors when they coexist with common orthopaedic conditions, *J Knee Surg* 32(4):296, 2019.

Hashimoto K, Nishimura S, Kakinoki R, Akagi M: Aggressive intraosseous lipoma of the intermediate phalanges of the thumb, *Mol Clin Oncol* 9(1):62, 2018.

Hattori T, Matsumine A, Uchida K, et al.: Benign fibrous histiocytoma of the talus: a case report, *J Foot Ankle Surg* 58(4):762, 2019.

Hauschild O, Lüdemann M, Engelhardt M, et al.: Aneurysmal bone cyst (ABC): treatment options and proposal of a follow-up regime, *Acta Orthop Belg* 82(3):474, 2016.

Hefti F, Donnan L, Krieg AH: Treatment of shepherd's crook deformity in patients with polyostotic fibrous dysplasia using a new type of custom made retrograde intramedullary nail: a technical note, *J Child Orthop* 11(1):64, 2017.

Hou HY, Wu K, Wang CT, et al.: Treatment of unicameral bone cyst: a comparative study of selected techniques, *J Bone Joint Surg* 92A:855, 2010.

Hou HY, Wu K, Wang CT, et al.: Treatment of unicameral bone cyst: surgical technique, *J Bone Joint Surg* 93A:92, 2011.

Hu J, He S, Yang J, et al.: Management of brown tumor of spine with primary hyperparathyroidism: a case report and literature review, *Medicine (Baltimore)* 98(14):e15007, 2019.

Hu W, Kan SL, Xu HB, et al.: Thoracic aggressive vertebral hemangioma with neurologic deficit: a retrospective cohort study, *Medicine (Baltimore)* 97(41):e12775, 2018.

Huang AJ: Radiofrequency ablation of osteoid osteoma: difficult-to-reach places, *Semin Musculoskelet Radiol* 20(5):486, 2016.

Ippolito E, Farsetti P, Boyce AM, et al.: Radiographic classification of coronal plane femoral deformities in polyostotic fibrous dysplasia, *Clin Orthop Relat Res* 472:1558, 2014.

Ippolito E, Farsetti P, Valentini MB, Potenza V: Two-stage surgical treatment of complex femoral deformities with severe coxa vara in polyostotic fibrous dysplasia, *J Bone Joint Surg Am* 97(2):119, 2015.

Ippolito E, Valentini MB, Lala R, et al.: Changing pattern of femoral deformity during growth in polyostotic fibrous dysplasia of the bone: an analysis of 46 cases, *J Pediatr Orthop* 36(5):488, 2016.

Jordan RW, Koc T, Chapman AW, Taylor HP: Osteoid osteoma of the foot and ankle – a systematic review, *Foot Ankle Surg* 21(4):228, 2015.

Jurik AG, Jørgensen PH, Mortensen MM: Whole-body MRI in assessing malignant transformation in multiple hereditary exostoses and enchondromatosis: audit results an literature review, *Skel Radiol*, 2019, https://doi.org/10.1007/s00256-019-03268-z.

Kadar A, Kleinstern G, Morsy M, et al.: Multiple enchondromas of the hand in children: long-term follow-up of mean 15.4 years, *J Pediatr Orthop* 38(10):543, 2018.

Kadhim M, Sethi S, Thacker MM: Unicameral bone cysts in the humerus: treatment outcomes, *J Pediatr Orthop* 36(4):392, 2016.

Kang DH, Kang BS, Sim HB, et al.: Periosteal chondroma with spinal cord compression in the thoracic spinal canal: a case report, *Skeletal Radiol* 45(8):1133, 2016.

Kang HS, Kim T, Oh S, et al.: Intraosseous lipoma: 18 years of experience at a single institution, *Clin Orthop Surg* 10(20):234, 2018.

Kay M, Counsel P, Wood D, Breidahl W: Cortical desmoid of the humerus: radiographic and MRI correlation, *Skeletal Radiol* 46(7):1011, 2017.

Kim HS, Lim KS, Seo SW, et al.: Recurrence of a unicameral bone cyst in the femoral diaphysis, *Clin Orthop Surg* 8(4):484, 2016.

King EA, Hanauer DA, Choi SW, et al.: Osteochondromas after radiation for pediatric malignancies: a role for expanded counseling for skeletal side effects, *J Pediatr Orthop* 34:331, 2014.

Klein C, Delcourt T, Salon A, et al.: Surgical treatment of enchondromas of the hand during childhood in Ollier disease, *J Hand Surg Am* 43(10):946, 2018.

Lafforgue P, Trijau S: Bone infarcts: unsuspected gray areas? *Joint Bone Spine* 83(5):495, 2016.

Laliotis NA, Bendoudi AS, Tsitouridis IA, et al.: Osteoid osteoma of the acetabulum: diagnosis and medical treatment, *J Pediatr Orthop B* 26(6):565, 2017.

Lassalle L, Campagna R, Corcos G, et al.: Therapeutic outcome of CT-guided radiofrequency ablation in patients with osteoid osteoma, *Skeletal Radiol* 46(7):949, 2017.

Lee DH, Hills JM, Jordanov MI, Jaffe KA: Common tumors and tumor-like lesions of the shoulder, *J Am Acad Orthop Surg* 27(7):236, 2019.

Leet AI, Boyce AM, Ibrahim KA, et al.: Bone-grafting in polyostotic fibrous dysplasia, *J Bone Joint Surg Am* 98(3):211, 2016.

Levy DM, Gross CE, Garras DN: Treatment of unicameral bone cysts of the calcaneus: a systematic review, *J Foot Ankle Surg* 54(4):652, 2015.

Li S, Sun C, Zhou X, et al.: Treatment of intraosseous ganglion cyst of the lunate: a systematic review, *Ann Plast Surg* 82(5):577, 2019.

Lubahn JD, Bachoura A: Enchondroma of the hand: evaluation and management, *J Am Acad Orthop Surg* 24(9):625, 2016.

Majoor BC, Peeters-Boef MJ, van de Sande MA, et al.: What is the role of allogeneic cortical strut grafts in the treatment of fibrous dysplasia of the proximal femur? *Clin Orthop Relat Res* 475(3):786, 2017.

Majoor BC, Peeters-Boef MJ, vande Sande MA, et al.: Erratum to: what is the role of allogeneic cortical strut grafts in the treatment of fibrous dysplasia of the proximal femur? *Clin Orthop Relat Res* 475(3):923, 2017.

Majoor BCJ, Traunmueller E, Mauerer-Ertl W, et al.: Pain in fibrous dysplasia: relationship with anatomical and clinical features, *Acta Orthop* 90(4):401, 2019.

Maione V, Stinco G, Errichetti E: Multiple enchondromas and skin angiomas: Maffucci syndrome, *Lancet* 388(10047):905, 2016.

Marić D, Djan I, Petković L, et al.: Osteoid osteoma: fluoroscopic guided percutaneous excision technique – our experience, *J Pediatr Orthop B* 20:46, 2011.

Marcocci C, Cianferotti L, Cetani F: Bone disease in primary hyperparathyroidism, *Ther Adv Musculoskelet Dis* 4:357, 2012.

Mascard E, Gomez-Brouchet A, Lambot K: Bone cysts: unicameral and aneurysmal bone cyst, *Orthop Traumatol Surg Res* 101(Suppl 1):S119, 2015.

Matcuk Jr GR, Chopra S, Menendez LR: Solid aneurysmal bone cyst of the humerus mimics metastasis or brown tumor, *Clin Imaging* 52:117, 2018.

Mavčič B, Saraph V, Gilg MM, et al.: Comparison of three surgical treatment options for unicameral bone cysts in humerus, *J Pediatr Orthop B* 28(1):51, 2019.

Mavrogenis AF, Rossi G, Calabrò T, et al.: The role of embolization for hemangiomas, *Musculoskelet Surg* 96:125, 2012.

May CJ, Bixby SD, Anderson ME, et al.: Osteoid osteoma about the hip in children and adolescents, *J Bone Joint Surg Am* 101(6):486, 2019.

McCabe MP, Heck RK: H*istoplasma* osteomyelitis simulating giant-cell tumor of the distal part of the radius: a case report, *J Bone Joint Surg* 92A:708, 2010.

McFarlane J, Knight T, Sinha A, et al.: Exostoses, enchondromatosis and metachondromatosis: diagnosis and management, *Acta Orthop Belg* 82(1):102, 2016.

Miller SF: Imaging features of juxtacortical chondroma in children, *Pediatr Radiol* 44:56, 2014.

Miszczyk L, Tukiendorf A: Radiotherapy of painful vertebral hemangiomas: the single center retrospective analysis of 137 cases, *Int J Radiat Oncol Biol Phys* 82:e173, 2012.

Mohapatra A, Patel V, Choudhury P, Phalak M: Intraosseous ganglion cyst of the distal tibia: a rare entity in a rare location, *BMJ Case Rep* 2018, pii:bcr-2018-224395.

Morassi LG, Kokkinis K, Evangelopoulos DS, et al.: Percutaneous radiofrequency ablation of spinal osteoid osteoma under CT guidance, *Br J Radiol* 87:1038, 2014.

Moretti VM, Slotcavage RL, Crawford EA, et al.: Curettage and graft alleviates athletic-limiting pain in benign lytic bone lesions, *Clin Orthop Relat Res* 469:283, 2011.

Most MJ, Sim FH, Inwards CY: Osteofibrous dysplasia and adamantinoma, *J Am Acad Orthop Surg* 18:358, 2010.

Mulligan ME: How to diagnose enchondroma, bone infarct, and chondrosarcoma, *Curr Probl Diagn Radiol* 48(3):262, 2019.

Muthusamy S, Subhawong T, Conway SA, Temple HT: Locally aggressive fibrous dysplasia mimicking malignancy: a report of four cases and review of the literature, *Clin Orthop Relat Res* 473(2):742, 2015.

Napoli A, Bastantuono M, Cavallo Marincola B, et al.: Osteoid osteoma: MR-guided focused ultrasound for entirely noninvasive treatment, *Radiology* 2167:514, 2013.

Napoli A, Bazzocchi A, Scipione R, et al.: Noninvasive therapy for osteoid osteoma: a prospective developmental study with MR imaging- guided high-intensity focused ultrasound, *Radiology* 285(1):186, 2017.

Nishida Y, Tsukushi S, Hosono K, et al.: Surgical treatment for fibrous dysplasia of femoral neck with mild but prolonged symptoms: a case series, *J Orthop Surg Res* 10:63, 2015.

Noh JH, Lee JW: Fibrous dysplasia in the epiphysis of the distal femur, *Knee Surg Relat Res* 29(1):69, 2017.

Noordin S, Allana S, Umer M, et al.: Unicameral bone cysts: current concepts, *Ann Med Surg (Lon)* 34:43, 2018.

Novais EN, Rose PS, Yaszemski MJ, Sim FH: Aneurysmal bone cyst of the cervical spine in children, *J Bone Joint Surg* 93A:1534, 2011.

Osagie L, Gallivan S, Wickham N, Umarji S: Intraosseous ganglion cysts of the carpus: current practice, *Hand (NY)* 10(4):598, 2015.

Özer D, Aycan AE, Er ST, et al.: Primary tumor and tumor-like lesions of bones of the foot: single-center experience of 166 cases, *J Foot Ankle Surg* 56(6):1180, 2017.

Park JW, Lee C, Han I, et al.: Optimal treatment of osteofibrous dysplasia of the tibia, *J Pediatr Orthop* 38(7):e404, 2018.

Park HY, Yang SK, Sheppard WL, et al.: Current management of aneurysmal bone cysts, *Curr Rev Musculoskelet Med* 9(4):435, 2016.

Park SH, Kong GM, Kwon YU, Park JH: Pathologic fracture of the femur in brown tumor induced in parathyroid carcinoma: a case report, *Hip Pelvis* 28(3):173, 2016.

Phan AQ, Pacifici M, Esko JD: Advances in the pathogenesis and possible treatments for multiple hereditary exostoses from the 2016 international MHE conference, *Connect Tissue Res* 59(1):85, 2018.

Pretell-Mazzini J, Murphy RF, Kushare I, Dormans JP: Unicameral bone cysts: general characteristics and management controversies, *J Am Acad Orthop Surg* 22:295, 2014.

Quraishi NA, Boriani S, Sabou S, et al.: A multicenter cohort study of spinal osteoid osteomas: results of surgical treatment and analysis of local recurrence, *Spine J* 17(3):401, 2017.

Rajeh MA, Diaz JJ, Facca S, et al.: Treatment of hand enchondroma with injectable calcium phosphate cement: a series of eight cases, *Eur J Orthop Surg Traumatol* 27(2):251, 2017.

Ramirez A, Abril JC, Touza A: Unicameral bone cyst: radiographic assessment of venous outflow by cystography as a prognostic index, *J Pediatr Orthop B* 21:489, 2012.

Rapp M, Grauel F, Wessel LM, et al.: Treatment outcome in 60 children with pathological fractures of the humerus caused by juvenile or aneurysmal bone cysts, *Acta Orthop Belg* 82(4):723, 2016.

Rapp TB, Ward JP, Alaia MJ: Aneurysmal bone cyst, *J Am Acad Orthop Surg* 20:233, 2012.

Raux S, Bouhamama A, Gaspar N, et al: Denosumab for treating aneurysmal bone cysts in children, *Orthop Traumatol Surg Res* 2019 Jul 26. Pii:S1877-0568(19)30208-7.

Reda B: Cystic bone tumors of the foot and ankle, *J Surg Oncol* 117(8):1786, 2018.

Reddy KI, Sinnaeve F, Gaston CL, et al.: Aneurysmal bone cysts: do simple treatments work? *Clin Orthop Relat Res* 472:1901, 2014.

Reid IR, Lyles K, Su G, et al.: A single infusion of zoledronic acid produces sustained remissions in Paget disease: data to 6.5 years, *J Bone Miner Res* 26:2261, 2011.

Reverte-Vinaixa MM, Velez R, Alvarez S, et al.: Percutaneous computed tomography-guided resection of nonspinal osteoid osteomas in 54 patients and review of the literature, *Arch Orthop Trauma Surg* 133:449, 2013.

Rimondi E, Mavrogenis AF, Rossi G, et al.: Radiofrequency ablation for nonspinal osteoid osteomas in 557 patients, *Eur Radiol* 22:181, 2012.

Robbins MM, Kuo S, Epstein R: Hereditary multiple exostoses, *Radiol Case Rep* 3(3):99, 2015.

Rossi G, Mavrogenis AF, Papagelopoulos PJ, et al.: Successful treatment of aggressive aneurysmal bone cyst of the pelvis with serial embolization, *Orthopedics* 35:e963, 2012.

Rui J, Guan W, Gu Y, Lao J: Treatment and functional result of desmoplastic fibroma with repeated recurrences in the forearm: a case report, *Oncol Lett* 11(2):1506, 2016.

Rybak LD, Gangi A, Buy X, et al.: Thermal ablation of spinal osteoid osteomas close to neural elements: technical considerations, *Am J Roentgenol* 195:W293, 2010.

Sakamoto A, Oda Y, Iwamoto Y: Intraosseous ganglia: a series of 17 treated cases, *Biomed Res Int*, 2013, https://doi.org/10.1155/2013/462730.

Salunke AA, Kanani H, Singh S, Sheth H: Intraosseous ganglion cyst of the scaphoid: a rare bone tumor, *J Cancer Res Ther* 12(1):426, 2016.

Salunke AA, Shah J, Warikoo V, et al.: Salvage of the proximal femur following pathological fractures involving benign bone tumors, *J Surg Oncol* 114(2):254, 2016.

Samir Barakat A, Alsinaby H, Shousha M, et al.: Early recurrence of a solid variant of aneurysmal bone cyst in a young child after resection: technique and literature review and two-year follow-up after corpectomy, *J Am Acad Orthop Surg* 26(10):369, 2018.

Sanders T, Wenger DE, Ashraf A, et al.: Treatment of pediatric osteoid osteomas not amenable to radiofrequency ablation: a retrospective review of surgical outcomes, *J Surg Orthop Adv Winger* 27(4):299, 2018.

Santiago E, Pauly V, Brun G, et al.: Percutaneous cryoablation for the treatment of osteoid osteoma in the adult population, *Eur Radiol* 28(6):2336, 2018.

Sasaki H, Nagano S, Shimada H, et al.: Diagnosing and discriminating between primary and secondary aneurysmal bone cysts, *Oncol Lett* 13(43):2290, 2017.

Sasaki H, Nagano S, Shimada H, et al.: Intraosseous epidermoid cyst of the distal phalanx reconstructed with synthetic bone graft, *J Orthop Surg (Hong Kong)* 25(1):2309499016684096, 2017.

Scholfield DW, Sadozai Z, Ghali C, et al.: Does osteofibrous dysplasia progress to adamantinoma and how should they be treated? *Bone Joint J* 99-B(3):409, 2017.

Sebaaly A, Ghostine B, Kreichati G, et al.: Aneurysmal bone cyst of the cervical spine in children: a review and a focus on available treatment options, *J Pediatr Orthop* 35(7):693, 2015.

Senthil V, Balaji S: Monostotic Paget disease of the lumbar vertebrae: a pathological mimicker, *Neurospine* 15(2):182, 2018.

Sferopoulos NK: Giant bone island of the tibia in a child, *Am J Orthop (Belle Mead NJ)* 45(1):38, 2016.

Shah JN, Cohen HL, Choudrhri AF, et al.: Pediatric benign bone tumors: what does the radiologist need to know?: pediatric imaging, *Radiographics* 37(3):1001, 2017.

Shimal A, Davies AM, James SL, Grimer RJ: Fatigue-type stress fractures of the lower limb associated with fibrous cortical defects/nonossifying fibromas in the skeletally mature, *Clin Radiol* 65:382, 2010.

Shooshtarizadeh T, Movahedinia S, Mostafavi H, et al.: Aneurysmal bone cyst: an analysis of 38 cases and report of four unusual surface ones, *Arch Bone Jt Surg* 4(2):166, 2016.

Silverman S: Paget disease of bone: therapeutic options, *J Clin Rheumatol* 14:299, 2008.

Simon K, Leithner A, Bodo K, Windhager R: Intraosseous epidermoid cysts of the hand skeleton: a series of eight patients, *J Hand Surg Eur* 36:376, 2011.

Skunda R, Puckett T, Martin M, et al.: 14-year-old boy with mild antecedent neck pain in setting of acute trauma: a rare case of benign fibrous histiocytoma of the spine, *Am J Orthop (Belle Mead NJ)* 45(3):e148, 2016.

Sorel JC, Facee Schaeffer M, Homan AS, et al.: Surgical hip dislocation according to Ganz for excision of osteochondromas in patients with multiple hereditary exostoses, *Bone Joint J* 98-B(2):260, 2016.

Stevens J, Moin S, Salter D, et al.: Desmoplastic fibroma: a rare pathological midshaft femoral fracture treated with resection, acute shortening, and re-lengthening: a case report, *JBJS Case Connect* 9(2):e0022, 2019.

Sugiyama H, Omonishi K, Yonehara S, et al.: Characteristics of benign and malignant bone tumors registered in the Hiroshima Tumor Tissue Registry, 1973-2012, *JBJS Open Access* 3(2):e0064, 2018.

Sunny G, Hoisala VR, Cicilet S, et al.: Multiple enchondromatosis: Olliers disease – a case report, *J Clin Diagn Res* 10(1):TD01, 2016.

Tan E, Mehlman C, Baker M: Benign osteolytic lesions in children with previously normal radiographs, *J Pediatr Orthop* 37(4):e282, 2017.

Tang C, Chan M, Fok M, et al.: Current management of hand enchondroma: a review, *Hand Surg* 20(1):191, 2015.

Tang H, Ahlawat S, Fayad LM: Multiparametric MR imaging of benign and malignant bone lesions, *Magn Reson Imaging Clin N Am* 26(4):559, 2018.

Temple HT, Central chondrosarcoma in patients with multiple osteochondromas: commentary on an article by Annemarie L. Loud, MD, PhD, et al.: "Intraosseous atypical chondroid tumor or chondrosarcoma grade 1 in patients with multiple osteochondromas", *J Bone Joint Surg Am* 97(1):e5, 2015.

Thompson MJ, Domson G, Dragoescu E: Review of the recent literature, *JBJS Case Connect* 5(3):368, 2015.

Toepfer A, Harrasser N, Recker M, et al.: Distribution patterns of foot and ankle tumors: University Tumor Institute experience, *BMC Cancer* 18(1):735, 2018.

Tong K, Liu H, Wang X, et al.: Osteochondroma: review of 431 patients from one medical institution in South China, *J Bone Oncol* 8:23, 2017.

Tscholl PM, Biedert RM, Gal I: Cortical desmoids in adolescent top-level athletes, *Acta Radiol Open* 4(5):2058460115580878, 2015.

Tutar S, Ulusoy OL, Ozturk E, et al.: Aggressive vertebral hemangioma of the thoracic spine, *Spine J* 16(8):e489, 2016.

Urrutia J, Postigo R, Larrondo R, Martin AS: Clinical and imaging findings in patients with aggressive spinal hemangioma requiring surgical treatment, *J Clin Neurosci* 18:209, 2011.

Vaishya R, Agarwal AK, Vijay V, Vaish A: A brown tumor of tibial diaphysis masquerading as malignancy, *Cureus* 9(6):e1319, 2017.

Wan J, Zhang C, Liu YP, He HB: Surgical treatment for shepherd's crook deformity in fibrous dysplasia: there is no best, only better, *Int Orthop* 43(3):719.

Wang EH, Marfori ML, Serrano MV, Rubio DA: Is curettage and high-speed burring sufficient treatment for aneurysmal bone cysts? *Clin Orthop Relat Res* 472:3438, 2014.

Wang B, Meng N, Zhuang H, et al.: The role of radiotherapy and surgery in the management of aggressive vertebral hemangioma: a retrospective study of 20 patients, *Med Sci Monit* 24:6840, 2018.

Wang L, Song Y: A rare case of symptomatic hemangioma of the lumbar spine involving the spinous process, *Spine J* 16(3):e191, 2016.

Westacott D, Kannu P, Stimec J, et al.: Osteofibrous dysplasia of the tibia in children: outcome without resection, *J Pediatr Orthop* 39(8):3614, 2019.

Woo T, Lalam R, Cassar-Pullicino V, et al.: Imaging of upper limb tumors and tumorlike pathology, *Radiol Clin North Am* 57(5):1035, 2019.

Yang C, Zhang R, Lin H, Wang H: Insights into the molecular regulatory network of pathomechanisms in osteochondroma, *J Cell Biochem* 120(10):16362, 2019.

Yang JS, Chu L, Li X, et al.: Multiple intraosseous vertebral lipomas with chronic back pain, *Spine J* 15(7):1676, 2015.

Yin H, Zhang D, Wu Z, et al.: Desmoplastic fibroma of the spine: a series of 12 cases and outcomes, *Spine J* 14:1622, 2014.

Yu X, Wang B, Yang S, et al.: Percutaneous radiofrequency ablation versus open surgical resection for spinal osteoid osteoma, *Spine J* 19(3):509, 2019.

Zenonos G, Jamil O, Governale LS, et al.: Surgical treatment for preliminary spinal aneurysmal bone cysts: experience from Children's Hospital Boston, *J Neurosurg Pediatr* 9:305, 2012.

Zhang P, Kang L, Hu Q, et al.: Treatment of diaphyseal pathological fractures in children with monostotic fibrous dysplasia using cortical strut allografts and internal plating: a retrospective clinical study, *Medicine (Baltimore)* 98(5):e14318, 2019.

Zhao Y, He S, Sun H, et al.: Symptomatic aneurysmal bone cysts of the spine: clinical features, surgical outcomes, and prognostic factors, *Eur Spine J* 28(6):1537, 2019.

Zhao JG, Wang J, Huang WJ, et al.: Interventions for treating simple bone cysts in the long bones of children, *Cochrane Database Syst Rev* 2:CD010847, 2017.

Zhou X, Zhao B, Keshav P, et al.: The management and surgical intervention timing of enchondromas: a 10-year experience, *Medicine (Baltimore)* 96(16):e6678, 2017.

Zheng K, Yu X, Xu S, Xu M: Periosteal chondroma of the femur: a case report and review of the literature, *Oncol Lett* 9(4):1637, 2015.

Zileli M, Isik HS, Ogut FE, et al.: Aneurysmal bone cysts of the spine, *Eur Spine J* 22:593, 2013.

The complete list of references is available online at Expert Consult.com.

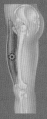

The aggressiveness of the lesions described in this chapter ranges between purely benign and frankly malignant. Although these lesions frequently are treated satisfactorily with intralesional procedures, such as curettage, they are sometimes very aggressive locally and require marginal or wide resection. Systemic involvement, although rare, must be evaluated and treated. Giant cell tumors and chondroblastomas can develop pulmonary metastases and in rare cases can be fatal. Langerhans cell histiocytosis (LCH) can involve multiple organ systems in addition to bone involvement and likewise in rare cases can be fatal. This chapter briefly describes the clinical, radiographic, and pathologic features of these lesions. A summary table is provided for quick reference (Table 9.1).

GIANT CELL TUMOR

According to a Mayo Clinic series, giant cell tumors represent 5% of neoplasms of bone. They typically occur in patients 20 to 40 years old, and there is a slight female predominance. The most common location for this tumor is the distal femur, followed closely by the proximal tibia. In the distal radius (the third most common location), these tumors frequently are more aggressive. Spinal involvement, other than the sacrum, is rare.

Giant cell tumors usually are solitary lesions; however, 1% to 2% may be synchronously or metachronously multicentric. It is unclear whether multicentric disease represents multiple primary lesions or simply bone metastases from a single primary lesion. Although these tumors typically are benign, pulmonary metastases occur in approximately 3% of patients. Some patients with pulmonary metastases have spontaneous regression or remain asymptomatic for many years. Others may have progressive pulmonary lesions, however, that lead to death despite the tumors remaining histologically benign. The overall mortality rate from disease for patients with pulmonary metastases is approximately 15%. Patients with recurrent lesions or primary lesions that appear aggressive radiographically (stage 3) are at higher risk for pulmonary metastases.

Malignant giant cell tumors represent less than 5% of cases and are classified as primary or secondary. Primary malignant giant cell tumors are extremely rare and are defined as sarcomas that occur within lesions that otherwise are typical of benign giant cell tumors. Secondary malignant giant cell tumors are sarcomas that occur at the sites of giant cell tumors that have been treated, usually with radiation.

Most patients with giant cell tumors have progressive pain that often is related to activity initially and only later becomes evident at rest. The pain is rarely severe, unless a pathologic fracture has occurred. In 10% to 30% of patients, pathologic fractures are evident at initial examination.

Radiographic findings often are diagnostic. The lesions are eccentrically located in the epiphyses of long bones and usually abut the subchondral bone. Although rare in skeletally immature patients, giant cell tumors arise in the metaphysis in this patient population. One theory suggests that these tumors originate in the metaphysis and later extend into the epiphysis after closure of the physes. Radiographically, the lesions are purely lytic. The zone of transition can be poorly defined on plain radiographs. In less aggressive tumors, a partial rim of reactive bone may be present. The lesion frequently expands or breaks through the cortex; however, intraarticular extension is rare because the subchondral bone usually remains intact. Matrix production usually is not evident within the bone but often is evident if there is soft-tissue extension, soft-tissue recurrence, or pulmonary metastases. Magnetic resonance imaging (MRI) is useful to determine the extent of the lesion within the bone and in the soft tissue. On MRI, the lesion usually is dark on T1-weighted images and bright on T2-weighted images. MRI also may reveal fluid-fluid levels typical of a secondary aneurysmal bone cyst, which occurs in 20% of patients.

Microscopically, giant cell tumors are composed of many multinucleated giant cells (typically 40 to 60 nuclei per cell) in a sea of mononuclear stromal cells. The nuclei of the mononuclear cells are identical to the nuclei of the giant cells, a feature that helps distinguish giant cell tumors from other tumors that may contain many giant cells. Areas of storiform spindle cell formation, reactive bone formation, or foamy macrophages may be seen. Secondary aneurysmal bone cysts also may be present. Many authors have attempted to grade these tumors histologically, but no grading system has proved to be of prognostic significance.

Giant cell tumors frequently are locally aggressive. Most manifest as stage 2 or stage 3 lesions. Historically, treatment consisted of simple curettage; however, subsequent recurrence rates were greater than 50%. Now, most published series document recurrence rates of 5% to 15%. The decrease in recurrence rates probably can be attributed to several factors. MRI now allows for more accurate assessment of the extent of lesions, and the technique of curettage has improved. It is important to create a cortical window that is at least as large as the lesion to prevent leaving residual tumor cells "around the corner" adjacent to the near-side cortex. Also, use of a power burr to enlarge the cavity 1 to 2 cm in all directions is now considered standard. Care should be taken, however, to avoid perforation through the subchondral bone into the joint.

TABLE 9.1

Summary of Tumor Characteristics

TUMOR	AGE (YR)	DEMOGRAPHICS	SITE	PRESENTATION	IMAGING	HISTOLOGY	TREATMENT	COMMENTS
Giant cell tumor	20–40	Slight female predominance	Distal femur Proximal tibia Distal radius	Pain Pathologic fracture (10%–30%)	Eccentrically located in epiphysis Purely radiolucent (no matrix formation) Usually no rim of reactive bone Abuts subchondral bone May exhibit cortical destruction with soft-tissue extension Metaphyseal in skeletally immature patients	Multinucleated giant cells in sea of mononuclear cells Nuclei of mononuclear cells identical to nuclei of giant cells	Extended curettage Resection if residual bone stock inadequate Consider radiation for spinal/sacral tumors Resection of pulmonary metastases	3% incidence of benign pulmonary metastases
Chondroblastoma	10–25	Male : female 2 : 1	Distal femur Proximal tibia Proximal humerus	Pain Symptoms can mimic chronic synovitis	Well-circumscribed lesion in epiphysis or apophysis May cross an open physis Frequently with rim of bone, 30%–50% with matrix calcification	Sheets of chondroblasts (polygonal cells with distinct cytoplasmic outlines) "chicken wire" calcification Multinucleated giant cells Secondary aneurysmal bone cyst in 20%	Extended curettage Resection of pulmonary metastases	1% incidence of benign pulmonary metastases
Chondromyxoid fibroma	10–30	Slight male predominance	Proximal tibia	Pain Can present with painless mass in hands and feet	Well-circumscribed bubbly lesion Thin rim of reactive bone (appearance similar to nonossifying fibroma)	Lobules of hypocellular myxoid cartilaginous tissue Lobules separated by cellular fibrous tissue	Extended curettage	Important to distinguish from chondrosarcoma
Osteoblastoma	10–30	Male : female 3 : 1	Posterior elements of spine Any bone	Pain Painful scoliosis Neurologic symptoms	Bone-forming lesion in posterior elements of spine Variable/nonspecific radiographic appearance outside of spine	Fibrovascular stroma Osteoid/woven bone Osteoblastic rimming Histologic appearance similar to osteoid osteoma	Extended curettage or resection Might require spinal stabilization	Important to distinguish from low-grade osteosarcoma
Langerhans cell histiocytosis	<20	Male : female 2 : 1	Vertebral bodies Flat bones Diaphysis of long bones	Bone lesions may be painful or asymptomatic Can mimic osteomyelitis (pain, fever, local signs)	Vertebra plana "hole within a hole" appearance in flat bones Aggressive, permeative appearance with periosteal reaction in long bones Radiographic appearance varies from very benign to very aggressive Can be multifocal Bone scan sometimes falsely negative	Large histiocytic cells with indented nucleus and abundant cytoplasm S-100 positive Clusters of eosinophils Birbeck granule seen on electron microscopy	Observation of asymptomatic lesions (usually resolve) Steroid injection for symptomatic lesions Curettage/grafting for impending fractures Chemotherapy for systemic disease	Hand-Schüller-Christian disease triad of skull lesions, exophthalmos, and diabetes insipidus Letterer-Siwe disease—fever, lymphadenopathy, hepatosplenomegaly, and multiple bone lesions

The use of adjuvants, such as liquid nitrogen, phenol, bone cement, electrocautery, or an argon beam coagulator, theoretically helps kill any remaining tumor cells. Also, preliminary studies suggest that bisphosphonates (administered systemically or locally) might help prevent recurrence.

To fill the defect after curettage, the surgeon has several options, including autograft bone, allograft bone, an artificial bone graft substitute, or methyl methacrylate bone cement. If an autograft is to be harvested from another site, separate gloves and instruments should be used because cross-contamination could lead to transplantation of tumor cells to the harvest site. A bone graft (or artificial substitute) has the theoretical advantage of restoring normal biomechanics to the joint surface to prevent future degenerative joint disease and restoring bone stock, which may help if future procedures are necessary. There are two main disadvantages, however, to using bone grafts: (1) the joint must be protected for an extended time to prevent a pathologic fracture and (2) tumor recurrence often is difficult or impossible to distinguish from graft resorption. These disadvantages may be overcome with the use of bone cement as a filling agent. Bone cement provides immediate stability, which aids in quicker rehabilitation; allows easier detection of recurrence, which is evident as an expanding radiolucency adjacent to the cement mantle; and may kill residual tumor cells through the heat of polymerization.

Our institution treats most giant cell tumors with aggressive, extended curettage followed by argon beam coagulation, which is easy to use, effective, and associated with few complications. Phenol or liquid nitrogen is not used as adjuvant treatment because of potential complications, such as pathologic fracture, wound healing problems, and nerve injury. Bone cement is chosen to fill the cavity because of its ease of application, immediate structural support, and ease with which local recurrence can be detected adjacent to the cement mantle. Screws placed in a crossed (Fig. 9.1) or divergent (Fig. 9.2) pattern are used to augment the cement mantle. Biomechanical studies performed at our institution have shown this method to significantly increase the strength of the reconstruction.

En bloc wide resection may be required in some stage 3 tumors, cases of local recurrence, and tumors recalcitrant to other methods of intervention. Around the knee, a hemicondylar osteoarticular allograft reconstruction or a rotating hinge endoprosthesis may be necessary (Fig. 9.3). For aggressive lesions of the distal radius, primary resection and reconstruction with a proximal fibular autograft (either as an arthroplasty or as an arthrodesis) may be indicated (Fig. 9.4). For lesions in expendable bones (e.g., the distal ulna, clavicle, or proximal fibula), primary resection without reconstruction may be indicated. For inoperable lesions in the spine or pelvis, irradiation or embolization (or both) may be used (Fig. 9.5); however, caution is advised because of the risk of sarcomatous change in patients treated with irradiation. In patients with pulmonary metastases, resection should be attempted. Chemotherapy has limited success, and irradiation should be reserved for symptomatic inoperable lesions.

There is clinical rationale for the use of bisphosphonates in treating giant cell tumor of bone, as these drugs inhibit osteoclastic activity and promote osteoclast apoptosis. Studies using systemic zoledronic acid in inoperable tumors have reported stabilization of both local and metastatic disease. Bisphosphonates have been proposed for use as a surgical adjuvant or as an option in unresectable tumors; however, high-level evidence is still lacking, and further investigation is required to validate its use.

Another new treatment under examination is the systemic administration of denosumab. Denosumab is a fully human monoclonal antibody that inhibits normal and tumor-associated bone lysis by limiting osteoclastic maturation (i.e., prevents activation of receptor activator of nuclear factor-kB [RANK]). This drug has approval from the US Food and Drug Administration for use in adults and skeletally mature patients who have an unresectable giant cell tumor or a condition in which surgical resection would result in severe morbidity. Early results are promising, with radiographic studies showing sclerosis and reconstitution of cortical bone with a subsequent decrease in clinical symptoms such as pain. Longer term data are still being collected.

Patients diagnosed with giant cell tumors require long-term follow-up. Most local recurrences and pulmonary metastases occur within 3 years but have been reported to occur 20 years later. Chest radiographs should be obtained at the time of diagnosis to stage the lesion. We routinely obtain a chest computed tomography (CT) scan as a baseline reference at this time. At minimum, patients should have radiographs of the primary tumor site and the chest at 3- to 4-month intervals for 2 years, at 6-month intervals for the following year, and annually thereafter. An abnormality on the chest radiograph should be evaluated further with CT. Bone recurrence usually is evident as an expanding lucency on the radiograph. Soft-tissue recurrences may be apparent as ossification or may be evident only as a palpable mass, in which case MRI is indicated.

Treatment of recurrent lesions is the same as for primary lesions. If biopsy shows that the tumor is still benign, repeat curettage or resection should be performed.

CHONDROBLASTOMA

Chondroblastoma, a rare neoplasm, typically occurs in patients 10 to 25 years old, with a 2 : 1 male predominance. According to the Mayo Clinic series, this tumor represents 1% of all primary bone tumors. Because of its rarity, no prospective and few retrospective studies have been reported in the literature. This tumor has a predilection for the epiphyses or apophyses of long tubular bones (e.g., distal femur, proximal humerus, and proximal tibia). Less frequently, chondroblastoma tends to occur in flat bones in older patients. Multicentric disease is exceedingly rare. Most patients complain of progressive pain that may mimic a chronic synovitis or other intraarticular pathologic conditions.

Radiographic findings usually are characteristic. This well-circumscribed lesion is usually centered in an epiphysis of a long bone; however, it may also be located in an apophysis, such as the greater tuberosity (Fig. 9.6) or the greater trochanter (Fig. 9.7). Often it has a surrounding rim of reactive bone (Fig. 9.8), and 30% to 50% exhibit matrix calcification. CT can be helpful in detecting subtle areas of calcification that may or may not be detectable on plain radiographs. MRI frequently demonstrates abundant surrounding edema. Soft-tissue extension is extremely rare. In children, a well-circumscribed epiphyseal lesion that crosses an open physis is highly suggestive of chondroblastoma but could also represent an infectious process. For adults, differential diagnoses for an epiphyseal lesion include giant cell tumor and clear

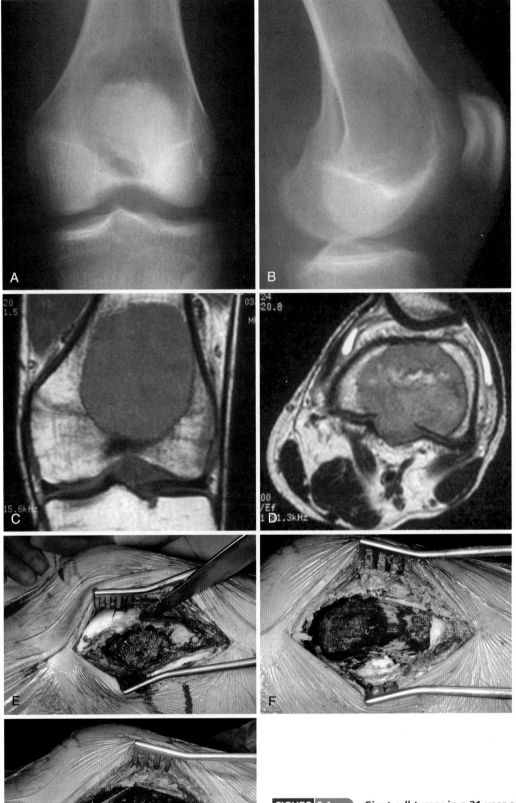

FIGURE 9.1 **Giant cell tumor in a 21-year-old man.** Patient complained of worsening left knee pain. **A** and **B,** Anteroposterior and lateral radiographs of left distal femur show lytic lesion with extension to articular surface. **C** and **D,** Coronal and axial MR images show extent of lesion within bone and soft tissue. **E,** Intra-operative photograph after creation of cortical window. **F,** Tumor removed and cavity enlarged with power burr. **G,** After treatment with argon beam coagulator, screws are placed to support cement mantle.

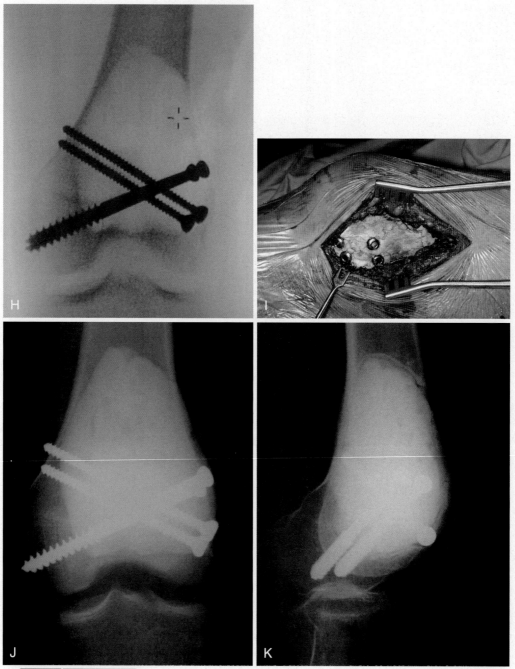

FIGURE 9.1, Cont'd   **H,** Placement of screws confirmed by image intensifier. **I,** Bone cement packed in cavity around screws. **J** and **K,** Anteroposterior and lateral postoperative radiographs. Fifteen years after surgery, the patient is currently asymptomatic and is employed as a construction worker.

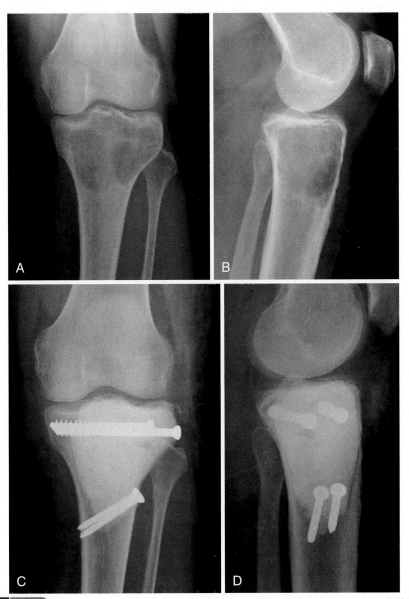

FIGURE 9.2 **A** and **B,** Anteroposterior and lateral radiographs of the proximal tibia of a 41-year-old woman with a giant cell tumor. The lesion is radiolucent without a sclerotic rim, is eccentric, and abuts subchondral bone. **C** and **D,** Anteroposterior and lateral radiographs of the proximal tibia after curettage and placement of cement and divergent screws.

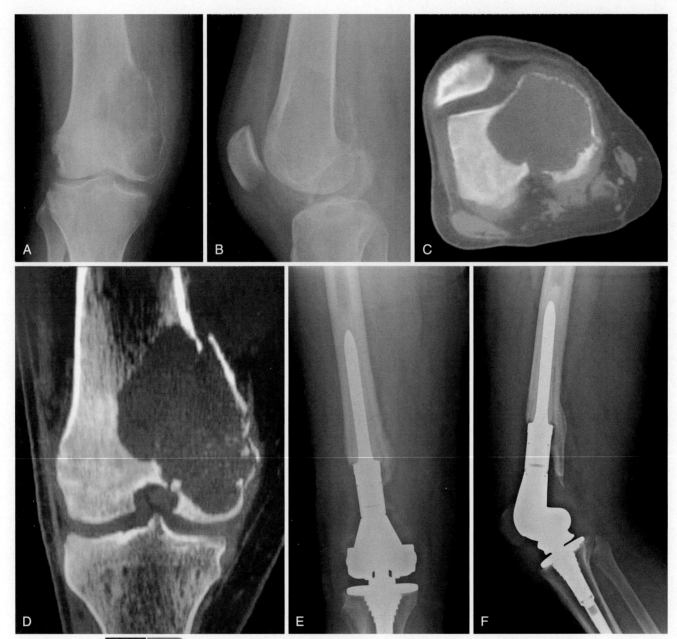

FIGURE 9.3   Anteroposterior **(A)** and lateral **(B)** radiographs of a 28-year-old man with a giant cell tumor of the right distal femur. Axial **(C)** and coronal **(D)** CT reconstructions demonstrate extensive bone destruction and an intraarticular pathologic fracture. The decision was made to proceed with en bloc resection and endoprosthetic reconstruction. Anteroposterior **(E)** and lateral **(F)** postoperative radiographs. Patient currently is doing well 8 years after surgery.

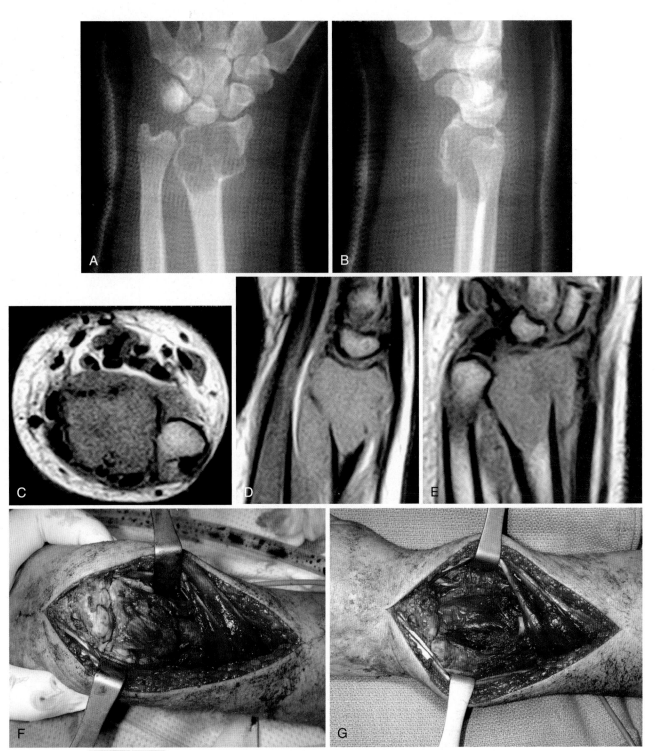

FIGURE 9.4　**A** and **B,** Anteroposterior and lateral radiographs of distal radius of 40-year-old woman with pathologic fracture through giant cell tumor. **C** to **E,** Axial **(C),** sagittal **(D),** and coronal **(E)** MR images of lesion. **F,** Intraoperative photograph of tumor in situ. **G,** Tumor has been resected en bloc.

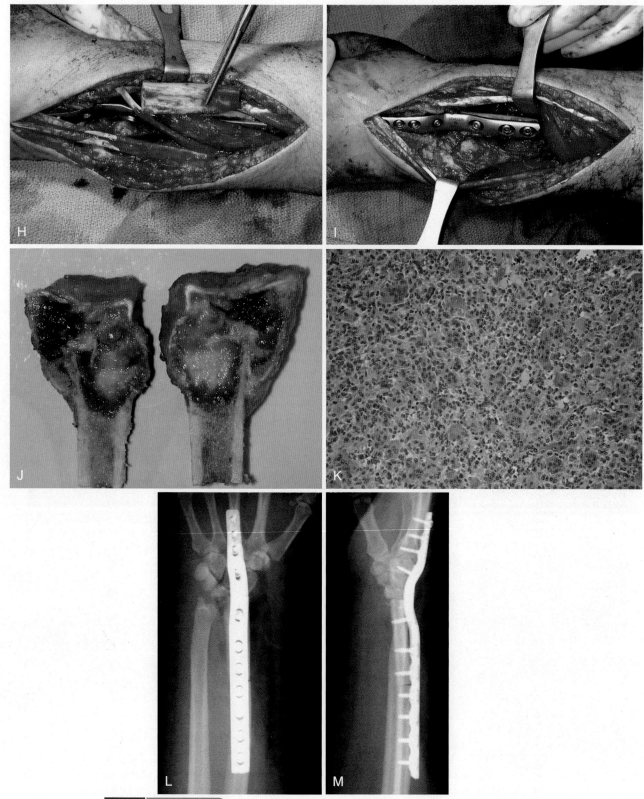

FIGURE 9.4, Cont'd   **H,** Contralateral proximal fibular autograft. **I,** Graft has been secured with wrist fusion plate. **J,** Photograph of resected specimen. **K,** Typical microscopic appearance of giant cell tumor. Nuclei of giant cells are identical to nuclei of mononuclear cells. **L** and **M,** Anteroposterior and lateral postoperative radiographs.

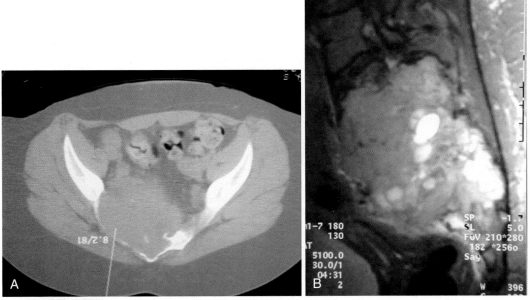

FIGURE 9.5 **Giant cell tumor in 23-year-old woman.** Patient had 1-year history of worsening low back pain that radiated down her right leg. **A,** CT scan. **B,** Sagittal T2-weighted MR image reveals large lesion in sacrum. CT-guided biopsy confirmed this to be giant cell tumor. Because of morbidity of surgical treatment of lesion in this location, the patient was referred for radiation therapy.

cell chondrosarcoma. In contrast to chondroblastomas, however, giant cell tumors usually do not have a rim of sclerotic bone or intralesional calcification and may have a soft-tissue component.

Microscopically, chondroblastoma consists of sheets of chondroblasts usually with a background of chondroid matrix. The cells are round to polygonal with distinct cytoplasmic outlines. Dystrophic calcification is frequently present and may surround individual cells, giving the classic "chicken wire" appearance. Multinucleated giant cells are abundant, and secondary aneurysmal bone cysts are present in 20% of patients. Histologic grading is of no prognostic significance.

Chondroblastomas usually present as stage 2 and, more rarely, as stage 3 lesions. Although they typically are not as aggressive as giant cell tumors, surgical management is warranted for almost all chondroblastomas owing to the slow progressive nature of the disease. Following biopsy to establish the diagnosis, treatment consists of extended curettage and bone grafting or placement of bone cement. This technique is associated with high chance of joint preservation and good functional outcomes. Adequate curettage always should take precedence over sparing the physis (Fig. 9.9). In cases where physeal growth arrest has been reported, it is not known whether the insult is from the chondroblastoma itself or the surgical intervention.

Radiographs of the primary site and of the chest should be obtained every 6 months for at least 3 years and annually thereafter. Recurrence occurs in 10% to 20% of patients and can be treated similar to a primary lesion. Benign pulmonary metastases occur in approximately 1% of patients and should be treated by resection. Malignant transformation of a chondroblastoma is extremely rare.

CHONDROMYXOID FIBROMA

Chondromyxoid fibroma is a rare lesion of cartilaginous origin, representing less than 0.5% of all bone tumors according to the Mayo Clinic series. Although chondromyxoid fibromas may occur at any age, most occur in patients 10 to 30 years old. Any bone may be involved, but the proximal tibia is the most common location (Figs. 9.10 and 9.11). Although patients typically complain of pain, if the tumor is in the hands or feet, a painless mass or swelling may be the chief complaint.

The radiographic appearance is that of a benign neoplasm. It usually is a well-circumscribed lesion with a rim of sclerosis in the metaphysis of a long bone and may have a bubbly appearance mimicking a nonossifying fibroma. In contrast to other cartilaginous lesions, radiographic evidence of intralesional calcification usually is absent (except in the rare instance of a surface lesion in which calcification may be abundant). Chondromyxoid fibroma rarely is included in the radiographic differential diagnosis of a lesion, unless it is in the proximal tibial metaphysis. Other diagnoses to include in the differential are chondrosarcoma, chondroblastoma, fibrous dysplasia, nonossifying fibroma, giant cell tumor, aneurysmal bone cyst, and simple bone cyst.

Microscopically, chondromyxoid fibroma appears lobulated. The center of the lobules contains loose myxoid tissue, and the periphery contains a more cellular fibrous tissue. The background often appears chondroid, although distinct areas of hyaline cartilage are rare. Microscopic calcification may be present. The lesion may contain areas with atypical pleomorphic hyperchromatic nuclei, but this should not lead to the erroneous diagnosis of chondrosarcoma if the lesion is

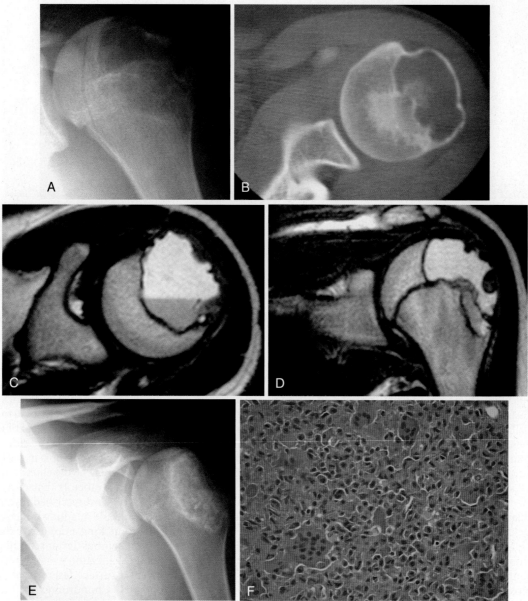

FIGURE 9.6   **Chondroblastoma in a 16-year-old boy.** Patient had left shoulder pain for 1 year. **A,** Anteroposterior radiograph of left shoulder reveals lytic lesion in proximal left humerus extending across open physis. **B,** CT scan shows calcification of lesion. **C** and **D,** MR images show fluid-fluid level. Incision biopsy confirmed diagnosis of chondroblastoma with secondary aneurysmal bone cyst. **E,** Anteroposterior radiograph after curettage and bone grafting. **F,** Typical microscopic appearance of chondroblastoma.

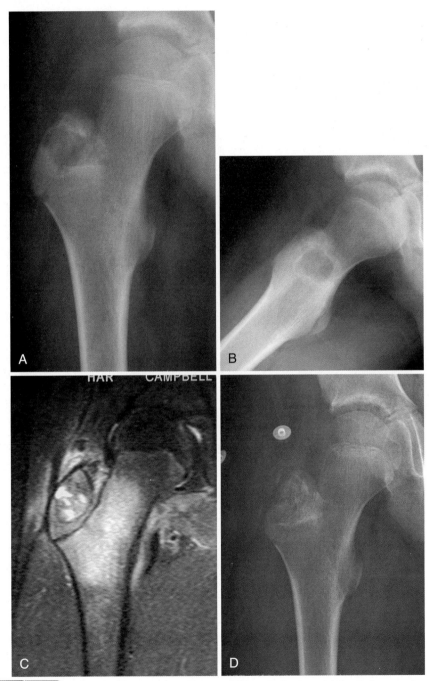

FIGURE **9.7**   **Chondroblastoma in a 12-year-old boy.** Patient complained of worsening right hip pain for several months. **A** and **B,** Anteroposterior and lateral radiographs of right hip show radiolucent lesion in greater trochanter. **C,** Coronal MR image shows lesion in greater trochanter with surrounding edema. **D,** Postoperative radiograph after curettage and grafting with allograft cancellous bone chips and demineralized bone matrix.

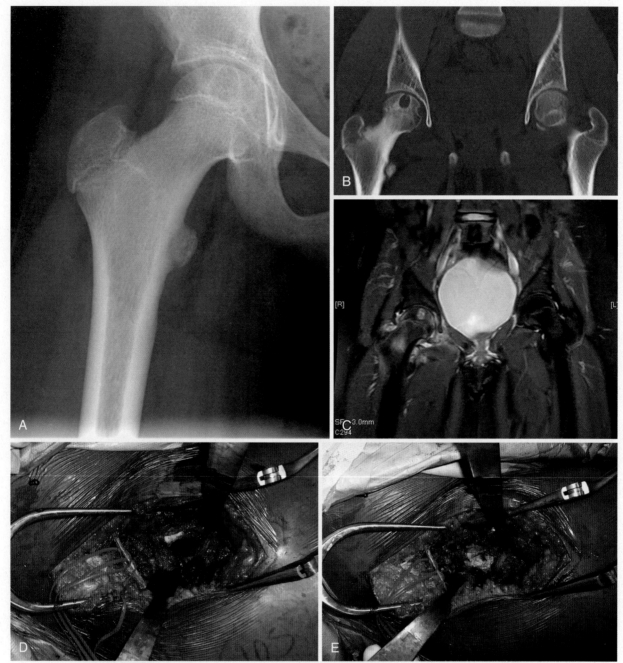

FIGURE 9.8 **A** and **B**, Anteroposterior radiograph and CT scan of a 16-year-old girl with a chondroblastoma of the femoral head. The lesion is epiphyseal and has a narrow zone of transition with a thin rim of reactive bone and a small amount of matrix mineralization. **C**, MR image demonstrates the lesion with extensive surrounding edema and an effusion. **D**, Extended curettage was performed through an anterior approach followed by the placement of a bone graft substitute (**E**).

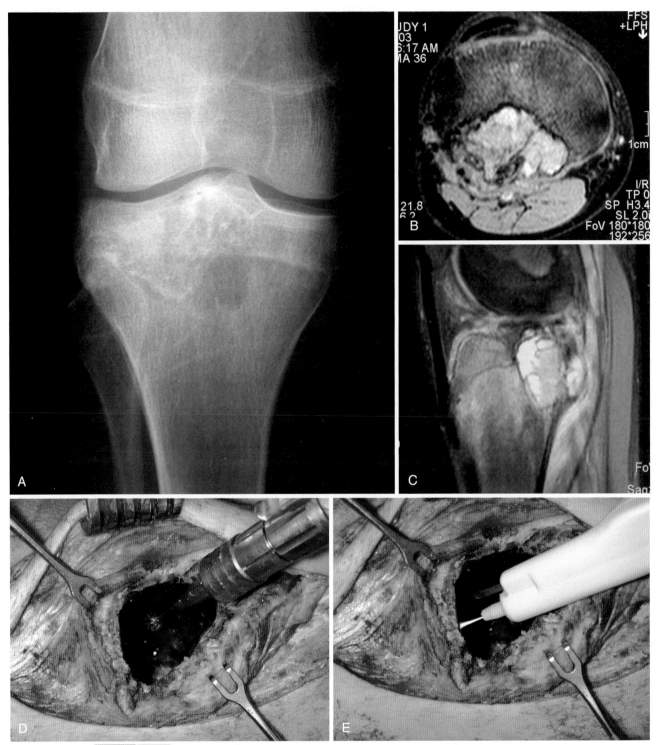

FIGURE 9.9 **A,** Anteroposterior radiograph demonstrates a chondroblastoma in the proximal tibial epiphysis of a 15-year-old boy. **B** and **C,** Coronal and sagittal MR images more clearly demonstrate the lesion and extensive surrounding edema. **D** and **E,** Lesion is treated with extended curettage with a power burr and argon beam coagulation.

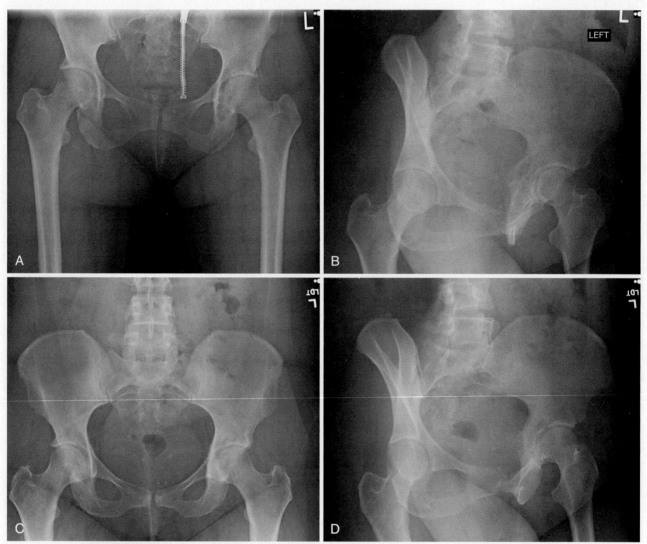

FIGURE 9.10   Anteroposterior **(A)** and Judet **(B)** views of the pelvis in a 31-year-old woman with a chondromyxoid fibroma of the posterior column of the left acetabulum. Anteroposterior **(C)** and Judet **(D)** views 3 years after extended curettage and grafting with freeze-dried cancellous allograft and demineralized bone matrix.

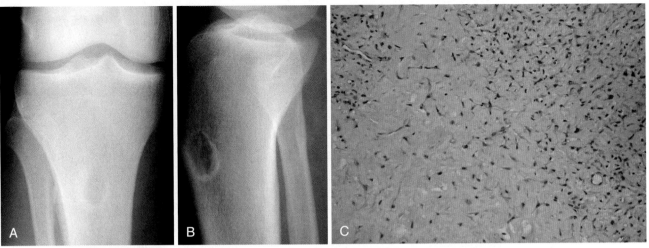

FIGURE 9.11 Chondromyxoid fibroma in a 36-year-old man. Patient had right knee pain for 1 year. **A** and **B,** Anteroposterior and lateral radiographs show chondromyxoid fibroma in its most common location, proximal tibial metaphysis. **C,** Typical microscopic appearance of chondromyxoid fibroma.

otherwise radiographically and histologically consistent with chondromyxoid fibroma.

Treatment consists of resection or extended curettage with bone grafting (Fig. 9.12). Wide resection is associated with a lower risk of recurrence than is intralesional curettage but results in a potentially larger functional deficit. Local recurrence occurs in about 20% of patients and is treated with repeat surgery. Malignant degeneration is rare.

OSTEOBLASTOMA

Osteoblastoma is a rare bone-forming neoplasm that represents less than 1% of bone tumors in the Mayo Clinic series. Most patients with osteoblastoma are 10 to 30 years old. There is a male predominance of 3:1. Although any bone may be involved, 40% to 50% of the lesions are in the spine. Pain, which is the most common symptom, may be similar to that produced by an osteoid osteoma (i.e., worse at night and relieved by nonsteroidal antiinflammatory drugs). In the spine, painful scoliosis or neurologic deficit may be present. In the lumbar spine, signs and symptoms of nerve root compression may be evident, whereas in the thoracic spine, cord compression is more common. The tumor usually is slow growing, and symptoms may be present for 1 to 2 years before a diagnosis is made.

The most common radiographic appearance is that of a bone-forming neoplasm in the posterior elements of the spine in a young patient (Figs. 9.13 and 9.14). The differential diagnoses include aneurysmal bone cyst and osteoid osteoma. Outside the spine, however, the radiographic appearance rarely reveals the diagnosis. The classic appearance of a mineralized central nidus with a surrounding radiolucent halo and reactive sclerosis is seen only occasionally (Fig. 9.15), in which case the differentiation of osteoblastoma from the more common osteoid osteoma is based on size because the nidus of an osteoid osteoma

is less than 1.5 cm. More often, the radiographic appearance is nonspecific. The lesion may be purely radiolucent (Fig. 9.16), sclerotic, or mixed. Lesions may be diaphyseal or metaphyseal, and they may be primarily cortical or intramedullary. In some cases, they may have a frankly malignant radiographic appearance. Extension into the soft tissue is rare except in the spine, where soft-tissue extension is common.

Microscopically, the lesion resembles an osteoid osteoma. It contains a fibrovascular stroma with the production of osteoid and primitive woven bone. Bony trabeculae are lined by a single layer of osteoblasts, which may be important in differentiating osteoblastoma from osteosarcoma. Other features favoring an osteoblastoma include sharp circumscription and a loose arrangement of the tissue. Features favoring a malignant diagnosis include permeation of surrounding tissue and sheets of osteoblasts without bone production.

Treatment consists of extended curettage or resection. Bone grafting of the defect may be necessary. In the spine, instrumented fusion may be necessary if resection causes instability. Some authors recommend adjuvant radiation therapy for spinal lesions because revision surgery for recurrences in this area is difficult. Other authors have noted that some incompletely removed lesions subsequently have remained quiescent. Most authors do not recommend radiation therapy unless absolutely necessary for symptomatic inoperable lesions.

Sarcomatous degeneration has been reported and may be more common in lesions previously treated with radiation. Many of these cases likely represent initial misdiagnoses of low-grade osteosarcomas. Regardless, it is apparent that some cases initially diagnosed as osteoblastoma have behaved aggressively later and occasionally have led to the death of the patients. As follow-up care, patients should have serial radiographs of the primary site and of the chest.

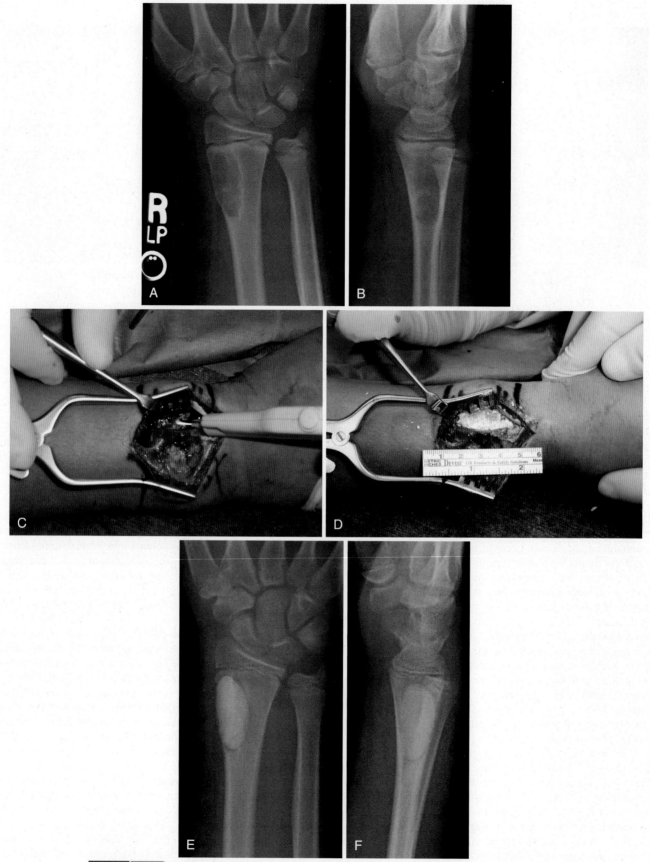

FIGURE 9.12 **Chondromyxoid fibroma in a 14-year-old boy.** Patient complained of right wrist pain after minor injury. **A** and **B,** Anteroposterior and lateral radiographs of right wrist show benign-appearing lesion in distal radial metaphysis. **C** After removal of tumor with curets and power burr, tumor cavity is treated with argon beam coagulation **D,** Cavity was packed with calcium phosphate bone graft substitute. **E** and **F,** Postoperative anteroposterior and lateral radiographs.

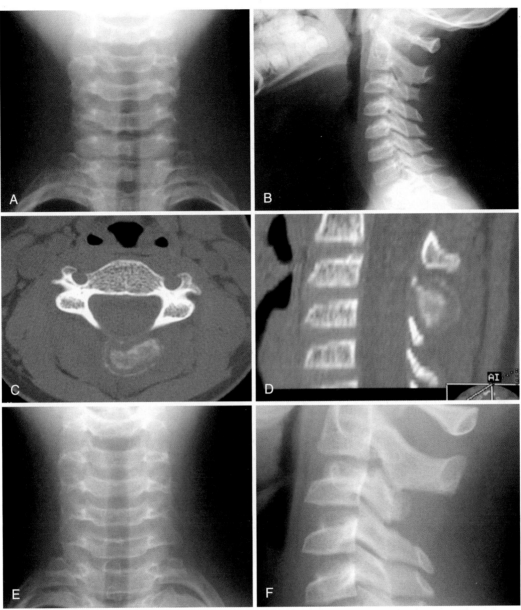

FIGURE 9.13 Ten-year-old boy with 1-month history of neck pain. **A** and **B**, Anteroposterior and lateral radiographs of cervical spine significant for lesion of C3 spinous process. **C** and **D**, Lesion, which proved to be osteoblastoma, is shown better with CT. **E** and **F**, Anteroposterior and lateral radiographs after marginal resection of lesion.

LANGERHANS CELL HISTIOCYTOSIS

Langerhans cell histiocytosis (LCH), previously called histiocytosis X because of its unknown etiology, refers to a group of diseases with similar pathologic features. Because the disease may affect virtually any organ system in the body, there is a wide range of clinical presentations. Whether LCH represents a reactive or a neoplastic process is still a matter of debate. The term *eosinophilic granuloma* refers to isolated bone lesions, and *Hand-Schüller-Christian disease* classically refers to the clinical triad of skull lesions, exophthalmos, and diabetes insipidus. Currently, however, some authors use the term *Hand-Schüller-Christian disease* simply to refer to any case of multisystemic LCH. *Letterer-Siwe disease*, another variation, usually has its onset before 3 years of age and is characterized

by fever, lymphadenopathy, hepatosplenomegaly, and multiple bone lesions. Letterer-Siwe disease frequently is rapidly fatal. Whether these terms represent different diseases or simply different manifestations of the same pathologic process is debatable. Because the pathogenesis is poorly understood, there is currently no optimal treatment protocol for multifocal involvement, and the reactivation rate is high. Diverse therapeutic modalities may be considered, depending on the organ system involved, including surgery, radiation, and chemotherapy. Risk factors for succumbing to LCH include multisystem involvement and diagnosis at an age younger than 2 years.

The orthopaedic surgeon is primarily concerned with eosinophilic granuloma of bone. Patients usually are 5 to 20 years old and usually have progressive pain. The clinical picture may be similar to that produced by osteomyelitis with pain at rest (and at night), fever, and local signs of inflammation. Any bone may be affected, but the most common locations are the vertebral bodies, the flat bones, and the diaphyses of long bones.

Radiographically, LCH can have various appearances. Marked flattening of the vertebral body, or vertebra plana, is a common manifestation. Although LCH is the most common cause of vertebra plana (Fig. 9.17), other disease processes should be considered in the differential diagnosis if the clinical situation warrants. Other causes of vertebra plana include Ewing sarcoma, lymphoma, leukemia, Gaucher disease, aneurysmal bone cyst, and infection. In flat bones, the lesions usually are well circumscribed, "punched-out," purely lytic lesions. The lesions may have a "hole within a hole" appearance because of different involvement of the two tables. In the diaphyses of long bones, the lesions may have an aggressive permeative appearance with periosteal reactive bone formation (Fig. 9.18). This appearance may resemble Ewing sarcoma, infection, or lymphoma. A bone scan may help identify additional lesions, but approximately 30% of scans may be falsely negative. A skeletal survey is more effective for this purpose.

Microscopically, the diagnosis is made by the identification of Langerhans cells. The Langerhans cell is a large histiocytic cell with an indented nucleus, a crisp nuclear membrane, and abundant eosinophilic cytoplasm. The cells stain positively for S-100 protein. The lesion also contains multinucleated giant cells and other inflammatory cells, including clusters of eosinophils. Electron microscopy may identify characteristic organelles in the Langerhans cell cytoplasm called Birbeck granules.

Biopsy is required to make the diagnosis. When the diagnosis is established, most of the orthopaedic manifestations of LCH can be treated conservatively. Simple skeletal lesions tend to resolve spontaneously over a period of months to years, and healing may be initiated from the biopsy itself. Other recommended treatments have included corticosteroid injections, radiation therapy, and curettage with or without

bone grafting. A few case reports have suggested that intravenous zoledronic acid may help resolve pain in symptomatic lesions, but the long-term sequelae are not well defined. If a lesion is asymptomatic, no treatment is necessary because lesions have been noted to regress spontaneously. Indications for treatment include pain, restriction of mobility, impending

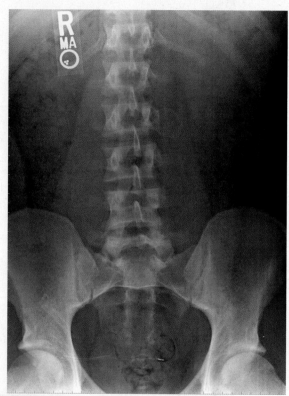

FIGURE 9.14 Anteroposterior radiograph of an 18-year-old boy with osteoblastoma of the left L2 transverse process.

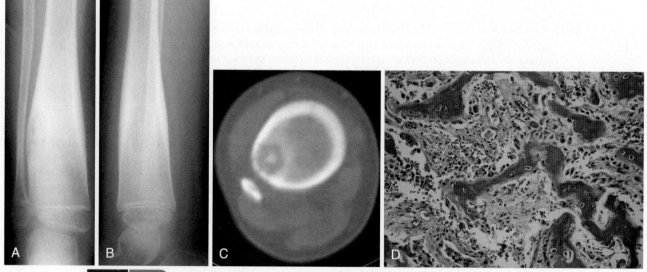

FIGURE 9.15 **Four-year-old boy with a 1-year history of right leg pain.** He walked with an antalgic gait. Right tibia measured 2 cm longer than left. **A** and **B,** Anteroposterior and lateral radiographs of tibia reveal lesion in distal metaphysis. Lesion has led to bowing of fibula, giving evidence of long history and benign nature. **C,** CT scan shows lesion more clearly; it proved to be osteoblastoma. **D,** Typical microscopic appearance of osteoblastoma.

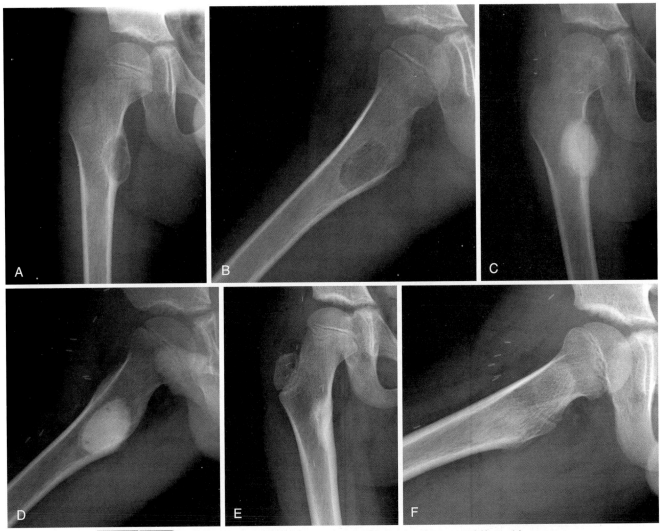

FIGURE 9.16 **A** and **B,** Anteroposterior and lateral radiographs of a 7-year-old boy with an osteo-blastoma of the right lesser trochanter. **C** and **D,** Anteroposterior and lateral radiographs immediately after curettage and placement of a calcium sulfate/calcium phosphate bone graft substitute. **E** and **F,** Lateral radiographs 2 years later demonstrate remodeling of the bone with no sign of recurrence.

pathologic fractures, and nerve compression (spinal or optic nerve). Intralesional injection of steroids is a relatively safe and effective treatment modality. Low-dose radiotherapy, however, should be reserved for involvement of spinal or optic nerve compression. If the diagnosis is established by open biopsy, the lesion can be curetted during the same procedure. Care must be taken, however, to rule out infection before placing corticosteroids or bone graft into a lesion.

Vertebra plana likewise may be treated conservatively because most lesions spontaneously regress. Vertebral height typically is partially restored with growth in skeletally immature patients. Temporary bracing may help relieve symptoms. Irradiation may be indicated for treatment of mild neurologic signs. Surgical decompression and fusion with instrumentation is indicated for rapidly progressive neurologic signs or cord compression that is not responsive to radiation therapy.

The overall prognosis for skeletal lesions is excellent with a very low rate of local recurrence and few complications. Systemic disease may be progressive, however, and may require chemotherapy.

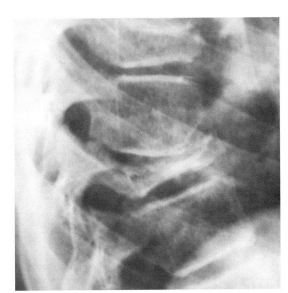

FIGURE 9.17 **Eosinophilic granuloma of vertebral body.** Compression of body may produce radiographic changes of vertebra plana. Patient had lesions involving several other bones.

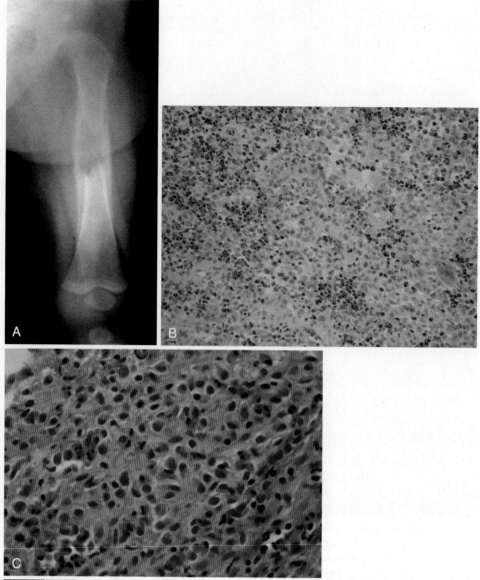

FIGURE 9.18   **A,** Solitary eosinophilic granuloma of femoral diaphysis causing severe periosteal reaction. **B** and **C,** Low-power and high-power photomicrographs demonstrate Langerhans cell histiocyte and eosinophils.

REFERENCES

GIANT CELL TUMOR

Amantullah DF, Clark TR, Lopez MJ, et al.: Giant cell tumor of bone, *Orthopedics* 37:112, 2014.

Balke M, Campanacci L, Gebert C, et al.: Bisphosphonate treatment of aggressive primary, recurrent, and metastatic giant cell tumour of bone, *BMC Cancer* 10:462, 2010.

Boriani S, Bandiera S, Casadei R, et al.: Giant cell tumor of the mobile spine: a review of 49 cases, *Spine (Phila Pa 1976)* 37:E37, 2012.

Branstetter DG, Nelson SD, Manivel JC, et al.: Denosumab induces tumor reduction and bone formation in patients with giant-cell tumor of bone, *Clin Cancer Res* 18:4415, 2012.

Caubere A, Harrosch S, Fioravanti M, et al.: Does curettage-cement packing for treating giant cell tumors at the knee lead to osteoarthritis? *Orthop Traumatol Surg Res* 103:1075, 2017.

Chan CM, Adler Z, Reith JD, Gibbs Jr CP: Risk factors for pulmonary metastases from giant cell tumor of bone, *J Bone Joint Surg Am* 97:420, 2015.

Chawla S, Henshaw R, Seeger L, et al.: Safety and efficacy of denosumab for adults and skeletally mature adolescents with giant cell tumour of bone: interim analysis of an open-label, parallel-group, phase 2 study, *Lancet Oncol* 14:901, 2013.

Chen CC, Liau CT, Chang CH, et al.: Giant cell tumors of bone with pulmonary metastasis, *Orthopedics* 39:e68, 2016.

Cheng DD, Hu T, Zhang HZ, et al.: Factors affecting the recurrence of giant cell tumor of bone after surgery: a clinicopathological study of 80 cases from a single center, *Cell Physiol Biochem* 36:1961, 2015.

Cornelis F, Truchetet ME, Amoretti N, et al.: Bisphosphonate therapy for unresectable symptomatic benign bone tumors: a long-term prospective study of tolerance and efficacy, *Bone* 58:11, 2014.

Domovitov SV, Healey JH: Primary malignant giant-cell tumor of bone has high survival rate, *Ann Surg Oncol* 17:694, 2010.

Federman N, Brien EW, Narasimhan V, et al.: Giant cell tumor of bone in childhood: clinical aspects and novel therapeutic targets, *Paediatr Drugs* 16:21, 2014.

Gao ZH, Yin JQ, Xie XB, et al.: Local control of giant cell tumors of the long bone after aggressive curettage with and without cement, *BMC Musculoskelet Disord* 15:330, 2014.

Gaston CL, Bhumbra R, Watanuki M, et al.: Does the addition of cement improve the rate of local recurrence after curettage of giant cell tumours in bone? *J Bone Joint Surg Br* 93:1665, 2011.

Goldschlager T, Dea N, Boyd M, et al.: Giant cell tumors of the spine: has denosumab changed the treatment paradigm? *J Neurosurg Spine* 22:526, 2015.

Gortzak Y, Kandel R, Deheshi B, et al.: The efficacy of chemical adjuvants on giant-cell tumour of bone. An in vitro study, *J Bone Joint Surg Br* 92:1475, 2010.

Kito M, Matusmoto S, Ae K, et al.: Pulmonary metastasis from giant cell tumor of bone: clinical outcome prior to the introduction of molecular target therapy, *Jpn J Clin Oncol* 47:529, 2017.

Klenke FM, Wenger DE, Inwards CT, et al.: Giant cell tumor of bone: risk factors for recurrence, *Clin Orthop Relat Res* 469:591, 2011.

Lenke FM, Wenter DE, Inwards CY, et al.: Recurrent giant cell tumor of long bones: analysis of surgical management, *Clin Orthop Relat Res* 469:1181, 2011.

Liede A, Bach BA, Stryker S, et al.: Regional variation and challenges in estimating the incidence of giant cell tumor of bone, *J Bone Joint Surg Am* 96:1999, 2014.

Luksanapruksa P, Buchowski JM, Singhatanadgige W, et al.: Management of spinal giant cell tumors, *Spine J* 16:259, 2016.

Ma Y, Xu W, Yin H, et al.: Therapeutic radiotherapy for giant cell tumor of the spine: a systematic review, *Eur Spine J* 24:1754, 2015.

Mak IW, Evaniew N, Popovic S, et al.: A translational study of the neoplastic cells of giant cell tumor of bone following neoadjuvant denosumab, *J Bone Joint Surg Am* 96:e127, 2014.

Malhotra R, Kiran Kumar GN, K Digge V, Kumar V: The clinical and radiological evaluation of the use of an allograft-prosthesis composite in the treatment of proximal femoral giant cell tumours, *Bone Joint J* 96-B:1106, 2014.

Martin-Broto J, Cleeland CS, Glare PA, et al.: Effects of denosumab on pain and analgesic use in giant cell tumor of bone: interim results from a phase II study, *Acta Oncol* 53:1173, 2014.

Mavrogenis AF, Igoumenou VG, Megaloijonomos PD, et al.: Giant cell tumor of bone revisited, *SICOT J* 3:54, 2017.

Mozaffarian K, Modjallal M, Vosoughi AR: Treatment of giant cell tumor of distal radius with limited soft tissue invasion: curettage and cementing versus wide excision, *J Orthop Sci* 23:174, 2018.

Nishisho T, Hanaoka N, Miyagi R, et al.: Local administration of zoledronic acid for giant cell tumor of bone, *Orthopedics* 38:e25, 2015.

Oguro S, Okuda S, Sugiura H, et al.: Giant cell tumors of the bone: changes in image features after denosumab administration, *Magn Reson Med Sci*, 2018 Feb 1. [Epub ahead of print].

Park SY, Lee MH, Lee JS, et al.: Ossified soft tissue recurrence of giant cell tumor of bone: four case reports with follow-up radiographs, CT, ultrasound, and MR images, *Skeletal Radiol* 43:1457, 2014.

Raskin KA, Schwab JH, Mankin HJ, et al.: Giant cell tumor of bone, *J Am Acad Orthop Surg* 21:118, 2013.

Rockberg J, Bach BA, Amelio J, et al.: Incidence trends in the diagnosis of giant cell tumor of bone in Sweden since 1958, *J Bone Joint Surg Am* 97:1756, 2015.

Rosario M, Kim HS, Yun JY, et al.: Suyrveillance for lung metastasis from giant cell tumor of bone, *J Surg Oncol* 116:907, 2017.

Rutkowski P, Gaston L, Borkowska A, et al.: Denosumab treatment of inoperable or locally advanced giant cell tumor of bone—multicenter analysis outside clinical trial, *Eur J Surg Oncol* 44:1384, 2018.

Salunke AA, Pathak S, Shah J, et al.: Wide resection versus curettage in giant cell tumor with pathologic fracture? A systematic review and meta-analysis, *J Clin Orthop Trauma* 9(Suppl 1):S15, 2018.

Savvidou OD, Bolia IK, Chloros GD, et al.: Denosumab: current use in the treatment of primary bone tumors, *Orthopedics* 40:204, 2017.

Siddiqui MA, Seng C, Tan MH: Risk factors for recurrence of giant cell tumours of bone, *J Orthop Surg (Hong Kong)* 22:108, 2014.

Singh AS, Chawla NS, Chawla SP: Giant-cell tumor of bone: treatment options and role of denosumab, *Biologics* 9:69, 2015.

Skubitz KM: Giant cell tumor of bone: current treatment options, *Curr Treat Options Oncol* 15:507, 2014.

van der Heijden L, Dijkstra PDS, Blay JY, et al.: Giant cell tumour of bone in the denosumab ear, *Eur J Cancer* 77:75, 2017.

van der Heijden L, Mastboom MJ, Dijkstera PD, van de Sande MA: Functional outcome and quality of life after the surgical treatment for diffuse-type giant-cell tumour around the knee: a retrospective analysis of 30 patients, *Bone Joint J* 96-B:1111, 2014.

van der Heijden L, van de Sande MA, Heineken AC, et al.: Mid-term outcome after curettage with polymethylmethacrylate for giant cell tumor around the knee: higher risk of radiographic osteoarthritis? *J Bone Joint Surg Am* 95:e159, 2013.

van der Heijden L, van der Geest IC, Schreuder HW, et al.: Liquid nitrogen or phenolization for giant cell tumor of bone?: A comparative cohort study of various standard treatments at two tertiary referral centers, *J Bone Joint Surg Am* 96:e35, 2014.

Wijsbek AE, Vazquez-Garcia BL, Grimer RJ, et al.: Giant cell tumour of the proximal femur: is joint-sparing management ever successful? *Bone Joint J* 96-B:127, 2014.

Xing R, Yang J, Kong Q, et al.: Giant cell tumour of bone in the appendicular skeleton: an analysis of 276 cases, *Acta Orthop Belg* 79:731, 2013.

Xu W, Wang Y, Wang J, et al.: Long-term administration of bisphosphonate to reduce local recurrence of sacral giant cell tumor after nerve-sparing surgery, *J Neurosurg Spine* 26:716, 2017.

Yi J, Lee YH, Kim SK, et al.: Response evaluation of giant-cell tumor of bone treated by denosumab: histogram and texture analysis of CT images, *J Orthop Sci* 23:570, 2018.

Zheng K, Yu XC, Hu YC, et al.: How to fill the cavity after curettge of giant cell tumors around the knee? A multicenter analysis, *Chin Med J (Engl)* 130:2541, 2017.

Zwolak P, Manivel JC, Jasinski P, et al.: Cytotoxic effect of zoledronic acid-loaded bone cement on giant cell tumor, multiple myeloma, and renal cell carcinoma cell lines, *J Bone Joint Surg Am* 92:162, 2010.

CHONDROBLASTOMA

Angelini A, Hassanni M, Mavrogenis AF, et al.: Chondroblastoma in adult age, *Eur J Orthop Surg Traumatol* 27:843, 2017.

Chen W, DiFrancesco LM: Chondroblastoma: an update, *Arch Pathol Lab Med* 141:867, 2017.

Cho HS, Park YK, Oh JH, et al.: Proximal tibia chondroblastoma treated with curettage and bone graft and cement use, *Orthopedics* 39:e80, 2016.

De Mattos CB, Angsanuntsukh C, Arkader A, Dormans JP: Chondroblastoma and chondromyoid fibroma, *J Am Acad Orthop Surg* 21:225, 2013.

Farfalli GL, Slullitel PA, Muscolo DL, et al.: What happens to the articular surface after curettage for epiphyseal chondroblastoma? A report on functional results, arthritis, and arthroplasty, *Clin Orthop Relat Res* 475:760, 2017.

Hapa O, Karakash A, Demirkiran N, et al.: Operative treatment of chondroblastoma: a study of 11 cases, *Acta Orthop Belg* 82:68, 2016.

Lalam RK, Cribb GL, Tins BJ, et al.: Image guided radiofrequency thermoablation therapy of chondroblastoma: should it replace surgery? *Skeletal Radiol* 43:513, 2014.

Lehner B, Witte D, Weiss S: Clinical and radiological long-term results after operative treatment of chondroblastoma, *Arch Orthop Trauma Surg* 131:45, 2011.

Mashhour MA, Abdel Rahman M: Lower recurrence rate in chondroblastoma using extended curettage and cryosurgery, *Int Orthop* 38:1019, 2014.

Strong DP, Grimer RJ, Carter SR, et al.: Chondroblastoma of the femoral head: management and outcome, *Int Orthop* 34:413, 2010.

Tiefenboeck TM, Stockhammer V, Panotopoulos J, et al.: Complete local tumor control after curettage of chondroblastoma—a retrospective analysis, *Orthop Traumatol Surg Res* 102:473, 2016.

Xiong Y, Lang Y, Yu Z, et al.: The effects of surgical treatment with chondroblastoma in children and adolescents in open epiphyseal plate of long bones, *World J Surg Oncol* 16:14, 2018.

Xu H, Nugent D, Monforte HL, et al.: Chondroblastoma of bone in the extremities: a multicenter retrospective study, *J Bone Joint Surg Am* 97:925, 2015.

CHONDROMYXOID FIBROMA

Bagewadi RM, Nerune SM, Hippargi SB: Chondromyxoid fibroma of radius: a case report, *J Clin Diagn Res* 10:ED01, 2016.

Bhamra JS, Al-Khateeb H, Dhinsa BS, et al.: Chondromyxoid fibroma management: a single institution experience of 22 cases, *World J Surg Oncol* 12:283, 2014.

Cappelle S, Pans S, Sciot R: Imaging features of chondromyxoid fibroma: report of 15 cases and literature review, *Br J Radiol*, 89(1064):20160088.

Kim HS, Jee WH, Ryu KN, et al.: MRI of chondromyxoid fibroma, *Acta Radiol* 52:875, 2011.

Minasian T, Claus C, Hariri OR, et al.: Chondromyxoid fibroma of the sacrum: a case report and literature review, *Surg Neurol Int* 7(Suppl 13):S370, 2016.

Roberts EJ, Meier MJ, Hild G, et al.: Chondromyxois fibroma of the calcaneus: two case reports and literature review, *J Foot Ankle Surg* 52:643, 2013.

OSTEOBLASTOMA

Atesok KI, Alman BA, Schemitsch EH, et al.: Osteoid osteoma and osteoblastoma, *J Am Acad Orthop Surg* 19:678, 2011.

Chen Q, Liu L, Song Y: Benign osteoblastoma of cervical spine, *Spine J* 15:e21, 2015.

Galgano MA, Goulart CR, Iwenofu H, et al.: Osteoblastomas of the spine: a comprehensive review, *Neurosurg Focus* 41(E4), 2016.

Jiang L, Liu XG, Wang C, et al.: Surgical treatment options for aggressive osteoblastoma in the mobile spine, *Eur Spine J* 24:1778, 2015.

Kadhim M, Binitie O, O'Toole P, et al.: Surgical resection of osteoid osteoma and osteoblastoma of the spine, *J Pediatr Orthop B* 26:362, 2017.

Koc K, Ilik MK: Surgical management of an osteoblastoma involving the entire C2 vertebra and a review of the literature, *Eur Spine J* 25(Suppl 1):220, 2016.

Li Z, Zhao Y, Hou S, et al.: Clinical features and surgical management of spinal osteoblastoma: a retrospective study in 18 cases, *PLoS* 8:e74635, 2013.

Ravindra VM, Eli IM, Schmidt MH, et al.: Primary osseous tumors of the pediatric spinal column: review of pathology and surgical decision making, *Neurosurg Focus* 41(E3), 2016.

Ruggieri P, Huch K, Mavrogenis AF, et al.: Osteoblastoma of the sacrum: report of 18 cases and analysis of the literature, *Spine (Phila Pa 1976)* 39:E97, 2014.

von Chamier G, Holl-Wieden A, Stenzel M, et al.: Pitfalls in diagnostics of hip pain: osteoid osteoma and osteoblastoma, *Rheumatol Int* 30:395, 2010.

Weber MA, Sprengel SD, Omlor GW, et al.: Clinical long-term outcome, technical success, and cost analysis of radiofrequency ablation for the treatment of osteoblastomas and spinal osteoid osteomas in comparison to open surgical resection, *Skeletal Radiol* 44:981, 2015.

Yin H, Zhou W, Yu Y, et al.: Clinical characteristics and treatment options for two types of osteoblastoma in the mobile spine: a retrospective study of 32 cases and outcomes, *Eur Spine J* 23:411, 2014.

LANGERHANS CELL HISTIOCYTOSIS

Angelini A, Mavrogenis AF, Rimondi E, et al.: Current concepts for the diagnosis and management of eosinophilic granuloma of bone, *J Orthop Traumatol* 18:83, 2017.

Baptista AM, Camargo AF, de Camargo OP, et al.: Does adjunctive chemotherapy reduce remission rates compared to cortisone alone in unifocal or multifocal histiocytosis of bone? *Clin Orthop Relat Res* 470:663, 2012.

Cantu MA, Lupo PJ, Bilgi M, et al.: Optimal therapy for adults with Langerhans cell histiocytosis bone lesions, *PLoS ONE* 7:e43257, 2012.

DiCaprio MR, Roberts TT: Diagnosis and management of Langerhans cell histiocytosis, *J Am Acad Orthop Surg* 22:643, 2014.

Di Felice F, Zaina F, Donzelli S, et al.: Spontaneous and complete regeneration of a vertebra plana after surgical curettage of an eosinophilic granuloma, *Eur Spine J* 26(Suppl 1):225, 2017.

Goo HW, Yang DH, Ra YS, et al.: Whole-body MRI of Langerhans cell histiocytosis: comparison with radiography and bone scintigraphy, *Pediatr Radiol* 36:1019, 2006.

Grana N: Langerhans cell histiocytosis, *Cancer Control* 21:328, 2014.

Haupt R, Minkov M, Astigarraga I, et al.: Langerhans cell histiocytosis (LCH): guidelines for diagnosis, clinical work-up, and treatment for patients till the age of 18 years, *Pediatr Blood Cancer* 60:175, 2013.

Huang WD, Yang XH, Wu ZP, et al.: Langerhans cell histiocytosis of spine: a comparative study of clinical, imaging features, and diagnosis in children, adolescents, and adults, *Spine J* 13:1108, 2013.

Kamath S, Akader A, Jubran RF: Outcomes of children younger than 24 months with Langerhans cell histiocytosis and bone involvement: a report from a single institution, *J Pediatr Orthop* 34:825, 2014.

Khung S, Budzik JF, Amzallag-Bellenger E, et al.: Skeletal involvement in Langerhans cell histiocytosis, *Insights Imaging* 4:569, 2013.

Kotecha R, Venkatramani R, Juban RF, et al.: Clinical outcomes of radiation therapy in the management of Langerhans cell histiocytosis, *Am J Clin Oncol* 37:592, 2014.

Laird J, Ma J, Chau K, et al.: Outcome after radiation therapy for Langerhans cell histiocytosis is dependent on site of involvement, *Int J Radiat Oncol Biol Phys* 100:670, 2018.

Lee JW, Shin HY, Kang HJ, et al.: Clinical characteristics and treatment outcome of Langerhans cell histiocytosis: 22 years' experience of 154 patients at a single center, *Pediatr Hematol Oncol* 31:293, 2014.

Morimoto A, Oh Y, Shioda Y, et al.: Recent advances in Langerhans cell histiocytosis, *Pediatr Int* 56:451, 2014.

Postini AM, Andreacchio A, Boffano M, et al.: Langerhans cell histiocytosis of bone in children: a long-term retrospective study, *J Pediatr Orthop B* 21:457, 2012.

Rivera JC, Wylie E, Dell'orfano S, et al.: Approaches to treatment of unifocal Langerhans cell histiocytosis: is biopsy alone enough? *J Pediatr Orthop* 34:820, 2014.

Sasaki H, Nagano S, Shimada H, et al.: Clinical course of the bony lesion of single-system single-site Langerhans cell histiocytosis – Is appropriate follow-up sufficient treatment? *J Orthop Sci* 23:168, 2018.

Song YS, Lee IS, Yi JH, et al.: Radiologic findings of adult pelvis and appendicular skeletal Langerhans cell histiocytosis in nine patients, *Skeletal Radiol* 40:1421, 2011.

Wang J, Wu X, Xi ZJ: Langerhans cell histiocytosis of bone in children: a clinicopathologic study of 108 cases, *World J Pediatr* 6:255, 2010.

Xu X, Han S, Jiang L, et al.: Clinical features and treatment outcomes of Langerhans cell histiocytosis of the spine, *Spine J*, 2018 Mar 2. [Epub ahead of print].

Zhong N, Xu W, Meng T, et al.: The surgical strategy for eosinophilic granuloma of the pediatric cervical spine complicated with neurologic deficit and/or spinal instability, *World J Surg Oncol* 14:301, 2016.

Zhou Z, Zhang H, Guo C, et al.: Management of eosinophilic granuloma in pediatric patients: surgical intervention and surgery combined with postoperative radiotherapy and/or chemotherapy, *Childs Nerv Syst* 33:583, 2017.

The complete list of references is available online at Expert Consult.com.

CHAPTER 10

MALIGNANT TUMORS OF BONE

Robert K. Heck Jr., Patrick C. Toy

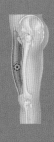

OSTEOSARCOMA

Osteosarcoma is a tumor characterized by the production of osteoid by malignant cells. It is the most common non-hematologic primary malignancy of bone. The incidence is 1:3 per 1 million per year. Onset can occur at any age; however, primary high-grade osteosarcoma occurs most commonly in the second decade of life. Parosteal osteosarcoma has a peak incidence in the third and fourth decades, and secondary osteosarcomas (e.g., those that occur in the setting of Paget disease or previous radiation therapy) are more common in older individuals. The incidence is slightly higher in males (with the exception of parosteal osteosarcoma, which is more common in females). There are no significant differences among races, and genetic factors rarely have been shown to play a role, although osteosarcoma may be more common in patients with the hereditary form of retinoblastoma, Rothmund-Thomson syndrome, and Li-Fraumeni syndrome. All skeletal locations can be affected; however, most primary osteosarcomas occur at the sites of the most rapid bone growth, including the distal femur, the proximal tibia, and the proximal humerus.

Almost all patients with high-grade osteosarcoma report progressive pain (patients with low-grade surface osteosarcomas may report a painless mass). Pain initially may improve with conservative measures and activity modifications, which can lead to a false sense of security for the patient and the physician. The pain eventually becomes severe if the diagnosis is delayed. Night pain may be an important clue to the true diagnosis; however, only about 25% of patients experience this phenomenon. Patients frequently are misdiagnosed with a more common musculoskeletal problem at the initial visit. The average delay from the onset of symptoms to the correct diagnosis was approximately 15 weeks in one study. This included the sum of the average patient delay of 6 weeks (the time between the onset of symptoms and initial physician encounter) and the average physician delay of 9 weeks (the time from the first visit to the correct diagnosis). The primary reasons for delay on the part of physicians included failure to obtain radiographs at the initial visit and, more important, failure to repeat the radiographs when a patient's symptoms persisted or worsened.

Although the radiographic appearance of osteosarcoma can vary, plain radiographs are the most valuable tools for making the correct diagnosis. The most common appearance is that of an aggressive lesion in the metaphysis of a long bone.

Approximately 10% are primarily diaphyseal, and less than 1% are primarily epiphyseal. Although the lesion can be either predominantly blastic or predominantly lytic, more commonly areas of bone production and bone destruction are present. The lesion usually is quite permeative, and the borders are ill defined. If the tumor has broken through the cortex, a soft-tissue mass may be present at the time of diagnosis. Periosteal reaction may take the form of a "Codman triangle," or it may have a "sunburst" or "hair-on-end" appearance. Magnetic resonance imaging (MRI) is the best imaging modality to measure the extent of the tumor within the bone and in the soft tissue and to determine the relationship of the tumor to nearby anatomic structures. A bone scan should be obtained to look for skeletal metastases, and radiography and computed tomography (CT) of the chest should be done to search for pulmonary metastases; the lungs are the most common sites of metastases. These tests should be done before biopsy.

Osteosarcomas are categorized as primary or secondary. Primary osteosarcomas are subcategorized as conventional osteosarcoma, low-grade intramedullary osteosarcoma, parosteal osteosarcoma, periosteal osteosarcoma, high-grade surface osteosarcoma, telangiectatic osteosarcoma, and small cell osteosarcoma.

Most osteosarcomas are classified as conventional osteosarcomas (Figs. 10.1 to 10.3) and have a radiographic appearance as previously described. These high-grade tumors begin in an intramedullary location but may break through the cortex and form a soft-tissue mass. Histologically, they may be primarily osteoblastic, fibroblastic, or chondroblastic; however, to establish the diagnosis, osteoid production from the tumor cells must be shown. The spindle cell component is high grade with hypercellularity, abundant mitotic figures, and marked nuclear pleomorphism.

Periosteal osteosarcoma (Fig. 10.4) is an intermediate-grade malignancy that arises on the surface of the bone. The most common locations are the diaphyses of the femur and tibia. It occurs in a slightly older and broader age group. Histological examination of periosteal osteosarcoma shows strands of osteoid-producing spindle cells radiating between lobules of cartilage.

Low-grade intramedullary osteosarcoma is a rare type characterized by an indolent course with relatively benign features on radiograph. In some patients, it can be mistaken radiographically and histologically for an osteoblastoma or

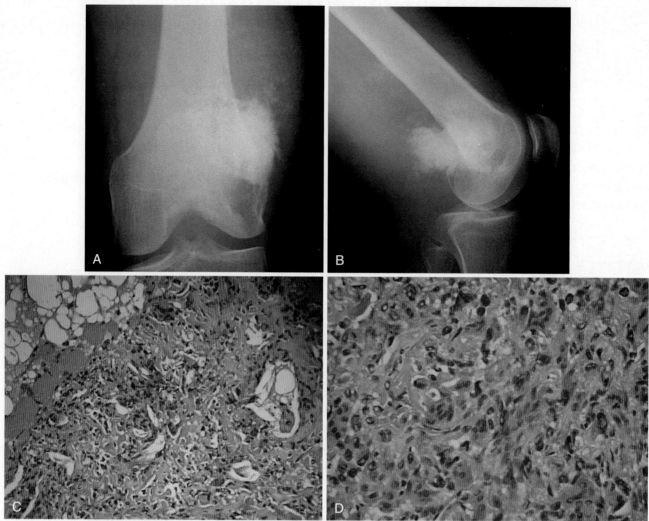

FIGURE 10.1   **A** and **B,** Anteroposterior and lateral radiographs show osteosarcoma in left distal femur of 31-year-old man. **C** and **D,** Low-power and high-power photomicrographs show malignant spindle cells producing osteoid. After preoperative chemotherapy, patient underwent wide resection and endoprosthetic reconstruction.

fibrous dysplasia. As the name implies, it is located in an intramedullary location. If left untreated, it may erode through the cortex very late in the disease process. Microscopically, it consists of slightly atypical spindle cells producing slightly irregular osseous trabeculae.

Parosteal osteosarcoma (Fig. 10.5) is also a rare, low-grade malignancy, but it arises on the surface of the bone and invades the medullary cavity only at a late stage. It has a peculiar tendency to occur as a lobulated ossified mass on the posterior aspect of the distal femur. CT may be helpful in differentiating this subtype of osteosarcoma from myositis ossificans or an osteochondroma. The ossification in myositis ossificans is more mature at the periphery of the lesion, whereas the center of a parosteal osteosarcoma is more heavily ossified. Parosteal osteosarcoma can be easily differentiated from an osteochondroma because the CT scan of an osteochondroma shows a medullary cavity containing marrow in continuity with the medullary canal of the involved bone. Microscopically, similar to a low-grade intramedullary osteosarcoma, parosteal osteosarcoma consists of slightly atypical spindle cells producing slightly irregular osseous trabeculae.

High-grade surface osteosarcoma is the least common type of osteosarcoma. As the name implies, it is an aggressive tumor arising on the outer aspect of the cortex. Radiographs show an invasive lesion with ill-defined borders. Similar to conventional osteosarcoma, the microscopic appearance is that of a high-grade tumor with hypercellularity, mitotic figures, and marked nuclear pleomorphism. In contrast to parosteal osteosarcoma, medullary involvement is common at the time of diagnosis.

Telangiectatic osteosarcoma is a purely lytic lesion. On a radiograph, it can have an invasive appearance, or it can have a ballooned appearance similar to that of an aneurysmal bone cyst. Grossly, it resembles a blood-filled cyst with only a very small solid portion. Microscopically, on low power, it most commonly resembles an aneurysmal bone cyst with blood-filled spaces separated by thin septa. On higher power magnification, however, the cells in the septa appear frankly malignant.

Small cell osteosarcoma, another rare variant, is a high-grade lesion that consists of small blue cells and may resemble Ewing sarcoma or lymphoma. If present in only a small quantity, the osteoid can be difficult to differentiate from the

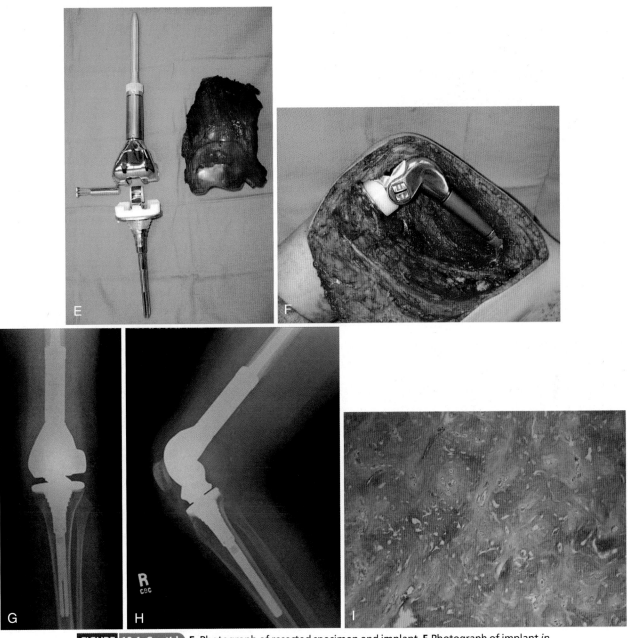

FIGURE 10.1, Cont'd **E**, Photograph of resected specimen and implant. **F**, Photograph of implant *in situ*. **G** and **H**, Postoperative anteroposterior and lateral radiographs. **I**, Photomicrograph showing complete tumor necrosis.

fibrin-like material that may be present in Ewing sarcoma. Cytogenetic and immunohistochemistry studies sometimes are needed to differentiate these lesions.

Secondary osteosarcomas occur at the site of another disease process. They rarely occur in young patients but constitute almost half of the osteosarcomas in patients older than 50 years. The most common factors associated with secondary osteosarcomas include Paget disease and previous radiation therapy. The incidence of osteosarcoma in Paget disease is approximately 1% and may be higher (5% to 10%) for patients with advanced polyostotic disease. Paget osteosarcoma most commonly occurs in patients in the sixth to eighth decades of life, and the pelvis is the most common location. Radiation-associated osteosarcoma occurs in approximately 1% of patients who have been treated with greater than 2500 cGy and can occur in unusual locations, such as the skull, spine, clavicle, ribs, scapula, and pelvis (Fig. 10.6). Although osteosarcoma is the most common radiation-associated sarcoma, fibrosarcoma and malignant fibrous histiocytoma (MFH) are also relatively common in this setting. The time to onset of the secondary osteosarcoma averages 10 to 15 years after radiation exposure but may occur 3 years to several decades after treatment. Other conditions that have been reported to be associated with secondary osteosarcomas include fibrous dysplasia, bone infarcts, osteochondromas, chronic osteomyelitis, melorheostosis, and osteogenesis imperfecta; however, secondary osteosarcomas are extremely rare in these settings, and a causal relationship has not been established.

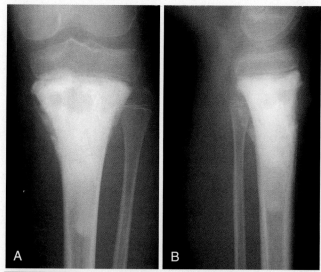

FIGURE 10.2 **A** and **B,** Anteroposterior and lateral radiographs of proximal tibia of 11-year-old boy with chondroblastic osteosarcoma.

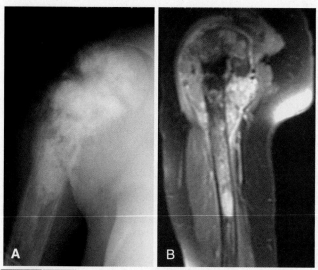

FIGURE 10.3 **A,** Anteroposterior view of proximal humerus of 8-year-old boy with osteoblastic osteosarcoma. **B,** MR image better shows extent of tumor within bone and soft tissue.

Before the advent of multiple-agent chemotherapy, the prognosis for patients with osteosarcoma was dismal. Despite treatment consisting of wide or radical amputation, approximately 80% of patients died as a result of distant metastases, usually within 2 years. With today's multiple-agent chemotherapy regimens and appropriate surgical treatment, most series report long-term survival of 60% to 75% for patients with high-grade osteosarcoma without metastases at initial presentation and 90% for those with low-grade lesions.

The most important prognostic factors at the time of diagnosis are the presence and location of metastases. Approximately 15% of patients with osteosarcoma have detectable pulmonary metastases at the time of diagnosis. As a group, these patients continue to have a poor prognosis, with less than 20% long-term survival. (Patients with one or a few resectable pulmonary metastases at presentation may have greater than

50% long-term survival, whereas patients with many, large, or unresectable pulmonary metastases have an extremely poor prognosis.) Patients with nonpulmonary metastases (e.g., bone metastases) have an even worse prognosis, with less than 5% long-term survival. Patients with "skip" metastases (i.e., a metastasis within the same bone as the primary tumor or across the joint from the primary tumor) have the same poor prognosis as patients with distant metastases.

The next most important prognostic feature is the grade of the lesion. Low-grade lesions rarely metastasize, and patients with low-grade lesions have a marked survival advantage over patients with high-grade lesions. Size of the primary tumor also appears to be of prognostic significance. Although authors differ on the specific criteria for what constitutes a large or a small tumor, most studies confirm that patients with large tumors have a worse prognosis than patients with smaller tumors. Skeletal location is also thought to be important because patients with more proximal tumors do worse than patients with more distal tumors. Size and location are likely interrelated variables, however, because most proximal tumors are larger at the time of diagnosis than most distal tumors. Paget osteosarcomas continue to have a poor prognosis, with less than 15% long-term survival. Radiation-associated osteosarcomas have been regarded as having a poor prognosis; however, this may be due primarily to their frequent occurrence in unusual locations where resection is difficult. Radiation-associated osteosarcomas in the extremities may have the same prognosis as any other high-grade osteosarcoma. Age at diagnosis and gender do not seem to be of prognostic significance.

As stated earlier, historically, patients with high-grade osteosarcoma were treated with immediate wide or radical amputation. Despite this treatment, 80% of patients with apparently isolated disease died of distant metastases. From this, it can be deduced that most patients with high-grade osteosarcoma have nondetectable micrometastases at presentation. The goal of adjuvant or neoadjuvant chemotherapy is to treat these micrometastases. Currently, at most musculoskeletal oncology centers, the treatment of high-grade osteosarcoma consists of neoadjuvant chemotherapy, wide or radical surgery (resection or amputation), and adjuvant chemotherapy. Pulmonary metastases likewise are resected if possible after neoadjuvant chemotherapy. The histologic response of the primary tumor to neoadjuvant chemotherapy has been shown to be a good predictor of long-term survival. Greater than 90% tumor necrosis indicates a very good prognosis. Low-grade osteosarcoma can be treated with wide resection or amputation without chemotherapy.

About 50% of patients with high-grade osteosarcoma have some type of relapse after the initial treatment. About 10% of patients have local recurrence after wide resection or wide amputation. Patients who have a local recurrence have a very poor prognosis and usually are treated with a radical amputation (if cure is the goal) and further chemotherapy. Late pulmonary metastases likewise are treated with surgery and chemotherapy. Poor prognostic factors include rapid relapse after completion of the initial treatment, many (more than eight) pulmonary nodules, large (>3 cm) pulmonary nodules, and unresectable pulmonary nodules. Patients with a few, small, resectable pulmonary nodules that occur late may have as high as a 60% chance of cure with aggressive treatment.

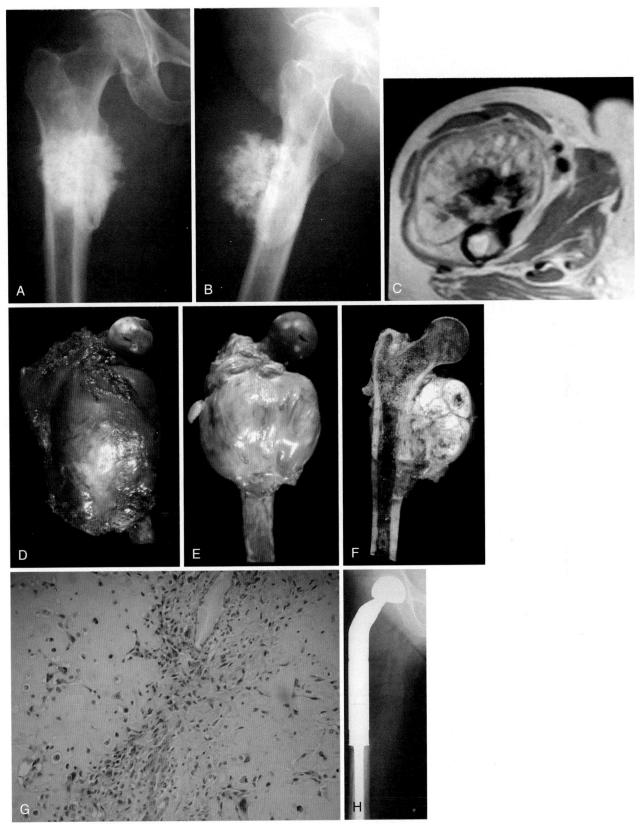

FIGURE 10.4   **A** and **B,** Anteroposterior and lateral radiographs of proximal femur of 67-year-old woman with periosteal osteosarcoma. **C,** MR image shows lesion arising from surface of bone. Marrow does not seem to be involved. **D,** Specimen after wide resection. **E,** Specimen after removal of surrounding muscle. **F,** Cut specimen. Lesion arises from surface of bone, and marrow cavity is not involved. **G,** Typical microscopic appearance of periosteal osteosarcoma. Lobules of malignant cartilage are separated by malignant spindle cells producing osteoid. **H,** Anteroposterior radiograph of reconstructed femur.

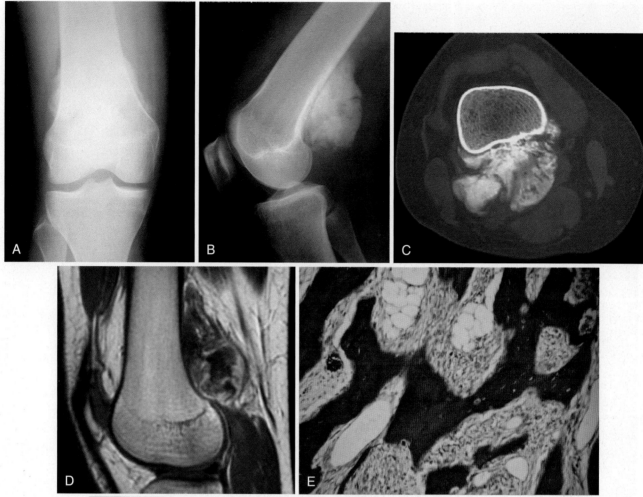

FIGURE 10.5 **A** and **B,** Anteroposterior and lateral radiographs of parosteal osteosarcoma arising in its most common location. **C** and **D,** CT scan and MR image show lesion arising from posterior surface of distal femur without involvement of marrow cavity. **E,** Typical microscopic appearance of parosteal osteosarcoma. Slightly atypical spindle cells produce relatively normal-appearing trabeculae.

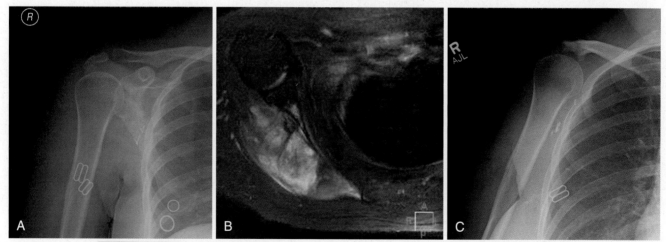

FIGURE 10.6 A 44-year-old woman complained of right shoulder pain 6 years after undergoing surgery, chemotherapy, and radiation treatment for metastatic melanoma involving right axilla. **A,** Anteroposterior radiograph of right shoulder revealing very subtle bony sclerosis along the lateral aspect of scapula. **B,** T2-weighted axial MRI demonstrating aggressive appearing lesion with large soft-tissue mass. Biopsy showed that the lesion was a conventional osteosarcoma. **C,** Right shoulder after chemotherapy and scapulectomy.

CHONDROSARCOMA

Chondrosarcoma has an incidence about half that of osteosarcoma. It is the second most common nonhematologic primary malignancy of bone. It occurs over a broad age range, with peaks between 40 and 60 years for primary chondrosarcoma and between 25 and 45 years for secondary chondrosarcoma. Chondrosarcoma can occur in any location; however, most are located in a proximal location such as the pelvis, proximal femur, and proximal humerus. Although chondrosarcomas rarely occur in the hand, they are the most common primary malignancy of bone in this location. Similar to most bone tumors, the incidence is slightly higher among males. Race predilection is not significant.

Clinically, most patients with primary chondrosarcomas report increasing pain. A palpable mass may also be present. Chondrosarcomas frequently are slow growing, and symptoms can be present for several years before a patient seeks medical attention. Pain in the absence of a pathologic fracture can be important in helping to differentiate an enchondroma from a low-grade chondrosarcoma. Frequently, patients are referred for evaluation of an asymptomatic cartilaginous lesion discovered as an incidental finding on a bone scan or radiograph obtained for another reason. (The radiographic abnormality usually is the sole reason the patient is referred to the orthopaedic oncologist.) Although an asymptomatic radiographic abnormality is common in a patient with an enchondroma, the diagnosis of chondrosarcoma would be extremely rare in this circumstance. A chondrosarcoma may occur in the area of a treated "enchondroma." In this circumstance, the original pathology specimen should be reviewed.

Secondary chondrosarcomas arise at the site of a preexisting benign cartilage lesion. They occur most frequently in the setting of multiple enchondromas and multiple hereditary exostoses. In Ollier disease (multiple enchondromas), the incidence of malignancy (most commonly chondrosarcoma) is approximately 25% by the age of 40 years, and in patients with Maffucci syndrome (multiple enchondromas with soft-tissue hemangiomas), the incidence may be even higher. Although data for osteochondromas are difficult to analyze, the lifetime incidence of secondary chondrosarcoma is estimated to be 5% for patients with multiple hereditary exostoses and approximately 1% for patients with solitary osteochondromas (Fig. 10.7). As discussed in other chapter, the true incidence of malignant degeneration of osteochondromas is unknown. Published estimates are likely too high, owing to the effect of referral bias on pathology data at tertiary referral centers. The true prevalence of osteochondromas in the general population is unknown. Whether or not a solitary benign enchondroma has the potential to give rise to a secondary chondrosarcoma is difficult to determine. If this does occur, the incidence is not high enough to warrant prophylactic treatment of asymptomatic enchondromas. Other conditions that have been reported to be associated with secondary chondrosarcoma include synovial chondromatosis, chondromyxoid fibroma, periosteal chondroma, chondroblastoma, previous radiation treatment, and fibrous dysplasia.

The radiographic appearance of chondrosarcoma frequently is diagnostic (Fig. 10.8). Similar to enchondroma, it is a lesion arising in the medullary cavity with irregular matrix calcification. The pattern of calcification has been described as "punctate," "popcorn," or "comma shaped." Compared with enchondroma, however, chondrosarcoma has a more aggressive appearance with bone destruction, cortical erosions, periosteal reaction, and a soft-tissue mass. CT can be helpful to show endosteal erosions or other evidence of a destructive lesion and to differentiate benign from malignant cartilage lesions. The site of the lesion must also be considered because lesions in the hand (the most common site for an enchondroma and a rare site for a chondrosarcoma) may appear aggressive and still be diagnosed as benign. The same amount of cortical destruction shown in a pelvic or proximal femoral lesion would be diagnostic of a chondrosarcoma. Finally, the size of the cartilaginous cap of an osteochondroma, as evaluated with CT or MRI, is important in evaluating the possibility of a secondary chondrosarcoma. If the cartilaginous cap is larger than 2 cm in a skeletally mature patient, a secondary chondrosarcoma must be considered.

Histologically, conventional chondrosarcomas are composed of malignant cells with abundant cartilaginous matrix. (If

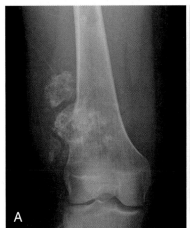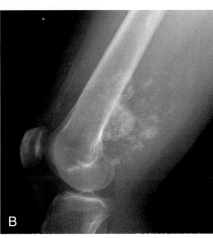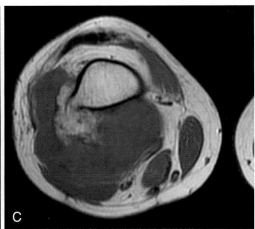

FIGURE 10.7 Anteroposterior (**A**) and lateral (**B**) radiographs of right distal femur of 25-year old man who complained of painful mass in right thigh. **C,** Axial T1-weighted MRI showing lesion arising from a previously existing osteochondroma. Biopsy proved that this was a secondary chondrosarcoma.

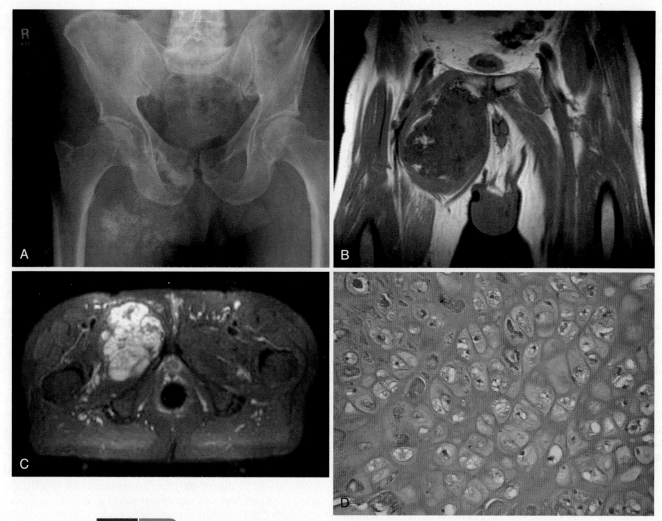

FIGURE 10.8   **A,** Anteroposterior view of pelvis of a 78-year-old man reveals a large tumor arising from the pubis with soft-tissue extension. The mass has punctate calcification consistent with a chondrosarcoma. Although plain radiography is more helpful for determining the diagnosis, MRI (**B** and **C**) better defines the extent of the soft-tissue mass and its relationship to adjacent anatomic structures. **D,** Typical microscopic appearance of conventional chondrosarcoma.

malignant osteoid is present even in small amounts, the diagnosis should be chondroblastic osteosarcoma; a tumor with different prognostic and therapeutic implications.) Differentiating a low-grade chondrosarcoma from an enchondroma can be difficult solely from a biopsy specimen. Factors that favor a malignant diagnosis include hypercellularity, plump nuclei, more than occasional binucleate cells, a permeative pattern, and entrapment of bony trabeculae (Fig. 10.9). As much tissue as possible should be obtained from the biopsy of a borderline lesion. Perhaps, in no other circumstance is correlation with the clinical and radiographic findings more important. Lesions in the setting of multiple enchondromas, periosteal chondromas, synovial chondromatosis, and enchondromas of the hand all may appear hypercellular and yet still can be benign. This same appearance in a biopsy specimen taken from a solitary large pelvic lesion with radiographically shown cortical erosions would be diagnostic of a chondrosarcoma.

Less common histologic subtypes of chondrosarcoma include dedifferentiated chondrosarcoma, clear cell chondrosarcoma, and mesenchymal chondrosarcoma. Together, these subtypes constitute less than 20% of all chondrosarcomas. Histologically, dedifferentiated chondrosarcoma consists of a high-grade spindle cell sarcoma (most commonly osteosarcoma followed in frequency by fibrosarcoma and MFH adjacent to an otherwise typical low-grade chondrosarcoma (Fig. 10.10). The radiographic features of a dedifferentiated chondrosarcoma often show a more aggressive radiolucent area juxtaposed on an otherwise typical chondrosarcoma.

Clear cell chondrosarcoma is a low-grade malignancy. As the name implies, it consists of round cells with abundant clear cytoplasm and distinct cytoplasmic borders with a background of cartilaginous matrix. Multinucleated giant cells usually are apparent. Clear cell chondrosarcoma has a strong tendency to arise in an epiphysis (especially the proximal femur). It may have benign radiographic features and can be confused with chondroblastoma or giant cell tumor.

Mesenchymal chondrosarcoma is a high-grade tumor consisting of small, round blue cells with islands of benign-appearing cartilage. The cellular portions often have a hemangiopericytomatous pattern of growth with "staghorn-like"

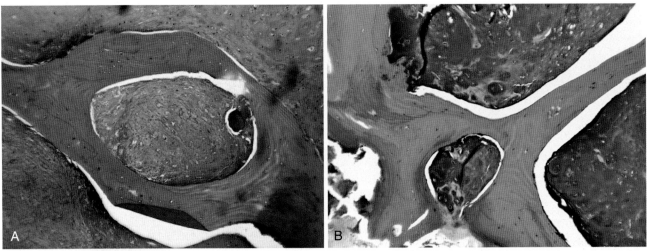

FIGURE 10.9 Low-power **(A)** and high-power **(B)** photomicrographs of a chondrosarcoma demonstrate entrapment of trabeculae.

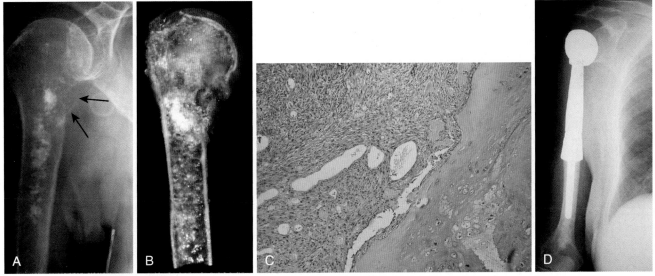

FIGURE 10.10 **A,** Anteroposterior view of right proximal humerus of 92-year-old woman with dedifferentiated chondrosarcoma shows aggressive-appearing area *(arrows)* adjacent to otherwise typical chondrosarcoma. **B,** Resected specimen shows these features. **C,** Typical microscopic appearance of dedifferentiated chondrosarcoma. High-grade spindle cell sarcoma is located adjacent to low-grade chondrosarcoma. **D,** Anteroposterior radiograph after reconstruction with endoprosthesis.

vessels. Radiographically, mesenchymal chondrosarcoma may look similar to a conventional chondrosarcoma (Fig. 10.11). More frequently, however, it has a nonspecific, aggressive radiographic appearance.

The treatment of low-grade chondrosarcoma is controversial, with many authors reporting excellent results after extended curettage with the use of intraoperative adjuvant treatments. Extended curettage is considered adequate treatment only for low-grade lesions that are confined within the medullary canal. Those with soft-tissue extension should be treated similar to high-grade lesions. The treatment of high-grade chondrosarcoma is wide or radical resection or amputation. Because cartilage is relatively avascular, the cells survive transplantation easily. The local recurrence rate after intraoperative tumor contamination is high. For lesions in

an expendable location, primary wide resection without a biopsy may be indicated to decrease the chance of tumor contamination. After wide resection, local recurrence is less than 10% and can be treated with repeat wide resection or wide amputation. Likewise, pulmonary metastases should be treated with surgical resection if possible. Chemotherapy has no role in the treatment of conventional chondrosarcoma but is frequently used for the treatment of dedifferentiated and mesenchymal chondrosarcomas. Radiation therapy likewise has a limited role and is used only as a palliative measure for surgically inaccessible lesions.

The prognosis for patients with chondrosarcoma depends mostly on the size, grade, and location of the lesion. If a high-grade lesion cannot be completely resected with wide or radical margins (usually because of its size or location), local recurrence

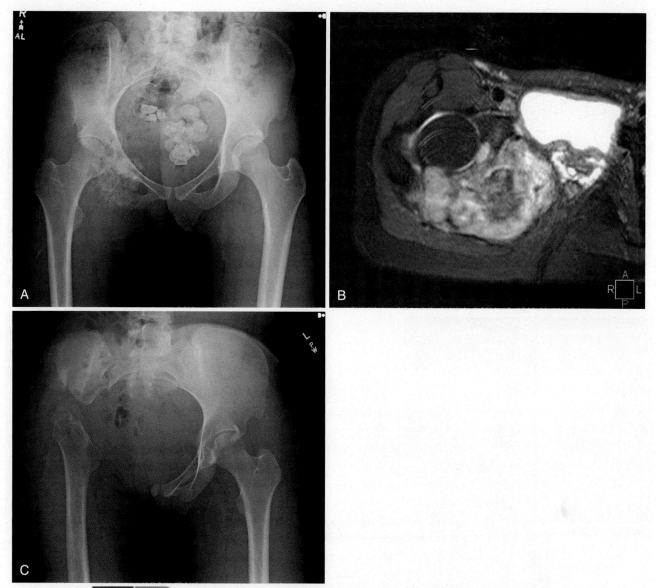

FIGURE 10.11   **A,** Anteroposterior radiograph of pelvis of 22-year-old woman with mesenchymal chondrosarcoma. **B,** Axial T2-weighted MRI demonstrating full extent of lesion within bone and soft tissue. **C,** Anteroposterior radiograph of pelvis after chemotherapy and resection.

is likely. Patients with low-grade lesions have been reported to have a greater than 90% 10-year survival rate, whereas patients with high-grade conventional chondrosarcoma are reported to have a 20% to 40% 10-year survival rate. The 5-year survival rate is 10% to 25% for patients with dedifferentiated chondrosarcoma, with most deaths occurring in the first 2 years. Because chondrosarcomas often are slow growing, local recurrences and pulmonary metastases may not be detected until years or decades after the primary procedure. A significant percentage of recurrences show a higher histologic grade than the original tumor. Long-term follow-up with regular imaging of the operative site and the chest is imperative so that treatment can be initiated promptly in the event of a recurrence.

EWING SARCOMA

Ewing sarcoma is the third most common nonhematologic primary malignancy of bone, but it is the second most common

(after osteosarcoma) in patients younger than 30 years and the most common in patients younger than 10 years. The incidence is less than one per 1 million per year. Ewing sarcoma has been reported to occur in a wide age range of patients from infants to the elderly, but most occur in patients aged 5 to 25 years. The most common locations include the metaphyses of long bones (often with extension into the diaphysis) and the flat bones of the shoulder and pelvic girdles (Figs. 10.12 and 10.13). Rarely, it occurs in the spine or in the small bones of the feet or hands. Similar to most sarcomas of bone, there is a slightly higher incidence in males. Ewing sarcoma is exceedingly rare in individuals of African descent. There are no known predisposing factors.

Pain is an almost universal complaint of patients with Ewing sarcoma. Usually, the onset is insidious, and the pain may be of long duration before the patient seeks medical attention. The pain may be only mild and intermittent initially and may respond to initial conservative treatment. The

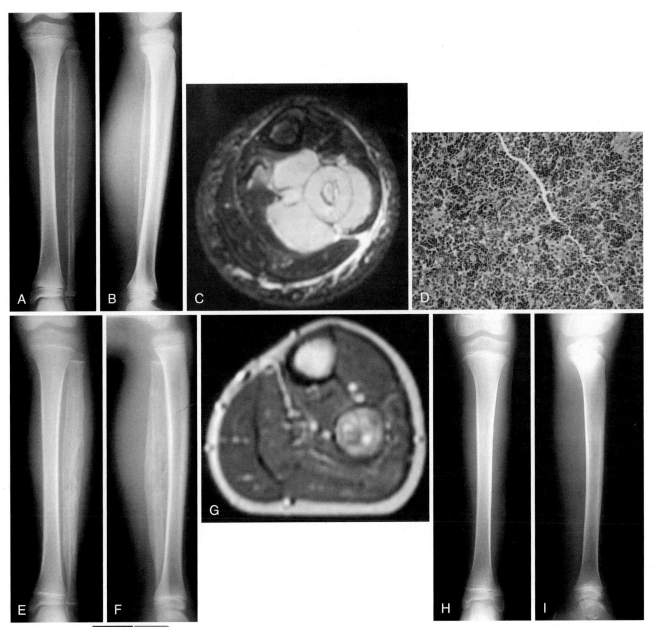

FIGURE 10.12 **A** and **B,** Anteroposterior and lateral radiographs of left fibula of 7-year-old girl with Ewing sarcoma. Involvement of large portion of bone (or even entire bone) is typical of Ewing sarcoma. **C,** MR image shows a large soft-tissue mass. **D,** Typical microscopic appearance of Ewing sarcoma. **E** and **F,** Anteroposterior and lateral radiographs after completion of neoadjuvant chemotherapy. Note increased ossification of lesion. **G,** Repeat MR image after neoadjuvant chemotherapy shows marked reduction in size of soft-tissue mass. **H** and **I,** Anteroposterior and lateral radiographs of left tibia after wide resection of tumor. Distal fibular physis was preserved. Wide resection avoids complications associated with radiation therapy in growing child.

average delay from the onset of symptoms to the diagnosis has been reported to be 34 weeks. The average patient delay in one study was 15 weeks from the onset of symptoms until the first medical appointment, and the average physician delay was 19 weeks from the initial visit to correct diagnosis. These numbers show the importance of radiographs at the initial visit and rechecking them at subsequent visits if the patient continues to have symptoms.

In addition to pain, patients may also have fever, erythema, and swelling, suggesting osteomyelitis. Laboratory

studies may reveal an increased white blood cell count, an elevated erythrocyte sedimentation rate, and an elevated C-reactive protein level. To complicate matters further, a needle aspirate of Ewing sarcoma may grossly resemble pus, and the tissue may be sent in its entirety to microbiology and none to pathology. (As a general rule, most biopsy specimens should be sent for culture and pathologic analysis.)

Classically, Ewing sarcoma appears radiographically as a destructive lesion in the diaphysis of a long bone with an "onion skin" periosteal reaction. In reality, Ewing sarcoma

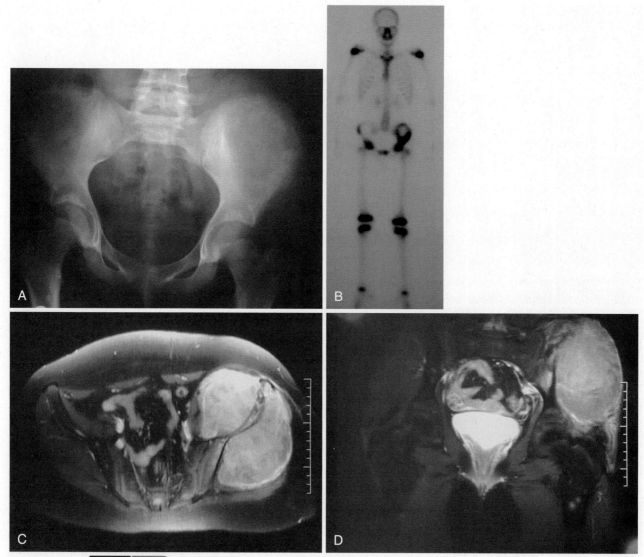

FIGURE 10.13   **A,** Anteroposterior radiograph of 13-year-old girl with Ewing sarcoma of left hemipelvis. **B,** Bone scan. **C** and **D,** Axial and coronal MR images show full extent of lesion. Because of morbidity associated with surgical management of large tumor in this location, the patient was treated with chemotherapy and radiation.

more often originates in the metaphysis of a long bone but frequently extends for a considerable distance into the diaphysis. Although "skip" metastases (similar to those that occur in osteosarcoma) are not reported in Ewing sarcoma, it is common for a large portion of the bone (or even the entire bone) to be involved. In flat bones, Ewing sarcoma appears as a nonspecific destructive lesion. Regardless of the location, MRI of the entire bone should be ordered to evaluate the full extent of the lesion, which typically extends beyond the abnormality apparent on plain films. MRI is also useful to evaluate the extent of the soft-tissue mass, which often is very large. All patients should have a baseline radiograph and CT of the chest because the lung is the most common site of metastases. A bone scan should be performed because bone is the second most common site of metastases. At some institutions, a bone marrow aspirate is performed as part of the staging of Ewing sarcoma to rule out diffuse systemic disease. Others have recommended FDG-PET/CT or whole-body MRI for this purpose.

Histologically, Ewing sarcoma consists of small blue cells with very little intercellular matrix. Cytogenetic or immunohistochemical studies often are required to differentiate Ewing sarcoma from other small blue cell tumors. The t(11;22)(q24;q12) is the most common translocation diagnostic of Ewing sarcoma and is present in more than 90% of cases. Other diagnostic translocations, including t(21;22)(q22;q12) and t(7;22)(p22;q12), have also been identified. Immunohistochemical staining for the *MIC-2* gene product has been reported to be specific for Ewing sarcoma. In addition, Ewing sarcomas usually are periodic acid–Schiff (PAS) positive (owing to intracellular glycogen) and reticulin negative. This is in contrast to lymphomas, which are PAS negative and reticulin positive. Lymphomas also stain positive for leukocyte common antigen and other T- and B-cell antigens. Embryonal rhabdomyosarcoma stains positive for desmin, myoglobin, and muscle-specific actins. Hemangiopericytomas stain positive for factor VIII, and small cell metastatic carcinomas and melanomas stain positive for cytokeratin.

The worst prognostic factor is the presence of distant metastases. Even with aggressive treatment, patients with metastases have only a 20% to 30% chance of long-term survival. The size of the primary lesion has been shown consistently to be of prognostic significance, although specific parameters have not been firmly established. Location has also been reported to be of prognostic significance, but it is difficult to differentiate the effects of location and size because most proximally located tumors are larger at presentation than distally located tumors. Histologic grade is of no prognostic significance because all Ewing sarcomas are considered high grade. Fever, anemia, and elevation of laboratory values (white blood cell count, erythrocyte sedimentation rate, and lactate dehydrogenase) have been reported to indicate more extensive disease and a worse prognosis. Older age at presentation (with a cutoff around the age of 12 to 15 years) and male gender have also been reported to be associated with a worse prognosis. The specific translocation, t(11;22) versus t(21;22), does not seem to affect the clinical course; however, secondary genetic alterations, such as aberrant TP53 expression, may prove to be important. As with osteosarcoma, histologic response to neoadjuvant chemotherapy has been shown to be prognostically important. Greater than 90% necrosis after preoperative chemotherapy indicates a good prognosis.

The treatment of Ewing sarcoma must include neoadjuvant or adjuvant chemotherapy, or both, to treat distant metastases that may or may not be readily apparent at the initial staging. Before the use of multiple-agent chemotherapy, long-term survival was less than 10%. Today, most centers report long-term survival rates of 60% to 75%.

Local treatment of the primary lesion is more controversial. Ewing sarcoma is radiosensitive, yet some authors report a decreased rate of local recurrence (<10%) and an increased rate of overall survival with wide resection of the primary tumor. These reports are difficult to interpret, however, because large, central, unresectable tumors often are treated with radiation, whereas smaller, more accessible lesions (which inherently have a better prognosis) are more likely to be treated with surgery. At this time, the choice between surgery and radiation for treatment of the primary lesion must be made on an individual basis. Repeat staging studies should be obtained after neoadjuvant chemotherapy. The repeat radiographs often show increased ossification, and repeat MRI often shows a marked decrease in the soft-tissue mass. At this point, if it appears that the lesion can be resected with wide margins with an acceptable functional deficit, surgery should be the treatment of the primary lesion. If wide margins would be difficult to obtain or if the functional deficit resulting from surgery would be unacceptable, radiation of the primary lesion is an acceptable alternative. Radiation can also be used as an adjuvant after a marginal resection or a contaminated wide resection. The treatment plan in each case is most appropriately made after long discussions with the patient and the family. The discussions should include expected function after amputation, limb salvage surgery, or radiation and the inherent short-term and long-term risks involved with each option.

Disease relapse is associated with a poor prognosis despite aggressive treatment of the relapse with further surgery, radiation, and chemotherapy. Patients with local recurrence have been reported to have about a 20% 5-year survival rate, whereas patients who relapse with distant metastases have approximately a 10% 5-year survival rate. As with osteosarcoma, time to relapse has prognostic significance. Patients who relapse within the first year after primary treatment have a worse prognosis than patients who have an extended disease-free interval.

CHORDOMA

Chordoma is a rare malignant neoplasm that arises from notochord remnants. Chordoma is the second most common primary malignancy in the spine (behind myeloma) and is the most common primary malignancy of the sacrum. Greater than 50% of chordomas arise in the sacrococcygeal area, and more than 30% arise at the base of the skull; the remainder are dispersed throughout the rest of the spine. Peak incidence for sacrococcygeal chordomas occurs in the fifth to seventh decades, whereas the peak for sphenooccipital lesions is the fourth to sixth decades. Most series show a marked male predominance (3:1), especially for sacrococcygeal tumors.

The presenting signs and symptoms vary according to the site of the lesion. Because most chordomas are slow growing, patients frequently have symptoms for more than a year before diagnosis. Patients with tumors in the sphenooccipital region may report headaches or symptoms related to cranial nerve compression. In the spine, symptoms can be caused by nerve root or cord compression. If an anterior mass exists with a cervical spine lesion, the symptoms may be similar to those caused by a retropharyngeal abscess. The most common presenting complaint for patients with sacrococcygeal tumors is low back pain. Bowel and bladder disturbance and sciatic pain are also common with sacral tumors. A palpable mass frequently is present on rectal examination.

Radiographically, chordomas appear as destructive lesions (Fig. 10.14). They virtually always arise from the midline. Sacrococcygeal lesions often are missed on the initial radiographic examination because of overlying bowel gas. They are usually seen more easily on a lateral view of the sacrum. Likewise, radioisotope accumulation in the bladder can obscure a sacral tumor on a bone scan. More than 50% of chordomas exhibit radiographically detectable calcification. CT may be better for detecting calcification (which may help with the diagnosis), but MRI is better for determining the full extent of the lesion and its relationship to other anatomic structures. A common pitfall in the evaluation of a patient with a chordoma and low back pain is ordering an MRI of only the lumbar spine; this study usually misses a sacrococcygeal chordoma because most arise below S3.

Microscopically, chordoma appears as lobules of cells separated by fibrous bands. The cells usually contain abundant vacuolated cytoplasm (physaliferous cells). The cells usually are arranged in long strands, or "cords," with a mucinous background. Most chordomas are low grade, although dedifferentiated chordomas exist. These dedifferentiated chordomas contain areas of a high-grade sarcoma (most frequently an MFH) and behave in a more aggressive manner.

The primary treatment is surgical resection with wide margins, even if this creates a neurologic deficit, because progressive growth of the tumor would create a neurologic deficit anyway and possibly metastatic disease. Resection that preserves the S3 nerve roots bilaterally results in relatively normal bowel and bladder function, whereas resection above this level results in incremental loss of bowel and bladder function. Resection of bilateral S2 nerve roots results in complete loss of control of bowel and bladder function. If wide margins

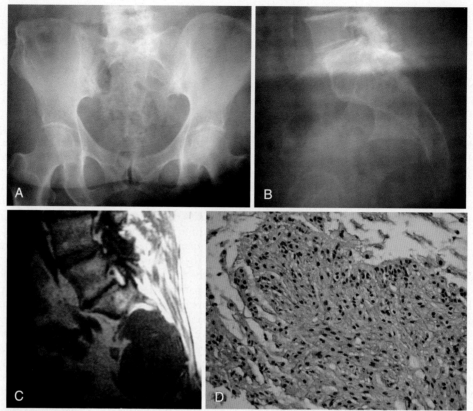

FIGURE 10.14 **A** and **B,** Anteroposterior and lateral views of sacrum of patient with sacrococcygeal chordoma. This lesion could be missed easily because of overlying bowel gas. **C,** MR image clearly shows lesion. **D,** Typical microscopic appearance of chordoma. Cells with abundant vacuolated cytoplasm (physaliferous cells) are arranged in cords with mucinous background.

cannot be obtained or if tumor contamination occurs intra-operatively, radiation may be beneficial. Radiation may also be beneficial for patients in whom resection is not feasible, although a cure is rarely, if ever, achieved in these patients. Chemotherapy is of no proven benefit. Likewise, distant metastases are treated surgically.

The 5-year overall survival rate for patients with chordomas is approximately 60% to 80%, but the survival rate continues to decline with longer follow-up because of late recurrences (25% to 60% 10-year survival). Local recurrences are common because of the difficulty encountered in achieving wide margins. Male gender and younger age at diagnosis have been reported to be associated with a favorable prognosis. A more distal location for sacral lesions is also associated with a better prognosis. Metastases are rare at initial presentation (<5%) but may occur later in 30% to 60%. In addition to the lungs, metastases are common in bone and have been reported and in unusual locations such as skin, eyelid, brain, liver, and other internal organs.

ADAMANTINOMA

Adamantinoma is a rare neoplasm representing less than 1% of all primary malignancies of bone. Adamantinoma has a wide age distribution, but most patients are in the second or third decade at the time of diagnosis. It has a peculiar predilection for occurring in the tibia (approximately 85%) and may also involve the ipsilateral fibula. It has been postulated

that adamantinoma arises from aberrant nests of epithelial cells, which would account for the fact that this tumor primarily occurs in bone that is in a subcutaneous location.

Pain is the most common symptom. The lesion is typically slow growing; therefore, the pain can be present for many years before the patient seeks medical attention. Because the lesion usually occurs in a subcutaneous location, a palpable mass may be present. Approximately 20% of patients have a pathologic fracture.

The most common radiographic appearance is that of multiple, sharply demarcated radiolucent lesions in the tibial diaphysis (Fig. 10.15). The radiolucent lesions are separated by areas of dense, sclerotic bone. Although the radiographic appearance is similar to that of osteofibrous dysplasia, adamantinoma usually has a more aggressive appearance. A large portion or even the entire tibia can be involved. Frequently, the fibula is also involved by direct extension of the tumor.

Microscopically, adamantinoma consists of islands of epithelial cells in a fibrous stroma. Some areas of the tumor can resemble fibrous dysplasia or osteofibrous dysplasia. (Some authors consider adamantinoma to be a malignant variant of osteofibrous dysplasia.) Nuclear atypia is minimal, and mitotic figures are rare. Immunohistochemical staining usually is positive for cytokeratins and vimentin. It generally is a low-grade lesion, and histologic features are not predictive of behavior.

The optimal treatment of adamantinoma is wide resection or amputation. The tumor generally is radioresistant and chemoresistant. Local recurrence occurs in approximately 25%

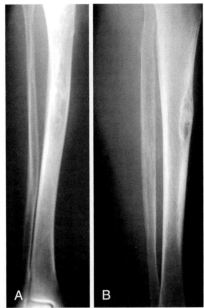

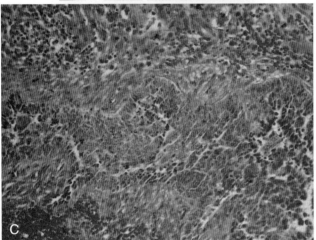

FIGURE 10.15 **A** and **B**, Anteroposterior and lateral radiographs of 79-year-old man with tibial adamantinoma. **C,** Typical microscopic appearance of adamantinoma. Islands of epithelioid cells are seen with fibrous background.

of patients, and amputation should be considered for these patients. Metastases are rare at presentation but may occur later in 30% of patients. Overall survival is approximately 85% at 10 years. Prognosis depends most on the adequacy of the surgical margin. Compared with patients who have marginal or intralesional surgical procedures, patients who have wide or radical procedures have significantly reduced rates of local recurrence and metastases (<10%). Because of the slow-growing nature of this lesion, local recurrence or metastasis may occur very late, reportedly 19 years after the initial treatment. The importance of long-term follow-up must be stressed.

MALIGNANT VASCULAR TUMORS

The terminology used to describe malignant vascular tumors in the literature is confusing. Multiple terms have been used interchangeably, including *hemangioendothelioma, hemangioendothelial sarcoma, hemangiosarcoma, angiosarcoma,* and others. Although not strictly defined, most authors use the term *hemangioendothelioma* to describe low-grade malignant vascular tumors and the term *angiosarcoma* to describe high-grade malignant vascular tumors.

These are rare tumors. After the first decade, they may occur at any age and in any bone. There is a slight male predominance but no significant race predilection. Stewart-Treves syndrome refers to the occurrence of angiosarcoma in the setting of chronic lymphedema (e.g., in the upper extremity of a patient who has previously undergone a radical mastectomy). Angiosarcomas have also been reported to occur adjacent to orthopaedic implants, although a causal relationship has not been firmly established.

Pain or, more rarely, pathologic fracture is the presenting complaint. Duration of symptoms varies depending on the grade of the tumor. The radiographic appearance of this lesion is also correlated with its grade. Low-grade tumors appear as well-demarcated lytic lesions that may or may not have surrounding reactive bone formation (Fig. 10.16). High-grade tumors have a more permeative appearance. Periosteal reaction is unusual. Malignant vascular tumors have a peculiar tendency to be multicentric at presentation regardless of grade. Most commonly, multiple lesions are found within the same bone or within multiple bones of the same extremity.

Microscopically, low-grade tumors show well-formed anastomosing vascular channels lined by plump endothelial cells. Well-differentiated hemangioendotheliomas can be difficult to differentiate from benign hemangiomas. High-grade lesions can be pleomorphic and may appear as an undifferentiated sarcoma or carcinoma. In some extremely pleomorphic lesions, the diagnosis can be made only through immunohistochemistry. Although metastatic carcinoma and malignant vascular tumors may be keratin positive, factor VIII–related antigen, CD31, and CD34 should be positive only in vascular tumors.

Treatment is individualized depending on the clinical situation. Solitary lesions are treated with wide resection if possible. Radiation can be used successfully in the treatment of surgically inaccessible lesions or in the treatment of multiple lesions. For high-grade lesions, adjuvant chemotherapy can be added to the treatment regimen. Prognosis depends most on grade. Patients with low-grade lesions may have better than an 80% chance for long-term survival, whereas patients with high-grade tumors have less than a 20% long-term survival rate.

MALIGNANT FIBROUS HISTIOCYTOMA AND FIBROSARCOMA

Although MFH and fibrosarcoma are described in the literature as being separate entities, the distinction is sometimes arbitrary. The presentation, prognosis, and treatment of these two entities are similar, and so they are discussed together.

Excluding the first decade, they occur at any age with comparable frequency. Both men and women are affected equally. There is a slight tendency for the lesion to occur in the distal metaphysis of the femur or the proximal metaphysis of the tibia; however, any bone may be involved. Approximately 25% of these tumors are considered to be secondary to a preexisting bone abnormality. The most commonly reported predisposing conditions include Paget disease, radiation, giant cell tumor, and bone infarction (Fig. 10.17). They may also occur as part of a dedifferentiated chondrosarcoma.

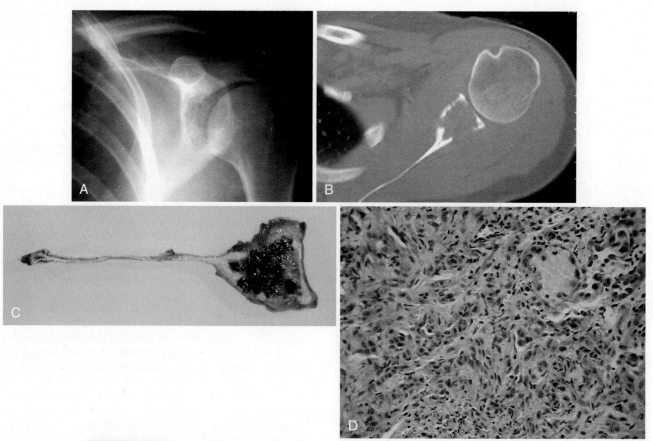

FIGURE 10.16 **A,** Anteroposterior view of left shoulder of 37-year-old woman with hemangioendothelioma reveals destructive lesion in left glenoid. **B,** CT better shows extent of lesion. **C,** Photograph of resected specimen. **D,** Typical microscopic appearance of hemangioendothelioma. Malignant endothelial cells produce anastomosing vascular channels. These cells stained positive for factor VIII–related antigen.

As is the case with other bone sarcomas, patients complain of pain at presentation. These patients have a higher incidence (approximately 20%) of pathologic fracture at presentation. Radiographically, these tumors have an aggressive appearance and are typically purely lytic with indistinct borders. They may appear as an area of bone destruction adjacent to an otherwise typical area of Paget disease or bone infarction. Periosteal reaction is absent, unless a pathologic fracture has occurred.

Histologically, the classic appearance of MFH is a high-grade spindle cell sarcoma arranged in a storiform or cartwheel pattern. The appearance can vary, however. Tumors may exhibit benign and malignant multinucleated cells, cells with a histiocytic appearance (large, indented nuclei with abundant, well-defined cytoplasm), cells with foamy cytoplasm, inflammatory cells, and variable amounts of fibrosis. The classic appearance of fibrosarcoma is that of a spindle cell neoplasm arranged in a herringbone pattern. Low-grade fibrosarcomas may exhibit abundant collagen production, whereas high-grade tumors are more cellular. MFH and fibrosarcoma are characterized by the lack of osteoid production. Even a small amount of osteoid production by the malignant cells would change the diagnosis to osteosarcoma.

At most institutions, the treatment of MFH of bone and fibrosarcoma of bone is similar to that of osteosarcoma. Most patients with high-grade lesions are treated with neoadjuvant chemotherapy, followed by surgery (wide resection or wide amputation) and adjuvant chemotherapy. Compared with osteosarcoma, however, MFH may be more radiosensitive. There are reports of long-term survivors of MFH of the spine who were treated with radiation alone. Radiation therapy may also be beneficial for patients with positive resection margins or intraoperative tumor contamination.

The prognosis is based on the presence or absence of metastases, the size and location of the tumor (as they relate to the ability of the surgeon to remove the tumor with wide margins), the grade of the tumor, and the histologic response to preoperative chemotherapy (as determined by percent necrosis). Reports have also shown older age to be associated with a worse prognosis; however, this may be caused partially by the inability of many older patients to tolerate chemotherapy. No difference in prognosis has been shown between patients with primary tumors and patients with tumors arising in a predisposing condition. Overall, the 5-year survival rate for patients with high-grade tumors of the extremities without metastases at presentation is approximately 65%.

MULTIPLE MYELOMA AND PLASMACYTOMA

Multiple myeloma is the most common primary malignancy of bone. Its peak incidence is in the fifth to seventh decades with a

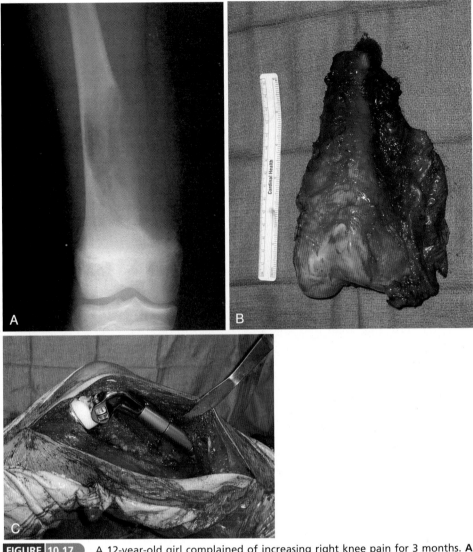

FIGURE 10.17   A 12-year-old girl complained of increasing right knee pain for 3 months. **A,** Anteroposterior radiograph of the right distal femur demonstrates a large, purely lytic, destructive lesion. After biopsy showed this to be a malignant fibrous histiocytoma, she underwent neoadjuvant chemotherapy, followed by wide resection **(B)** and endoprosthetic reconstruction **(C)**.

2:1 male predominance. Multiple myeloma and metastatic carcinoma should be included in the differential diagnosis for any patient older than 40 years with a new bone tumor.

Bone pain is the most common complaint for patients with multiple myeloma or with a solitary plasmacytoma. In contrast to most bone tumors, however, other systemic problems, such as weakness, weight loss, anemia, thrombocytopenia, peripheral neuropathy (especially with the osteosclerotic type of multiple myeloma), hypercalcemia, or renal failure, frequently are present at the time of diagnosis of multiple myeloma. Symptoms usually are of short duration because of the aggressive nature of the disease. Pathologic fractures are relatively common. The spine is the most common location, followed by the ribs and pelvis.

Radiographically, multiple myeloma appears as multiple, "punched-out," sharply demarcated, purely lytic lesions without any surrounding reactive sclerosis (Fig. 10.18). The lack of reactive bone formation is also shown by the fact that most lesions are negative on bone scan. (A less common variant of multiple

myeloma is characterized by extensive sclerosis.) Occasionally, myeloma is characterized by marked bone expansion, giving rise to a "ballooned" appearance.

The diagnosis usually can be confirmed by serum immunoelectrophoresis, which shows a monoclonal gammopathy. In addition to a complete blood cell count and serum chemistries, staging studies include a skeletal survey and a bone marrow biopsy. Occasionally, biopsy of the bone lesion is required to establish the diagnosis.

Histologically, multiple myeloma appears as sheets of plasma cells. These are small, round blue cells with "clock face" nuclei and abundant cytoplasm with a perinuclear clearing or "halo." Amyloid production can be abundant. With the exception of patients on long-term hemodialysis, the presence of amyloid in bone usually means a diagnosis of multiple myeloma. In patients with a solitary plasmacytoma, the pathologic differential diagnosis may include chronic osteomyelitis with abundant plasma cells (Fig. 10.19). In this situation, immunohistochemistry can be helpful. Plasmacytoma exhibits

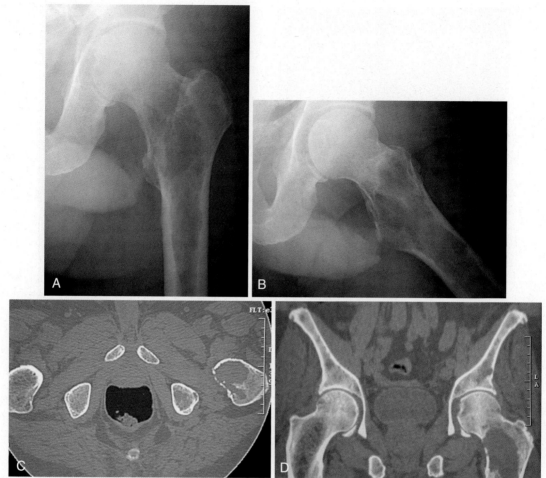

FIGURE 10.18   **A** and **B,** Anteroposterior and lateral radiographs of proximal femur of 61-year-old man with multiple myeloma show multiple lytic lesions. **C** and **D,** CT better shows extent of lesions and need for prophylactic fixation.

monoclonal κ or λ light chains, whereas the plasma cells of chronic osteomyelitis are polyclonal. Also, myeloma cells usually stain positive for the natural killer antigen CD56, whereas reactive plasma cells usually do not. Immunohistochemistry can also be helpful in poorly differentiated cases when lymphoma could be in the differential diagnosis. Lymphoma cells usually stain positive for CD45 (leukocyte common antigen) and CD20 (a B-cell marker), whereas myeloma cells usually are negative.

The primary treatment of multiple myeloma is chemotherapy. Symptomatic bone lesions usually respond rapidly to radiation therapy. Bisphosphonates have also been shown to be of benefit in the prevention of skeletally related events. The orthopaedic surgeon most commonly is consulted to treat impending or actual pathologic fractures of the spine, acetabulum, proximal femur, or proximal humerus. Every effort should be made to perform the operation that would allow the earliest resumption of full activity. This may include debulking the tumor and using internal fixation augmented with methacrylate. If this method would not allow immediate full weight bearing, cemented total joint arthroplasty or hemiarthroplasty should be considered. In most patients, local radiation therapy should be instituted 2 to 3 weeks after surgery or when the wound appears to be healed. The treating surgeon should keep in mind, however, that patients with myeloma

are at higher risk for perioperative complications (e.g., infection, deep vein thrombosis, or renal failure) when compared with most orthopaedic patients.

Patients who present with a solitary plasmacytoma without evidence of systemic involvement (i.e., negative bone marrow biopsy and negative skeletal survey) have a better prognosis. Although more than half of patients who present with a solitary plasmacytoma eventually go on to develop multiple myeloma, some patients have a considerable disease-free interval, and a few remain continuously free of disease. Until recently, long-term survival for patients with multiple myeloma was very rare. Currently, however, some centers are reporting greater than 60% long-term survival with aggressive treatment.

LYMPHOMA

Lymphoma may involve bone primarily or secondarily. Lymphoma can occur at any age but becomes more common in the sixth and seventh decades of life. The male-to-female ratio is approximately 1.5:1. The femur is the most common bone involved, followed by the pelvis, spine, and ribs.

Most patients complain of localized pain or swelling. Patients with spinal involvement may have nerve root or cord compression. The symptoms can be mild or severe. Some

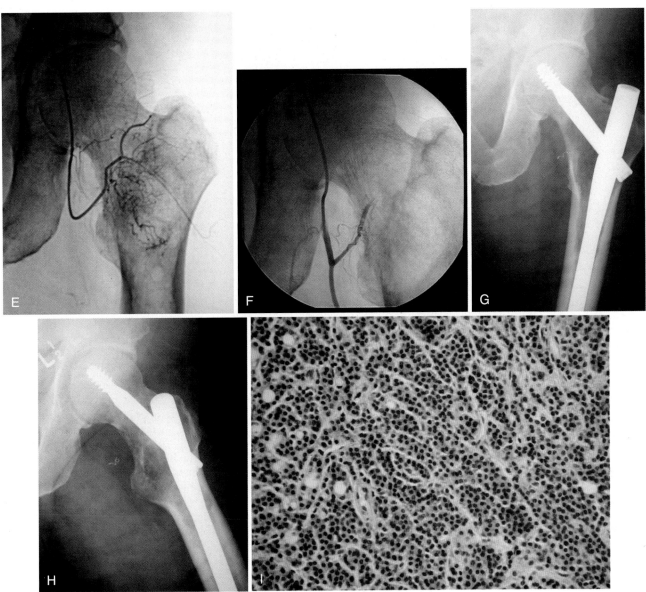

FIGURE 10.18, Cont'd   **E** and **F,** Preoperative embolization was done to minimize intraoperative blood loss, which can be extensive with multiple myeloma. **G** and **H,** Radiographs after prophylactic fixation with long gamma nail. **I,** Typical microscopic appearance of multiple myeloma with sheets of plasma cells.

patients have symptoms for several years before seeking medical attention. In contrast to patients with multiple myeloma, patients with lymphoma usually feel otherwise healthy.

Radiographically, lymphoma usually appears as an ill-defined area of bone destruction (frequently diaphyseal) and often has a permeative appearance. The cortex may be thickened, but a periosteal reaction rarely is seen. Frequently, a large portion of the bone or even the entire bone can be involved. The extent of the lesion may appear large compared with the patient's symptoms. Radiographs can be entirely normal despite extensive involvement of the medullary canal as seen on bone scan or MRI (Fig. 10.20). (Lymphoma usually should be included in the differential diagnosis of a patient who has bone pain and an abnormal bone scan or MRI with normal radiographs.) The soft-tissue mass can also be extensive. Staging studies should include a complete blood cell count and serum chemistries; bone scan; CT of the chest, abdomen, and pelvis; and a bone marrow biopsy. Whole body PET/CT is also useful for staging as well as for evaluation of response to treatment.

Microscopically, osseous lymphomas are composed of a mixture of large and small lymphoid cells with cleaved and noncleaved nuclei (Fig. 10.21). Some may appear sarcomatoid, and others may be difficult to distinguish from Ewing sarcoma or an undifferentiated carcinoma. Immunohistochemistry (specifically, positive staining for lymphoid markers, positive reticulin stain, negative keratin, and negative PAS) frequently is helpful in these cases.

A discussion of the classification of lymphomas is beyond the scope of this text. In general, however, patients with primary lymphoma of bone have a better prognosis (approximately 50% to 80% 5-year survival) than patients with systemic disease. The primary treatment of lymphoma is chemotherapy (Fig. 10.22). Local control usually is attained with radiation therapy.

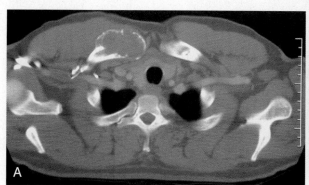
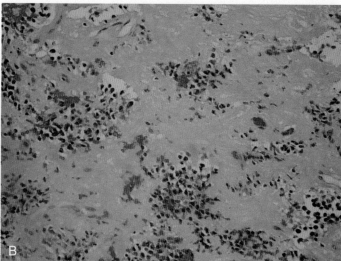

FIGURE 10.19 **A,** CT scan of 39-year-old man with solitary plasmacytoma of right medial clavicle. **B,** Biopsy specimen revealed monoclonal plasma cells with abundant amyloid. With exception of patients on long-term renal dialysis, amyloid production in bone usually is associated with diagnosis of myeloma.

Surgical intervention is rarely needed but may be indicated for treatment of impending or actual pathologic fractures.

METASTATIC CARCINOMA

Metastatic carcinoma is the most common malignancy treated by orthopaedic surgeons. Although only about 8000 new sarcomas are diagnosed in the United States each year, more than 1 million new carcinomas are diagnosed. It is estimated that 50% to 80% of patients with carcinoma have bone metastases at the time of death. As treatment for primary tumors improves, longer survival time is being reported after diagnosis of bone metastases. The orthopaedic surgeon should not approach these patients with a fatalistic attitude. Proper orthopaedic care is crucial for many of these patients to minimize pain, maintain function, maintain their independence, and improve their overall quality of life.

If a patient has a known history of a carcinoma, even in the remote past, a newly discovered bone lesion is most likely to be a metastasis. In any patient older than 40 years, even without a history of malignancy, a newly discovered, aggressive-appearing bone lesion is most likely to be metastatic carcinoma or multiple myeloma. The proper workup of a patient with suspected metastases of unknown origin is discussed in detail in other chapter.

Briefly, the workup consists of a history and physical examination, including breast or prostate; basic laboratory tests, including serum protein electrophoresis and possibly prostate-specific antigen; a radiograph of the entire involved bone; a chest radiograph; a bone scan to look for other sites of disease; and CT of the chest, abdomen, and pelvis. Failure to complete this workup before biopsy can lead to serious errors in patient care. This simple approach identifies the primary lesion in more than 85% of patients who have metastases of unknown origin. After the workup is complete, a biopsy can be performed. Even if a patient has a known history of carcinoma, a biopsy of the first site of bone disease must be performed to establish a firm relationship between the primary carcinoma and the suspected metastasis. This biopsy must be done in the same manner as a biopsy for a suspected primary sarcoma because, in rare instances, it may prove to be a primary sarcoma (Fig. 10.23). Subsequent bone metastases can be treated without biopsy confirmation.

Most carcinomas metastatic to bone are from the breast and prostate, followed by the lung, kidney, thyroid, and gastrointestinal tract in order of decreasing frequency. For patients who have suspected metastases of unknown origin, however, the most common primary malignancies are in the lung or kidney. Breast and prostate are uncommon sites of primary disease for this group of patients. This phenomenon has several possible explanations. First, the primary lesions in patients with breast cancer or prostate cancer may be detected more easily early in the disease course. Second, breast cancer and prostate cancer may not metastasize to bone until relatively late. Finally, lung and kidney cancer may escape detection until very late in the disease course and may metastasize to bone relatively earlier.

The radiographic appearance of metastatic carcinoma varies. The appearance usually is aggressive, suggesting malignancy. The lesions may be lytic, blastic, or mixed. Breast cancer and prostate cancer typically produce blastic lesions. Kidney cancer and thyroid cancer usually are purely lytic. Lung cancer may produce a mixed appearance. If the lesion is distal to the elbow or knee, lung cancer is the most likely primary lesion. In addition, metastatic lung cancer may have the distinct appearance of a "bite" taken out of the cortex.

The microscopic appearance of metastatic carcinoma usually is similar to that of the primary lesion. In well-differentiated cases, the biopsy easily yields the correct diagnosis. In some cases, such as a sarcomatoid kidney cancer, immunohistochemistry may be required to reveal epithelial markers.

The treatment of carcinoma metastatic to bone is multimodal. Systemic treatment with cytotoxic agents is directed by the medical oncologist. Hormone manipulation may

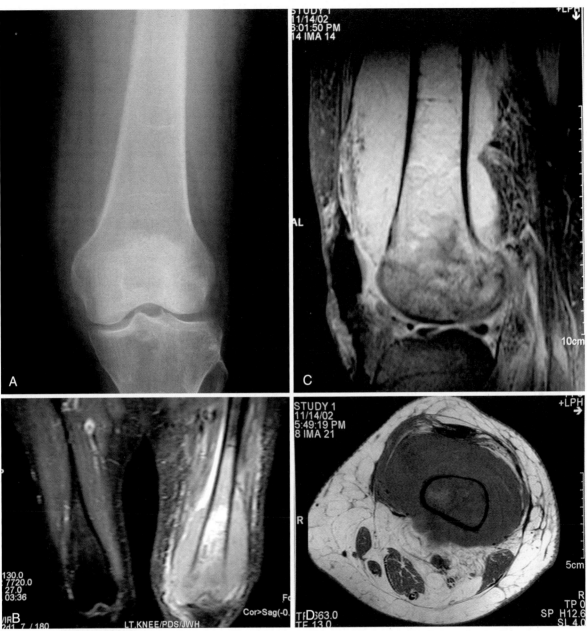

FIGURE 10.20 An 83-year-old woman complained of mild pain and a thigh mass that had been increasing in size over the past year. **A,** An anteroposterior radiograph of the knee is relatively unremarkable. **B-D,** MRI, however, demonstrates a large lesion that permeates through the bone with a large, circumferential soft-tissue mass. These findings are typical of lymphoma. Lymphoma should usually be considered when MRI demonstrates a large bone lesion despite relatively normal radiographs.

be beneficial for patients with breast or prostate cancer. Radioactive iodine may be beneficial for some patients with metastatic thyroid cancer. Bisphosphonates have a role in preventing new metastatic bone lesions from forming and slow the growth of existing lesions by inhibiting osteoclast resorption of bone. Most symptomatic bone metastases are responsive to radiation. Some carcinomas, especially kidney cancer, are typically radioresistant. Some of these lesions can be treated with radiofrequency ablation or cryoablation. Surgery is required for treatment of impending or actual pathologic fractures.

Precisely defined indications for prophylactic fixation of impending pathologic fractures have been debated. Parameters that have been suggested include pain that has not responded to radiation therapy, a lesion larger than 2.5 cm, a lesion that has destroyed more than 50% of the cortex, and an avulsion fracture of the lesser trochanter. Mirels devised a scoring system that evaluates the risk of pathologic fracture on the basis of the site, size, and lytic or blastic nature of the lesion, as well as the presence and quality of associated pain (Table 10.1). According to this system, prophylactic internal fixation should be considered for any patient with a score of 8

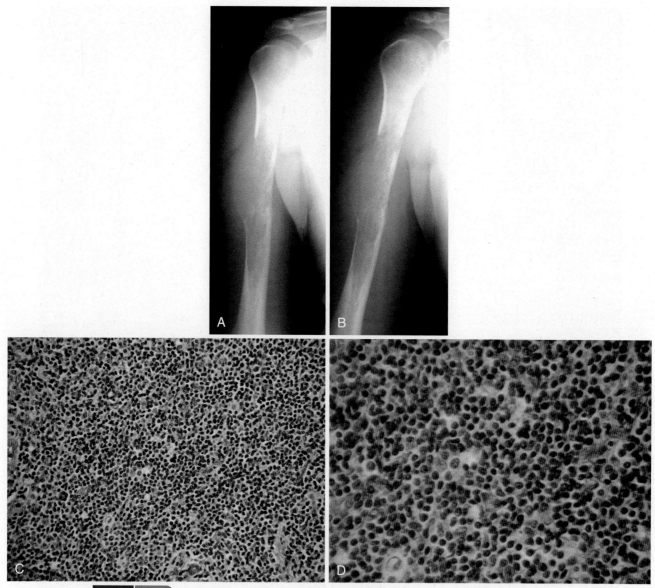

FIGURE 10.21 **A** and **B,** Anteroposterior and lateral views of right humerus of 36-year-old man with primary lymphoma of bone. Despite extensive bone destruction and large soft-tissue mass, patient's symptoms were mild. Low-power **(C)** and high-power **(D)** microscopic appearance of lymphoma. Lymphoma usually should be considered in differential diagnosis of patient with relatively mild symptoms compared with large size of lesion and also should be considered in the differential diagnosis of destructive-appearing diaphyseal lesions.

or higher. Although each of these guidelines aids in the decision-making process, none serves as an absolute criterion. Each patient should be evaluated individually while keeping two generally accepted principles in mind. First, prophylactic internal fixation of an impending fracture is technically easier than fixation of an actual pathologic fracture. Second, patient morbidity is decreased with prophylactic fixation compared with fixation after the fracture.

The prognosis of patients with metastatic carcinoma continues to improve. Although most patients with a pathologic fracture from metastatic lung cancer die within 6 months, length of survival is not always predictable. We have treated multiple patients who have survived with good quality of life

4 to 5 years after sustaining pathologic fractures secondary to metastatic lung cancer. Patients with breast, prostate, and kidney cancer commonly live many years after diagnosis of bone metastases. An isolated bone metastasis from kidney cancer can be treated with curative intent with wide resection (Fig. 10.24).

The unpredictability of survival makes proper surgical care more challenging. The fixation must be stable enough to allow immediate full weight bearing so that a patient would not have to endure an unnecessarily prolonged rehabilitation period when he or she may have only several months to live. Conversely, the reconstruction should be durable enough to last for many years if the patient happens to do well. In general, the tumor should be debulked before internal fixation. The

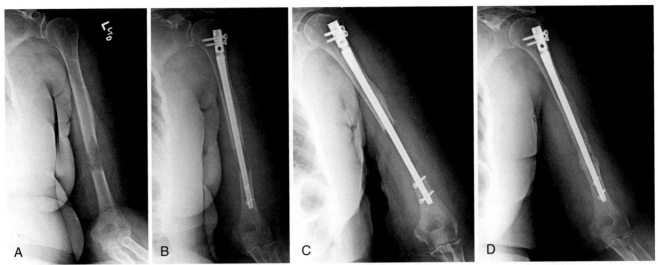

FIGURE 10.22 **A,** Anteroposterior radiograph of left humerus of 75-year-old woman who complained of left arm pain. Examination revealed lesion to be primary lymphoma of bone. **B,** After stabilization with intramedullary nail. **C,** Left humerus 2 months after surgery demonstrating local progression as patient had refused all other treatment. **D,** Left humerus after treatment with chemotherapy and radiation demonstrating consolidation of bone.

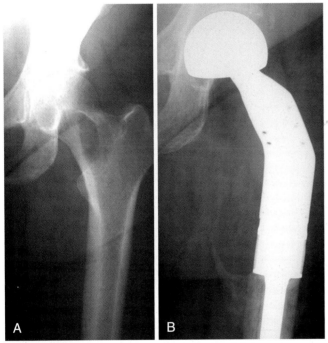

FIGURE 10.23 **A,** Anteroposterior view of left hip of 50-year-old woman with history of breast cancer. She had been disease free for 2 years. Lytic lesion is seen in femoral neck. Although the most likely diagnosis for this lesion is metastatic carcinoma, biopsy must be performed in appropriate fashion. This lesion proved to be malignant fibrous histiocytoma. **B,** Anteroposterior view of left hip after wide resection and endoprosthetic reconstruction. If this patient had been treated with prophylactic fixation of presumed metastatic carcinoma, her outcome would have been severely compromised.

TABLE 10.1

Scoring System for Predicting Pathologic Fracture

	SCORE		
VARIABLE	**1**	**2**	**3**
Site	Upper limb	Lower limb	Peritrochanter
Pain	Mild	Moderate	Functional
Size	<1/3	1/3–2/3	>2/3
Lesion	Blastic	Mixed	Lytic

From Mirels H: Metastatic disease in long bones: a proposed scoring system for diagnosing impending pathologic fractures, *Clin Orthop Relat Res* 249:256–264, 1989.

cavity can be filled with methacrylate to augment the fixation. The entire bone should be protected with intramedullary fixation in most cases (Figs. 10.25 to 10.31). If this approach would not provide the stability required for immediate full weight bearing, resection and prosthetic reconstruction should be considered. Lesions of the femoral neck should be considered for hemiarthroplasty or total hip arthroplasty. Arthroplasty components frequently are fixed with cement because the bone usually is treated with radiation. Recent studies, however, have shown that modern press-fit implants, especially those made with trabecular metal appear to obtain adequate fixation in this setting. Radiation therapy usually is administered to the entire operative field beginning 2 to 3 weeks after surgery if the wound has healed. Due to the general medical condition of these patients, as well as the extent of the procedures combined with chemotherapy and radiation treatment, infection risk is relatively high. Surgeons should consider a prolonged course of postoperative antibiotics, although specific protocols need further study to prove efficacy.

A summary of the characteristics of malignant tumors of bone is presented in Table 10.2.

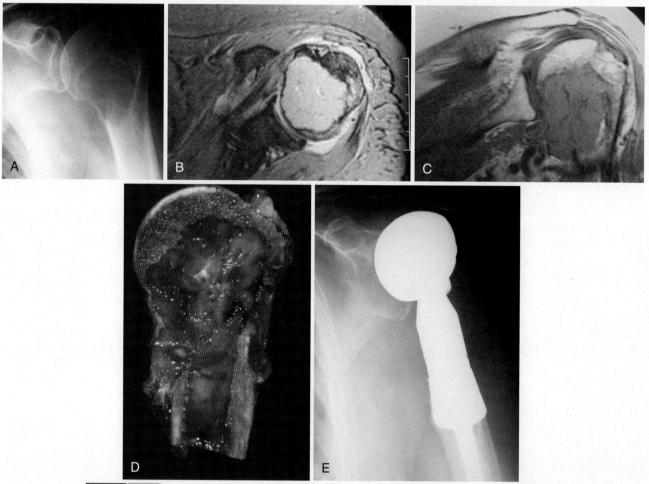

FIGURE 10.24   **A,** Anteroposterior radiograph of 77-year-old woman with renal cancer metastatic to left proximal humerus. **B** and **C,** MRI shows extent of lesion. This was the only site of metastatic disease, so the patient was treated with wide resection and endoprosthetic reconstruction. **D,** Photograph of resected specimen. **E,** Anteroposterior view of left shoulder after endoprosthetic reconstruction.

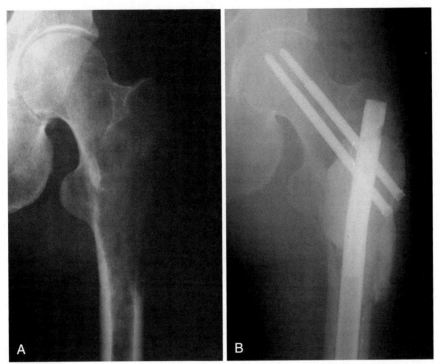

FIGURE 10.25 **A,** Anteroposterior radiograph of 41-year-old man with metastatic squamous cell carcinoma with impending pathologic femoral fracture. Patient was admitted for prophylactic fixation. His femur fractured when he rolled over in bed the night before his scheduled surgery. **B,** Anteroposterior radiograph after fixation with reconstruction nail and bone cement.

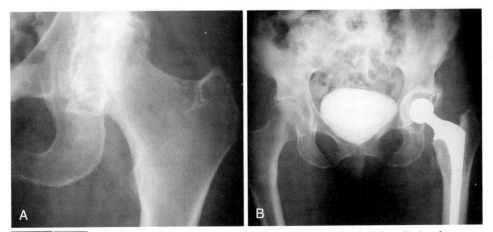

FIGURE 10.26 **A,** Anteroposterior view of left hip of patient treated with radiation for metastatic breast cancer. She subsequently developed osteonecrosis of femoral head. **B,** Anteroposterior view of pelvis after treatment with cemented total hip arthroplasty. Because bone had been irradiated, femoral and acetabular components were cemented.

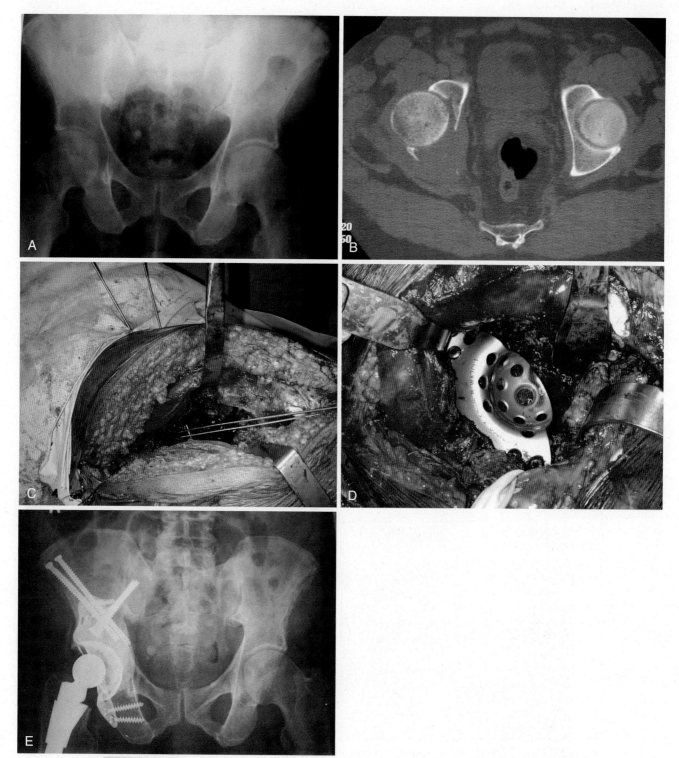

FIGURE 10.27 **A,** Anteroposterior radiograph of 66-year-old man with metastatic lung cancer in right acetabulum. **B,** Computed tomography better shows destruction of posterior column and wall. Patient was treated with preoperative embolization to help minimize intraoperative blood loss. **C,** Intraoperative photograph after curettage of lesion. Two guidewires were placed from the defect to the posterior ilium. Two more guidewires were placed from the anterior iliac crest to the defect. Cannulated screws were placed over guidewires to help support cement mantle. **D,** Acetabular cage was placed. Tumor defect was filled with bone cement as acetabular cup was cemented into cage. **E,** Postoperative radiograph.

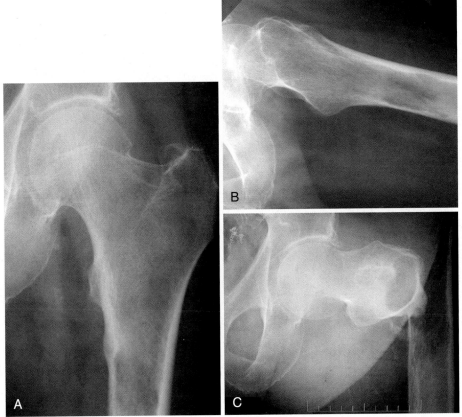

FIGURE 10.28   **A** and **B,** Anteroposterior and lateral radiographs of proximal femur of 82-year-old man with metastatic kidney cancer reveal multiple lytic lesions. Patient failed to respond to radiation. Prophylactic internal fixation was scheduled; however, operation was canceled because the patient was considered medically unstable for surgery. **C,** Anteroposterior view of left hip of same patient several weeks later after sustaining pathologic fracture. Surgery is now more difficult, and patient has experienced greater morbidity.

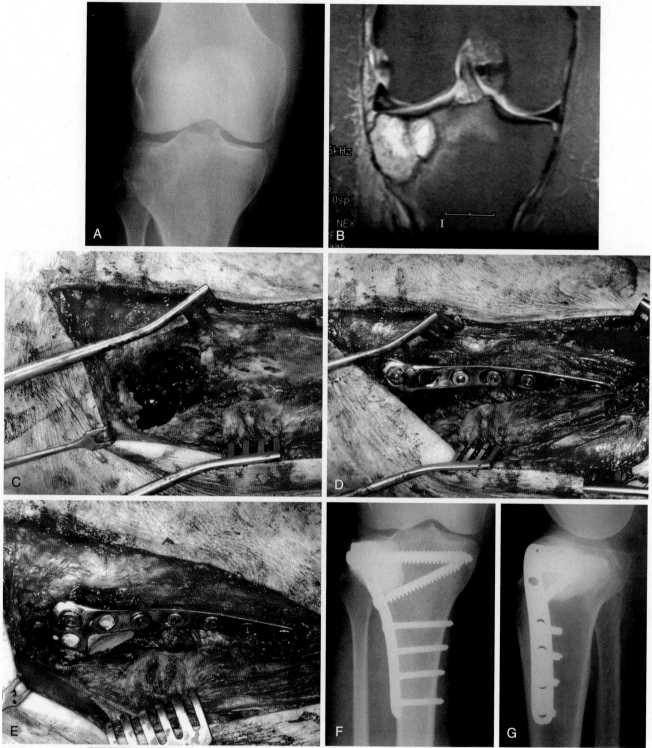

FIGURE **10.29** Anteroposterior radiograph **(A)** and coronal MR image **(B)** of 70-year-old woman with metastatic lung cancer in right proximal tibia who was unable to bear weight. **C,** Intraoperative photograph after curettage of tumor. Plate was placed **(D),** and cavity was packed with bone cement to allow immediate ambulation **(E). F** and **G,** Postoperative anteroposterior and lateral radiographs.

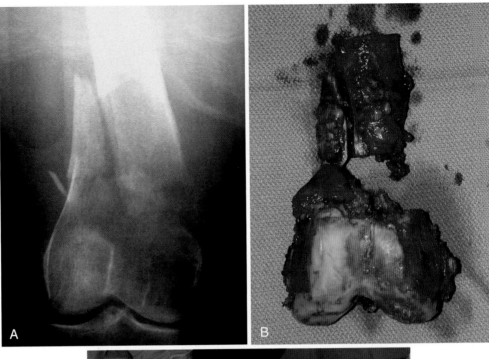

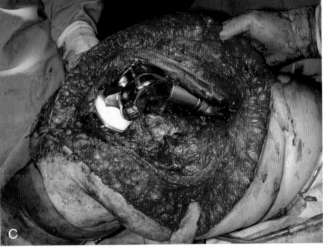

FIGURE 10.30 **A,** Pathologic fracture of right distal femur secondary to hepatobiliary carcinoma in 71-year-old woman. Because of extensive bone destruction, the decision was made to proceed with endoprosthetic reconstruction to allow full weight bearing. **B,** Photograph of resected bone fragments. **C,** Photograph of prosthesis in situ.

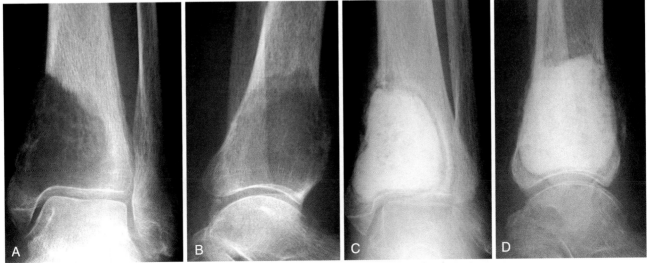

FIGURE 10.31 **A** and **B,** Anteroposterior and lateral radiographs of left ankle of 78-year-old woman with metastatic kidney cancer. **C** and **D,** Anteroposterior and lateral views after extended curettage and packing of defect with methacrylate. Patient was able to resume immediate full weight bearing with relief of her pain.

TABLE 10.2

Malignant Tumors of the Bone

TUMOR	AGE	DEMOGRAPHICS	SITE	PRESENTATION	IMAGING	HISTOLOGY	TREATMENT	COMMENTS
OSTEOSARCOMA								
Conventional osteosarcoma	2nd decade	Slight male predominance	Metaphyseal Distal femur Proximal tibia Proximal humerus	Progressive pain	Mixed lytic and blastic appearance Cortical destruction Periosteal reaction (Codman triangle or hair-on-end) Soft-tissue mass	Osteoid production from malignant spindle cells Marked nuclear pleomorphism Abundant mitotic figures	Chemotherapy and wide resection	Rarely associated with hereditary form of retinoblastoma, Rothmund–Thomson syndrome, or Li-Fraumeni syndrome
Periosteal osteosarcoma	2nd-3rd decades	Slight female predominance	Diaphysis femur and tibia	Pain Mass	Diaphyseal lesion Lesion sits in depression on surface of bone Irregular ossification blends into soft tissue	Strands of osteoid radiating among lobules of cartilage	Wide resection Chemotherapy controversial	
Parosteal osteosarcoma	3rd-4th decades	Slight female predominance	Posterior aspect of distal femur	Painless mass	Lobulated ossified mass on posterior surface of distal femur	Slightly atypical spindle cells Slightly atypical trabeculae	Wide resection alone	
Telangiectatic osteosarcoma	2nd decade	Slight male predominance	Distal femur Proximal tibia	Progressive pain	Purely lytic May have ballooned/cystic appearance (similar to aneurysmal bone cyst)	Blood-filled spaces separated by thin septa Spindle cells in septa frankly malignant	Chemotherapy and wide resection	
Secondary osteosarcoma	6th-8th decades	Male:female 2:1, Paget osteosarcoma Male:female 1:2, radiation osteosarcoma	Axial location (sites of previous radiation or Paget disease)	Progressive pain	Mixed lytic and blastic appearance Cortical destruction	Similar to high-grade conventional osteosarcoma	Chemotherapy and wide resection	Poor prognosis Paget osteosarcoma more common in patients with advanced polyostotic disease Radiation osteosarcoma usually occurs 10-15 years after radiation treatment

CHONDROSARCOMA

Tumor	Age	Sex	Location	Symptoms	Imaging	Histology	Treatment	Other
Conventional chondrosarcoma	5th-7th decades	Slight male predominance	Pelvis, Proximal femur, Proximal humerus	Progressive pain	Punctate calcification, Cortical erosion, Soft-tissue mass	Cartilaginous matrix, Binucleate cells, Grade related to degree of hypercellularity, Entrapment of bony trabeculae	Wide resection (extended curettage for low-grade intramedullary tumors), No role for chemotherapy or radiation	Important to correlate symptoms, radiographic findings, and histology
Dedifferentiated chondrosarcoma	5th-8th decades	Slight male predominance	Pelvis, Proximal femur, Proximal humerus	Progressive pain	Aggressive radiolucent area adjacent to an otherwise typical chondrosarcoma	High-grade spindle cell sarcoma adjacent to a low-grade cartilaginous neoplasm	Chemotherapy and wide resection	Very poor prognosis
Clear cell chondrosarcoma	Wide age range	Male predominance	Epiphyseal, Proximal femur, Proximal humerus	Pain may be of long duration	Well-circumscribed radiolucent epiphyseal lesion, May have rim of reactive bone, Imaging findings can appear benign	Round cells with abundant clear cytoplasm, Distinct cytoplastic borders, Cartilaginous matrix	Wide resection	Extremely rare
Mesenchymal chondrosarcoma	2nd-5th decades	Slight male predominance	Wide distribution	Pain	Nonspecific destructive lesion, May have features of conventional chondrosarcoma	Small round blue cells, Islands of cartilage, "Staghorn" vessels	Chemotherapy and wide resection	Rare
Ewing sarcoma	1st-3rd decades	Male predominance	Flat bones, Metadiaphysis of long bones	Pain and swelling, May have systemic complaints	Permeative bone destruction, Large soft-tissue mass, "Onion skin" periosteal reaction	Small round blue cells, MIC-2 positive	Chemotherapy, Surgery and/or radiation for local control	t(11,22)
Chordoma	5th-7th decades	Male:female 3:1	Sacrum, Base of skull	Pain, Neurologic signs/symptoms	Midline lesion, Soft-tissue mass anterior to sacrum	Cells arranged in long strands or "cords", Mucinous background, Vacuolated cytoplasm—physaliferous cells	Wide resection	

Continued

TABLE 10.2

Malignant Tumors of the Bone—cont'd

TUMOR	AGE	DEMOGRAPHICS	SITE	PRESENTATION	IMAGING	HISTOLOGY	TREATMENT	COMMENTS
Adamantinoma	2nd-3rd decades	Male = female	Tibial diaphysis	Pain of long duration	Sharply demarcated radiolucent lesions in tibial diaphysis based in anterior cortex	Islands of epithelial cells in a fibrous stroma	Wide resection	Rare
Malignant vascular tumors	After 1st decade	Slight male predominance	Any bone Slight tendency toward axial location	Pain	Lytic lesions Low-grade tumors may have partial sclerotic rim High-grade tumors appear more destructive Frequently multifocal within same bone or adjacent bones	Low-grade tumors well-formed vascular channels with plump endothelial cells High-grade tumors—pleomorphic spindle cells CD31, CD34, and factor VIII–related antigen positive	Wide resection if possible Irradiation for multifocal or surgically inaccessible lesions Chemotherapy for high-grade lesions	Rare Stewart-Treves syndrome—angiosarcoma occurring in the setting of chronic lymphedema
Malignant fibrous histiocytoma (MFH)/fibrosarcoma	After 1st decade	Male = female	Distal femur Proximal tibia	Pain 20% with pathologic fracture	Purely lytic Destructive	Pleomorphic spindle cells MFH—storiform pattern Fibrosarcoma—herringbone pattern	Chemotherapy and wide resection	25% are secondary to preexisting condition such as Paget disease, radiation, giant cell tumor, or bone infarct

	Age	Sex	Location	Symptoms	Radiographic appearance	Histology	Treatment	Comments
Plasmacytoma/ multiple myeloma	6th–7th decades	Male:female 2:1	Axial location Proximal femur Proximal humerus	Pain Systemic complaints	Multiple purely lytic sharply demarcated "punched out" lesions	Sheets of plasma cells	Chemotherapy Irradiation for symptomatic bone lesions Surgery for impending or actual pathologic fractures	Diagnosis often made by serum or urine protein electrophoresis, which demonstrates a monoclonal gammopathy
Lymphoma	6th–7th decades	Male:female 1.5:1	Femur Pelvis Spine Ribs	Pain	Variable radiographic appearance—can be very destructive or can have relatively normal radiographs Extent of tumor on MRI can be much greater than the apparent extent on radiographs	Mixture of large and small lymphoid cells Reticulin positive, PAS negative Stain positive for lymphoid markers	Chemotherapy and radiation Surgery for impending or actual pathologic fractures	Lymphoma should be considered in the differential diagnosis of a patient with normal radiographs despite a large bone lesion with soft-tissue mass on MRI
Metastatic carcinoma	5th–8th decades	Male = female	Axial location Proximal femur Proximal humerus	Pain Symptoms referable to the primary lesion	Blastic—breast, prostate Lytic—kidney, thyroid Mixed—lung	Histology usually similar to the primary tumor	Systemic treatment for the primary tumor Irradiation for symptomatic bone lesions Surgery for impending or actual pathologic fractures	Breast and prostate most common Kidney and lung most common if patient presents with bone metastases and no known primary tumor

MRI, Magnetic resonance imaging; *PAS*, periodic acid–Schiff.

REFERENCES

OSTEOSARCOMA

Aggerholm-Pedersen N, Maretty-Nielsen K, Keller J, et al.: The importance of standardized treatment in high-grade osteosarcoma: 30 years of experience from a hospital-based database, *Acta Oncol* 54(1):17, 2015.

Angeloini A, Drago G, Trovarelli G, et al.: Infection after surgical resection for pelvic bone tumors: an analysis of 270 patients from one institution, *Clin Orthop Relat Res* 472:349, 2014.

Arkader A, Yang CH, Tolo VT: High long-term local control with sacrectomy for primary high-grade bone sarcoma in children, *Clin Orthop Relat Res* 470:1491, 2012.

Ayerza MA, Farfalli GL, Aponte-Tinao L, Luis Muscolo D: Does increased rate of limb-sparing surgery affect survival in osteosarcoma? *Clin Orthop Relat Res* 468:2854, 2010.

Bertrand TE, Cruz A, Binitie O, et al.: Do surgical margins affect local recurrence and survival in extremity, nonmetastatic, high-grade osteosarcoma? *Clin Orthop Relat Res* 474:677, 2016.

Bus MP, Dijkstra PD, van de Sande MA, et al.: Intercalary allograft reconstructions following resection of primary bone tumors: a nationwide multicenter study, *J Bone Joint Surg* 96A:e26, 2014.

Cates JM, Schoenecker JG: Proximal location in extremity long bones is a poor prognostic factor for osteosarcoma: a retrospective cohort study of 153 patients, *Acta Oncol* 55(8):1036, 2016.

Chung SW, Han I, Oh JH, et al.: Prognostic effect of erroneous surgical procedures in patients with osteosarcoma: evaluation using propensity score matching, *J Bone Joint Surg* 96A:e60, 2014.

Cipriano C, Griffin AM, Ferguson PC, Wunder JS: Developing an evidence-based followup schedule for bone sarcomas based on local recurrence and metastatic progression, *Clin Orthop Relat Res* 475:830, 2017.

Cipriano CA, Gruzinova IS, Frank RM, et al.: Frequent complications and severe bone loss associated with the repiphysis expandable distal femoral prosthesis, *Clin Orthop Relat Res* 473:831, 2015.

Corradi D, Wenger DE, Bertoni F, et al.: Multicentric osteosarcoma: clinicopathologic and radiographic study of 56 cases, *Am J Clin Pathol* 136:799, 2011.

Craft AW: Osteosarcoma: the European Osteosarcoma Intergroup (EOI) perspective, *Cancer Treat Res* 152:263, 2010.

Dotan A, Dadia S, Bickels J, et al.: Expandable endoprosthesis for limb-sparing surgery in children: long-term results, *J Child Orthop* 4:391, 2010.

Durnali A, Alkis N, Cangur S, et al.: Prognostic factors for teenage and adult patients with high-grade osteosarcoma: an analysis of 240 patients, *Med Oncol* 30:624, 2013.

Eleutério SJ, Senerchia AA, Aimeida MT, et al.: Osteosarcoma in patients younger than 12 years old without metastases have similar prognosis as adolescent and young adults, *Pediatr Blood Cancer* 62(7):1209, 2015.

Ferrari S, Palmerini E, Staals EL, et al.: The treatment of nonmetastatic high grade osteosarcoma of the extremity: review of the Italian Rizzoli experience. Impact on the future, *Cancer Treatment Res* 152:275, 2010.

Fuchs B, Hoekzema N, Larson DR, et al.: Osteosarcoma of the pelvis: outcome analysis of surgical treatment, *Clin Orthop Relat Res* 467:510, 2009.

Gaston CL, Nakamura T, Reddy K, et al.: Is limb salvage surgery safe for bone sarcomas identified after a previous surgical procedure? *Bone Joint J* 96-B:665, 2014.

Guo W, Sun X, Ji T, Tang X: Outcome of surgical treatment of pelvic osteosarcoma, *J Surg Oncol* 106:406, 2012.

Haddox CL, Han G, Anijar L, et al.: Osteosarcoma in pediatric patients and young adults: a single institution retrospective review of presentation, therapy, and outcome, *Sarcoma* 2014:402509, 2014.

Han G, Bi WZ, Xu M, et al.: Amputation versus limb-salvage surgery in patients with osteosarcoma: a meta-analysis, *World J Surg* 40(8):2016, 2016.

Hernberg MM, Kivioja AH, Böhling TO, et al.: Chemoradiotherapy in the treatment of inoperable high-grade osteosarcoma, *Med Oncol* 2010, [Epub ahead of print].

Isakoff MS, Barkauskas DA, Ebb D, et al.: Poor survival for osteosarcoma of the pelvis: a report from the Children's Oncology Group, *Clin Orthop Relat Res* 470:2007, 2012.

Iwata S, Ishii T, Kawai A, et al.: Prognostic factors in elderly osteosarcoma patients: a multi-institutional retrospective study of 86 cases, *Ann Surg Oncol* 21:263, 2014.

Jaffe N: Osteosarcoma: review of the past, impact on the future. The American Experience, *Cancer Treat Res* 152:239, 2010.

Jeon DG, Song WS, Kong CB, et al.: MFH of bone and osteosarcoma show similar survival and chemosensitivity, *Clin Orthop Relat Res* 469:584–590, 2011.

Jeys LM, Thorne CJ, Parry M, et al.: A novel system for the surgical staging of primary high-grade osteosarcoma: the Birmingham classification, *Clin Orthop Relat Res* 475:842, 2017.

Kager L, Zoubek A, Dominkus M, et al.: Osteosarcoma in very young children: experience of the cooperative osteosarcoma study group, *Cancer* 116:5316, 2010.

Kim W, Han I, Lee JS, et al.: Postmetatasis survival in high-grade extremity osteosarcoma: a retrospective analysis of prognostic factors in 126 patients, *J Surg Oncol* 117:1223, 2018.

Laitinen M, Parry M, Albergo JI, et al.: The prognostic and therapeutic factors which influence the oncological outcome of parosteal osteosarcoma, *Bone Joint J* 97-B:1698, 2015.

Leary SE, Wozniak AW, Billups CA, et al.: Survival of pediatric patients after relapsed osteosarcoma: the St. Jude children's research hospital experience, *Cancer* 119:2645, 2013.

Li J, Wang Z, Guo Z, et al.: Precise resection and biological reconstruction under navigation guidance for young patients with juxta-articular bone sarcoma in lower extremity: preliminary report, *J Pediatr Orthop* 34:101, 2014.

Li X, Moretti VM, Ashana AO, Lackman RD: Perioperative infection rate in patients with osteosarcomas treated with resection and prosthetic reconstruction, *Clin Orthop Relat Res* 469:2889, 2011.

Malagelada F, Tarrago LT, Tibrewal S, et al.: Pathological fracture in osteosarcoma: is is always an indication for amputation? *Ortop Traumatol Rehabil* 16:67, 2014.

Mavrogenis AF, Abati CN, Romagnoli C, Riggieri P: Similar survival but better function for patients after limb salvage versus amputation of distal tibia osteosarcoma, *Clin Orthop Relat Res* 470:1735, 2012.

Mei J, Zhu XZ, Wang ZYU, Cai XS: Functional outcomes and quality of life in patients with osteosarcoma treated with amputation versus limb-salvage surgery: a systematic review and meta-analysis, *Arch Orthop Trauma Surg* 134:1507, 2014.

Morris CD, Teot LA, Bernstein ML, et al.: Assessment of extent of surgical resection of primary high-grade osteosarcoma by treating institutions: a report from the children's oncology group, *J Surg Oncol* 113:351, 2016.

Ottaviani G, Jaffe N: The epidemiology of osteosarcoma, *Cancer Treat Res* 152:3, 2010.

Ottaviani G, Robert RS, Huh WW, et al.: Sociooccupational and physical outcomes more than 20 years after the diagnosis of osteosarcoma in children and adolescents: limb salvage versus amputation, *Cancer* 119:3727, 2013.

Parry MC, Laitinen M, Albergo J, et al.: Osteosarcoma of the pelvis, *Bone Joint J* 98-B(4):555, 2016.

Picci P, Mercuri M, Ferrari S, et al.: Survival in high-grade osteosarcoma: improvement over 21 years at a single institution, *Ann Oncol* 21:1366, 2010.

Pradhan A, Reddy KI, Grimer RJ, et al.: Osteosarcomas in the upper distal extremities: are their oncological outcomes similar to other sites? *Eur J Surg Oncol* 41(3):407, 2015.

Puri A, Pruthi M, Gulia A: Outcomes after limb sparing resection in primary malignant pelvic tumors, *Eur J Surg Oncol* 40:27, 2014.

Reddy KI, Wafa H, Gaston CL, et al.: Does amputation offer any survival benefit over limb salvage in osteosarcoma patients with poor chemonecrosis and close margins? *Bone Joint J* 97-B(1):115, 2015.

Rothermundt C, Seddon BM, Dileo P, et al.: Follow-up practices for high-grade extremity osteosarcoma, *BMC Cancer* 16:301, 2016.

Ruggieri P, Mavrogenis AF, Pala E, et al.: Outcome of expandable prostheses in children, *J Pediatr Orthop* 33:244, 2013.

Sherman CE, O'Connor MI, Sim FH: Survival, local recurrence, and function after pelvic limb salvage at 23 to 38 years of followup, *Clin Orthop Relat Res* 470:712, 2012.

Song WS, Cho WH, Jeon DG, et al.: Pelvis and extremity osteosarcoma with similar tumor volume have an equivalent survival, *J Surg Oncol* 101:611, 2010.

Takeuchi A, Lewis VO, Satcher RL, et al.: What are the factors that affect survival and relapse after local recurrence of osteosarcoma? *Clin Orthop Relat Res* 472:3188, 2014.

Thompson MJ, Shapton JC, Punt SE, Johnson CN, et al.: MRI identification of the osseous extent of pediatric bone sarcomas, *Clin Orthop Relat Res* 476:559-564.

Wong KC, Kumta SM: Joint-preserving tumor resection and reconstruction using image-guided computer navigation, *Clin Orthop Relat Res* 471:762, 2013.

Xie L, Guo W, Li Y, et al.: Pathologic fracture does not influence local recurrence and survival in high-grade extremity osteosarcoma with adequate surgical margins, *J Surg Oncol* 106:820, 2012.

Xu J, Xie L, Guo W: Neoadjuvant chemotherapy followed by delayed surgery: is it necessary for all patients with nonmetastatic high-grade pelvic osteosarcoma? *Clin Orthop Relat Res* 476:2177, 2018.

CHONDROSARCOMA

Albergo JI, Gaston CL, Jeys LM, et al.: Management and prognostic significance of pathological fractures through chondrosarcoma of the femur, *Int Orthop* 39(5):943, 2015.

Andreaou D, Ruppin S, Fehlberg S, et al.: Survival and prognostic factors in chondrosarcoma: results in 115 patients with long-term follow-up, *Acta Orthop* 82:749, 2011.

Arshi A, Sharim J, Park DY, et al.: Chondrosarcoma of the osseous spine: an analysis of epidemiology, patient outcomes, and prognostic factors using the SEER registry from 1973 to 2012, *Spine* 42(9):644, 2017.

Bishop MW, Somerville J, Bahrami A, et al.: Mesenchymal chondrosarcoma in children and young adults: a single institution retrospective review, *Sarcoma* 2015:6082789, 2015.

Bus MPA, Capanacci DA, Albergo JI, et al.: Conventional primary central chondrosarcoma of the pelvis: prognostic factors and outcome of surgical treatment in 162 patients, *J Bone Joint Surg Am* 100(4):316, 2018.

Capanacci DA, Scoccianti G, Franchi A, et al.: Surgical treatment of central grade 1 chondrosarcoma of the appendicular skeleton, *J Orthop Traumatol* 14:101, 2013.

Chen X, Yu LJ, Peng HM, et al.: Is intralesional resection suitable for central grade 1 chondrosarcoma: a systematic review and updated meta-analysis, *Eur J Surg Oncol* 43(9):1718, 2017.

Czajka CM, DiCaprio MR: What is the proportion of patients with multiple hereditary exostoses who undergo malignant degeneration? *Clin Orthop Relat Res* 473(7):2355, 2015.

De Aroim Berstein K, Liebsch N, Chen YL, et al.: Clinical outcomes for patients after surgery and radiation therapy for mesenchymal chondrosarcomas, *J Surg Oncol* 114(8):982, 2016.

De Camargo OP, Baptista AM, Atanásio MJ, Waisberg DR: Chondrosarcoma of bone: lessons from 46 operated cases in a single institution, *Clin Orthop Relat Res* 468:2969–2975, 2010.

Dhinsa BS, DeLisa M, Pollock R, et al.: Dedifferentiated chondrosarcoma demonstrating osteosarcomatous differentiation, *Oncol Res Treat* 41(7-8):456, 2018.

Dierselhuis EF, Gerbers JG, Ploegmakers JJ, et al.: Local treatment with adjuvant therapy for central atypical carilaginous tumors in the long bones: analysis of outcome and complications in one hundred and eight patients with a minimum follow-up of two years, *J Bone Joint Surg Am* 98(4):303, 2016.

Donati D, Colangeli S, Colangeli M, et al.: Surgical treatment of grade I central chondrosarcoma, *Clin Orthop Relat Res* 468:581, 2010.

Fei L, Ngoh, Porter DE: Chondrosarcoma transformation in hereditary multiple exostoses: a systematic review and clinical and cost-effectiveness of a proposed screening model, *J Bone Oncol* 13:114, 2018.

Fromm J, Klein A, Baur-Melnyk A, et al.: Survival and prognostic factors in conventional central chondrosarcoma, *BMC Cancer* 18(1):849, 2018.

Goud AL, Suyts W, Bessems J, et al.: Intraosseous atypical chondroid tumor or chondrosarcoma grade 1 in patients with multiple osteochondromas, *J Bone Joint Surg Am* 97(1):24, 2015.

Guo W, Li D, Tang X, Ji T: Surgical treatment of pelvic chondrosarcoma involving periacetabulum, *J Surg Oncol* 101:160, 2010.

Hodel S, Laux C, Farei-Capagna J, et al.: The impact of biopsy sampling errors and the quality of surgical margins on local recurrence and survival in chondrosarcoma, *Cancer Manag Res* 10:3765, 2018.

Kim HS, Bindiganavile SS, Han I: Oncologic outcome after local recurrence of chondrosarcoma: analysis of prognostic factors, *J Surg Oncol* 111(8):957, 2015.

Laitinen MK, Stevenson JD, Parry MC, et al.: The role of grade in local recurrence and the disease-specific survival in chondrosarcomas, *Bone Joint J* 100-B(5):662, 2018.

Lex JR, Evans S, Stevenson JD, et al.: Dedifferentiated chondrosarcoma of the pelvis: clinical outcomes and current treatment, *Clin Sarcoma Res* 8:23, 2018.

Mavrogenis AF, Angelini A, Drago G, et al.: Survival analysis of patients with chondrosarcomas of the pelvis, *J Surg Oncol* 108:19, 2013.

Mavrogenis AF, Gambarotti M, Angelini A, et al.: Chondrosarcomas revisited, *Orthopedics* 35:e379, 2012.

Meftah M, Schult P, Henshaw RM: Long-term results of intralesional curettage and cryosurgery for treatment of low-grade chondrosarcoma, *J Bone Joint Surg* 95:1358, 2013.

Nota SP, Braun Y, Schwab JH, et al.: The identification of prognostic factors an survival statistics of conventional central chondrosarcoma, *Sarcoma* 2015:623746, 2015.

Roitman PD, Farfalli GL, Ayerza MA, et al.: Is needle biopsy clinically useful in preoperative grading of central chondrosarcoma of the pelvis and long bones? *Clin Orthop Relat Res* 475(3):808, 2017.

Song K, Shi X, Liang X, et al.: Risk factors for metastasis at presentation with conventional chondrosarmoa: a population-based study, *Int Orthop* 42(12):2941, 2018.

Song K, Shi X, Wang H, et al.: Can a nomogram help to predict the overall and cancer-specific survival of patients with chondrosarcoma, *Clin Orthop Relat Res* 476(5):987, 2018.

Souna BS, Gelot N, Duval H, et al.: No recurrences in selected patients after curettage with cryotherapy for grade I chondrosarcomas, *Clin Orthop Relat Res* 468:1956, 2010.

Stevenson JD, Laitinen MK, Parry MC, et al.: The role of surgical margins in chondrosarcoma, *Eur J Surg Oncol* 44(9):1412, 2018.

Streitbuerger A, Ahrens H, Gosheger G, et al.: The treatment of locally recurrent chondrosarcoma: is extensive further surgery justified? *J Bone Joint Surg* 94B:122, 2012.

Strotman PK, Reif TJ, Kliwthermes SA, et al.: Dedifferentiated chondrosarcoma: a survival analysis of 159 cases from the SEER database (2001-2011), *J Surg Oncol* 116(2):252, 2017.

Stihsen C, Panotopoulos J, Puchner SE, et al.: The outcome of the surgical treatment of pelvic chondrosarcoma: a competing risk analysis of 58 tumours from a single centre, *Bone Joint J* 99-B(5):686, 2017.

Temple HT: Central chondrosarcoma in patients with multiple osteochondromas: commentary on an article by Annemarie L. Goud, MD, PhD, et al: "Intraosseous atypical chondroid tumor or chondrosarcoma grade 1 in patients with multiple osteochondromas, *J Bone Joint Surg Am* 97(1):35, 2015.

Van Maldegem A, Conley AP, Rutkowski P, et al.: Outcome of first-line systemic treatment for unresectable conventional, dedifferentiated mesenchymal, and clear cell chondrosarcoma, *Oncologist* 24(1):110, 2019.

van Praag Veroniek VM, Rueten-Budde AJ, Ho V, et al.: Incidence, outcomes and prognostic factors during 25 years of treatment of chondrosarcomas, *Surg Oncol* 27(3):402, 2018.

Verdegaal SH, Brouwers HF, van Zwet EW, et al.: Low-grade chondrosarcoma of long bones treated with intralesional curettage followed by application of phenol, ethanol, and bone-grafting, *J Bone Joint Surg* 94A:1201, 2012.

Verdegaal SH, van Rijswijk CS, Brouwers HF, et al.: MRI appearances of atypical cartilaginous tumour/grade I chondrosarcoma after treatment by curettage, phenolisation and allografting: recommendations for follow-up, *Bone Joint J* 98-B:1674, 2016.

Xu J, Li D, Xie L, et al.: Mesenchymal chondrosarcoma of bone and soft tissue: a systematic review of 107 patients in the past 20 years, *PloS One* 10(4):30122216, 2015.

Zamora T, Urrutia J, Schweitzer D, et al.: Do orthopaedic oncologists agree on the diagnosis and treatment of cartilage tumors of the appendicular skeleton? *Clin Orthop Relat Res* 475(9):2176, 2017.

Zoccali C, Baldi J, Attala D, et al.: Intralesional versus extralesional procedures for low-grade central chondrosarcoma: a systematic review of the literature, *Arch Orthop Trauma Surg* 138(7):929, 2018.

EWING SARCOMA

Albergo JI, Gaston CL, Laitinen M, et al.: Ewing's sarcoma: only patients with 100% of necrosis after chemotherapy should be classified as having a good response, *Bone Joint J* 98-B(8):1138, 2016.

Albergo JI, Gaston CLL, Parry MC, et al.: Risk analysis factors for local recurrence in Ewing's sarcoma: when should adjuvant radiotherapy be administered? *Bone Joint J* 100-B(2):247, 2018.

Bailly C, Lefoestier R, Campion L, et al.: Prognostic value of FDG-PET indices for the assessment of histological response to neoadjuvant chemotherapy and outcome in pediatric patients with Ewing sarcoma and osteosarcoma, *PloS One* 12(8):3e0183841, 2017.

Biswas B, Rastogi S, Khan SA, et al.: Outcomes and prognostic factors for Ewing-family tumors of the extremities, *J Bone Joint Surg* 96A:841, 2014.

Bosma SE, Ayu O, Fiocco M, et al.: Prognostic factors for survival in Ewing sarcoma: a systematic review, *Surg Oncol* 27(4):603, 2018.

Brasme JF, Chalumeau M, Oberlin O, et al.: Time to diagnosis of Ewing tumors in children and adolescents is not associated with metastasis or survival: a prospective multicenter study of 436 patients, *J Clin Oncol* 32:1935, 2014.

Charest-Morin R, Dirks MS, Patel S, et al.: Ewing sarcoma of the spine: prognostic variables for survival and local control in surgically treated patients, *Spine* 43(9):622, 2018.

Campbell K, Shulman D, Janeway KA, DuBois SG: Comparison of epidemiology, clinical features, and outcomes of patients with reported Ewing sarcoma and PNET over 40 years justifies current WHO classification and treatment approaches, *Sarcoma* 2018:1712964, 2018.

Dramis A, Grimer RJ, Malizos K, et al.: Non-metastatic pelvic Ewing's sarcoma: oncologic outcomes and evaluation of prognostic factors, *Acta Orthop Belg* 82(2):216, 2016.

DuBois SG, Krailo MD, Gebhardt MC, et al.: Comparative evaluation of local control strategies in localized Ewing sarcoma of bone: a report from the Children's Oncology Group, *Cancer* 121:467, 2015.

Duchman KR, Gao Y, Miller BJ: Prognostic factors for survival in patients with Ewing's sarcoma using the Surveillance, Epidemiology, and End Results (SEER) program database, *Cancer Epidemiol* 39(2):189, 2015.

Friedman DN, Chastain K, Chou JF, et al.: Morbidity and mortality after treatment of Ewing sarcoma: a single-institution experience, *Pediatr Blood Cancer* 64(11), 2017, Epub ahead of print.

Gaspar N, Hawkins DS, Dirksen U, et al.: Ewing sarcoma: current management and future approaches through collaboration, *J Clin Oncol* 33(27):3036, 2015.

Gorlick R, Janeway KA, Adamson PC: Dose intensification improves the outcome of Ewing sarcoma, *J Clin Oncol* JCO2018793489, 2018.

Heinemann M, Ranft A, Langer T, et al.: Recurrence of Ewing sarcoma: is detection by imaging follow-up protocol associated with survival advantage? *Pediatr Blood Cancer* 65(7):327011, 2018.

Henninger B, Glodny B, Rudisch A, et al.: Ewing sarcoma versus osteomyelitis: differential diagnosis with magnetic resonance imaging, *Skeletal Radiol* 42:1097, 2013.

Kadhim M, Womer RB, Dormans JP: Surgical treatment of pelvic sarcoma in children: outcomes for twenty six patients, *Int Orthop* 41(10):2149, 2017.

Kasalak Ö, Glaudemans AWJM, Overbosch J, et al.: Can FDG-PET/CT replace blind bone marrow biopsy of the posterior iliac crest in Ewing sarcoma? *Skeletal Radiol* 47(3):363, 2018.

Kopp LM, Hu C, Rozo B, et al.: Utility of bone marrow aspiration and biopsy in initial staging of Ewing sarcoma, *Pediatr Blood Cancer* 62:12, 2015.

Krakorova DA, Kubackova K, Dusek L, et al.: Advantages in prognosis of adult patients with Ewing sarcoma: 11-years experiences and current treatment management, *Pathol Oncol Res* 24(3):623, 2018.

Kreyer J, Ranft A, Timmermann B, et al.: Impact of the interdisciplinary tumor board of the cooperative Ewing sarcoma study group on local therapy and overall survival of Ewing sarcoma patients after induction therapy, *Pediatr Blood Cancer* 65(12):327384, 2018.

Kridis WB, Toumi N, Chaari H, et al.: A review of Ewing sarcoma treatment: is it still a subject of debate? *Rev Recent Clin Trials* 12(1):19, 2017.

Li Y, Yang X, Zhang WB, et al.: Clinical implications of six inflammatory biomarkers as prognostic indicators in Ewing sarcoma, *Cancer Manag Res* 9:443, 2017.

Lin AY, Hall ET: Second malignancies in Ewing sarcoma survivors, *Cancer* 123(2):4075, 2017.

Lin TA, Ludmir EB, Kiao KP, et al.: Timing of local therapy impacts survival in Ewing sarcoma, *Int J Radiat Oncol Biol Phys* pii:S0360-3016(18)34198-1, 2018.

Lopez JL, Cabrera P, Ordonez R, et al.: Role of radiation therapy in the multidisciplinary management of Ewing's Sarcoma of bone in pediatric patients: an effective treatment for local control, *Rep Pract Oncol Radiother* 16:103, 2011.

Marina N, Granowetter L, Grier HE, et al.: Age, tumor characteristics, and treatment regimen as event predictors in Ewing: a children's oncology group report, *Sarcoma* 2015:927123, 2015.

Miller BJ, Gao Y, Duchman KR: Does surgery or radiation provide the best overall survival in Ewing's sarcoma? a review of the National Cancer Database, *J Surg Oncol* 116(3):384, 2017.

Miller BJ, Lynch CF, Buckwalter JA: Conditional survival is greater than overall survival at diagnosis in patients with osteosarcoma and Ewing's sarcoma, *Clin Orthop Relat Res* 471:3398, 2013.

Ng VY, Jones R, Bompadre V, et al.: The effect of surgery with radiation on pelvic Ewing sarcoma survival, *J Surg Oncol* 112(8):861, 2015.

Puri A, Gulia A, Jambhekar NA, Laskar S: Results of surgical resection in pelvic Ewing's sarcoma, *J Surg Oncol* 106:417, 2012.

Raciborska A, Bilska K, Drabko K, et al.: Validation of a multi-modal treatment protocol for Ewing sarcoma—a report from the Polish pediatric oncology group, *Pediatr Blood Cancer* 61:2170, 2014.

Raciborska A, Bilska K, Rychlowska-Pruszynska M, et al.: Internal hemipelvectomy in the management of pelvic Ewing sarcoma—are outcomes better than with radiation therapy? *J Pediatr Surg* 49:1500, 2014.

Sari N, Togral G, Cetindag MF, et al.: Treatment results of the Ewing sarcoma of bone and prognostic factors, *Pediatr Blood Cancer* 54:19, 2010.

Tenneti P, Ahid U, Iftikhar A, et al.: Role of high-dose chemotherapy and autologous hematopoietic cell transplantation for children and young adults with relapsed Ewing's sarcoma: a systematic review, *Sarcoma* 2018:2640674, 2018.

Thévenin-Lemoine C, Destombes L, Vial J, et al.: Planning for bone excision in Ewing sarcoma: post-chemotherapy MRI more accurate than pre-chemotherapy MRI assessment, *J Bone Joint Surg Am* 100(1):13, 2018.

Thiel U, Wawer A, von Luettichau I, et al.: Bone marrow involvement identifies a subgroup of advanced Ewing sarcoma patients with fatal outcome irrespective of therapy in contrast to curable patients with multiple bone metastases but unaffected marrow, *Oncotarget* 7(43):70959, 2016.

Werier J, Yao X, Caudrelier JM, et al.: A systematic review of optimal treatment strategies for localized Ewing's sarcoma of bone after neoadjuvant chemotheraopy, *Surg Oncol* 25(1):16–23, 2016.

Whelan J, Le Deley MC, Dirksen U, et al.: High-dose chemotherapy and blood autologous stem-cell rescue compared with standard chemotheraopy in localized high-risk Ewing sarcoma: results of Euro-E.W.I.N.G.99 and Ewing-2008, *J Clin Oncol* JC0201882516, 2018.

Worch J, Matthay KK, Neuhaus J, et al.: Ethnic and racial differences in patients with Ewing sarcoma, *Cancer* 116:983, 2010.

CHORDOMA

Ahmed AT, Abdel-Rahman O, Morsy M, et al.: Management of sacrococcygeal chordoma: a systematic review and meta-analysis of observational studies, *Spine* 43(19):e1157, 2018.

Ailon T, Torabi R, Fisher CG, et al.: Management of locally recurrent chordoma of the mobile spine and sacrum: a systematic review, *Spine* 41(Suppl 20):S193, 2016.

Angelini A, Pala E, Calabró T, et al.: Prognostic factors in surgical resection of sacral chordoma, *J Surg Oncol* 112(4):344, 2015.

Asavamongkolkul A, Waikakul S: Wide resection of sacral chordoma via a posterior approach, *Int Orthop* 36:607, 2012.

Bakker SH, Jacobs WCH, Pondaag W, et al.: Chordoma: a systematic review of the epidemiology and clinical prognostic factors predicting progression-free and overall survival, *Eur Spine J* 27(12):3043, 2018.

Carey K, Bestic J, Attia S, et al.: Diffuse skeletal muscle metastases from sacral chordoma, *Skeletal Radiol* 43:985, 2014.

Chen KW, Yang HL, Lu J, et al.: Prognostic factors of sacral chordoma after surgical therapy: a study of 36 patients, *Spinal Cord* 48:166, 2010.

Colangeli S, Muratori F, Bttini L, et al.: Surgical treatment of sacral chordoma: en bloc resection with negative margins is a determinant of the long-term outcome, *Surg Technol Int* 33:343, 2018.

D'Amore T, Boyce B, Mesfin A: Chordoma of the mobile spine and sacrum: clinical management and prognosis, *J Spine Sug* 4(3):546, 2018.

De Amorim Berstein K, DeLaney T: Chordomas and chondrosarcomas: the role of radiation therapy, *J Surg Oncol* 114(5):564, 2016.

Denaro L, Berton A, Ciuffreda M, et al.: Surgical management of chordoma: a systematic review, *J Spinal Cord Med Jul* 26:1, 2018.

Ferraresi V, Nuzzo C, Zoccali C, et al.: Chordoma: clinical characteristics, management, and prognosis of a case series of 25 patients, *BMC Cancer* 10:22, 2010.

Frezza AM, Botta L, Trama A, RARECARE Working Group, et al.: Chordoma: update on disease, epidemiology, biology and medical therapies, *Curr Opin Oncol* 31(2):114, 2019.

Gokaslan ZL, Zadnik PL, Sciubba DM, et al.: Mobile spine chordoma: results of 166 patients from the AO spine knowledge forum tumor database, *J Neurosurg Spine* 24(4):644, 2016.

Holliday EB, Mitra HS, Somerson JS, et al.: Postoperative proton therapy for chordomas and chondrosarcomas of the Spine: adjuvant versus salvage radiation therapy, *Spine* 40(8):544, 2015.

Housari G, González M, Calero P, et al.: Sacral chordoma: management of a rare disease in a tertiary hospital, *Clin Transl Oncol* 15:327, 2013.

Jawaed MU, Scully SP: Surgery significantly improves survival in patients with chordoma, *Spine* 35:117, 2010.

Ji T, Guo W, Yang R, et al.: What are the conditonal surgical and functional outcomes after surgical treatment of 115 patients with sacral chordoma? *Clin Orthop Relat Res* 475(3):620, 2017.

Kayani B, Hanna SA, Sewell MD, et al.: A review of the surgical management of sacral chordoma, *Eur J Surg Oncol* 40:1412, 2014.

Kayani B, Sewell MD, Tan KA, et al.: Prognostic factors in the operative management of sacral chordomas, *World Neurosurg* 84(5):1354, 2015.

Lau CS, Mahendraraj K, Ward A, Chamberlain RS: Pediatric chordomas: a population-based clinical outcome study involving 86 patients from the Surveillance, Epidemiology, and End Result (SEER) database (1973-2011), *Pediatr Neursurg* 51(3):127, 2016.

Lee IJ, Lee RJ, Fahim DK: Prognostic factors and survival outcome in patients with chordoma in the United States: a population-based analysis, *World Neurosurg* 104:346, 2017.

Osaka S, Osaka E, Kojima T, et al.: Long-term outcome following surgical treatment of sacral chordoma, *J Surg Oncol* 109:184, 2014.

Ozger H, Eralp L, Sungur M, Atalar AC: Surgical management of sacral chordoma, *Acta Orthop Belg* 76:243, 2010.

Pillai S, Govender S: Sacral chordoma: a review of literature, *J Orthop* 15(2):679, 2018.

Radaelli S, Stacchiotti S, Ruggieri P, et al.: Sacral chordoma: long-term outcome of a large series of patients surgically treated at two reference centers, *Spine* 41(12):1049, 2016.

Rotondo RL, Folkert W, Liebsch NJ, et al.: High-dose proton-based radiation therapy in the management of spine chordomas: outcomes and clinicopathological prognostic factors, *J Neurosurg Spine* 23(6):788, 2015.

Ruosi C, Colella G, Di Donato SL, et al.: Surgical treatment of sacral chordoma: survival and prognostic factors, *Eur Spine J* 24(Suppl 7):912, 2015.

Stacchiotti S, Casali PG, Lo Vullo S, et al.: Chordoma of the mobile spine and sacrum: a retrospective analysis of a series of patients surgically treated at two referral centers, *Ann Surg Oncol* 17:211, 2010.

Stacchiotti S, Gronchi A, Fossati, et al.: Best practices for the management of local-regional recurrent chordoma: a position paper by the Chordoma Global Consensus Group, *Ann Oncol* 28(6):1230, 2017.

Tauziéde-Espariat A, Bresson D, Polivka M, et al.: Prognostic and therapeutic markers in chordomas: a study of 287 tumors, *J Neuropathol Ex Neurol* 75(2):111, 2016.

Tharmabala M, LaBrash D, Kanthan R: Acute cauda equina syndrome secondary to lumbar chordoma: case report and literature review, *Spine J* 13:e35, 2013.

Tsitouras V, Wang S, Dirks P, et al.: Management and outcome of chordomas in the pediatric population: the Hospital for Sick Children experience and review of the literature, *J Clin Neurosci* 34:169, 2016.

van Wullften Palthe O, Jee KW, Bramer JAM, et al.: What is the effect of high-dose radiation on bone in patients with sacral chordoma? A CT study, *Clin Orthop Relat Res* 476(3):520, 2018.

van Wullften Plathe ODR, Tromp I, Ferreira A, et al.: Sacral chordoma: a clinical review of 101 cases with 30-year experience in a single institution, *Spine J* 19(5):869, 2019.

Walcott BP, Nahed BV, Mohyeldin A, et al.: Chordoma: current concepts, management, and future directions, *Lancet Oncol* 13:e69, 2012.

Williams BJ, Raper DM, Godbout E, et al.: Diagnosis and treatment of chordoma, *J Natl Compr Canc Netw* 11:726, 2013.

Xie C, Whalley N, Adasonla K, et al.: Can local recurrence of a sacral chordoma be treated by further surgery? *Bone Joint J* 97-B(5):711, 2015.

Young VA, Curtis KM, Temple HT, et al.: Characteristics and patterns of metastatic disease from chordoma, *Sarcoma* 2015:517657, 2015.

Yu E, Koffer PP, DiPetrillo TA, Kinsella TJ: Incidence, treatment and survival patterns for sacral chordoma in the United States, 1974-2011, *Front Oncol* 6:203, 2016.

Zhong N, Yang X, Yang J, et al.: Surgical consideration for adolescents and young adults with cervical chordoma, *Spine* 42(10):E609, 2017.

Zou MX, LvGH, Wang XB, Li J: Prognostic factors in spinal chordoma: an update of current systematic review and meta-analysis, *J Surg oncol* 115(4):497, 2017.

Zhou J, Yang B, Wang X, Jing Z: Comparison of the effectiveness of radiotherapy with photons and particles for chordoma after surgery: a meta-analysis, *World Neurosurg* 117:46, 2018.

Zuckerman SL, Bilsky MH, Laufer I: Chordomas of the skull base, mobile spine, and sacrum: an epidemiologic investigation of presentation, treatment, and survival, *World Neurosurg* 113:e618, 2018.

ADAMANTINOMA

Angelini A, Mavrogenis AF, Gambarotti M, et al.: Surgical treatment and results of 62 patients with epithelioid hemangioendothelioma of bone, *J Surg Oncol* 109:791, 2014.

Errani C, Vanel D, Gambarotti M, et al.: Vascular bone tumors: a proposal of a classification based on clinicopathological, radiographic and genetic features, *Skeletal Radiol* 41:1495, 2012.

Hart JL, Edgar MA, Gardner JM: Vascular tumors of bone, *Semin Diagn Pathol* 31:30, 2014.

Houdek MT, Sherman CE, Inwards CY, et al.: Adamantinoma of bone: long-term follow-up of 46 consecutive patients, *J Surg Oncol* 118(7):1150, 2018.

Most MJ, Sim FH, Inwards CY: Osteofibrous dysplasia and adamantinoma, *J Am Acad Orthop Surg* 18:358, 2010.

Puchner SE, Varga R, Hobusch GM, et al.: Long-term outcome following treatment of adamantinoma and osteofibrous dysplasia of long bones, *Orthop Traumatol Surg Res* 102(7):925, 2016.

Scholfield DW, Dadozai Z, Ghali C, et al.: Does osteofibrous dysplasia progress to adamantinoma and how should they be treated? *Bone Joint J* 99-B(3):409, 2017.

Scott MT, Indelicato DJ, Morris CG, et al.: Radiation therapy for hemangioendothelioma: the University of Florida experience, *Am J Clin Oncol* 37:360, 2014.

Tharmabala M, Kandapur V, Senger JL, Kanthan R: Diagnostic pitfalls in tibial adamantinoma: two cases with a clinicopathological review, *Clin Pract* 1:3138, 2011.

Verbeke SL, Bovée JV: Primary vascular tumors of bone: spectrum of entities? *Int J Clin Exp Pathol* 14:541, 2011.

MALIGNANT VASCULAR TUMORS

Davis AT, Guo AM, Phillips NJ, Greenberg DD: A novel treatment for bone lesions of multifocal epithelioid sarcoma-like hemangioendothelioma, *Skeletal Radiol* 44(7):1013, 2015.

Kelahan LC, Sandhu FA, Sayah A: Multifocal hemangioendothelioma of the lumbar spine and response to surgical resection and radiations, *Spine J* 15(11):e49, 2015.

Saste A, Cabrera Fernandez DF, Gulati R, Gamalski S: A trimodality approach in the management of metastatic low-grade epithelioid hemangioendothelioma of bone, *BMJ Case Rep* 2015, July 16; 2015, bcr2015210196.

Schenker K, Blumer S, Jaramillo D, et al.: Epithelioid hemangioma of bone: radiological and magnetic resonance imaging characteristics with histopathological correlation, *Pediatr Radiol* 47(12):1631, 2017.

Scorletti F, Hammill A, Patel M, et al.: Malignant tumors misdiagnosed as benign vascular anomalies, *Pediatr Blood Cancer* 65(7):e27051, 2018.

Shen CJ, Parzuchowski AS, Kummerlowe MN, et al.: Combined modality therapy improves overall survival for angiosarcoma, *Acta Oncol* 56(9):1235, 2017.

Terrando S, Sambri A, Bianchi G, et al.: Angiosarcoma around total hip arthroplasty: case series and review of the literature, *Musculoskelet Surg* 102(1):21, 2018.

Van Ijzendoorn DGP, Bovée JVMG: Vascular tumors bone: the involvement of a classification based on molecular developments, *Surg Pathol Clin* 10(3):621, 2017.

Zhang H, Fu Y, Ye Z: Bone multicentric epithelioid hemangioendothelioma of the lower and upper extremities with pulmonary metastases: a case report, *Oncol Lett* 9(5):2177, 2015.

Zhu W, Feng B, Ma Q, et al.: Angiosarcoma around hip joint prosthesis, *Chin Med J* 29(21):2642, 2016.

MALIGNANT FIBROUS HISTIOCYTOMA AND FIBROSARCOMA

Koplas MC, Lefkowitz RA, Bauer TW, et al.: Imaging findings, prevalence and outcome of de novo and secondary malignant fibrous histiocytoma of bone, *Skeletal Radiol* 39:791, 2010.

Özkurt B, Başarir K, Yildiz YH, et al.: Primary malignant fibrous histiocytoma of long bones: long-term follow-up, *Eklem Hastalik Cerrahisi* 27(2):94, 2016.

PDQ Pediatric Treatment Editorial Board: Osteosarcoma and malignant fibrous histiocytoma of bone treatment (PDQ®): Health Professional version, PDQ Cancer Information Summaries [Internet]. Bethesda MD; National Cancer Institute (US); 2002-2018 Nov 12.

MULTIPLE MYELOMA

Barzenje DA, Kolstad A, Ghanima W, Holte H: Long-term outcome of patients with solitary plasmacytoma treated with radiotherapy: a populaton-based, single-center study with median follow-up of 13.7 years, *Hematol Oncol* 36(1):217, 2018.

Chafey DH, Lewis VO, Satcher RL, et al.: Is cephalomedullary nail durable treatment for patients with metastatic peritrochanteric disease? *Clin Orthop Relat Res* 476(12):2392, 2018.

Ferraro R, Agarwal A, Martin-Macintosh EL, et al.: MR imaging and PET/CT in diagnosis and management of multiple myeloma, *Radiographics* 35(2):438, 2015.

Fonseca R, Abouzaid S, Bonafede M, et al.: Trends in overall survival and costs of multiple myeloma, 2000-2014, *Leukemia* 31(9):1915, 2017.

Fotiou D, Dimopoulos MA, Kastritis E: How we manage patients with plasmacytomas, *Curr Hematol Malig Rep* 13(3):227, 2018.

Fujisawa M, Suehara Y, Kukumoto K, et al.: Changes in survival rate of multiple myeloma after the introduction of bortezomib: a single institutional experience over 20 years, *Ann Hematol* 95(1):63, 2016.

Goyal G, Bartley AC, Funni S, et al.: Treatment approaches and outcomes in plasmacytomas: analysis using a national dataset, *Leukemia* 32(6):1414, 2018.

Groot OQ, Ogink PT, Hansswen SJ, et al.: High risk of venous thromboembolism after surgery for long bone metastases: a retrospective study of 682 patients, *Clin Orthop Relat Res* 476(10):2052, 2018.

Hameed A, Brady JJ, Dowling P, et al.: Bone disease in multiple myeloma: pathophysiology and management, *Cancer Growth Metastasis* 7:33, 2014.

Menendez ME, Park KJ, Barnes CL: Early postoperative outcomes after total joint arthroplasty in patients with multiple myeloma, *J Arthroplasty* 31(8):1645, 2016.

Meyu Uj, Leitner C, Driessen C, et al.: Improved survival of older patients with multiple myeloma in the era of novel agents, *Hematol Oncol* 34(4):217, 2016.

Mhaskar R, Djulbegovic B: Bisphosphonates for patients diagnosed with multiple myeloma, *JAMA* 320(14), 2018.

Navarro SM, Matcuk GR, Patel DB: Musculoskeletal imaging findings of hematologic malignancies, *Radiographics* 37(3):881, 2017.

Ohana N, Rouvio O, Nailbandyan K, et al.: Classification of solitary plasmacytoma. is it more intricate than presently suggested? A commentary, *J Cancer* 9(21):3894, 2018.

Papamerkouriou YM, Kenanidis E, Gamie Z, et al.: Treatment of multiple myeloma bone disease: experimental and clinical data, *Expert Opin Biol Ther* 15(2):213, 2015.

Park KJ, Menendez ME, Mears SC, Barnes CL: Patients with multiple myeloma have more complications after surgical treatment of hip fractures, *Geriatr Orthop Surg Rehabil* 7(3):158, 2016.

Rajkumar SV: Multiple myeloma: 2016 update on diagnosis, risk stratification, and management, *Am J Hematol* 91(7):719, 2016.

Sakellariou VI, Mavrogenis AF, Savvidou O, et al.: Reconstruction of multiple myeloma lesions around the pelvis and acetabulum, *Eur J Orthop Surg Traumatol* 25:643, 2015.

Rasche L, Anguaco EJ, Alpe TL, et al.: The presence of large focal lesions is a stong independent prognostic factor in multiple myeloma, *Blood* 132(1):59, 2018.

Shen J, Du X, Zhao L, et al.: Comparative analysis of the surgical treatment results for multiple myeloma bone disease of the spine and the long bone/soft tissue, *Oncol Lett* 15(6):10017, 2018.

Surgeon's Committee of the Chinese Myeloma Working Group of the International Myeloma Foundation: Consensus on surgical management of myeloma bone disease, *Orthop Surg* 8(3):263, 2016.

Terpos E, Berenson J, Cook RJ, et al.: Prognostic variables for survival and skeletal complications in patients with multiple myeloma osteolytic bone disease, *Leukemia* 24:1043, 2010.

Tsang RW, Campbell BA, Goda JS, et al.: Radiation therapy for solitary plasmacytoma and multiple myeloma: guidelines from the international lymphoma radiation oncology group, *Int J Radiat Oncol Biol Physc* 101(4):794, 2018.

Wildes TM, Rosko A, Tuchman SA: Multiple myeloma in the older adult: better prospects, more challenges, *J Clin Oncol* 32:2531, 2014.

LYMPHOMA

Alencar A, Pitcher D, Byrne G, Lossos IS: Primary bone lymphoma—the University of Miami experience, *Leuk Lymphoma* 51:39, 2010.

Bhristie D, Dear K, Le T, et al.: Limited chemotherapy and shrinking field radiotherapy for osteolymphoma (primary bone lymphoma): results from the Trans-Tasman Radiation Oncology Group 99.04 and Australian Leukaemia and Lymphoma Group LY02 prospective trial, *Int J Radiat Oncol Biol Phys* 80:1164, 2010.

Chisholm KM, Ohgami RS, Tan B, et al.: Primary lymphoma of bone in the pediatric and young adult population, *Hum Pathol* 60:1, 2017.

Hayase E, Kurosawa M, Suzuki H, et al.: Primary bone lymphoma: a clinical analysis of 17 patients in a single institution, *Acta Haematol* 134(2):80, 2015.

Ibrahim I, Haughom BD, Fillingham Y, Gitelis S: Is radiation necessary for treatment of non-Hodgkin's lymphoma of bone? Clinical results with contemporary therapy, *Clin Orthop Relat Res* 473:719, 2016.

Messina C, Christie D, Zucca E, et al.: Primary and secondary bone lymphomas, *Cancer Treat Rev* 41(3):235, 2015.

Milks KS, McLean TW, Anthony EY: Imaging of primary pediatric lymphoma of bone, *Pediatr Radiol* 46(8):1150, 2016.

Murphey MD, Kransdorf MJ: Primary musculoskeletal lymphoma, *Radiol Clin North Am* 54(4):785, 2016.

Pilorge S, Harel S, Ribrag V, et al.: Primary bone diffuse large B-cell lymphoma: a retrospective evaluation on 76 cases from French institutional and LYSA studies, *Leuk Lymphoma* 57(12):2820, 2016.

Tao R, Allen PK, Rodriguez A, et al.: Benefit of consolidative radiation therapy for primary bone diffuse large B-cell lymphoma, *Int J Radiat Oncol Biol Phys* 92(1):122, 2015.

Wang LJ, Wu HB, Wang M, et al.: Utility of F-18 FDG PET/CT on the evaluation of primary bone lymphoma, *Eur J Radiol* 84(11):2275, 2015.

Jawad MU, Schneiderbauer MM, Min ES, et al.: Primary lymphoma of bone in adult patients, *Cancer* 116:871, 2010.

Steffner RJ, Jang ES, Danford NC: Lymphoma of bone, *JBJS Ref* 6(1):e1, 2018.

Zhang X, Zhu J, Song Y, et al.: Clinical characterization and outcome of primary bone lymphoma: a retrospective study of 61 chinese patients, *Sci Rep* 6:28834, 2016.

METASTATIC CARCINOMA

Ahmad I, Ahmed MM, Ahsraf NF, et al.: Pain management in metastatic bone disease: a literature review, *Cureus* 10(9):e3286, 2018.

Angelini A, Trovarelli G, Berizzi A, et al.: Treatment of pathologic fractures of the proximal femur, *Injury* 49(Suppl 3):S77, 2018.

Biermann JS, Holt GE, Lewis VO, et al.: Metastatic bone disease: diagnosis, evaluation, and treatment, *Instr Course Lect* 59:593, 2010.

Creek AT, Ratner DA, Porter SE: Evaluation and treatment of extremity metastatic disease, *Cancer Treat Res* 162:151, 2014.

Durfee RA, Sabo SA, Letson GD, et al.: Percutaneous acetabuloplasty for metastatic lesions to the pelvis, *Orthopedics* 40(1):3170, 2017.

Filippiadis D, Mavrogenis AF, Mazioti A, et al.: Metastatic bone disease from breast cancer: a review of minimally invasive techniques for diagnosis and treatment, *Eur J Orthop Surg Traumatol* 27(6):729, 2017.

Forsberg JA, Wedin R, Boland PJ, Healey JH: Can we estimate short-and intermediate- term survival in patients undergoing surgery for metastatic bone disease? *Clin Orthop Relat Res* 475(4):1252, 2017.

Fottner A, Szalantzy M, Wirthmann L, et al.: Bone metastases from renal cell carcinoma patient survival after surgical treatment, *BMC Musculoskelet Disord* 11:145, 2010.

Gardner CS, Ensor JE, Ahrar K, et al.: Cryoablation of bone metastases from renal cell carcinoma for local tumor control, *J Bone Joint Surg Am* 99(22):1916, 2017.

Hattori H, Mibe J, Yamamoto K: Modular megaprosthesis in metastatic bone disease of the femur, *Orthopedics* 34:3871, 2011.

Hettwer WH, Horstmann PF, Hovgaard TB, et al.: Low infection rate after tumor hip arthroplasty for metastatic bone disease in a cohort treated with extended antibiotic prophylaxis, *Adv Orthop* 2015:428985, 2015.

Higuchi T, Yamamoto N, Hayashi K, et al.: Long-term patient survival after the surgical treatment of bone and soft-tissue metastases from renal cell carcinoma, *Bone Joint J* 100-B(9):1241, 2018.

Hosaka S, Katagiri H, Niwakawa M, et al.: Radiotherapy combined with zoledronate can reduce skeletal-related events in renal cell carcinoma patients with bone metastasis, *Int J Clin Oncol* 23(6):1127, 2018.

Hovgaard TB, Horstmann PF, Petersen MM, Sørensen MS: Patient survival following joint replacement due to metastatic bone disease – comparison of overall patient and prostheses survival between cohorts treated in two different time-periods, *Acta Oncol* 57(6):839, 2018.

Howard EL, Shepherd KL, Cribb G, Cool P: The validity of the Mirels score for predicting impending pathological fractures of the lower limb, *Bone Joint J* 100-B(8):1100, 2018.

Hwang N, Nandra R, Grimer R, et al.: Massive endoprosthetic replacement for bone metastases resulting from renal cell carcinoma: factors influencing patient survival, *Eur J Surg Oncol* 40:429, 2014.

Jernigan EW, Tennant JN, Esther RJ: Not all patients undergoing stabilization of impending pathologic fractures for renal cell carcinoma metastases to the femur need preoperative embolization, *Clin Orthop Relat Res* 476(3):528, 2018.

Johnson CN, Gurich Jr RW, Pavey GJ, Thompson MJ: Contemporary management of appendicular skeletal metastasis by primary tumor type, *J Am Acad Orthop Surg* 27(10):345, 2019.

Kendal JK, Abbott A, Kooner S, et al.: A scoping review on the surgical management of metastatic bone disease of the extremities, *BMC Musculoskelt Disord* 19(1):279, 2018.

Kim YI, Kang HG, Kim JH, et al.: Closed intramedullary nailing with percutaneous cement augmentation for long bone metastases, *Bone Joint J* 98-B(5):703, 2016.

Kimura T: Multidisciplinary approach for bone metastasis: a review, *Cancers (Basel)* 10(6):E156, 2018.

Kirkinis MN, Lyne CJ, Wilson MD, Choong PF: Metastatic bone disease: a review of survival, prognostic factors and outcomes following surgical treatment of the appendicular skeleton, *Eur J Surg Oncol* 42(12):1787, 2016.

Kotian RN, Puvanesarajah V, Rao S, et al.: Predictors of survival after intramedullary nail fixation of completed or impending pathologic femur fractures from metastatic disease, *Surg Oncol* 27(3):462, 2018.

Lipton A, Cook R, Brown J, et al.: Skeletal-related events and clinical outcomes in patients with bone metastases and normal levels of osteolysis: exploratory analyses, *Clin Oncol (R Coll Radiol)* 25:217, 2013.

Laitinen M, Parry M, Ratasvuori M, Wedin R, et al.: Survival and complications of skeletal reconstructions after surgical treatment of bony metastatic renal cell carcinoma, *Eur J Surg Oncol* 41(7):886, 2015.

Macedo F, Ladeira K, Pinho F, et al.: Bone metastases: an overview, *Oncol Rev* 11(1):321, 2017.

Mac Niocaill RF, Quinlan JF, Stapleton RD, et al.: Inter and intra-observer variability associated with the use of the Mirels' scoring system for metastatic bone lesions, *Int Orthop* 35:83–86, 2011.

Miller BJ, Soni EE, Gibbs CP, Scarborough MT: Intramedullary nails for long bone metastases: why do they fail? *Orthopedics* 34, 2011. https://doi.org/10.3928/01477447-20110228-12.

Müller DA, Capanna R: The surgical treatment of pelvic bone metastases, *Adv Orthop* 2015:525363, 2015.

Nooh A, Goulding K, Isler MH, et al.: Early improvement in pain and functional outcome but not quality of life after surgery for metastatic long bone disease, *Clin Orthop Relat Res* 476(3):535, 2018.

Piccioli A, Maccauro G, Rossi B, et al.: Surgical treatment of pathologic fractures of the humerus, *Injury* 41:1112, 2010.

Piccioli A, Maccauro G, Spinelli MS, et al.: Bone metastases of unknown origin: epidemiology and principles of management, *J Orthop Traumatol* 16(2):81, 2015.

Price SL, Farukhi MA, Jones KB, et al.: Complications of cemented long-stem hip arthroplasty in metastatic bone disease revisited, *Clin Orthop Relat Res* 471:3303, 2013.

Quinn RH, Randall RL, Benevenia J, et al.: Contemporary management of metastatic bone disease: tips and tools of the trade for general practitioners, *Instr Course Lect* 63:431, 2014.

Raphael B, Hwang S, Lefkowitz RA, et al.: Biopsy of suspicious bone lesions in patients with a single know malignancy: prevalence of a secondary malignancy, *AJR Am J Roentgenol* 201:1309, 2013.

Scolaro JA, Lackman RD: Surgical management of metastatic long bone fractures: principles and techniques, *J Am Acad Orthop Surg* 22:90, 2014.

Scott E, Klement MR, Brigman BE, Eward WC: Beyond mirels: factors influencing surgical outcome of metastasis to the extremities in the modern era, *J Surg Orthop Adv* 27(3):178, 2018.

Sevelda F, Waldstein W, Panotopoulos J, et al.: Is total femur replacement a realiable treatment option for patients with metastatic carcinoma of the femur? *Clin Orthop Relat Res* 475(5):977, 2018.

Shepherd KL, Cool P, Cribb G: Prognostic indicators of outcome for patients with skeletal metastases from carcinoma of the prostate, *Bone Joint J* 100-B(12):1647, 2018.

Sørensen MS, Gerds TA, Hindsø K, Petersen MM: External validation and optimization of the SPRING model for prediction of survival after surgical treatment of bone metastases of the extremities, *Clin Orthop Relat Res* 476(8):1591, 2018.

Sørensen MS, Gerds TA, Hindsø K, Petersen MM: Prediction of survival after surgery due to skeletal metastases in the extremities, *Bone Joint J* 98-B(2):271, 2016.

Stevenson JD, McNair M, Cribb GL, Cool WP: Perognostic factors for patients with skeletal metastases from carcinoma of the breast, *Bone Joint J* 98-B(2):266, 2016.

van der Vliet QM, Paulino Pereira NR, Janssen SJ, et al.: What factors are associated with quality of life, pain interference, anxiety and depression in patients with metastatic bone disease? *Clin Orthop Relat Res* 475(2):498, 2017.

Vermesan D, Prejbeanu R, Haragus H, et al: Case series of patients with pathological diaphyseal fractures from metastatic bone disease, *Int Orthop* 41(10):2199, 2017.

Weber K: Metastatic carcinoma and orthopedists, *Orthopedics* 36:454, 2013.

Wisanuyotin T, Sirichativapee W, Sumnanoont C, et al.: Prognostic and risk factors in patients with metastatic bone disease of the upper extremity, *J Bone Oncol* 13:71, 2018.

Wolanczyk MJ, Fakhrian K, Adamietz IA: Radiotherapy, bisphosphonates and surgical stabilization of complete or impending pathologic fractures in patients with metastatic bone disease, *J Cancer* 7(1):121, 2016.

The complete list of references is available online at Expert Consult.com.

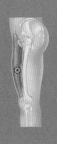

CHAPTER 11

SOFT-TISSUE TUMORS

Patrick C. Toy, Robert K. Heck Jr.

The evaluation of patients with musculoskeletal neoplasms was discussed in detail in other chapter, but certain points warrant repetition and elaboration. In contrast to bone tumors, the presence or absence of pain does not help to distinguish benign from malignant soft-tissue tumors because most patients with soft-tissue malignancies have minimal pain and consult a physician because of the presence of a mass. The mass, typically, is not invasive and grows in a centripetal fashion, pushing normal anatomic structures away. Careful physical examination of the mass, the involved part, and the lymph nodes draining the area is necessary. Standard radiographs provide little useful information about soft-tissue tumors but may show phleboliths (hemangiomas), calcification (synovial sarcoma), or fat-density radiolucencies (lipomas). Magnetic resonance imaging (MRI) may suggest a specific diagnosis in certain cases, such as lipoma, hemangioma, and pigmented villonodular synovitis. MRI should be obtained for all soft-tissue masses that are greater than 5 cm and/or deep to the fascia. More often, MRI characteristics are nonspecific, but MRI is useful in evaluating the size and anatomic relationships of the tumor. Soft-tissue sarcomas generally demonstrate low-signal intensity on T1-weighted images and high-signal intensity on T2-weighted images. Computed tomography (CT) can also be used for this purpose when a patient is unable to undergo MRI, but MRI is a superior imaging study in this circumstance. CT may help elucidate patterns of mineralization (i.e., calcification vs. ossification) found within the mass. Technetium bone scans or positron emission tomography (PET) scans do not usually provide significant benefit in the evaluation of the soft-tissue mass but may be useful in select cases to assess local and distant bone involvement (Fig. 11.1). For patients with malignant soft-tissue tumors, a CT scan of the lungs should be obtained to look for metastases (Fig. 11.2). Abdominal and pelvic CT scans are useful to detect retroperitoneal metastases in patients with myxoid liposarcomas and lymphatic spread in such lesions as synovial sarcoma, epithelioid sarcoma, and rhabdomyosarcoma. Biopsy is often required to establish the diagnosis and can be performed by core needle biopsy or by open incisional biopsy. Tissue sampling should be delayed until imaging studies are completed (biopsy will alter the study) and should be planned carefully according to the principles outlined in other chapter. Interpretation of the biopsy results may be facilitated by correlation with the clinical and imaging data. Staging can be performed using the Enneking system (see Table 7.1) or the American Joint Committee on Cancer system (see Table 7.2). Most soft-tissue tumors are initially sampled with core needle biopsy or fine needle aspiration. The resulting small sample may present a challenge in making an accurate diagnosis. Pathologists examine the characteristic architectural, stromal, and vascular features in an attempt to establish the specific diagnosis. Distinguishing benign from malignant tumors is critical when planning surgical excision and the desired margin (i.e., marginal or wide excision). Histologic grade also plays an important role in deciding adjuvant treatments such as radiation and/or chemotherapy.

Most benign soft-tissue tumors can be treated by observation or marginal resection. Observation is a feasible option when the imaging and clinical characteristics are strongly suggestive of a benign diagnosis. Some benign soft-tissue tumors can be locally aggressive (e.g., desmoid tumors) and may require wide resection or multimodal management for local control. Low-grade soft-tissue sarcomas are usually treated with wide resection alone or resection combined with radiation if margins are close. High-grade soft-tissue sarcomas are usually treated with combined surgery and radiation.

Several controversies exist regarding the management of soft-tissue sarcomas. Although surgery remains the primary treatment of these tumors, controversy still exists about which patients would benefit from the addition of radiation treatment for local control. It is also debatable as to whether the radiation is best delivered preoperatively or postoperatively. Preoperative irradiation is associated with an increased risk of wound-healing complications after surgery but may be more effective because of the available oxygenation in the virgin tissues. However, postoperative radiation can be done after the surgical wound has healed but requires an increased exposure area to ensure adequate coverage. Brachytherapy (radioactive seeds or sources placed in or near the tumor itself, giving a high radiation dose to the tumor while reducing the radiation exposure in the surrounding healthy tissues) is used extensively at some institutions but only rarely at others. Finally, the use of chemotherapy as adjuvant treatment for these patients continues to spark debate. Although chemotherapy protocols are in place at most cancer centers for adjuvant treatment of large, high-grade soft-tissue sarcomas, it is still unclear which patients actually benefit from this treatment.

In-depth discussion of these controversial issues is beyond the scope of this text. This chapter briefly describes the clinical presentation, imaging findings, and treatment options for some common soft-tissue tumors.

BENIGN TUMORS AND TUMOR-LIKE LESIONS (TABLE 11.1)
FATTY TUMORS

Lipomas are probably the most common benign tumors of connective tissue, resulting in clinicians often presuming malignant tumors to be benign lipomas. Although rare in children, they can occur at any age and in either sex, but are slightly more common in men than women. The true incidence of lipomas is likely underestimated because of the lack of medical attention secondary to an absence of symptoms. These tumors usually develop subcutaneously but may involve the deeper structures. They occasionally affect the synovium (lipoma arborescens) and rarely the periosteum. Clinically, they are soft, circumscribed, movable masses that are painless and slow growing. A knee effusion is characteristically the presenting complaint in patients with lipoma arborescens. On radiographs, large masses appear as discrete radiolucent areas within soft tissue, known as the "Bufalini sign." MRI usually provides a definitive diagnosis because lipomas are uniformly bright on T1-weighted images and are dark on fat-suppressed sequences like the surrounding subcutaneous tissue (Fig. 11.3). Lipomas can be defined as determinate because MRI characteristics allow diagnosis and preclude tissue sampling before treatment. The presence of heterogeneous signal intensity, absence of isointense signal with surrounding subcutaneous tissue, and necrosis are features that may suggest consideration of other diagnoses. Grossly, a lipoma is a well-encapsulated nodule of fat that may contain fibrous tissue. Microscopically, it is composed of mature fat cells with flattened nuclei, and mitotic activity is absent (Fig. 11.4). Some lipomas have a prominent vascular pattern and are appropriately referred to as angiolipomas. Angiolipomas are sometimes associated with pain. Focal areas with finely vacuolated cells of the brown fat type may be seen.

Occasionally, lipomas are multifocal, and in rare instances they are symmetric. A variant of multiple lipomatosis is Dercum disease, which is characterized by painful fatty infiltrations; the cause of the pain is poorly understood. Another variant of lipoma occurs in muscle and infiltrates between the muscle fibers; this apparent invasion may suggest malignancy, but usually the tumor is easily controlled. Still another variant is the rare hibernoma, or fetal fat cell lipoma. It is composed of large, finely vacuolated foam cells, is lobulated, and simulates the hibernating organs of some animals. It has a distinctive brown appearance and may become quite large. Angiomyolipoma is a type of lipoma usually found in the kidney. It is composed of smooth muscle, blood vessels, and fat. This tumor is occasionally

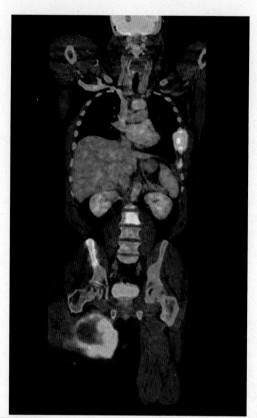

FIGURE 11.1 PET scan shows sarcoma in right thigh of a patient with metastatic disease.

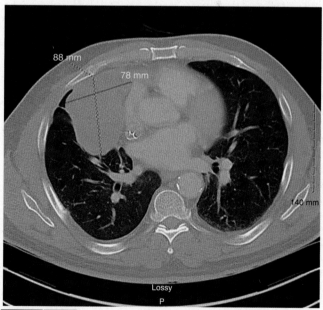

FIGURE 11.2 Axial CT of lungs shows mass in right lung field consistent with metastatic disease from a soft-tissue tumor.

associated with changes of tuberous sclerosis in the brain. A fatty tumor known as myelolipoma, containing bone marrow elements, may occur within the adrenal medulla. As an incidental finding at autopsy, this tumor is not rare but only occasionally becomes large enough to be of clinical significance. Rarely, a similar tumor may be found in the presacral region or the mediastinum. Lipoblastomatosis, another

TABLE 11.1

Benign Soft-Tissue Tumors

TUMOR	AGE	DEMOGRAPHICS	SITE	PRESENTATION	IMAGING	HISTOLOGY	TREATMENT	COMMENTS
FATTY TUMORS								
Lipoma	Any age; more common in adults, rare in children	Male = female	Any Most often subcutaneous	Painless mass Lipoma arborescens: knee effusion	MRI: homogeneous and isointense to host subcutaneous tissue	Mature adipocytes	Observation Marginal excision: recurrence rare	Dercum disease: multiple painful fatty infiltration Hibernoma: fetal fat cell lipoma (brown fat)
NERVE SHEATH TUMORS								
Neurilemmoma (schwannoma)	Usually adults	Male-female 40:60	Any	Usually painless mass Referred pain in distribution of involved nerve. May have symptoms associated with nerve compression Positive Tinel sign.	MRI: fusiform mass along course of nerve Split fat sign: rims of fat around tumor. Target sign: relatively decreased T2 signal in central portion with increased T2 signal peripherally	Biphasic tissue Antoni A— palisading spindle cells Antoni B— hypocellular loose myxomatous tissue Verocay bodies	Observation if asymptomatic Marginal excision with nerve sparing	S-100 positive in nuclear and cytoplasmic staining Malignant degeneration rare
Neurofibroma	Any age	Male = female	Any cranial or spinal peripheral nerve	Varies depending on involvement Cutaneous: localized nodule Diffuse: infiltrative mass Localized: solitary mass Plexiform: multiple fascicles involved: "bag of worms"	Similar to schwannoma Target sign: peripheral T2 hyperintensity	Hypocellular with disorganized bundles of collagen Spindle cells with wavy nuclei Rare mitotic figures	Local excision: sacrifices function of host nerve if tumor cannot be separated from nerve	Neurofibroma: von Recklinghausen disease (NF1) Autosomal dominant: mutation in *NF1* gene; chromosome 17q Other manifestations: cafe-au-lait spots, axillary freckling, Lisch nodules, optic gliomas, pheochromocytoma Osseous lesions: tibial pseudarthrosis, scoliosis, sphenoid wing dysplasia Small risk of degeneration to MPNST

Continued

TABLE 11.1

Benign Soft-Tissue Tumors—cont'd

TUMOR	AGE	DEMOGRAPHICS	SITE	PRESENTATION	IMAGING	HISTOLOGY	TREATMENT	COMMENTS
SYNOVIAL LESIONS								
Synovial chondromatosis	Adults	Male predominance	Hip and knee most common Hand, wrist, elbow, shoulder less common	Mechanical symptoms in joint due to loose bodies Limited range of motion Effusion	Plain radiographs: small calcified intraarticular nodules Advanced disease shows periarticular bone erosion and extension into soft tissues	Nodules of moderately cellular hyaline cartilage	Observation if asymptomatic Arthroscopic or open synovectomy; recurrence more common with arthroscopic synovectomy	Differential diagnosis includes myositis ossificans, synovial chondrosarcoma, synovial sarcoma
Giant cell tumor of tendon sheath	Adults		Hand, wrist	Slowly enlarging painless mass	Plain radiographs may show erosion of adjacent cortex	Similar to PVNS	Observation; Marginal excision	Second most common benign soft-tissue mass of hand and wrist
Pigmented villonodular synovitis	Young adults most common May be seen in children and elderly		Knee most common, but other joints possible	Diffuse type: monarticular pain and swelling Localized form: may cause mechanical symptoms Aspiration yields blood-tinged fluid	Plain radiographs may show periarticular erosions in advanced stages MRI: intraarticular mass hypointense on both T1- and T2-weighted sequences	Bland fibrous tissue containing histiocytes, giant cells, and hemosiderin	Localized form: local excision Diffuse form: arthroscopic or open synovectomy, arthroplasty, arthrodesis, amputation	External beam radiation may be considered in patients with recurrent disease
VASCULAR LESIONS								
Hemangioma (intramuscular)	Children, any age	Male-female 1:2, intramuscular hemangioma	Any; head and neck most common	Painful episodes associated with warmth and swelling, increased with activity Size increases in dependent position	Plain radiographs may show phleboliths (chronic calcified thrombi) MRI: not well circumscribed; T1 weighting shows fatty replacement of muscle fibers; T2 hyperintensity secondary to blood-filled channels	Multiple thin-walled dilated vessels	Observation if asymptomatic Compression treatment if symptomatic Local excision if small Sclerotherapy or embolization if not resectable	Klippel-Trenaunay syndrome associated with venous-lymphatic malformations, varicosities, cutaneous nevus flammeus (port wine stain) and hypertrophy of bone and associated soft tissues Maffucci syndrome: enchondromatosis combined with hemangiomatosis

TABLE 11.1

Benign Soft-Tissue Tumors—cont'd

	Age	Gender	Location	Clinical	Imaging	Histology	Treatment	Associated/Notes
Glomus tumor (glomangioma)	Children and young adults	Solitary: F > M Multiple: M > F	Most common in hands and feet Any location where a glomus body is found	Blue-red lesion that causes pain out of proportion to its size	May be well-circumscribed lytic lesion in distal phalanx	Epithelial-appearing cells that lie outside of vessels	Marginal excision is curative	Glomus body regulated blood flow and temperature through autonomic control of smooth muscle in arterial wall

FIBROUS LESIONS

	Age	Gender	Location	Clinical	Imaging	Histology	Treatment	Associated/Notes
Nodular fasciitis	Young adults	Male = female	Most commonly extremities; upper extremity 50%-75% Flank and back	Rapidly expanding mass for several weeks	Radiographs usually normal MRI: not necessarily characteristic but mass is associated with fascia and extends into subcutaneous tissue (most common) or underlying muscle	Uniform, immature, spindled fibroblasts without atypia	Local excision is curative	
Desmoid tumors (aggressive fibromatosis)	Young adults	Female predominance	Abdominal wall: pregnant and postpartum women Intraabdominal: pelvis and mesentery Extraabdominal: shoulder girdle, chest wall, arms, thighs	Slow growth with invasion of contiguous structures	MRI: hypointensity on both T1- and T2-weighted images	Abundant collagen with sparse spindle cells; not well encapsulated; no atypia	Wide excision if possible Radiation therapy in unresectable locations Systemic modalities: NSAIDs, hormone therapy, low-dose chemotherapy	Dupuytren disease: fibromatosis of palmar aponeurosis Ledderhose disease: fibromatosis of plantar fascia Peyronie disease: growth of fibrous plaques in soft tissue of penis Gardner syndrome: desmoids tumors, skull osteomas, epidermal cysts, intestinal adenomatosis

MPNST, Malignant peripheral nerve sheath tumor; *MRI*, magnetic resonance images; *NSAID*, nonsteroidal antiinflammatory drug; *PVNS*, pigmented villonodular synovitis.

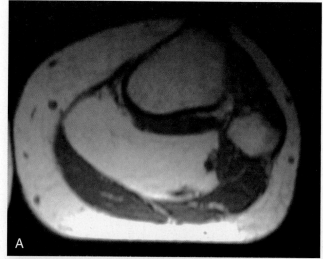

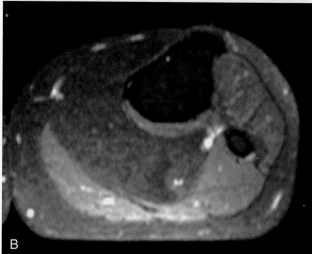

FIGURE 11.3 T1-weighted **(A)** and fat-suppressed **(B)** images of intramuscular lipomas in deep compartment of left leg. The magnetic resonance imaging signal of lipomas is identical to subcutaneous fat on all sequences.

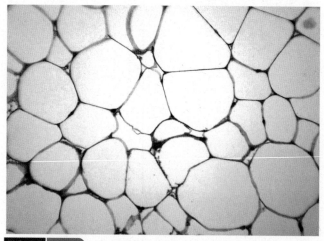

FIGURE 11.4 Lipoma. Photomicrograph shows mature adipocytes without aggressive features.

variant of lipoma, consists of embryonal fat and occurs more often in infants and young children. This tumor resembles some types of liposarcoma but has a distinct lobular pattern and no atypical nuclei. Chondroid lipoma contains tissue that resembles cartilage. It must be distinguished from liposarcoma and myxoid chondrosarcoma, which it superficially resembles.

Because there is almost no risk for malignant transformation, lipomas can be treated by observation. Marginal resection is considered in patients who have a mass that is clinically symptomatic or growing in size, and the decision for surgery should be individualized to each patient. Recurrence is rare. Some large lipomas must be studied carefully microscopically to avoid confusion with a well-differentiated lipoma-like liposarcoma; however, there is a large sampling error associated with large fatty tumors.

NERVE SHEATH TUMORS

Neurilemmoma (schwannoma) is typically a solitary encapsulated lesion that may be cystic when it is 3 to 4 cm in diameter. Any nerve may be involved, but it usually involves one of the larger peripheral nerves (Fig. 11.5); the sacral plexus or the sciatic nerve may be involved within the pelvis. Patients may report symptoms consistent with compression of associated nerve fascicles and a positive Tinel sign on physical examination. These findings are extremely rare in association with other soft-tissue masses except nerve sheath tumors. MRI often shows a fusiform mass along the course of a major peripheral nerve. The nerve may be visualized entering and exiting the mass on the coronal or sagittal MRI sequences. A "split fat sign" refers to a rim of fat that may be observed specifically on the T1-weighted MR image of schwannomas. A "target sign" is seen in approximately half of schwannomas and describes a relatively decreased T2 signal in the central portion of the mass with increased T2 signal peripherally (Fig. 11.6). This MRI finding suggests a benign diagnosis. However, MRI characteristics still remain nonspecific for this tumor. Microscopically, the tumor consists of two types of tissue: Antoni A and Antoni B. Antoni A tissue is more typical of the tumor and consists of compact collections of spindle cells that show marked palisading. Antoni B tissue is myxomatous and degenerative, and within it are cystic spaces and, often, thick-walled blood vessels. Verocay bodies are characteristically found in schwannomas and consist of an arrangement of two rows of palisading nuclei separated by fibrillary material (Fig. 11.7). Nuclear and cytoplasmic staining of the S-100 protein are not always required but help support the diagnosis. Often, the lesion simply spreads the nerve fibers apart without anatomical or functional interruption, allowing the tumor to be removed by careful blunt dissection after a longitudinal incision in the perineurium. There may be little, if any, dysfunction of the nerve after surgery. Occasionally, the tumor may recur, but usually the lesion or recurrent lesion can be removed without sacrificing numerous nerve fibers. Because the tumor grows without infiltrating the adjacent fascicles, excision that interrupts the continuity of the nerve should be avoided. Transient neurologic deficits occur on average in 32.4%, with a reported incidence ranging from 1.5% to 80%. Risk for neurologic injury increases with tumors larger than 3 cm, patient age of more than 50 years, and a longer history of symptoms. Malignant degeneration has been described but rarely occurs. Characteristics that suggest malignancy include size increase, peripheral enhancement pattern, peri-lesional soft-tissue edema, cystic change within the tumor, and increased uptake on fluorodeoxyglucose (FDG)-PET scan.

Neurofibroma is characterized by a much greater production of collagen than is neurilemmoma, and it, too, may occur as an isolated lesion (Fig. 11.8). It is much more likely than neurilemmoma to arise from a nerve branch too small to be identified, however. Neurofibromas also occur as a manifestation of von Recklinghausen disease (neurofibromatosis type 1), in which many such tumors may be found associated with *café-au-lait* spots and various other lesions (e.g., axillary/inguinal freckling, optic glioma, iris hamartomas). Most neurofibromas are found in individuals who do not have the *NF1* marker (gene

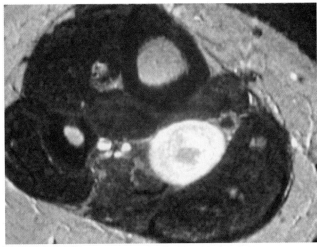

FIGURE 11.6 Target sign in axial MRI of schwannoma in posterior leg.

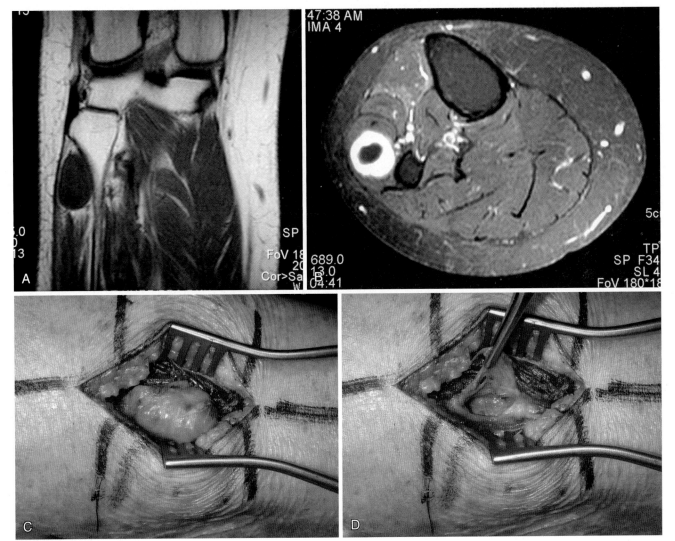

FIGURE 11.5 **A,** T1-weighted coronal magnetic resonance imaging shows a 3 cm fusiform mass along peroneal nerve. **B,** Contrast-enhanced, fat-suppressed axial image shows a high signal at the periphery of the lesion with a low signal in the center. The patient complained of pain radiating to the dorsum of the foot whenever she "bumped" the mass. All of these findings are typical of benign nerve sheath tumor. **C,** Intraoperative photograph shows neurilemmoma of the peroneal nerve. **D,** After incising the epineurium, the tumor was easily separated from the nerve fibers using blunt dissection.

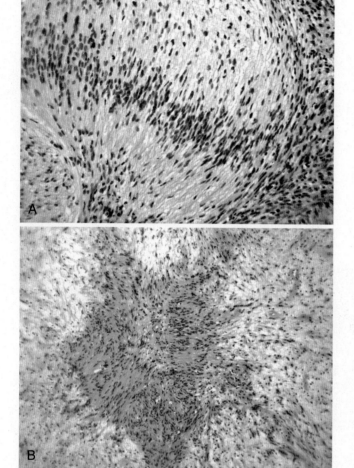

FIGURE 11.7   Neurilemmoma. Photomicrographs (H&E, ×20) show compact spindle cells with nuclear palisading **(A)** and Antoni A (compact collections of spindle cells with marked palisading) and Antoni B (loose myxomatous) patterns **(B)**.

SYNOVIAL LESIONS

Synovial chondromatosis is a benign, monarticular, synovial, proliferative disease in which cartilaginous or osteocartilaginous metaplasia occurs within the synovial membrane of joints, bursae, or tendon sheaths. The disease has been classified into three phases: (1) early, with synovial chondrometaplasia but no loose bodies; (2) transitional, with active synovial disease and loose bodies; and (3) late, with loose bodies but no synovial disease. Routine radiographs may show multiple loose bodies, and joint erosions may be present in late stages. MRI is often useful in establishing the diagnosis. Synovial chondromatosis is most common in the knee (70%) and hip, but almost any joint, bursa, or tendon sheath may be affected. This disease process predominantly affects males and occurs most commonly in the third to fifth decades of life. Pain and swelling are often the presenting symptoms, and mechanical symptoms from the loose bodies may develop slowly over years, necessitating surgical intervention. Treatment consists of arthroscopic or open synovectomy and removal of the loose bodies (Fig. 11.10). Recurrence after surgery is common, and there are rare reports of malignant transformation to chondrosarcoma. Histologically, synovial chondromatosis consists of moderately cellular hyaline cartilage arranged in nodules within the synovium (Fig. 11.11). Binucleate cells may be observed, and cells are usually crowded and clumped within the nodule.

Giant cell tumor of tendon sheath is a relatively common benign tumor usually involving the tendon sheaths of adult fingers (Fig. 11.12). It first appears as a slowly enlarging but painless mass. Occasionally, a radiograph shows bony erosion of adjacent cortices. The histology is characteristic, with foam cells (histiocytes), fibrous tissue, giant cells, and hemosiderin deposition similar to that seen in pigmented villonodular synovitis (Fig. 11.13). Treatment is by marginal excision, which may prove technically difficult in larger lesions. Recurrences are frequent if the excision is incomplete.

Pigmented villonodular synovitis may occur in a localized or diffuse form. The localized form is commonly referred to as focal nodular synovitis and is a solitary pedunculated lesion that is histologically identical to giant cell tumor of tendon sheath. The diffuse form also appears to be identical histologically to the localized form, but it involves the entire synovium of the affected joint. The diffuse form most commonly affects the knee, but the hip, ankle, shoulder, wrist, and other joints can be involved (Fig. 11.14). The patient usually presents with monarticular pain and swelling. Intraarticular lesions may cause mechanical symptoms, and a mass may be palpable. These non-specific symptoms may result in a delay in diagnosis. Aspiration of the joint characteristically reveals serosanguineous or blood-tinged fluid. Routine radiographs are often normal but may show bony erosion, especially if the hip is involved. MRI is frequently diagnostic, showing intraarticular masses that are dark on the T1-weighted and T2-weighted images. Additionally, the extent of the disease process may be further delineated with MRI. Goals of treatment include alleviation of symptoms, minimizing recurrence, and, ultimately, preservation of the joint.

located at chromosome 17q11.2). Sometimes, a neurofibroma occurs in which multiple fascicles of a peripheral nerve are involved; this is referred to as a "plexiform neurofibroma," and excising it completely may be impossible without sacrificing the nerve and its associated function. A patient presenting with a plexiform neurofibroma without a known history of neurofibromatosis should be evaluated for neurofibromatosis type 1. Other manifestations of neurofibromatosis include hypertrophy of soft tissue, including the skin; hypertrophy of bone; scoliosis; bone cysts; and other abnormalities. Microscopically, neurofibromas have low cellularity with disorganized bundles of collagen. The nuclei of the spindle-shaped cells are wavy, and mitotic figures are rare (Fig. 11.9). Because neurofibromas are difficult to separate from the host nerve, axons may be observed histologically within the tumor cells. Even though the risk of malignant degeneration is low, increased pain or change in the size of the mass should serve as warning signs of a possible malignant peripheral nerve sheath tumor.

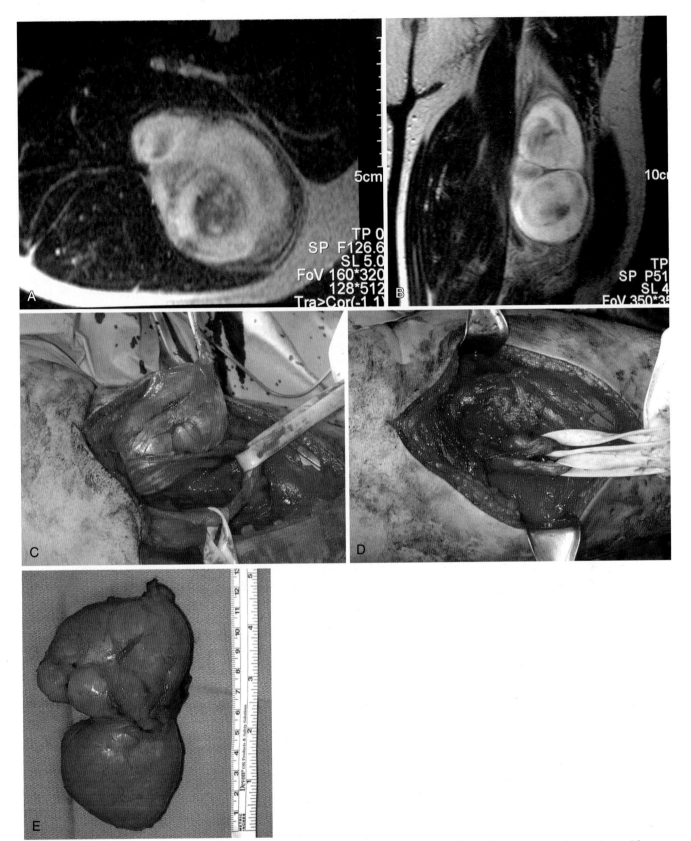

FIGURE 11.8 Axial (**A**) and coronal (**B**) magnetic resonance images show large tumor along the sciatic nerve in a patient with neurofibromatosis. Biopsy confirmed this to be a neurofibroma. **C,** After incising epineurium, nerve fibers were bluntly dissected away from tumor. **D,** Tumor has been removed with preservation of tibial and peroneal divisions of sciatic nerve. **E,** Photograph of specimen.

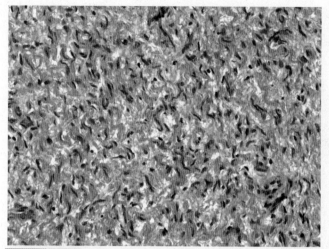

FIGURE 11.9 Neurofibroma. Photomicrograph (H&E, ×20) demonstrates disorganized bundles of collagen with wavy nuclei. Mucoid material separates the cells and collagen.

Recommended treatment for the localized form is marginal excision and for the diffuse form is total synovectomy. The localized form of PVNS often can be treated by arthroscopic excision, with reported recurrence rate of 0% to 8%. If there are significant secondary degenerative changes of the joint surfaces, arthroplasty should be strongly considered. Radiotherapy in the diffuse lesion may be justified if surgery fails to control the process.

VASCULAR LESIONS

Hemangiomas are common, and many types are present at birth. Their classification is currently unsatisfactory; the distinction between telangiectatic lesions, true neoplasms, and arteriovenous malformations is sometimes obscure.

The type of hemangioma composed of cellular masses of closely packed endothelial cells with many mitotic figures is often called a "strawberry hemangioma" or a "benign hemangioendothelioma." It is found at birth or shortly thereafter, is deep red, and may grow rapidly during the first few months of life. This type usually stops growing, however, and, in most

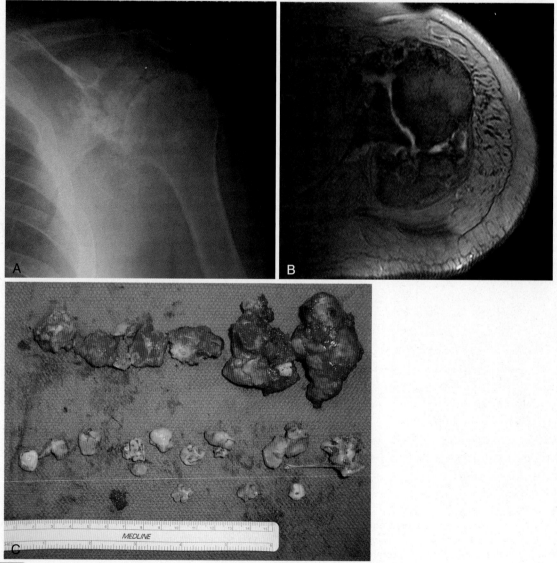

FIGURE 11.10 Anteroposterior radiograph **(A)** and axial MR image **(B)** of left shoulder of patient with synovial chondromatosis show multiple intraarticular ossified loose bodies and secondary degenerative changes. The patient underwent anterior and posterior synovectomy. **C,** Photograph of resected loose bodies.

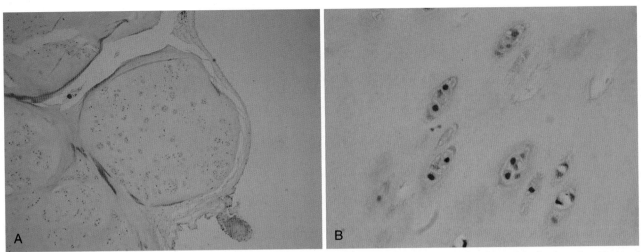

FIGURE 11.11 Synovial chondromatosis. **A,** Photomicrograph shows nodules of hypercellular cartilage within the synovium. **B,** Atypical cells are often seen in a clumped arrangement.

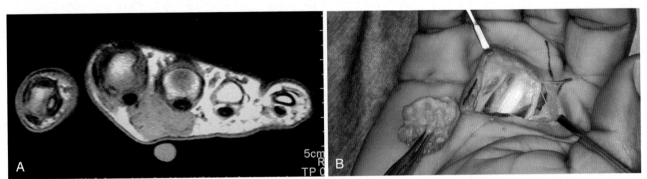

FIGURE 11.12 **A,** T1-weighted axial MR image shows mass in palm of right hand on flexor tendons of middle finger. **B,** Intraoperative photograph of giant cell tumor of tendon sheath.

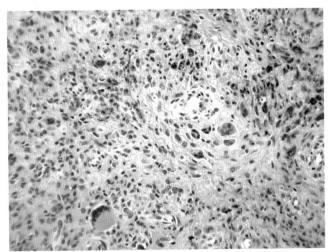

FIGURE 11.13 Pigmented villonodular synovitis. Photomicrograph (H&E, ×20) demonstrates bland polyhedral cells surrounded by collagen. Giant cells and hemosiderin are present.

instances, eventually disappears. Only occasionally does one require surgery. The port wine type often occurs on the face, neck, and upper trunk and is also present at birth. It grows at about the same rate as the patient but may become quite large. This lesion does not disappear spontaneously, and removal is quite difficult. Microscopically, it consists of thin-walled dilated vessels superficial in the skin.

Capillary hemangiomas consist of a network of newly formed capillaries. Cavernous hemangiomas consist of widely dilated vessels or thicker vessels that may resemble veins; these occur quite often in the liver. Hemangiomas also occur deep in skeletal muscle and other soft tissues of the extremities and trunk (Fig. 11.15). Intramuscular hemangiomas can be painful. The pain is often associated with the increased blood flow that occurs during increased activity or when the limb is in a dependent position. Radiographs, generally, are normal but may demonstrate phleboliths or calcifications in the soft tissues. Hemangiomas characteristically have increased fat content, as may be shown on MRI. The T2-weighted sequences will show increased signal secondary to the hyperemic vascular channels. Asymptomatic lesions can be observed. Multiple treatment options exist for painful lesions. Symptoms can frequently be controlled with compression hose. Surgical resection can be performed for small or well-defined lesions, although recurrence is common. Some intramuscular hemangiomas are infiltrative and extremely difficult to resect except by radical surgery. In these cases, treatment options include embolization or injection with sclerosing agents. Rarely, symptoms are refractory to all treatment options, in which case amputation could be considered.

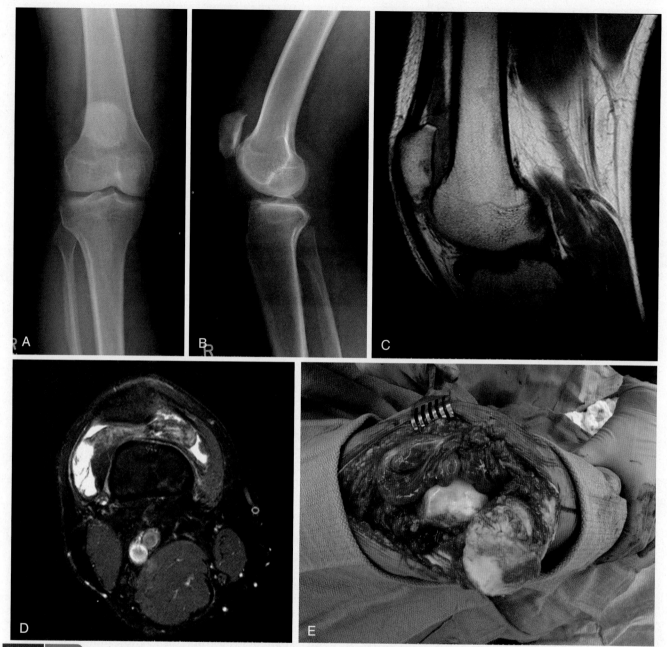

FIGURE 11.14 **A** and **B,** Plain radiographs of a patient with pigmented villonodular synovitis do not show any soft-tissue abnormality. T1-weighted (sagittal) **(C)** and T2-weighted (axial) **(D)** MR images demonstrate a diffuse intraarticular process that is dark on both sequences. **E,** Intraoperative photograph shows diffuse pigmented villonodular synovitis of the knee.

Glomus tumor, or glomangioma, is a rare but painful lesion. The skin and subcutaneous tissue of the hands and feet are usually affected, but a tumor may develop in any location in which a glomus body is found. A glomus body serves to control blood flow and temperature through the autonomic control of the smooth muscle of the arterial wall. The subungual area of the fingers is a characteristic site of involvement, especially in women. Exquisite point tenderness and hypersensitivity are invariably present. Because of this tumor's rarity and small size, the diagnosis may not be readily apparent. When visible, the lesion usually appears as a small, bluish red discoloration of the skin, and 2% to 3% of glomus tumors are multiple. Multiple lesions are more common in men.

Microscopically, this tumor consists of collections of round to oval uniform cells that appear epithelial and lie along the outside of abundant vessels (Fig. 11.16). Some smooth muscle may also be seen, and nonmyelinated nerve fibers may be shown via special stains. Glomus tumors are cured by marginal excision.

FIBROUS LESIONS

Several lesions have been described that microscopically consist of cellular tissue, often with bizarre cells and numerous mitotic figures, and that clinically have not behaved in a malignant fashion. One such lesion is nodular fasciitis (pseudosarcomatous fasciitis, subcutaneous pseudosarcomatous

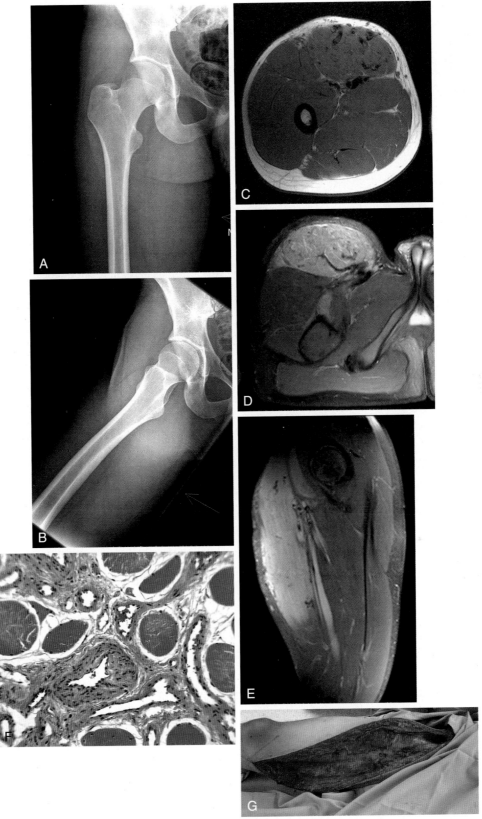

FIGURE 11.15 **A** and **B,** Plain radiographs of the hip show soft-tissue density of a large intramuscular hemangioma. **C** to **E,** T1- and T2-weighted axial and sagittal MR images demonstrate the intramuscular hemangioma of the sartorius muscle. **F,** Photomicrograph (H&E) shows dilated vascular spaces interspersed with skeletal muscle. **G,** Intraoperative photograph after resection. Dissection is along anatomic distribution of the sartorius muscle.

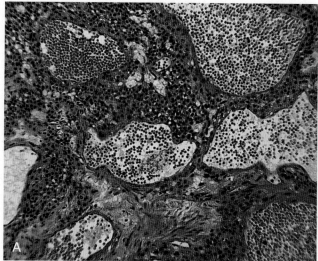

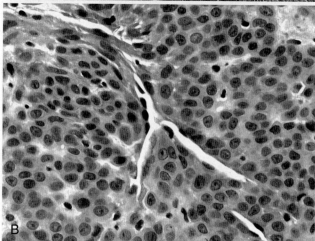

FIGURE 11.16 Glomus tumor. **A,** Photomicrograph (H&E) shows fibrous tissue containing groups of round-to-oval homogenous cells surrounded by vascular channels. **B,** Bland appearance of homogeneous round-to-oval cells.

fibromatosis), which consists of bland proliferating immature fibroblasts in a myxoid stroma with a predominantly vascular pattern (Fig. 11.17). Typically, it is found in young adults, most frequently in the forearm, but it has been reported in a variety of ages and locations. The deep fascia is usually involved, with the lesion protruding into the subcutaneous tissue or, less often, into the underlying muscle. At its periphery, the lesion contains many capillaries and, often, inflammatory cells, and resembles granulation tissue. Most lesions are relatively small (2 to 3 cm in diameter), but occasionally a larger one is found. Patients usually complain of a rapidly expanding mass that has been present for several weeks. Treatment is by marginal resection. Recurrence is rare.

Desmoid tumors (aggressive fibromatosis) are locally aggressive lesions of connective tissue origin that infiltrate surrounding tissues and have a marked propensity for persistence or recurrence. Although most authorities regard this lesion as benign, it can be locally very aggressive. These lesions occur most frequently in the anterior abdominal wall of women who have borne children; lesions in other locations are often known as extraabdominal desmoids. Microscopically, they contain abundant collagen with uniform elongated spindle cells (Fig. 11.18). Atypia and mitoses are scant, and the mass is not well encapsulated, often infiltrating the surrounding host soft tissues. Grossly, they are dense, hard, rubbery, and grayish white. Extraabdominal desmoids occur most frequently in the shoulder girdle, arm, thigh, neck, pelvis, forearm, and popliteal fossa (Fig. 11.19). Superficial fibromatoses of the palmar aponeurosis (Dupuytren contracture) and plantar fascia (Ledderhose disease) are commonly seen by the orthopaedist. The natural history of untreated lesions is unpredictable. Some patients experience a slow, relentless growth with invasion of contiguous structures. Spontaneous regression has also been reported. Metastases have been reported but are extremely rare. Most institutions currently recommend wide resection alone or marginal resection followed by adjuvant radiation therapy. For cases in which resection would involve unacceptable morbidity, radiation can be used alone. Subsequent resections for recurrence may prove arduous because of the

FIGURE 11.17 Nodular fasciitis. Photomicrograph (H&E) shows bland immature fibroblasts in a myxoid stroma.

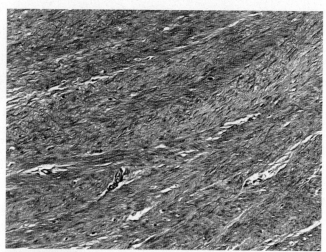

FIGURE 11.18 Desmoid tumor. Photomicrograph (H&E, ×10) demonstrates bland homogeneous spindle cells separated by abundant collagen.

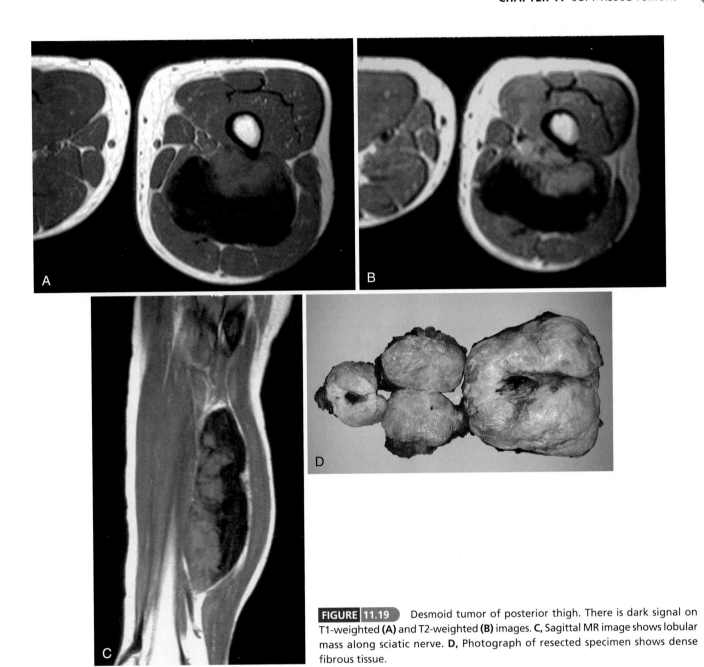

FIGURE 11.19 Desmoid tumor of posterior thigh. There is dark signal on T1-weighted **(A)** and T2-weighted **(B)** images. **C,** Sagittal MR image shows lobular mass along sciatic nerve. **D,** Photograph of resected specimen shows dense fibrous tissue.

difficulty in differentiating tumor from scar tissue. Other treatment options that have had reported success include systemic modalities such as tamoxifen, nonsteroidal antiinflammatory drugs, and low-dose cytotoxic agents.

MALIGNANT TUMORS (TABLE 11.2)
MALIGNANT FIBROUS HISTIOCYTOMA/ UNDIFFERENTIATED PLEOMORPHIC SARCOMA

Literature regarding malignant fibrous histiocytoma (MFH) can be extremely difficult to interpret. Although MFH was formerly regarded as the most commonly diagnosed soft-tissue sarcoma, many authorities currently question whether it should be considered a distinct pathologic entity. Many authors believe that MFH has become

a meaningless diagnosis used to describe a heterogeneous group of tumors with no distinct line of differentiation. Careful investigation frequently allows many of these tumors to be reclassified to more specific diagnoses. The latest World Health Organization (WHO) sarcoma classification does not recognize MFH as a discrete entity. Rather, MFH is now referred to as undifferentiated pleomorphic sarcoma (UPS).

Conventionally, UPS describes a pleomorphic soft-tissue sarcoma with a storiform (irregularly whorled pattern) histologic pattern of growth (Fig. 11.20). It most commonly occurs in patients 50 to 70 years old; however, all age groups can be affected. At the initial examination, most patients have a large (>5 cm) painless mass. The thigh is the most common location. Conventional radiographs may show a soft-tissue density but are usually normal. MRI usually shows a well-circumscribed mass that is

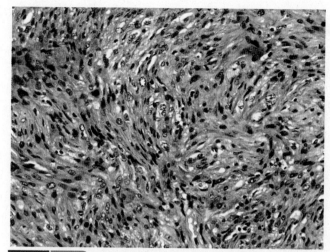

FIGURE 11.20 Malignant fibrous histiocytoma.

dark on T1-weighted images and bright on T2-weighted images (Fig. 11.21). Central necrosis is frequently evident on MRI of larger tumors. UPS has been subclassified into storiform-pleomorphic, giant cell, and inflammatory histiocytoma subtypes. Biologic behavior is better predicted by histologic grade, however.

Treatment is wide resection. Radiation can be used as adjuvant treatment for large tumors or for any case in which the margins are close, and can be administered preoperatively or postoperatively. Use of preoperative radiation should be strongly considered for tumors that are initially thought to be unresectable. Considerable controversy still exists regarding the use of chemotherapy. Although most cancer centers have established chemotherapy protocols for patients with large, high-grade soft-tissue sarcomas, it is still unclear exactly which patients benefit from this treatment. With multimodal treatment, local recurrence should be less than 10%. Metastases usually occur in the lungs and should be resected if possible. Patients should be followed with serial physical examinations, imaging of the tumor site, and imaging of the chest. Five-year survival is approximately 60%. Poor prognostic indicators include high grade, large tumor size, deep location, and presence of metastases.

LIPOSARCOMA

Liposarcoma is the second most commonly diagnosed soft-tissue sarcoma. Similar to UPS, most patients are adults older than 50 years and complain of a large, painless, deep-seated mass located proximally in the extremities. Plain radiographs are usually normal. MRI is nonspecific except for well-differentiated tumors in which fat signal is shown (Fig. 11.22). Histologic subtypes include atypical lipomatous tumor (ALT), well-differentiated liposarcoma (WDL), myxoid liposarcoma (Fig. 11.23), round cell liposarcoma, and pleomorphic liposarcoma (Fig. 11.24).

The terms *ALT* and *WDL* represent tumors that are identical histologically but different in anatomic location and clinical outcomes. Evans et al. further distinguished these two tumors into those occurring in the extremities (ALT) and those in the retroperitoneum (WDL). That difference was noted because of the relative ease of resection of extremity tumors as opposed to those of the retroperitoneum.

The World Health Organization reserves the term *ALT* for extremity and superficial trunk masses and the term *WDL* for masses in the retroperitoneum, mediastinum, or paratesticular locations. Treatment of an ALT is by surgery alone. Patients with ALTs are at risk for local recurrence; however, metastases are rare and long-term survival is excellent. Local recurrence occurs on average 6 to 8 years after resection. Treatment of other types of liposarcoma is similar to that described for UPS. Similar to UPS, metastases usually occur in the lungs and should be resected when possible. Myxoid liposarcomas are unique in that they have a tendency to occur in the retroperitoneum. Patients with myxoid liposarcomas should be staged and followed with CT of the chest, abdomen, and pelvis. Patients with high-grade tumors have a 60% 5-year survival rate. Poor prognostic indicators include high grade, large size, proximal or deep location, and the presence of metastases.

SYNOVIAL SARCOMA (MALIGNANT SYNOVIOMA)

Synovial sarcomas can occur across a wide age range and are the third most common extremity soft-tissue sarcoma. Compared with other "adult-type" soft-tissue sarcomas, synovial sarcomas have several unique clinical features. There is a greater tendency for synovial sarcomas to occur in young adults (median age of 35 years) compared with the older population affected by other soft-tissue sarcomas. Synovial sarcomas are relatively common in the distal extremities (80% are in extremities), including the hand, and are the most common soft-tissue sarcoma of the foot. They frequently have an indolent course initially, and the mass may be present for several years before coming to medical attention. Finally, synovial sarcomas are frequently relatively small (<5 cm) at presentation. This may be attributed to the fact that many patients complain of pain rather than an enlarging mass.

The term *synovial sarcoma* is a misnomer. The term originates from the histologic appearance of the cells, which can resemble synovial cells. The tumors do not arise from synovial tissue, however. An intraarticular location or even continuity with the joint capsule is extremely rare (<10%). Intraarticular synovial sarcomas are often confused with localized pigmented villonodular synovitis. Features that may help establish synovial sarcoma as the diagnosis are tumor size larger than 3 cm, absence of effusion, and male predominance. Plain radiographs frequently show amorphic calcification within the tumor (Fig. 11.25). Microscopically, the tumors frequently show a biphasic growth pattern with nests of epithelioid cells surrounded by malignant spindle cells (Fig. 11.26). A specific gene translocation t(X:18) is found in 90% of patients with synovial sarcomas. This translocation between the *SYT* gene on chromosome 18 and one of the three *SSX* genes on chromosome X produces an *SYT-SSX* fusion gene that is believed to underlie synovial sarcoma pathogenesis through dysregulation of gene expression. Patient evaluation and treatment are similar to that described for UPS. Chemotherapy has been shown to be useful in the treatment of this particular type of soft-tissue sarcoma, but curative resection should not be delayed for chemotherapy. Lymph node metastasis is relatively common (10% to 12%) and should be evaluated carefully on physical examination. Prognosis is similar to that described for UPS and depends on size, location (appendicular faring better than axial), and tumor type.

TABLE 11.2

Malignant Tumors

TUMOR	AGE	DEMOGRAPHICS	SITE	PRESENTATION	IMAGING	HISTOLOGY	TREATMENT	COMMENTS
Malignant fibrous histiocytoma, undifferentiated pleomorphic sarcoma	Older adults	No sex predilection	Any; thigh most common location	Large, deep painless mass	Well-circumscribed mass dark on T1-weighted images and bright on T2-weighted images Central necrosis may be present	Hypercellular spindle cell neoplasm, pleomorphic, mitotic figures	Wide excision combined with radiation therapy Chemotherapy controversial	High grade has increased metastatic potential
Atypical lipomatous tumor (ALT); Well-differentiated liposarcoma (WDL)	Adults	Middle age adults; equally found in males and females	Any; ALT—extremity based (most commonly the thigh) or superficial trunk location. WDL—retroperitoneum, mediastinum, or paratesticular locations.	Slow-growing, nonpainful mass	MRI: mass is isointense to surrounding subcutaneous tissue and may be difficult to distinguish from lipoma	Low grade with mature adipocytes, intervening hyperchromatic stromal cells	Wide excision No radiation therapy or chemotherapy indicated	Low metastatic potential; FISH marker (MDM2)
Myxoid liposarcoma	Adults	No sex predilection	Any but most commonly found in the lower extremity; May be found in retroperitoneum	Large deep painless mass	MRI: nonspecific, heterogeneous signal pattern	Myxoid stroma, chicken wire capillaries, stellate cells, signet ring lipoblasts	Wide excision combined with radiation therapy	Staging should include CT chest/abdomen/pelvis to rule out retroperitoneal involvement Translocation (12;16) FISH marker (FUS)
Pleomorphic liposarcoma	Adults	Slight male predilection	Any	Large, deep, rapidly growing mass; 25% arise in the subcutaneous tissue	MRI: nonspecific, findings suggestive of soft-tissue sarcoma, hypointense on T1-weighted image, hyperintense on T2-weighted image	Pleomorphic lipoblasts in spindle cell background	Wide excision combined with radiation therapy Chemotherapy in selected patients	Poor prognosis; Size, retroperitoneal location, and advanced age are associated with worse prognosis

Continued

TABLE 11.2

Malignant Tumors—cont'd

TUMOR	AGE	DEMOGRAPHICS	SITE	PRESENTATION	IMAGING	HISTOLOGY	TREATMENT	COMMENTS
Synovial sarcoma	Young adults	Male predominance	Juxtaarticular locations; only 10% intra-articular	Slow-growing mass; may be painful	Radiographs may show soft-tissue calcification MRI: nonspecific, findings suggestive of soft-tissue sarcoma, hypointense on T1-weighted image, hyperintense on T2-weighted image	Biphasic: nests of epithelioid cells surrounded by malignant spindle cells	Wide excision combined with radiation therapy Chemotherapy shown to be beneficial	Translocation (x;18): fusion product of *SYT* with *SSX1* or *SSX2* May spread via lymph nodes Most common soft-tissue sarcoma of foot FISH marker (SS18)
Fibrosarcoma	Adults	No sex predilection	Any Deep in extremities	Large, deep, painless mass	MRI: nonspecific, findings suggestive of soft-tissue sarcoma, hypointense on T1-weighted image, hyperintense on T2-weighted image	Malignant spindle cells in a herringbone pattern	Wide excision combined with radiation therapy Chemotherapy is controversial	
Epithelioid sarcoma	Adolescents and young adults	No sex predilection	Distal upper extremities	Slow-growing mass; may be associated with ulceration	MRI: nonspecific, findings suggestive of soft-tissue sarcoma, hypointense on T1-weighted image, hyperintense on T2-weighted image	Polyhedral cells with dense eosinophilic cytoplasm	Wide excision or amputation, combined with radiation therapy	May spread via lymph nodes Most common soft-tissue sarcoma of hand
Dermatofibrosarcoma protuberans	Young adults	Male predominance	Trunk and proximal extremities	Slow-growing (years) mass just beneath epidermis	MRI: nonspecific, findings suggestive of soft-tissue sarcoma, hypointense on T1-weighted image, hyperintense on T2-weighted image	Hypercellular well-differentiated fibroblasts, low to intermediate grade	Wide excision	High rate of local recurrence

TABLE 11.2
Malignant Tumors—cont'd

	Age/Incidence	Association	Location	Clinical	Imaging	Histology	Treatment	Prognosis
Rhabdomyosarcoma	Children and young adults; peak incidence age 1-5 years		Alveolar type usually involves muscles of extremities or trunk, more aggressive type	Fast-growing painful lump in muscle; may be misdiagnosed as injury	MRI: usually isointense to skeletal muscle on T1-weighted images, high signal intensity on T2-weighted images	Variable cell population; small, round tumor cells with hyperchromatic nuclei; large, polygonal-shaped cells with abundant eosinophilic cytoplasm	Resection, chemotherapy irradiation	70%-90% 5-year survival rate depending on site, type and size of tumor, extent of disease after resection FISH marker for alveolar type (FOX01)
Malignant peripheral nerve sheath tumor	2nd-5th decades	Up to 50% in patients with neurofibromatosis type 1	Large peripheral nerves (sciatic, brachial plexus, sacral plexus)	Enlarging, palpable mass. Pain variable, muscle weakness, paresthesias	MRI: fusiform shape, longitudinal orientation in direction of nerve; invasion of fat planes, heterogeneity, ill-defined margins, surrounding edema	Dense cellular fascicles alternating with myxoid regions (marbleized pattern); spindle-shaped cells with irregular contours	Resection (wide margins) Radiation therapy	20%-80% survival depending on tumor grade, extent of excision, size of tumor; high rates of local recurrence and distant metastases
Extraskeletal osteosarcoma	4th-6th decades	Male predominance	Thigh, upper extremity	Slow-growing painful mass, usually large (average 9 cm) History of trauma common	Radiographs: large soft-tissue mass with focal to massive areas of mineralization MRI: high-signal intensity on T2-weighted images	Variable amounts of neoplastic bone, cartilage, osteoid	Wide surgical excision or amputation Chemotherapy Radiation therapy	Poor prognosis (<40% survival) Metastases frequent (lungs, lymph nodes, bones)
Extraskeletal Ewing sarcoma	Adolescents, young adults (>80% <20 years)		Trunk, extremities Diaphyseal/metaphyseal area of long bones Paravertebral region	Rapidly growing, painful mass	CT: hypodensity, unclear margins MRI: isointense to muscle on T1-weighted images, hyperintense on T2-weighted images	Solid sheets of small uniform primitive cells with round nuclei and scanty cytoplasm	Wide resection Chemotherapy	Overall 5-year survival 60%-80% High recurrence rate Distant metastases common (lung, bone) FISH marker (EWSR1)
Extraskeletal chondrosarcoma	4th-5th decades	Male-female 2:1	Deep soft tissues, extremities or trunk	Deep-seated, slowly growing mass Pain variable Large tumors may cause skin ulceration	Radiographs: nodular, radiolucent mass, pseudocapsule MRI: nonspecific, intermediate to high intensity on T1-weighted images	Multilobulated mass of uniform rounded or elongated cells, small nuclei, small amount of eosinophilic cytoplasm	Wide resection Radiation therapy	Overall 5-year survival rate ~80% High rates of local recurrence and distant metastases

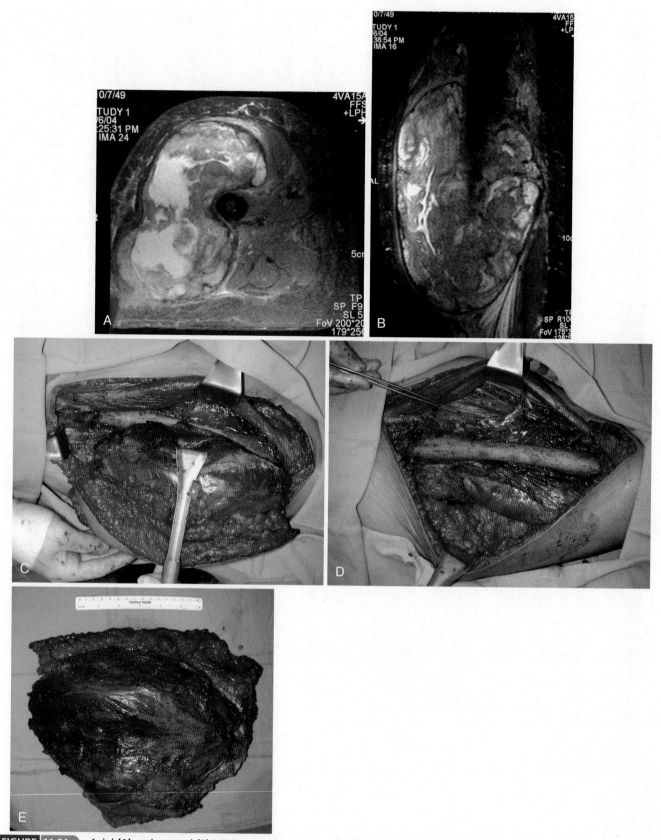

FIGURE **11.21**   Axial **(A)** and coronal **(B)** MR images show large soft-tissue mass in thigh with mixed-signal intensity that proved to be malignant fibrous histiocytoma. **C,** Intraoperative photograph shows tumor being resected with wide margins. Biopsy track is kept in continuity with tumor. **D,** Tumor bed after resection. **E,** Photograph of resected specimen. Plane of dissection is through normal muscle.

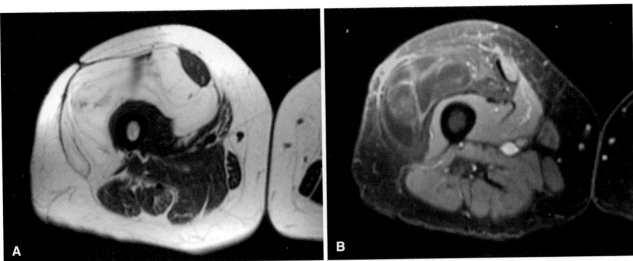

FIGURE 11.22 T1-weighted **(A)** and contrast-enhanced, fat-suppressed axial **(B)** MR images of well-differentiated lipoma-like liposarcoma (atypical lipoma) of thigh. Lesion is similar to lipoma with exception of multiple, thick, enhancing septa.

FIBROSARCOMA

Fibrosarcoma is rarely diagnosed at this institution. Diagnostic criteria are subjective and it has become a diagnosis of exclusion. The characteristic microscopic appearance of fibrosarcoma consists of spindle cells arranged in a herringbone pattern (Fig. 11.27). The typical presentation is a 5- to 10 cm, slow-growing, painless mass in the deep soft tissues of the lower extremity in adults 30 to 50 years old. Imaging characteristics, treatment, and prognosis are similar to those described for UPS.

EPITHELIOID SARCOMA

Epithelioid sarcoma is a rare soft-tissue sarcoma with several unusual clinical features. It is a slow-growing malignant tumor usually occurring in adolescents and young adults and frequently involves the distal upper extremities, including the hands and fingers. It is the most common sarcoma in the hand. It frequently presents as a small (average 3 cm), superficial, soft-tissue mass. The overlying skin may be ulcerated. Because of its indolent growth, it is frequently misdiagnosed, initially, as a carcinoma or a benign skin lesion. Patients commonly undergo surgical procedures with inadequate surgical margins before the correct diagnosis is made. The recommended treatment is wide resection or amputation. Similar to synovial sarcoma, lymph node metastases are relatively common. Microscopically, epithelioid sarcoma consists of polyhedral cells with dense eosinophilic cytoplasm. There is a predominant epithelial appearance. Despite its slow growth, the aggressive nature of the tumor is evidenced by a high local recurrence rate (>50% in some series). The 5-year survival rate is approximately 70%, but survival declines to 50% at 10 years owing to the high incidence of late metastases. Prognosis is worse for patients with tumors larger than 3 cm or tumors in proximal locations.

DERMATOFIBROSARCOMA PROTUBERANS

Dermatofibrosarcoma protuberans is a rare sarcoma of intermediate malignancy that arises just beneath the epidermis as one or several nodules and eventually may grow to form a large, bulky mass. Often, the tumor initially manifests as a firm plaque-like lesion of the skin with surrounding blue or red discoloration. The overlying skin may become atrophic and easily traumatized. The tumor grows slowly but is quite likely to recur after excision because of its infiltrative nature. It occurs more often on the trunk than on the extremities and most frequently in the early to middle decades of life. Microscopically, the tissue is well differentiated but cellular and the cells resemble fibroblasts. The cells may have a distinctive storiform pattern (Fig. 11.28). Pleomorphic nuclei are sparse and there is low to moderate mitotic activity. More than 90% of these tumors are characterized by a t(17;22) translocation. This translocation produces a platelet-derived growth factor beta (PDGF-β)/collagen type 1A1 fusion gene, which leads to the constitutive production of collagen. The treatment of choice is wide resection (Fig. 11.29). Recurrence is common and is usually the result of failure to excise enough adjacent normal tissue to include the pseudocapsule and occult finger-like projections. Rarely, after several recurrences, a lesion becomes less well differentiated and may metastasize.

RHABDOMYOSARCOMA

Rhabdomyosarcoma varies considerably in frequency and type among different age groups. Microscopically, it can be subdivided into three main types: embryonal, alveolar, and pleomorphic. Some tumors have mixed features. The embryonal and alveolar types occur in children and adolescents and are among the more common malignant tumors in these age groups. The classic pleomorphic type occurs in adults and is rare. Rhabdomyosarcoma is usually found within a muscle but may secondarily involve the skin. Its origin from some of the smaller muscles may not be obvious.

Embryonal rhabdomyosarcomas are usually located in the head or neck or in the genitourinary tract. They are often soft and gelatinous and are microscopically composed of long spindle cells with hyperchromatic nuclei and abundant cytoplasm. The cells may be arranged in parallel bundles, and myxoid areas may be prominent. Giant cells may be present but not in abundance. A variation of this tumor, botryoid sarcoma, is often found in the genitourinary tract; it is located beneath the epithelial surface and is polypoid.

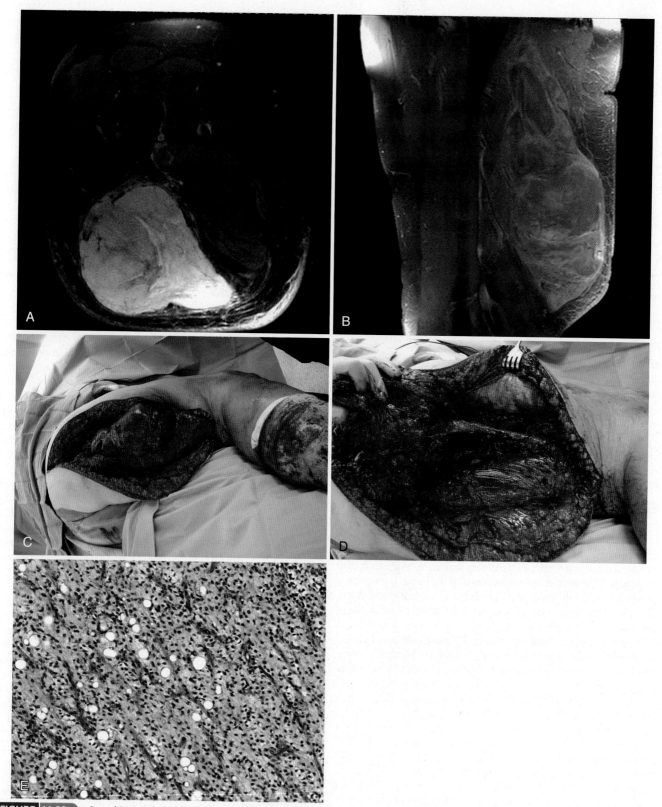

FIGURE **11.23** **A** and **B**, Axial and sagittal T2-weighted MR images show biopsy-proved myxoid liposarcoma of the posterior thigh. **C** and **D**, Intraoperative photographs of resection show that the sciatic nerve passed through the tumor and had to be sacrificed. **E**, Photomicrograph (H&E, ×10) shows bland cells in a myxoid matrix with a surrounding capillary network.

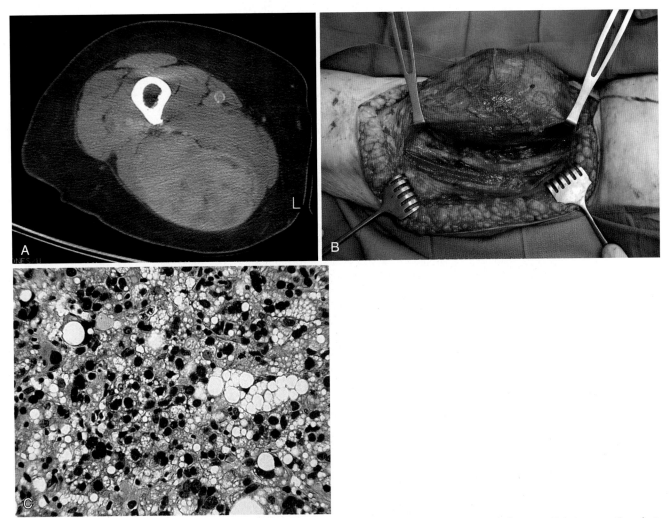

FIGURE 11.24 **A,** CT of thigh of 73-year-old patient with pleomorphic liposarcoma adjacent to sciatic nerve. **B,** Intraoperative photograph of wide resection. **C,** Photomicrograph demonstrates pleomorphic cells, mitotic figures, and bizarre lipoblasts.

Alveolar rhabdomyosarcoma usually occurs in the head, neck, or extremities and is typically firmer and less myxoid than the embryonal type. Microscopically, the predominant cell is round and has scanty eosinophilic cytoplasm. An occasional cell that looks like a typical rhabdomyoblast is seen, and multinucleated giant cells are present but are usually inconspicuous. The latter cells may grow diffusely and in some parts of the tumor produce an alveolar pattern by their tendency to line connective tissue septa.

The pleomorphic type of rhabdomyosarcoma usually occurs on the extremities and is much less common than either of the other types. Microscopically, it is composed of spindle-shaped cells arranged in parallel and interlacing bundles. Multinucleated giant cells are prominent and the typical strap- and racquet-shaped cells are often seen; mitotic activity is prominent (Fig. 11.30).

Rhabdomyosarcoma frequently has a rapid and aggressive clinical course. Metastases occur in the lungs, lymph nodes, and bone marrow. Treatment is multimodal, consisting of surgery, radiation, and chemotherapy. In contrast to adult soft-tissue sarcomas, a dramatic improvement in patient survival has been observed with the use of multiple-agent chemotherapy. The overall 5-year survival rate is approximately 65%.

MALIGNANT PERIPHERAL NERVE SHEATH TUMOR

Malignant peripheral nerve sheath tumor (malignant schwannoma, neurofibrosarcoma) is the malignant counterpart of neurofibroma and is rare (Fig. 11.31). About 25% of patients with this tumor have neurofibromatosis. Approximately 5% of patients who have neurofibromatosis develop malignant change in a neurofibroma, and pain should alert the clinician to the possibility of transformation. It was originally thought that patients with neurofibromatosis had a worse prognosis than other patients with malignant peripheral nerve sheath tumor; however, when other prognostic factors (e.g., size and location) are considered, the underlying diagnosis of neurofibromatosis becomes less important. Common locations of occurrence include close proximity to nerve roots and bundles of the extremities and pelvis, including the sciatic nerve, brachial plexus, and sacral plexus. These tumors typically arise in adults 30 to 50 years old, but patients with neurofibromatosis experience malignant transformation at younger ages (mean age 28 years). At the initial examination, most patients have a painless mass. Some patients complain of pain in the distribution of the involved nerve, and the complaint of pain is more prevalent in those with

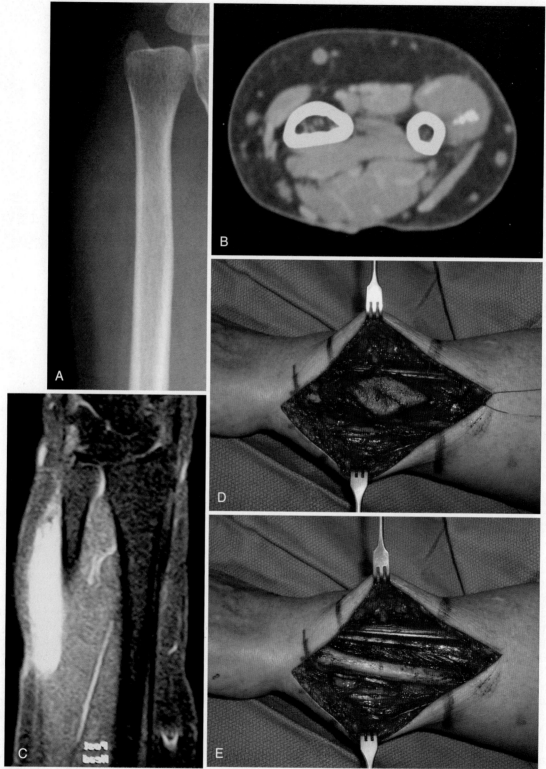

FIGURE 11.25   A, Anteroposterior radiograph of wrist of 67-year-old patient shows irregular calcifications within soft-tissue mass (synovial sarcoma). B, CT scan better shows calcifications within mass. C, MR image shows extent of mass. D, Intraoperative photograph during wide resection. E, Intraoperative photograph of tumor bed after resection.

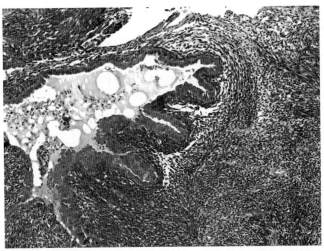

FIGURE 11.26 Biphasic synovial sarcoma. Photomicrograph shows biphasic pattern of malignant spindle cells and columnar cells forming gland-like spaces.

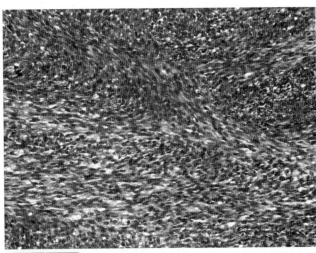

FIGURE 11.27 Fibrosarcoma. Photomicrograph (H&E, ×20) shows spindle cells arranged in fascicles resembling a herringbone pattern.

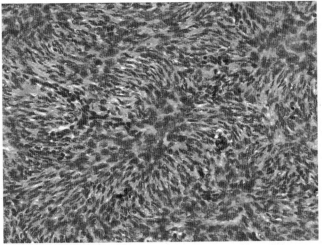

FIGURE 11.28 Dermatofibrosarcoma protuberans. Photomicrograph (H&E, ×20) shows spindle cells arranged in a storiform pattern.

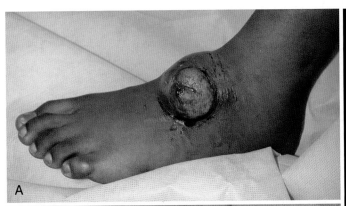

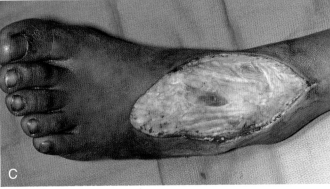

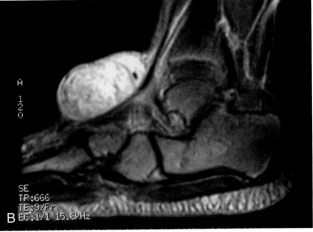

FIGURE 11.29 **A,** Dermatofibrosarcoma protuberans in 15-year-old boy. **B,** MRI shows that tumor has remained very superficial. **C,** Treatment consisted of wide resection and split-thickness skin graft.

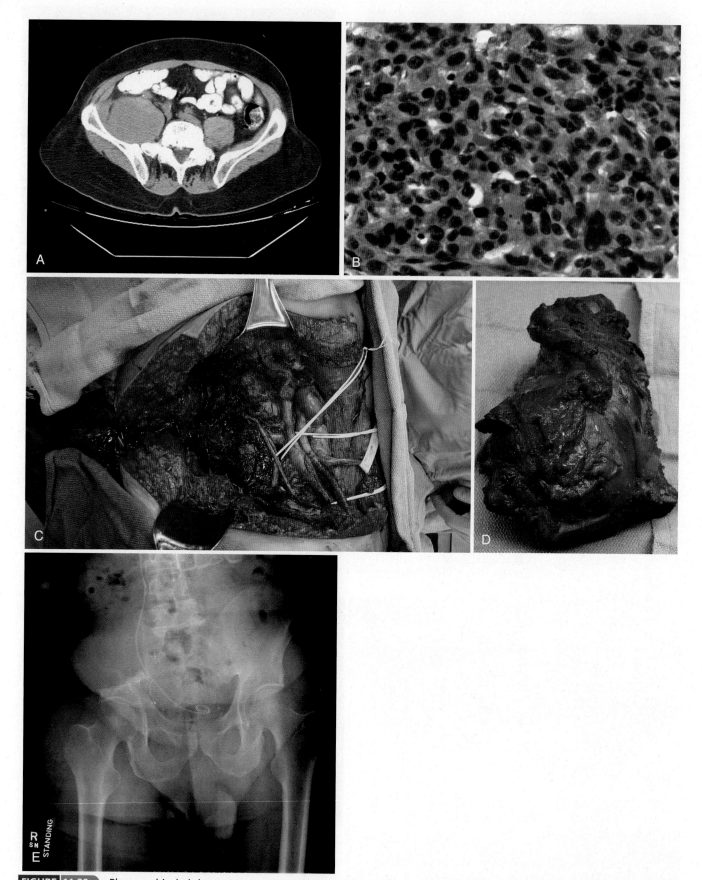

FIGURE 11.30 Pleomorphic rhabdomyosarcoma. **A,** Axial CT scan shows deep-seated tumor along the right ilium. **B,** Photomicrograph (H&E, ×40) shows hyperchromatic nuclei, marked pleomorphism, and mitotic figures. **C,** Intraoperative photograph shows tumor bed after resection. **D,** Resected specimen. **E,** Postoperative radiograph.

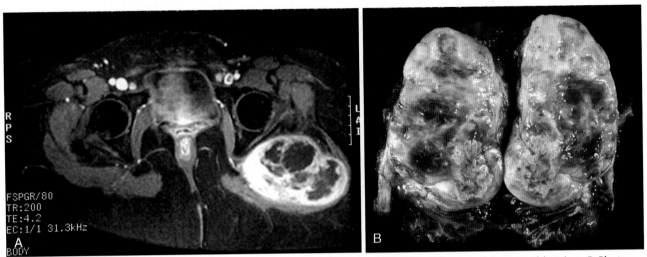

FIGURE 11.31 **A,** Axial MR image shows malignant peripheral nerve sheath tumor of sciatic nerve in 36-year-old patient. **B,** Photograph of resected specimen. Note sciatic nerve entering *(bottom left)* and exiting *(right)* tumor.

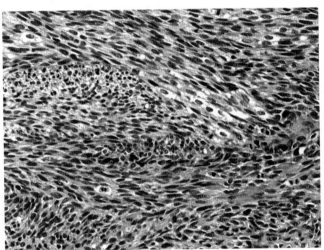

FIGURE 11.32 Malignant peripheral nerve sheath tumor. Photomicrograph (H&E, ×40) shows spindle cells arranged in a swirling pattern. Multiple mitoses are seen throughout the field.

neurofibromatosis type 1. Paresthesias and neurologic deficits may also be observed. Microscopic diagnosis of early malignant change in a neurofibroma may be difficult. The tumors have a similar microscopic appearance as a fibrosarcoma; however, the spindle cells tend to have irregular contours (Fig. 11.32). Treatment consists of wide resection and radiation. Chemotherapy should be considered for young patients with large, high-grade tumors. Local recurrence is high in some series because the tumor can extend along the perineurium of the involved nerve for some distance. This diagnosis generally carries a poor prognosis, and the overall 5-year survival is approximately 50%.

EXTRASKELETAL OSTEOSARCOMA

Extraskeletal osteosarcoma is extremely rare, accounting for approximately 1% of all soft tissue sarcomas. Similar to osteosarcoma of bone, it is a malignant spindle cell neoplasm marked by the production of osteoid. In contrast to osteosarcoma of bone, extraskeletal osteosarcoma generally affects adults older than 40 years and the lower extremity is the most common location. The clinical course varies. Patients complain of an enlarging mass of variable duration that may or may not be painful. Any site can be affected; however, the deep soft tissue of the thigh is the most common location. Imaging studies usually show immature ossification within the mass (Fig. 11.33). The histology is similar to that of osteosarcoma of bone. There is no universally accepted treatment algorithm because of its rare occurrence. Treatment is multimodal, including wide resection, radiation, and multiple-agent chemotherapy. Compared with osteosarcoma of bone and other soft-tissue sarcomas, prognosis has generally been poor, with an average 5-year survival rate of 25%.

EXTRASKELETAL EWING SARCOMA

Extraskeletal Ewing sarcoma is similar to Ewing sarcoma of bone. This tumor generally affects adolescents and young adults, who typically complain of a rapidly enlarging soft-tissue mass. The most common locations include the paravertebral musculature and the chest wall. Imaging studies are nonspecific. The pathologic findings are similar to those of Ewing sarcoma of bone. It is a small, round, blue cell tumor. Most tumors show an 11;22 translocation and most stain positively for the *MIC2* gene product. Treatment protocols are similar to those outlined for Ewing sarcoma of bone and include surgery, radiation, and multiple-agent chemotherapy.

EXTRASKELETAL CHONDROSARCOMA

Extraskeletal myxoid chondrosarcoma is a low- to intermediate-grade soft-tissue sarcoma that generally affects adults older than 35 years. It typically presents as a deep-seated, slowly enlarging mass. Imaging studies are nonspecific, although the tumors are frequently lobular. Treatment consists of wide resection (Fig. 11.34). Radiation is used if margins are close. The slow-growing nature of this tumor is evidenced by the fact that late recurrences are relatively common. Five-year survival rates are approximately 90%; however, this number declines to approximately 70% at 10 years and 60% at 15 years.

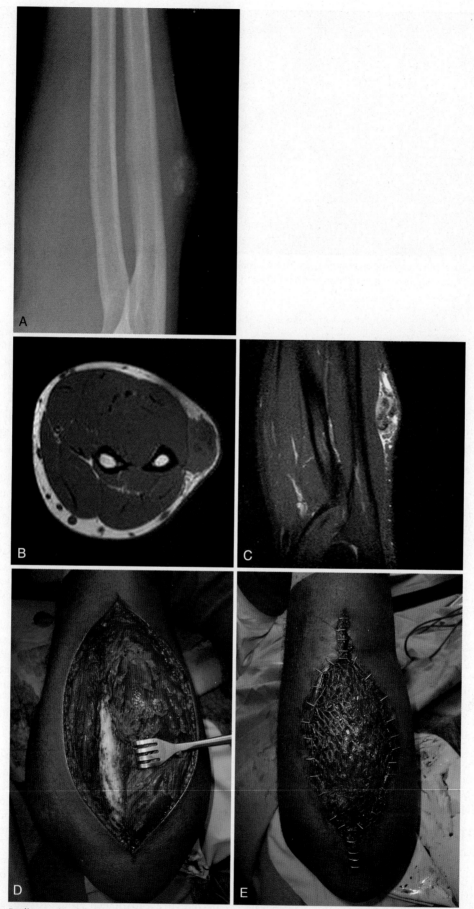

FIGURE 11.33 **A,** Radiograph of forearm of 33-year-old patient shows immature ossification in soft-tissue mass that proved to be extraskeletal osteosarcoma. Axial **(B)** and sagittal **(C)** MR images show extent of lesion. Tumor was treated with wide resection **(D)** and split-thickness skin grafting **(E).**

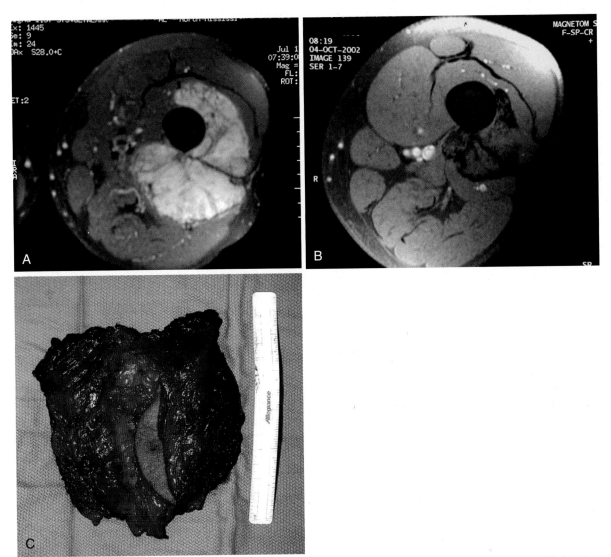

FIGURE 11.34 **A,** Axial MR image shows large lobulated soft-tissue mass that proved to be extraskeletal myxoid chondrosarcoma. **B,** Axial MR image after preoperative radiation treatment shows dramatic decrease in size of mass, making resection technically much easier. **C,** Photograph of specimen after wide resection. Biopsy track is resected en bloc with tumor, and plane of dissection is entirely through normal tissue.

Extraskeletal mesenchymal chondrosarcoma is a rare, high-grade tumor that generally affects patients who are 15 to 35 years old. The most common locations include the head and neck. Treatment consists of wide resection, radiation, and chemotherapy. The prognosis has generally been poor.

REFERENCES

Abolghasemian M, Gharanizadeh K, Kuzyk P, et al.: Hips with synovial chondromatosis may display the features of femoroacetabular impingement, *J Bone Joint Surg Am* 96:e11, 2014.

Alamanda VK, Moore DC, Song Y, et al.: Obesity does not affect survival outcomes in extremity soft tissue sarcoma, *Clin Orthop Relat Res* 472:2799, 2014.

Armah HB, Parwani AV: Epithelioid sarcoma, *Arch Pathol Lab Med* 133:814, 2009.

Aurégan JC, Klouche S, Bohu Y, et al.: Treatment of pigmented villonodular synovitis of the knee, *Arthroscopy* 30:1327, 2014.

Bagatur AE, Yalcinkaya M, Dogan A, et al.: Surgery is not always necessary in intraosseous lipoma, *Orthopedics* 33:306, 2010.

Bains R, Magdum A, Bhat W, et al.: Soft tissue sarcoma—a review of presentation, management and outcomes in 110 patients, *Surgeon* 14:129, 2016.

Barbier O, Anract P, Plout E, et al.: Primary or recurring extra-abdominal desmoid fibromatosis: assessment of treatment by observation only, *Orthop Traumatol Surg Res* 96:884, 2010.

Brennan MF, Antonescu CR, Moraco N, Singer S: Lessons learned from the study of 10,000 patients with soft tissue sarcomas, *Ann Surg* 260:416, 2014.

Briand S, Barbier O, Biau D, et al.: Wait-and-see policy as a first-line management for extra-abdominal desboid tumors, *J Bone Joint Surg Am* 96:631, 2014.

Chao AH, Mayerson JL, Chandawarkar R, Scharschmidt TJ: Surgical management of soft tissue sarcomas: extremity sarcomas, *J Surg Oncol* 111:540, 2015.

Choi LE, Healey JH, Kuk D, Brennan MF: Analysis of outcomes in extraskeletal osteosarcoma: a review of fifty-three cases, *J Bone Joint Surg Am* 96:e2, 2014.

Christoforou D, Strauss EJ, Abramovici L, Posner MA: Benign extraosseous cartilage tumours of the hand and wrist, *J Hand Surg Eur* 37(8), 2012.

Coyle J, White LM, Dickson B, et al.: MRI characteristics of nodular fasciitis of the musculoskeletal system, *Skeletal Radiol* 42:975, 2013.

de Sa D, Horner NS, MacDonald A, et al.: Arthroscopic surgery for synovial chondromatosis of the hip: a systematic review of rates and predisposing factors for recurrence, *Arthroscopy* 30:1499, 2014.

Doyle LA: Sarcoma classification: an update based on the 2013 World Health Organization classification of tumors of soft-tissue and bone, *Cancer* 120:1763, 2014.

Errani C, Zhang L, Panicek DM, et al.: Epithelioid hemangioma of bone and soft tissue: a reappraisal of a controversial entity, *Clin Orthop Relat Res* 470:1498, 2012.

Evenski AJ, Stensby JD, Rosas S, et al.: Diagnostic imaging and management of common intra-articular and peri-articular soft tissue tumors and tumorlike conditions of the knee, *J Knee Surg* 32:322, 2019.

Farid M, Demicco EG, Garcia R, et al.: Malignant peripheral nerve sheath tumors, *Oncol* 19:193, 2014.

Felderhof JM, Creutzberg CL, Putter H, et al.: Long-term clinical outcome of patients with soft tissue sarcomas treated with limb-sparing surgery and postoperative radiotherapy, *Acta Oncol* 52:745, 2013.

Fletcher CDM, Bridge JA, Gofendoorn PCW, et al.: *WHO classification of tumours of soft tissue and bone*, ed 4, Herndon, Virginia, 2013, Stylus Publishing, pp 19–42.

Gu HF, Zhang SJ, Zhao C, et al.: A comparison of open and arthroscopic surgery for treatment of diffuse pigmented villonodular synovitis of the knee, *Knee Surg Sports Traumatol Arlthrosc* 22:2830, 2014.

Guha D, Davidson B, Nadi M, et al.: Management of peripheral nerve sheath tumors: 17 years of experience at Toronto Western Hospital, *J Neurosurg* 128:1226, 2018.

Hirai T, Kobayashi H, Akiyama T, et al.: Predictive factors for complications after surgical treatment of schwannomas of the extremities, *BMC Musculoskelet Disord* 20:166, 2019.

Ho YY, Choueka J: Synovial chondromatosis of the upper extremity, *J Hand Surg Am* 38:804, 2013.

Houdek MT, Rose PS, Kakar S: Desmoid tumors of the upper extremity, *J Hand Surg [Am]* 39:1761, 2014.

Johnson CN, Has AS, Chen E, et al.: Lipomatous soft-tissue tumors, *J Am Acad Orthop Surg* 26:779, 2018.

King DM, Hackbarth DA, Kirkpatrick A: Extremity soft tissue sarcoma resections: how wide do you need to be? *Clin Orthop Relat Res* 470:692, 2012.

Kneisl JS, Coleman MM, Raut CP: Outcomes in the management of adult soft tissue sarcomas, *J Surg Oncol* 11:527, 2014.

Kok KY, Telisinghe PU: Lipoblastoma: clinical features, treatment, and outcome, *World J Surg* 34:1517, 2010.

Koplas MC, Lefkowitz RA, Bauer TW, et al.: Imaging findings, prevalence and outcome of de novo and secondary malignant fibrous histiocytoma of bone, *Skeletal Radiol* 39:791, 2010.

Krych A, Odland A, Rose P, et al.: Oncologic conditions that simulate common sports injuries, *J Am Acad Orthop Surg* 22:223, 2014.

Levi AD, Ross AL, Cuartas E, et al.: The surgical management of symptomatic peripheral nerve sheath tumors, *Neurosurgery* 66:833, 2010.

Ma X, Shi G, Xia C, et al.: Pigmented villonodular synovitis: a retrospective study of seventy five cases (eighty one joints), *Int Orthop* 37:1165, 2013.

Mankin HJ, Hornicek FJ, Springfield DS: Extra-abdominal desmoid tumors: a report of 234 cases, *J Surg Oncol* 102:380, 2010.

Mankin H, Trahan C, Hornicek F: Pigmented villonodular synovitis of joints, *J Surg Oncol* 103:386, 2011.

Maretty-Nkielsen K, Aggerholm-Pedersen N, Safwat A, et al.: Prognostic factors for local recurrence and mortality in adult soft tissue sarcoma of the extremities and trunk wall: a cohort study of 922 consecutive patients, *Acta Orthop* 85:323, 2014.

Miller ED, Xu-Welliver M, Haglund KE: The role of modern radiation therapy in the management of extremity sarcomas, *J Surg Oncol* 111:599, 2015.

Nazerani S, Motamedi MH, Keramati MR: Diagnosis and management of glomus tumors of the hand, *Tech Hand Up Extrem Surg* 14:8, 2010.

Neumann JA, Garrigues GE, Brigman BE, et al.: Synovial chondromatosis, *JBJS Rev* 4:pii: 01874474-201605000-00005, 2016.

Nordemar D, Oberg J, Brosjo O, et al.: Intra-articular synovial sarcomas: incidence and differentiating features from localized pigmented villonodular synovitis, *Sarcoma* 2015:903873, 2015.

Ng VY, Louie P, Punt S, et al.: Malignant transformation of synovial chondromatosis: a systematic review, *Open Orthop J* 11:517, 2017.

Potter BK, Hwang PF, Forsberg JA, et al.: Impact of margin status and local recurrence on soft-tissue sarcoma outcomes, *J Bone Joint Surg Am* 95:e151, 2013.

Pourbagher A, Pourbagher MA, Karan B, Ozkoc G: MRI manifestations of soft-tissue haemangiomas and accompanying reactive bone changes, *Br J Radiol* 84:1100, 2011.

Prodinger PM, Rechl H, Keller M, et al.: Surgical resection and radiation therapy of desmoid tumours of the extremities: results of a supra-regional tumour centre, *Int Orthop* 37:1987, 2013.

Rougraff BT, Lawrence J, Davis K: Length of symptoms before referral: prognostic variable for high-grade soft tissue sarcoma? *Clin Orthop Relat Res* 470:706, 2012.

Sawamura C, Matsumoto S, Shimoji T, et al.: What are risk factors for local recurrence of deep high-grade soft-tissue sarcomas? *Clin Orthop Relat Res* 470:700, 2012.

Schwartz A, Rebecca A, Smith A, et al.: Risk factors for significant wound complications following wide resection of extremity soft tissue sarcomas, *Clin Orthop Relat Res* 471:3612, 2013.

Siqueira MG, Socolovsky M, Martins RS, et al.: Surgical treatment of typical peripheral schwannomas: the risk of new postoperative deficits, *Acta Neurochir (Wien)* 155:1745, 2013, 2013.

Sluijmer HC, Becker SJ, Bossen JK, Ring D: Excisional biopsy of suspected benign soft tissue rumors of the upper extremity: correlation between preoperative diagnosis and actual pathology, *Hand (N Y)* 9:351, 2014.

Stevenson JD, Jaiswal A, Gregory JJ, et al.: Diffuse pigmented villonodular synovitis (diffuse-type giant cell tumour) of the foot and ankle, *Bone Joint Lett J* 95:384, 2013.

Su CH, Hung JK, Chang IL: Surgical treatment of intramuscular, infiltrating lipoma, *Int Surg* 96:56, 2011.

Teng H, Xinghai Y, Wei H, et al.: Malignant fibrous histiocytoma of the spine: a series of 13 clinical case reports and review of 17 published cases, *Spine (Phila Pa 1976)* 36:E1453, 2011.

Thakur NA, Daniels AH, Schiller J, et al.: Benign tumors of the spine, *J Am Acad Orthop Surg* 20:715, 2012.

Thampi S, Matthay KK, Boscardin WJ, et al.: Clinical features and outcomes differ between skeletal and extraskeletal osteosarcoma, *Sarcoma*, 2014:902620, 2014.

Vasileios KA, Eward WC, Brigman BE: Surgical treatment and prognosis in patients with high-grade soft tissue malignant fibrous histiocytoma of the extremities, *Arch Orthop Trauma Surg* 132:955, 2012.

Verspoor FG, Zee AA, Hannink G, et al.: Long-term follow-up results of primary and recurrent pigmented villonodular synovitis, *Rheumatology (Oxford)* 53:2063, 2014.

Wachtel M, Runge T, Leuschner I, et al.: Subtype and prognostic classification of rhabdomyosarcoma by immunohistochemistry, *J Clin Oncol* 24:816, 2006.

Walczak BE, Irwin RB: Sarcoma chemotherapy, *J Am Acad Orthop Surg* 21:480, 2013.

Williams J, Hodari A, Janevski P, Siddiqui A: Recurrence of giant cell tumors in the hand: a prospective study, *J Hand Surg [Am]* 35:451, 2010.

Woltsche N, Gilg MM, Fraissler L, et al.: Is wide resection obsolete for desmoid tumors in children and adolescents? Evaluation of histological margins, immunohistochemical markers, and review of literature, *Pediatr Hematol Oncol* 32:60, 2015.

Yoon PW, Yoo JJ, Koo KH, et al.: Joint space widening in synovial chondromatosis of the hip, *J Bone Joint Surg Am* 93:303, 2011.

The complete list of references is available online at ExpertConsult.com.